T2-CSE-982

MODERN
Essentials™

A Contemporary Guide to the Therapeutic Use of Essential Oils

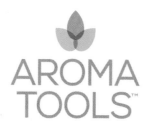

AROMA TOOLS™

www.aromatools.com

Published and Distributed by:

AromaTools®
144 W. 1900 North
Spanish Fork, UT 84660

Phone: 1-866-728-0070 • 801-798-7921

Internet: www.AromaTools.com

E-mail: Webmaster@AromaTools.com

Copyright:

© **2018 AromaTools®**. 10th Edition, 1st Printing, September 2018. All rights reserved. No part of this book may be reproduced or transmitted in any form or by any means, electronic or mechanical, including photocopying, recording, or by any other information storage or retrieval system, without written permission from AromaTools®.

ISBN Number:

978-1-937702-88-5

Disclaimer:

This book has been designed to provide information to help educate the reader in regard to the subject matter covered. It is sold with the understanding that the publisher and the authors are not liable for the misconception and misuse of the information provided. It is not provided in order to diagnose, prescribe, or treat any disease, illness, or injured condition of the body. The authors and publisher shall have neither liability nor responsibility to any person or entity with respect to any loss, damage, or injury caused, or alleged to be caused, directly or indirectly by the information contained in this book. The information presented herein is in no way intended as a substitute for medical counseling. Anyone suffering from any disease, illness, or injury should consult a qualified health care professional.

Printed and Bound in the U.S.A.

AromaTools®, is a true third-party company that does not profit from the sales of essential oils, and is not sponsored by, affiliated with, or endorsed by any essential oil company. We present this material as a third-party, unbiased presentation about oils and products sold by one of the leading essential oil suppliers and producers in the world. Product names throughout this book are trademarks or registered trademarks of dōTERRA® Holdings, LLC. AromaTools is not sponsored by, affiliated with, or endorsed by dōTERRA® Holdings, LLC.

Table of Contents

My Usage Guide

The Basics of Essential Oils

Essential Oils

Essential Oil Blends

Essential Supplements

Personal Care & Spa

Essential Living

EO Science in Depth

Appendix

Index

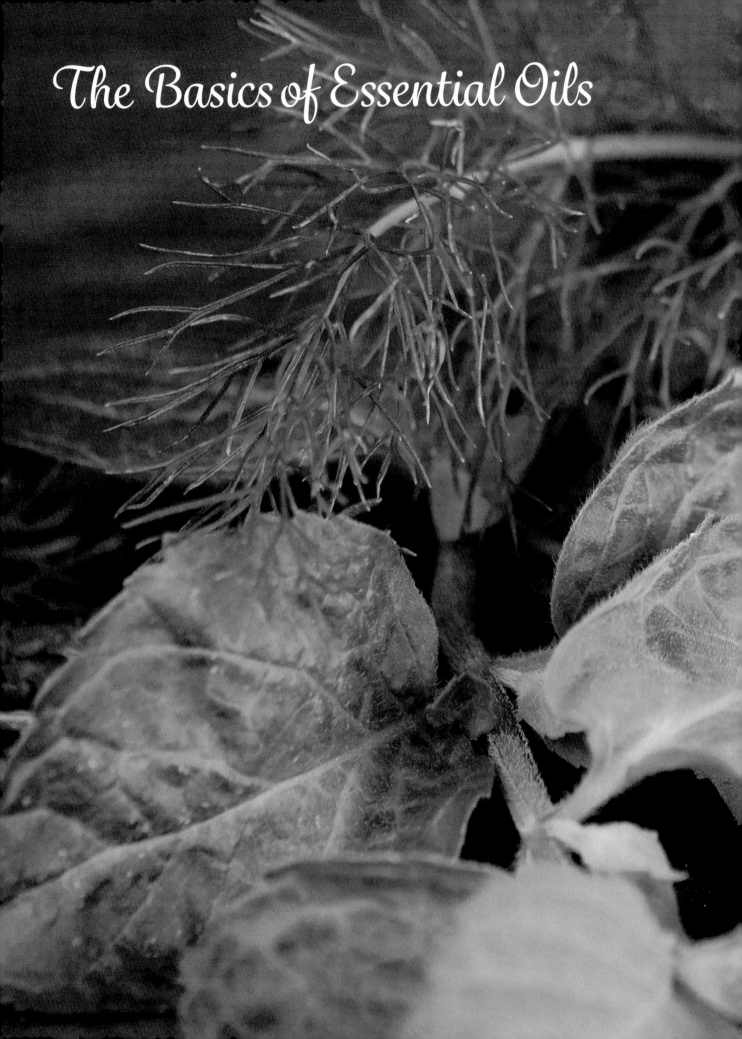

The Basics of Essential Oils

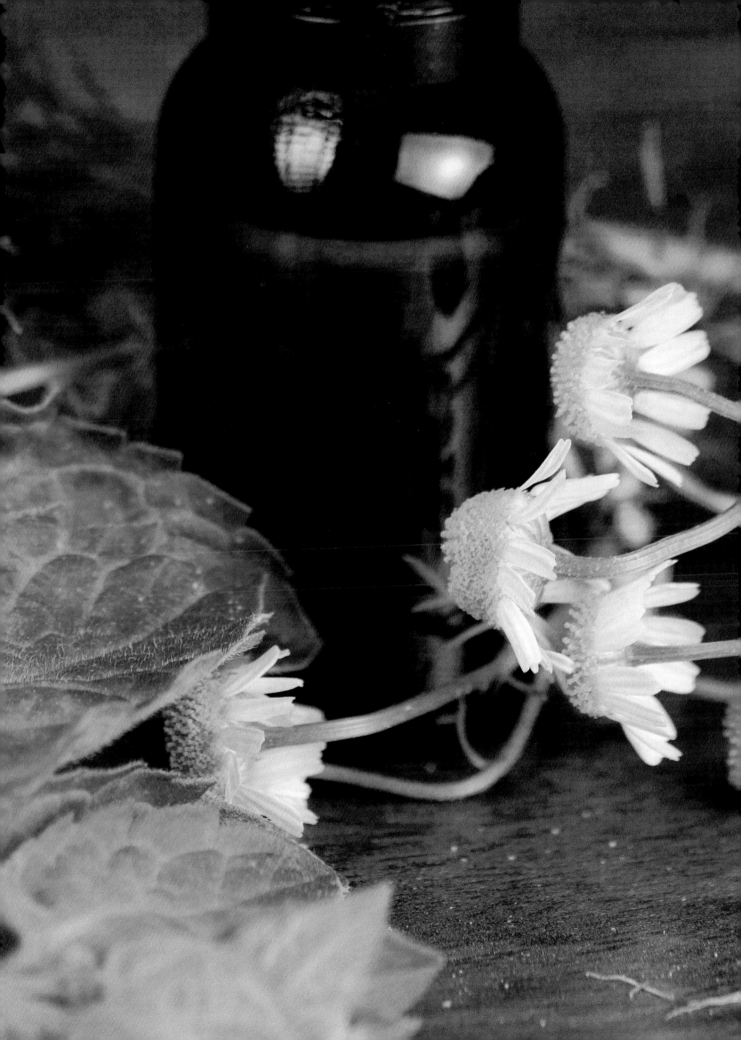

An Introduction to Essential Oils

What are essential oils?

Essential oils are the volatile liquids that are distilled from plants (including their respective parts such as seeds, bark, leaves, stems, roots, flowers, fruit, etc.). One of the factors that determines the purity and therapeutic value of an oil is its chemical constituents. These constituents can be affected by a vast number of variables: the part(s) of the plant from which the oil was produced, soil condition, fertilizer (organic or chemical), geographic region, climate, altitude, harvest season and method, and distillation process (Andradea et al., 2011; Sell, 2006; Pengelly, 2004). For example, common thyme, or thyme vulgaris, produces several different chemotypes (biochemical specifics or simple species) depending on the conditions of its growth, climate, and altitude (Thompson et al., 2003). High levels of thymol depend on the time of year in which the oil is distilled. If distilled during mid-summer or late fall, there can be higher levels of carvacrol, which can cause the oil to be more caustic or irritating to the skin (Hudaib et al., 2002). For more information on how plants create essential oils, see the section "Plants and Essential Oils" starting on page 431.

As we begin to understand the power of essential oils in the realm of personal holistic healthcare, we comprehend the absolute necessity of obtaining pure, therapeutic-grade essential oils. No matter how costly pure, therapeutic-grade essential oils may be, there can be no substitute. Chemists can replicate some of the known individual constituents (Sell, 2006); but it would be difficult, if not impossible, to successfully recreate complete essential oils in the laboratory.

The information in this book is based on the use of pure, therapeutic-grade essential oils. Those who are beginning their journey into the realm of aromatherapy and essential oils must actively seek for the purest quality and highest therapeutic-grade oils available. Anything less may not produce the desired results and can, in some cases, be extremely toxic.

Why is it so difficult to find pure, therapeutic-grade essential oils?

Producing the purest of oils can be very costly because it may require several hundred pounds, or even several thousand pounds, of plant material to extract one pound of pure essential oil. For example, one pound of pure melissa oil sells for thousands of dollars. Although this sounds quite expensive, one must realize that three tons of plant material are required to produce that single pound of oil. Because the vast majority of all the oils produced in the world today are used by the perfume industry, the oils are being purchased for their aromatic qualities only. Unnecessary high pressure and high temperature, rapid processing, and the use of chemical solvents are often employed during the distillation process so that a greater quantity of oil can be produced at a faster rate. These oils may smell just as good and cost much less, but they will lack most, if not all, of the chemical constituents necessary to produce the expected therapeutic results.

What benefits do pure, therapeutic-grade essential oils provide?

Essential oils embody the regenerating, protective, and immune-strengthening properties of plants.

Essential oil constituents are both small in molecular size and are also lipid soluble, allowing many of them to easily and quickly penetrate the skin (Onocha et al., 2011; Kohlert et al., 2000). The lipid solubility of essential oil constituents also allows the constituents to penetrate cell membranes, even if these membranes have hardened because of an oxygen deficiency (Onocha et al., 2011). In fact, essential oil constituents have the potential to affect every cell of the body within 20 minutes and then be metabolized like other nutrients (Jager et al., 1992; Jager et al., 1996).

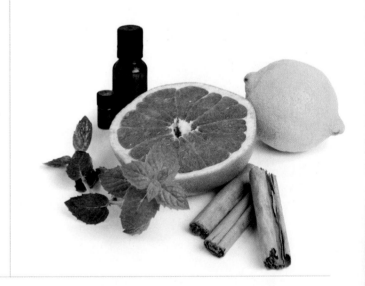

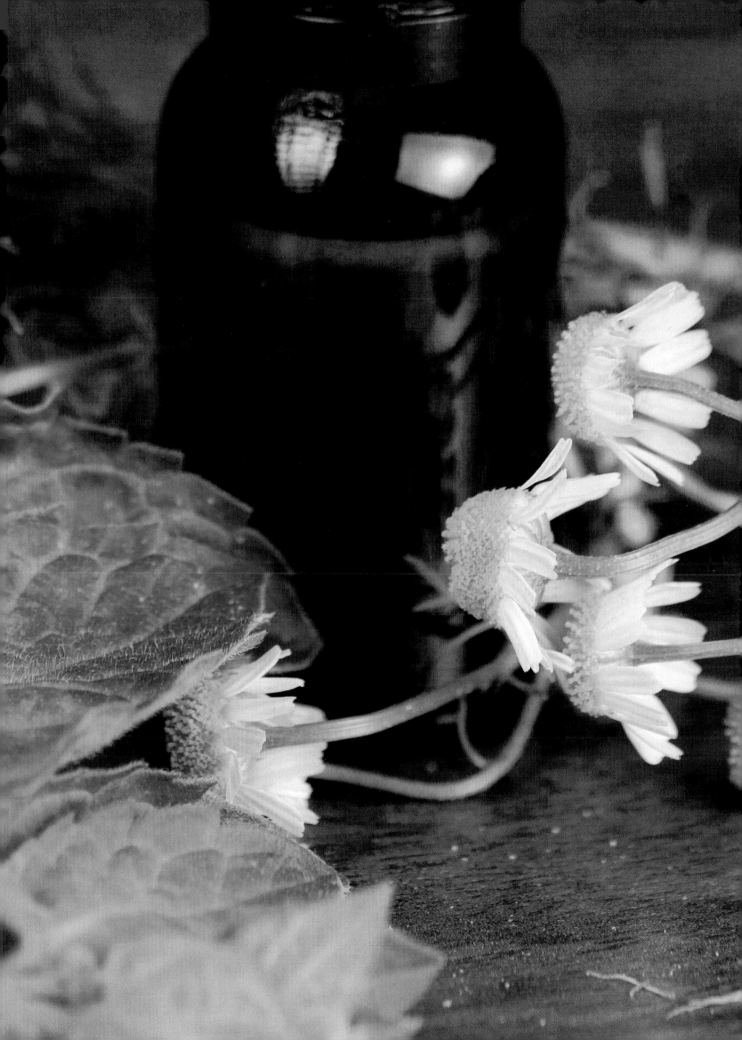

An Introduction to Essential Oils

What are essential oils?

Essential oils are the volatile liquids that are distilled from plants (including their respective parts such as seeds, bark, leaves, stems, roots, flowers, fruit, etc.). One of the factors that determines the purity and therapeutic value of an oil is its chemical constituents. These constituents can be affected by a vast number of variables: the part(s) of the plant from which the oil was produced, soil condition, fertilizer (organic or chemical), geographic region, climate, altitude, harvest season and method, and distillation process (Andradea et al., 2011; Sell, 2006; Pengelly, 2004). For example, common thyme, or thyme vulgaris, produces several different chemotypes (biochemical specifics or simple species) depending on the conditions of its growth, climate, and altitude (Thompson et al., 2003). High levels of thymol depend on the time of year in which the oil is distilled. If distilled during mid-summer or late fall, there can be higher levels of carvacrol, which can cause the oil to be more caustic or irritating to the skin (Hudaib et al., 2002). For more information on how plants create essential oils, see the section "Plants and Essential Oils" starting on page 431.

As we begin to understand the power of essential oils in the realm of personal holistic healthcare, we comprehend the absolute necessity of obtaining pure, therapeutic-grade essential oils. No matter how costly pure, therapeutic-grade essential oils may be, there can be no substitute. Chemists can replicate some of the known individual constituents (Sell, 2006); but it would be difficult, if not impossible, to successfully recreate complete essential oils in the laboratory.

The information in this book is based on the use of pure, therapeutic-grade essential oils. Those who are beginning their journey into the realm of aromatherapy and essential oils must actively seek for the purest quality and highest therapeutic-grade oils available. Anything less may not produce the desired results and can, in some cases, be extremely toxic.

Why is it so difficult to find pure, therapeutic-grade essential oils?

Producing the purest of oils can be very costly because it may require several hundred pounds, or even several thousand pounds, of plant material to extract one pound of pure essential oil. For example, one pound of pure melissa oil sells for thousands of dollars. Although this sounds quite expensive, one must realize that three tons of plant material are required to produce that single pound of oil. Because the vast majority of all the oils produced in the world today are used by the perfume industry, the oils are being purchased for their aromatic qualities only. Unnecessary high pressure and high temperature, rapid processing, and the use of chemical solvents are often employed during the distillation process so that a greater quantity of oil can be produced at a faster rate. These oils may smell just as good and cost much less, but they will lack most, if not all, of the chemical constituents necessary to produce the expected therapeutic results.

What benefits do pure, therapeutic-grade essential oils provide?

Essential oils embody the regenerating, protective, and immune-strengthening properties of plants.

Essential oil constituents are both small in molecular size and are also lipid soluble, allowing many of them to easily and quickly penetrate the skin (Onocha et al., 2011; Kohlert et al., 2000). The lipid solubility of essential oil constituents also allows the constituents to penetrate cell membranes, even if these membranes have hardened because of an oxygen deficiency (Onocha et al., 2011). In fact, essential oil constituents have the potential to affect every cell of the body within 20 minutes and then be metabolized like other nutrients (Jager et al., 1992; Jager et al., 1996).

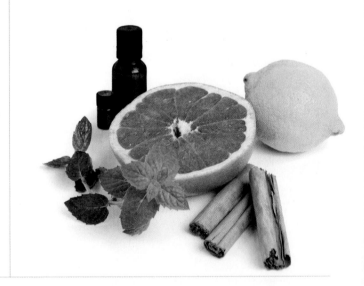

Percent of Essential Oil–
Producing Plants on Earth

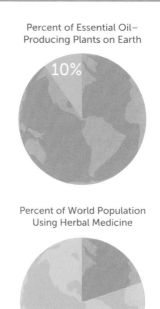

10%

Percent of World Population
Using Herbal Medicine

80%

How Do Essential Oils Benefit Plants?

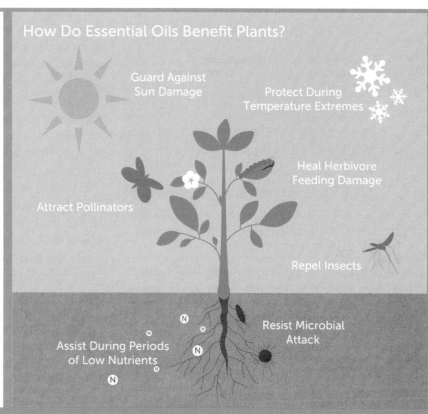

Guard Against
Sun Damage

Protect During
Temperature Extremes

Attract Pollinators

Heal Herbivore
Feeding Damage

Repel Insects

Assist During Periods
of Low Nutrients

Resist Microbial
Attack

How Can Essential Oils Support the Body?

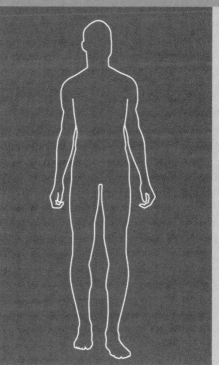

Promote Relaxation

Support Healthy Immune Function

Calm Tension and Nerves

Promote Healthy Metabolism

Uplift Mood

Promote Emotional Health

Help Reduce Occasional
Stomach Upset

Support Muscle and Joint Function

Increase Positive Feelings

Help Decrease Stress

Protect Against Environmental
and Seasonal Threats

Improve Appearance of the Skin

Provide Antioxidants

Maintain Healthy Circulation

Repel Insects

Promote Healthy Digestion

Purify the Body's Systems

Support Healthy
Respiratory Function

Soothe Occasional
Skin Irritations

Simple Diffusion Across the Cell Membrane

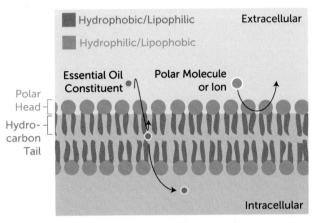

When water and oil are mixed together in a cup, they eventually separate, forming two layers. A similar phenomenon results in the formation of the cell membrane. The hydrocarbon tails of the lipid membrane form an oily barrier separating extracellular fluid from the intracellular fluid of the cell. Essential oils are able to penetrate the oily barrier because the barrier and the essential oil have similar lipophilic properties. Hydrophilic molecules, like ions, are reluctant to enter the lipophilic interior created by the hydrocarbon tails (Alberts et al., 2013). The smaller the molecule and the more lipophilic, or nonpolar, it is, the more rapidly it will diffuse across the membrane (Alberts et al., 2013).

Essential oils can be powerful antioxidants. Antioxidants neutralize or quench free radicals (Lobo et al., 2010). Free radicals are atoms with at least one unpaired electron and are created naturally by the body during metabolism. The body uses free radicals to perform important roles in gene transcription, cell signal-ing, and other regulatory functions (Fang et al., 2002). Free radicals can also be created by environmental factors such as pollution, radiation, and cigarette smoke. In these situations, free radicals outnumber the body's natural antioxidants and may cause cell injury and death (Fang et al., 2002). This imbalance between free radicals and antioxidants is called oxidative stress and occurs when antioxidants are unable to neutralize free radicals (Urso et al., 2003). If a free radical is not properly managed, it can cause "domino-like" damage by creating new free radicals out of normal atoms. Consequences of oxidative stress may include damage to proteins, DNA, and tissue, as well as the triggering of a number of human diseases (Fang et al., 2002; Lobo et al., 2010). Essential oils, omega-3 fatty acids found in fish oil, and certain vitamins have been shown to act as inhibitors of free radical generation (Fang et al., 2002) and can help diminish oxidative stress and harmful free radical production, helping the body fight disease and damage.

Many essential oil constituents have antibacterial, antifungal (Aguiar et al., 2014), anti-infectious, antimicrobial, antitumor, antiparasitic, antiviral, and antiseptic properties. Essential oils have been shown to destroy many harmful bacteria and viruses while simultaneously providing immune system support (Serafino et al., 2008).

Some essential oils can support the liver in detoxifying the blood. For example, rosemary essential oil constituents have been shown to induce enzyme activity in the liver,

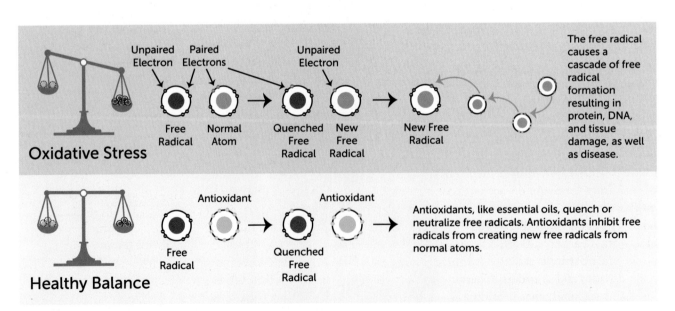

Oxidative stress, an imbalance between free radicals and antioxidants, causes damage and disease. Free radicals, atoms with an unpaired electron, steal electrons away from normal atoms. Normal atoms are then transformed into free radicals. Essential oils and other antioxidants can inhibit free radical damage by donating an electron to a free radical. Antioxidants do not become free radicals because they are stable in either form.

Percent of Essential Oil–
Producing Plants on Earth

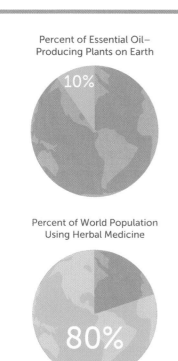

10%

Percent of World Population
Using Herbal Medicine

80%

How Do Essential Oils Benefit Plants?

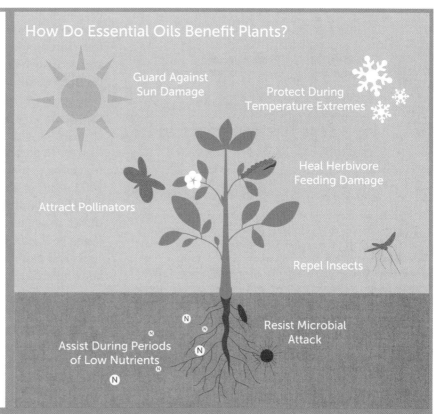

Guard Against
Sun Damage

Protect During
Temperature Extremes

Heal Herbivore
Feeding Damage

Attract Pollinators

Repel Insects

Resist Microbial
Attack

Assist During Periods
of Low Nutrients

How Can Essential Oils Support the Body?

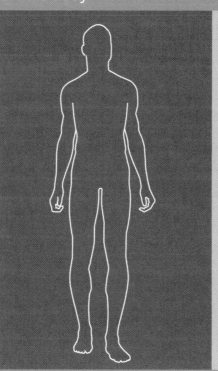

Promote Relaxation

Support Healthy Immune Function

Calm Tension and Nerves

Promote Healthy Metabolism

Uplift Mood

Promote Emotional Health

Help Reduce Occasional
Stomach Upset

Support Muscle and Joint Function

Increase Positive Feelings

Help Decrease Stress

Protect Against Environmental
and Seasonal Threats

Improve Appearance of the Skin

Provide Antioxidants

Maintain Healthy Circulation

Repel Insects

Promote Healthy Digestion

Purify the Body's Systems

Support Healthy
Respiratory Function

Soothe Occasional
Skin Irritations

Simple Diffusion Across the Cell Membrane

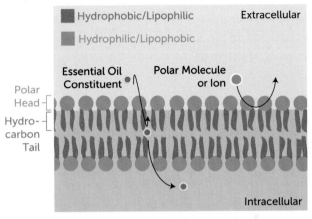

When water and oil are mixed together in a cup, they eventually separate, forming two layers. A similar phenomenon results in the formation of the cell membrane. The hydrocarbon tails of the lipid membrane form an oily barrier separating extracellular fluid from the intracellular fluid of the cell. Essential oils are able to penetrate the oily barrier because the barrier and the essential oil have similar lipophilic properties. Hydrophilic molecules, like ions, are reluctant to enter the lipophilic interior created by the hydrocarbon tails (Alberts et al., 2013). The smaller the molecule and the more lipophilic, or nonpolar, it is, the more rapidly it will diffuse across the membrane (Alberts et al., 2013).

Essential oils can be powerful antioxidants. Antioxidants neutralize or quench free radicals (Lobo et al., 2010). Free radicals are atoms with at least one unpaired electron and are created naturally by the body during metabolism. The body uses free radicals to perform important roles in gene transcription, cell signal-

ing, and other regulatory functions (Fang et al., 2002). Free radicals can also be created by environmental factors such as pollution, radiation, and cigarette smoke. In these situations, free radicals outnumber the body's natural antioxidants and may cause cell injury and death (Fang et al., 2002). This imbalance between free radicals and antioxidants is called oxidative stress and occurs when antioxidants are unable to neutralize free radicals (Urso et al., 2003). If a free radical is not properly managed, it can cause "domino-like" damage by creating new free radicals out of normal atoms. Consequences of oxidative stress may include damage to proteins, DNA, and tissue, as well as the triggering of a number of human diseases (Fang et al., 2002; Lobo et al., 2010). Essential oils, omega-3 fatty acids found in fish oil, and certain vitamins have been shown to act as inhibitors of free radical generation (Fang et al., 2002) and can help diminish oxidative stress and harmful free radical production, helping the body fight disease and damage.

Many essential oil constituents have antibacterial, antifungal (Aguiar et al., 2014), anti-infectious, antimicrobial, antitumor, antiparasitic, antiviral, and antiseptic properties. Essential oils have been shown to destroy many harmful bacteria and viruses while simultaneously providing immune system support (Serafino et al., 2008).

Some essential oils can support the liver in detoxifying the blood. For example, rosemary essential oil constituents have been shown to induce enzyme activity in the liver,

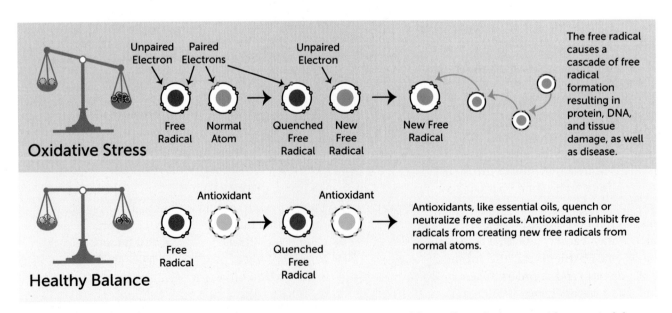

Oxidative stress, an imbalance between free radicals and antioxidants, causes damage and disease. Free radicals, atoms with an unpaired electron, steal electrons away from normal atoms. Normal atoms are then transformed into free radicals. Essential oils and other antioxidants can inhibit free radical damage by donating an electron to a free radical. Antioxidants do not become free radicals because they are stable in either form.

suggesting a possibility of increased ability to remove toxins (Debersac et al., 2001).

Many essential oils possess powerful air-purifying properties (Tyagi et al., 2010). When vaporized, some essential oils, including peppermint, produce stronger antimicrobial properties than when used in the liquid phase (Tyagi et al., 2010). This increased antimicrobial action occurs because vaporized essential oils combine with negative ions in the air for synergistic air purification and disinfection (Tyagi et al., 2010). Furthermore, essential oils fill the air with a fresh aromatic scent while destroying odors.

Essential oils help promote emotional, physical, and spiritual healing.

How long have essential oils been around?

From the beginning of early civilization, aromatic plants have been used for their therapeutic properties. Egyptian papyri and Chinese manuscripts describe the medicinal use of aromatics employed thousands of years ago. The Egyptians placed a great value on aromatic oils and even included 35 alabaster jars for the oils in King Tutankhamen's tomb. Similarly, the Greeks attributed the invention of perfumes to the gods and believed all aromatic plants to be of divine origin. Additionally, there are many references to aromatics, ointments, and incenses (such as frankincense, myrrh, rosemary, etc.) in the Bible and Torah. For more on the history of essential oils, please refer to the history section on page 12.

How do essential oils affect the brain?

The blood-brain barrier is the filtering mechanism between the circulating blood and the brain that prevents certain damaging substances from reaching brain tissue and cerebrospinal fluid. A common misconception is that all small molecules cross the blood-brain barrier. However, an astounding 98% of small molecule drugs cannot cross the blood-brain barrier (Pardridge, 2009). Dr. William M. Pardridge, an expert in blood-brain barrier research, determined that "the development of new drugs for the brain has not kept pace with progress in the molecular neurosciences, because the majority of new drugs discovered do not cross the blood-brain barrier" (2003). The ability to cross the blood-brain barrier is essential for the treatment of brain diseases and disorders. Chemical constituents known as sesquiterpenes—commonly found in essential oils such as frankincense and sandalwood—are known to be able to go beyond the blood-brain barrier

The Limbic System

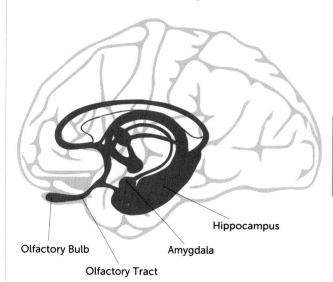

The limbic system is closely tied to the olfactory (smelling) nerves, allowing smells to greatly affect emotions and long term memory.

(Wang et al., 2012; Zhang et al., 2009). Therefore, sesquiterpenes can directly interact with brain cells, unlike most pharmaceutical drugs, and can impact the brain therapeutically. In fact, sesquiterpenes are known to interact with neurotransmitter receptors, specifically glycine, dopamine, and serotonin receptors (Wang et al., 2012; Okugawa et al., 2000).

Even if the chemical constituents of an essential oil cannot cross the blood-brain barrier, the essential oil can still affect the brain through activation of the olfactory bulb. Odors and emotions are processed in similar brain structures located in the limbic system (Pause et al., 2003). The limbic system is a group of related structures in the brain that are responsible for processing emotion, memory, and smell. The sense of smell is unique in the fact that "no other sensory system makes this kind of direct and intense contact with the neural substrates of emotion and memory, which may explain why odor-evoked memories are unusually emotionally potent" (Herz et al., 1996).

Also present in the limbic system of the brain is a gland called the amygdala. In the 1980s, it was discovered that the amygdala plays a major role in the storing and releasing of emotional trauma (LeDoux, 2003; LeDoux et al., 1988; Iwata et al., 1986; LeDoux et al., 1989). One way to stimulate this gland is with fragrance or the sense of smell (Kadohisa, 2013). Therefore, essential oils can be a powerful key to help unlock and release emotional trauma.

How are essential oils able to have so many different benefits?

The benefits of an essential oil depend greatly on the oil's diversity of chemical constituents—and not only on the existence of specific constituents but also on their amounts in proportion to other constituents present in the same oil. Some individual oils may have hundreds of different chemical constituents (Miguel, 2010; Sell, 2006). Many of these constituents have yet to be identified. Although not everything is known about all the different constituents, most of them can be grouped into a few distinct families, each with some dominant characteristics. The essential oil constituent section beginning on page 443 provides greater insights into these constituent families.

How are essential oils extracted?

There are two ways in which pure, therapeutic-grade essential oils are extracted:

—Steam Distillation

In order to understand why and how steam distillation works, it is important to be aware of two central characteristics of essential oils: First, essential oils are volatile. This means that they evaporate easily when exposed to the air. And second, essential oils are hydrophobic, which means that they do not mix with water.

Steam distillation is the method most commonly used to extract essential oils; in fact, 93% of essential oils are extracted by steam distillation (Masango, 2005). In this method, plant material is placed in an extraction chamber and then steam (produced by boiling water in another chamber) is released into the bottom of the extraction chamber where the plant material is. As the steam passes through the plant material, both the steam and the essential oil rise to the top (this is because essential oils are volatile). The steam and essential oil are directed to another chamber where they are allowed to cool. Since essential oils are hydrophobic, as the oil/steam mixture cools, the essential oil rises to the top of the chamber, while the water stays at the bottom. The essential oil can then be easily separated from the water.

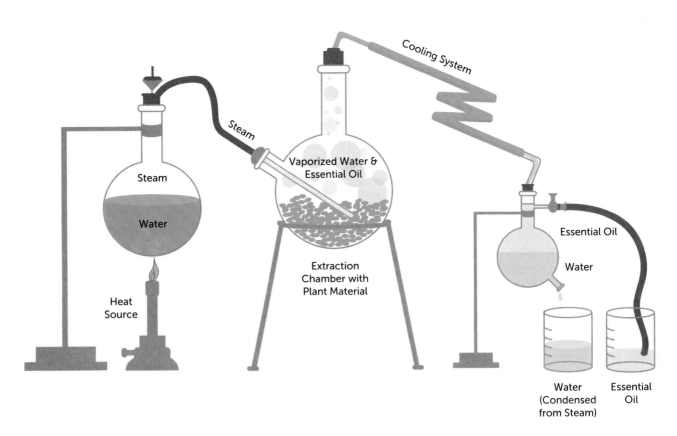

Schematic of the steam distillation of plant material to produce essential oil.

—Expression

Cold expression, or cold pressing, is the method most commonly used for extracting essential oils from citrus fruits. Mechanical pressure is used to "press" the oils out of the plant material—most often from the peel or rind.

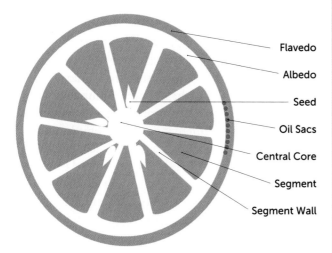

Flavedo

Albedo

Seed

Oil Sacs

Central Core

Segment

Segment Wall

Orange essential oil is contained in oil sacs found in the peel. The peel consists of a thin colored outer layer called the flavedo and a thicker fibrous inner layer called the albedo. The oil sacs are located in the flavedo of the peel. Expression requires the breaking of these oil sacs in order to release the essential oil they contain.

A Brief History of Essential Oils

Aromatic plants have long played an important role in human civilizations. They have been a part of religion, marriage ceremonies, dating and courtship, cosmetics, funerary services, medicine, and many other aspects of human life. Although the use of essential oils has evolved over the years, the basic principles remain the same. From the beginning of time, oils extracted from aromatic plants have been recognized as the most effective medicine known to mankind.

Egypt

The Egyptians are among the earliest to use essential oils. Although there is still some debate, most historians believe that the oils used in ancient Egypt were not identical to the steam-distilled essential oils used today. Rather, the oils used by the ancient Egyptians appear to be animal fats and vegetable oils into which the aromatic essential oils from the plants had been extracted—typically by steeping the plant material in the hot oils or fats (Tisserand 22). Although not as concentrated as the steam-distilled oils used at present, they were, nonetheless, used for their aromatic and therapeutic properties and are considered the precursors to pure essential oils.

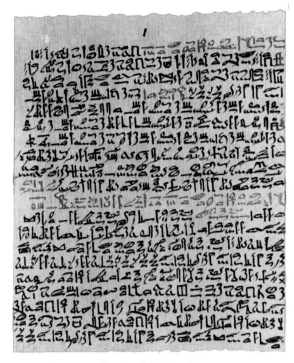

—*Portion of the Ebers Papyrus*

For the Egyptians, the distinction between medicines and perfumes was not always clear. Often a single scented oil served both purposes. Common aromatics of the time included frankincense, myrrh, cedarwood, spikenard, juniper, coriander, bitter almond, henna, calamus, and origanum (Tisserand 22).

One of the oldest and best-preserved documents that we know of, the Ebers Papyrus, documents the Egyptians' use of frankincense and other aromatics in treating a variety of different ailments. This papyrus is thought to have been composed somewhere between 1553 and 1550 BC (Hill 44).

When Herodotus and Democrates visited Egypt in the fourth century BC, they declared that the people were "masters of the art of perfumery" (Tisserand 25).

In 1922, archeologist Howard Carter and his team discovered the tomb of the ancient Egyptian king Tutankhamen. Despite evidence of some robbery and the tomb having been resealed, the majority of the original treasures remained in the tomb (Carter 33–44).

As Carter surveyed the contents of the tomb, he discovered 35 alabaster jars that had been used to hold scented oils and unguents, but every single one of them had been emptied. It soon became evident to Carter that two separate robberies had taken place in the tomb—the first robbery was for precious metals, and the second robbery was for the oils and unguents (Carter 248-50). Carter marveled that in the presence of so many other precious objects the thieves would have chosen to steal the oils. The only thing Carter could conclude was that "the greases, or oils, that they contained had, no doubt, a far greater value in those days than possibly we imagine" (Carter 249).

China

The ancient Chinese are also believed to have been masters of the use of aromatic plants for healing. Some speculate that the Chinese may have begun studying aromatics at the same time as the Egyptians did—or even before. An ancient Chinese text, "Pen T'Sao," which is believed to have been written by Emperor Shen Nung around 2500 BC, identifies medicinal uses for over 300 different plants (Petrovska 1–5). Chinese aromatherapists believed that extracting a plant's fragrance represented freeing the plant's soul (Keville, 2012).

The Chinese upper classes used fragrances lavishly during the T'ang dynasty, scenting their homes, clothing, temples, ink, paper, and cosmetics with aromatics. Huge statues of Buddha were even carved from fragrant camphor wood (Keville, 2012).

Greece

Hydrodistillation of plant materials to extract aromatics dates back to at least 1850 B.C. on the island of Crete. Archaeological discoveries on the island of Crete have provided evidence that the people of ancient Crete distilled scents from plants such as lavender, rosemary, coriander, and bergamot using earthenware stills (Belgiorno).

The Greeks believed all aromatic plants to be of divine origin, and they attributed the invention of perfumes to the gods (Tisserand 25).

The Greek physician Marestheus recognized that aromatic plants had either stimulating or sedative properties. He identified rose and hyacinth as refreshing and invigorating. Another Greek, Theophrastus, wrote that he wasn't surprised that perfumes should have medicinal properties when taking into consideration the other virtues of perfumes (Tisserand 27).

Without fully understanding the composition or chemical processes of essential oils, the Greeks were still able to profit from the antiseptic properties of the oils. Hippocrates used aromatic essences to fumigate the city of Athens to fight off the plague epidemic. Hippocrates also suggested that the key to good health is found in taking a daily aromatic bath and receiving a daily scented massage (Gawronski 142).

Rome

The Romans also used aromatics—even more lavishly than the Greeks did. They used aromatics to scent everything—their hair, their clothes, their beds, their bodies, their military flags, the walls of their houses, and everything else they could think of. They also used the oils and unguents in massage and baths (Tisserand 28).

The Romans, who were famous for their preoccupation with public health and for their public baths, were said to have embraced aromatherapy. Roman soldiers were also known to carry pouches filled with the seeds of aromatic plants on their military campaigns (Gawronski 142).

Israel

The value of aromatics to the ancient people of Israel is clearly evident throughout many historical texts.

The writings of the Old Testament/Torah contain numerous references to aromatics, ointments, and incenses that were used by the ancient Israelites.

The New Testament also includes additional references to the use of aromatics and aromatic ointments by the Israelites, including the gifts of frankincense and myrrh given by the wise men who came to worship the Christ child (St. Matthew 2:11) and the use of spikenard for anointing (St. John 12:3–5).

Arabia

Between 1000 BC and 400 BC, Arabia was the center of a lucrative spice trade route. During this time, frankincense was by far the biggest trade commodity and brought great wealth to Arabia. The trade route extended from the Dhofar region of Omar to Petra in Jordan—approximately 2400 miles—and was commonly referred to as the Frankincense Trail. This trail was used so many times that modern day satellite images still show faint marks on the ground where the camel caravans passed over (Hill 44–46).

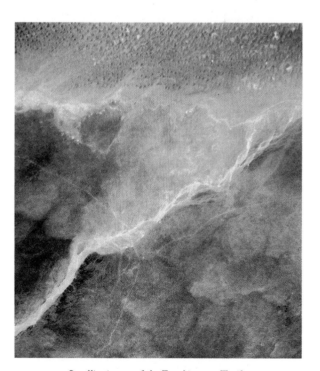

—Satellite image of the Frankincense Trail

Persia

The Persians are credited with being the first to discover steam distillation as a method of extracting essential oils from plants around 1000 AD. The Persian physician 'Abu 'Ali al-Husian Ibn 'Abd Allah Ibn Sina, more commonly known as Avicenna, is said to be the inventor of this method of distillation. Avicenna distilled both essences and aromatic waters (Tisserand 30).

Europe

With the invention of distillation, the use of aromatic essential oils in perfumes quickly migrated to Europe, and by the end of the twelfth century, the Europeans were distilling their own essential oils and manufacturing their own perfumes (Tisserand 30).

When the Great Plague became widespread in Europe, fumigations with aromatics were often employed to try and drive the sickness from the cities. It was found that those who were most in contact with aromatics, especially the perfumers, were virtually immune to the plague while so many died around them (Tisserand 38–39). In London, houses and workplaces were fumigated on a daily basis to try and keep away the plague. Frankincense was among the aromatics used (Porter 42).

By the 1500s physicians such as Hieronymus Brunschwig (who wrote one of the earliest printed books on essential oil distillation and use, *Liber de Arte Distillandi*) were distilling and using essential oils for their medicinal benefits.

The Reintroduction of Essential Oils

Essential oils regained popularity in the mid-19th century largely because of their desirable fragrances. As the cosmetic, soap, and food industries grew, so did the demand for essential oils to be used to scent and flavor these products (Başer et al. 184). These essential oils weren't necessarily of a therapeutic grade, but they did call back the attention to essential oils.

With the help of research and several key individuals, essential oils became recognized once again for their therapeutic and medicinal properties, and aromatherapy and pure, therapeutic-grade essential oils were reintroduced to the general public.

—René-Maurice Gattefossé

René-Maurice Gattefossé was a French chemist born in 1881. He is known as the "father of aromatherapy" because of his extensive research of essential oils and is credited with coining the term "aromatherapy" (Gattefossé 134).

Gattefossé is most famous for his work and personal experience with lavender essential oil. While working in his laboratory one day, there was an explosion that covered Gattefossé with "burning substances," which he extinguished by rolling on the grass outside. Gattefossé says of the experience, "Both my hands were covered with a rapidly developing gas gangrene. Just one rinse with lavender essence stopped 'the gastification of the tissue.' This treatment was followed by profuse sweating and healing began the next day" (Gattefossé 87). Gattefossé was only partly surprised by the healing power of the lavender essential oil because Gattefossé had been researching essential oils long enough to know of their powerful antiseptic and healing properties (Tisserand 41–42).

Although René-Maurice Gattefossé was not the first to use essential oils, nor was he the first to write about their therapeutic use, his vision was

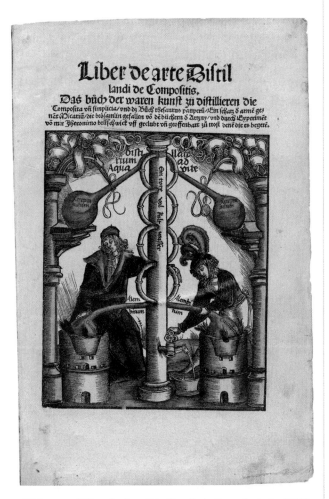

—*Title page of* Liber de Arte Distillandi, *by Brunschwig (c. 1512)*

unlike that of any of his contemporaries. Gattefossé saw aromatherapy as a discipline of its own and recognized the great value of essential oils in healthcare. There were others researching essential oils at the same time as Gattefossé, but none of them equaled Gattefossé in their enthusiasm and dedication to the subject (Gattefossé v). Gattefossé was instrumental in helping essential oils to be seen for their therapeutic properties, and not just for their pleasant smell.

—Jean Valnet

Jean Valnet, MD, was a French army physician and surgeon. During World War II in Tonkin, China, Valnet used his limited supply of essential oils in the treatment of injured soldiers and was very satisfied with the consistency of the results he achieved (Valnet 66).

Valnet recognized the drawbacks of modern medications and antibiotics with their harmful side effects and the need to continually increase their dosages as the body's tolerance increases (Valnet 49–50), and for this reason he turned to essential oils as a natural alternative.

Valnet very strongly believed that there was always something more that could be done for a patient before condemning him or her to death (Valnet 227), and essential oil use was that "something more" that Valnet turned to.

—Robert B. Tisserand

Robert Tisserand searched for 20 years to obtain a copy of *Gattefossé's Aromatherapy*. After searching for so long, Tisserand began to doubt that the book even existed (Gattefossé v). Once he found the book, he edited it and added his own introduction to the 1993 printing. He calls *Gattefossé's Aromatherapy* the "missing link for 20th century aromatherapy" (Gattefossé vi).

Tisserand's own research delves into the history, use, properties, and therapeutic benefits of essential oils. Tisserand was also instrumental in making information about the therapeutic use of essential oils available to the general public.

Essential Oils Today

Today, scientists, physicians, researchers, and many individuals concerned with managing their own personal health are just beginning to explore and discover some of the amazing benefits pure, therapeutic-grade essential oils have to offer.

Essential Oil Application Methods: Topical

Topical application is the process of placing an essential oil on the skin, hair, mouth, teeth, nails, or mucous membranes of the body. Applying essential oils directly on the body without any kind of dilution is commonly referred to as applying the oil "neat." Since essential oils are so potent, and because some essential oils may irritate the skin or other areas of the body, they are often diluted with a pure vegetable oil (usually called a "carrier oil") such as fractionated coconut oil, almond oil, olive oil, jojoba oil, etc. Several topical application methods are outlined below.

Direct Application:

Direct application is applying the oils directly on the area of concern. Because essential oils are so potent, more is not necessarily better. To achieve the desired results, 1–3 drops of oil are usually adequate. A few guidelines for direct application of the oils are as follow:

- The feet are the second fastest area of the body to absorb oils because of the large pores. Other quick-absorbing areas include behind the ears and on the wrists.

- To produce a feeling of peace, relaxation, or energy, 3–6 drops per foot are adequate.

- When massaging a large area of the body, always dilute the oils by 15%–30% with fractionated coconut oil.

- When applying oils to infants and small children, dilute with fractionated coconut oil. Use 1–3 drops of an essential oil to 1 Tbs. (15 ml) of fractionated coconut oil for infants and 1–3 drops of an essential oil to 1 tsp. (5 ml) fractionated coconut oil for children ages 2–5.

- Use caution when creating blends for topical therapeutic use. Commercially available blends have been specially formulated by someone who understands the chemical constituents of each oil and which oils blend well. The chemical properties of the oils can be altered when mixed improperly, resulting in some undesirable reactions.

- Layering individual oils is preferred over mixing your own blends for topical use. Layering refers to the process of applying one oil, rubbing it in, and then applying another oil. There is no need to wait more than a couple of seconds between each oil, as absorption occurs quite rapidly. If dilution is necessary, fractionated coconut oil may be applied on top. The layering technique is not only useful in physical healing but also in emotional clearing.

Massage:

Massage is the stimulation of muscle, skin, and connective tissues using various techniques to help promote healing, balance, and connection. Massages can be invigorating, relaxing, stimulating, or soothing, and essential oils applied using massage can help enhance these benefits. There are many different massage techniques currently in use, and to explore all of the various techniques would be beyond the scope of this book.

Unless you are a certified massage therapist and have a thorough understanding of anatomy, it is best to use only light to medium massage strokes for applying oils and to avoid the spine and other sensitive areas of the body. Extreme caution must also be used when massaging pregnant women and others with certain health conditions.

To create a simple massage oil that includes the benefits of essential oils, combine 3–10 drops of your desired essential oil or blend with 1 Tbs. (15 ml) of fractionated coconut oil or another carrier oil. Apply a small amount of this mixture on location, and massage it into the skin using light to medium-light strokes of the hand or fingers.

Reflexology/Reflex Therapy:

Reflex therapy is a simple method of applying oils to contact points (or nerve endings) in the feet or hands. A series of hand rotation movements at those control points create a vibrational healing energy that carries the oils along the neuroelectrical pathways. The oils either help remove any blockage along the pathways or travel the length of the pathway to benefit the particular organ. Refer to the reflex hand and foot charts on the following pages for more details.

Auricular Therapy

Auricular therapy is a method of applying the oils to various points on the rim of the ears to effect changes on internal body parts. Small amounts of the oil are applied to the point, and then the point is stimulated with the fingers or with a glass probe. See the Auricular Body Points chart on the following page for more details.

Compresses

1. Basin. Fill a wash basin with 8 cups (2 L) of hot or cold water, and add the desired essential oils. Stir the water vigorously; then lay a towel on top of the water. Since the oils will float to the top, the towel will absorb the oils with the water. After the towel is completely saturated, wring out the excess water (leaving much of the oils in the towel), and place the towel over the area needing the compress. For a hot compress, cover with a dry towel and a hot water bottle. For a cold compress, cover with a piece of plastic or plastic wrap. Finally, put another towel on top, and leave for as long as possible (1–2 hours is best).

2. Massage. Apply a hot, wet towel and then a dry towel on top of an already massaged area. The moist heat will force the oils deeper into the tissues of the body.

Baths

1. Bathwater. Begin by adding 3–6 drops of oil to the bathwater while the tub is filling. Because the individual oils will separate as the water calms down, the skin will quickly draw the oils from the top of the water. Some people have commented that they were unable to endure more than 6 drops of oil. Such individuals may benefit from adding the oils to a bath and shower gel base first. Soak for 15 minutes.

2. Bath and Shower Gel. Begin by adding 3–6 drops of oil to 1 Tbs. (15 ml) of a bath and shower gel base; add to the water while the tub is filling. Adding the oils to a bath and shower gel base first allows one to obtain the greatest benefit from the oils as they are more evenly dispersed throughout the water and not allowed to immediately separate.

3. Bath Salts. Combine 3–10 drops essential oil with ¼–½ cup (50–125 g) of bath salts or Epsom salt. Dissolve the salt mixture in warm bathwater before bathing.

4. Washcloth. When showering, add 3–6 drops of oil to a bath and shower gel base before applying to a washcloth and using to wash the body.

5. Body Sprays. Fill a small spray bottle with distilled water, and add 10–15 drops of your favorite oil blend or single oils. Shake well, and spray onto the entire body just after taking a bath or shower.

Auricular Internal Body Points

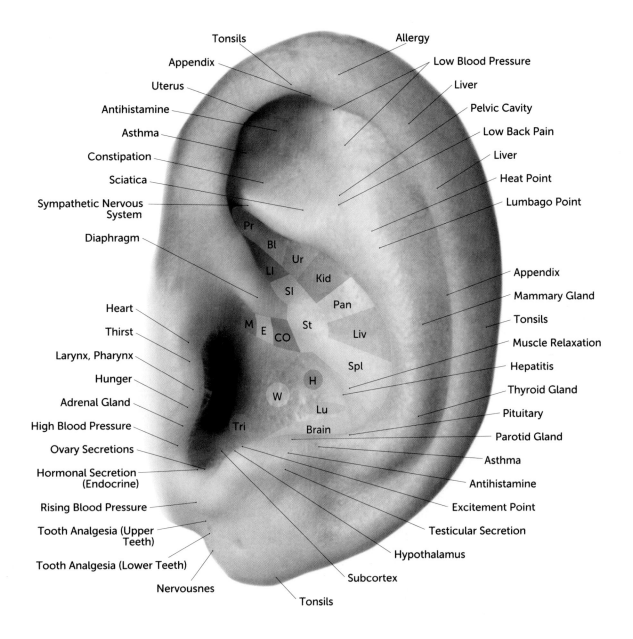

Tonsils
Appendix
Uterus
Antihistamine
Asthma
Constipation
Sciatica
Sympathetic Nervous System
Diaphragm

Allergy
Low Blood Pressure
Liver
Pelvic Cavity
Low Back Pain
Liver
Heat Point
Lumbago Point

Pr
Bl
Ur
LI
Kid
SI
Pan
M E St
CO Liv
Spl
H
W Lu
Tri Brain

Heart
Thirst
Larynx, Pharynx
Hunger
Adrenal Gland
High Blood Pressure
Ovary Secretions
Hormonal Secretion (Endocrine)
Rising Blood Pressure
Tooth Analgesia (Upper Teeth)
Tooth Analgesia (Lower Teeth)
Nervousnes

Appendix
Mammary Gland
Tonsils
Muscle Relaxation
Hepatitis
Thyroid Gland
Pituitary
Parotid Gland
Asthma
Antihistamine
Excitement Point
Testicular Secretion
Hypothalamus
Subcortex
Tonsils

Bl: Bladder	Liv: Liver	Spl: Spleen
CO: Cardiac Orifice	Lu: Lungs	St: Stomach
E: Esophagus	M: Mouth	Tri: Triple Warmer
H: Heart	Pan: Pancreas	Ur: Ureter
Kid: Kidney	Pr: Prostate	W: Windpipe/Trachea
LI: Large Intestine	SI: Small Intestine	

Reflex Therapy Hand Chart

Reflex points on this hand chart correspond to those on the feet. Occasionally the feet can be too sensitive for typical reflex therapy. Working with the hands will not only affect the specific body points but may also help to provide some pain relief to the corresponding points on the feet.

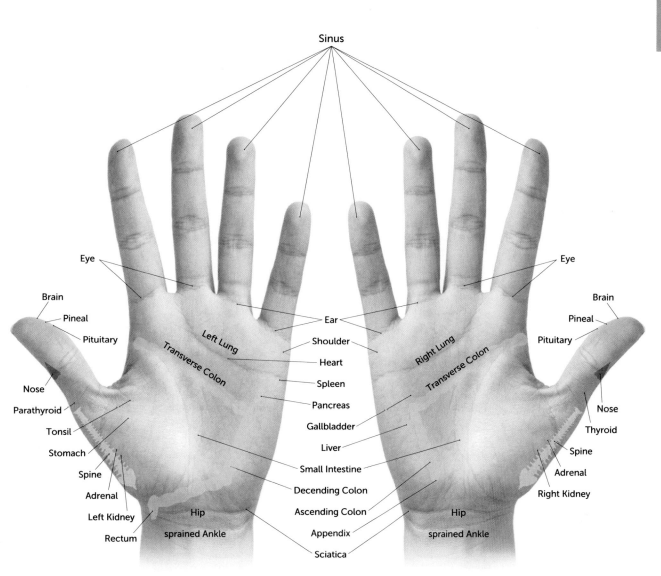

Reflex Therapy Feet Charts

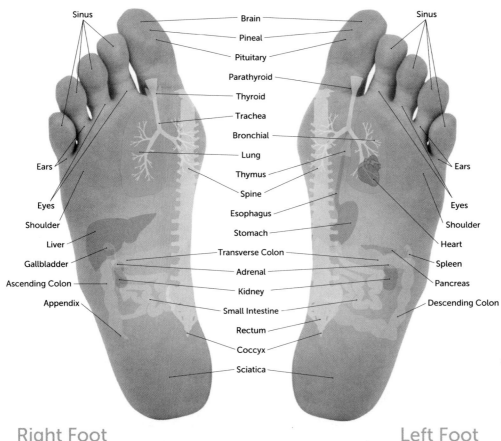

Sinus — Brain — Sinus
Pineal
Pituitary
Parathyroid
Thyroid
Trachea
Bronchial
Ears — Lung — Ears
Thymus
Eyes — Spine — Eyes
Shoulder — Esophagus — Shoulder
Liver — Stomach — Heart
Gallbladder — Transverse Colon — Spleen
Ascending Colon — Adrenal — Pancreas
Appendix — Kidney — Descending Colon
Small Intestine
Rectum
Coccyx
Sciatica

Right Foot   Left Foot

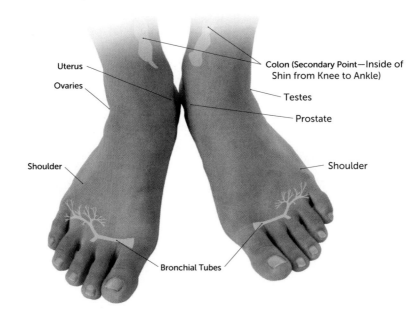

Uterus
Ovaries
Colon (Secondary Point—Inside of
Shin from Knee to Ankle)
Testes
Prostate
Shoulder — Shoulder
Bronchial Tubes

Aroma Touch Technique

This technique is a simple, yet effective, way that both beginners and experts alike can apply essential oils with meaningful results.

This effective technique utilizes eight individual essential oils and oil blends that have demonstrated profound effects on four conditions that constantly challenge the ability of the body's systems to function optimally: stress, increased toxin levels, inflammation, and autonomic nervous system imbalance.

This system is comprised of simple application methods that enable these powerful essential oils to reach the optimal areas within the body where they are able to help combat stress, enhance immune function, decrease inflammation, and balance the autonomic nervous system within the recipient.

Stress:

Stress refers to the many systemic changes that take place within the body as it responds to challenging situations. Stress comes not only from difficult, new, and pressured circumstances but also from the body being challenged to cope with things such as abnormal physical exertion, a lack of proper nutrients in the diet, disease-causing microorganisms, and toxic chemicals that make their way into the body. While the systems within a healthy body can typically deal with most short-term challenges, having constant or chronic stress on these systems can overly fatigue them, limiting their abilities to respond to future challenges.

Toxic Insult:

The body is constantly working to cope with a vast array of toxins that continually bombard it. These toxins can come from many different sources, including chemical-laden foods, pollution in the air and water, and pathogenic microorganisms that invade the body. As the environment of the world becomes increasingly saturated with toxins and a rising number of resistant pathogens, the cells, tissues, and systems of the body are forced to work harder to process and eliminate these threats in order to maintain health.

Inflammation:

Inflammation is an immune system response that allows the body to contain and fight infection or to repair damaged tissue. This response dilates the blood vessels and increases vascular permeability to allow more blood to flow to an area with injured or infected tissue. It is characterized by redness, swelling, warmth, and pain. While a certain amount of inflammation can be beneficial in fighting disease and healing injuries, chronic inflammation can actually further injure surrounding tissues or cause debilitating levels of pain.

Autonomic Imbalance:

The autonomic nervous system is comprised of nerves that are connected to the muscles, organs, tissues, and systems that don't require conscious effort to control. The autonomic system is divided into two main parts that each have separate, balancing functions: the sympathetic nervous system and the parasympathetic nervous system. The sympathetic nervous system functions to accelerate heart rate, increase blood pressure, slow digestion, and constrict blood vessels. It activates the "fight or flight" response in order to deal with threatening or stressful situations. The parasympathetic nervous system functions to slow heart rate, store energy, stimulate digestive activity, and relax specific muscles.

Maintaining a proper balance within the autonomic nervous system is important for optimal body function and maintenance.

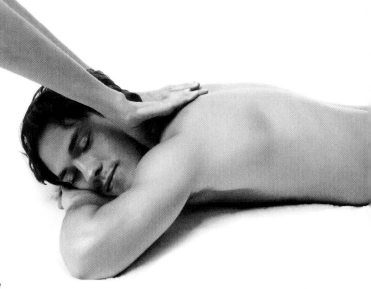

Oils Used in the Balancing Touch Technique:

For additional information on the oils and blends used in this technique, see the Single Essential Oils and Essential Oil Blends sections of this book.

Stress-Reducing Oils:

Balance: is an oil blend formulated from oils that are known to bring a feeling of calmness, peace, and relaxation. It can aid in harmonizing the various physiological systems of the body and promote tranquility and a sense of balance.

Lavender: has been used for generations for its calming and sedative properties.

Immune Enhancement Oils:

Melaleuca: has potent antifungal, antibacterial, and anti-inflammatory properties.

On Guard: is a blend of oils that have been studied for their strong abilities to kill harmful bacteria, mold, and viruses.

Inflammatory Response–Reducing Oils:

AromaTouch: is a blend of oils that were selected specifically for their ability to relax, calm, and relieve the tension of muscles, soothe irritated tissue, and increase circulation.

Deep Blue: is a blend containing oils that are well known and researched for their abilities to soothe inflammation, alleviate pain, and reduce soreness.

Autonomic Balancing Oils:

Orange: has antidepressant properties and is often used to relieve feelings of anxiety and stress. Its aroma is uplifting to both the body and mind.

Peppermint: has invigorating and uplifting properties.

Applying the Oils: Step One—Stress Reduction

Balance:

Apply Oil: Apply Balance from the base (top) of the sacrum to the base of the skull, distributing the oil evenly along the spine. Use the pads of your fingers to lightly distribute the oils over the length of the spine.

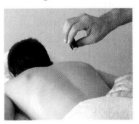

Palm Circles and Connection: With the palms down and fingers overlapping, make three clockwise circles over the heart area; hold the hands briefly in that area, and then slide one hand to the base of the sacrum and the other hand to the base of the skull.

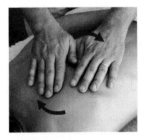

Hold as long as necessary to form a connection, balance, and feeling of trust.

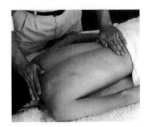

Lavender

Apply Oil: Apply lavender oil from the base of the sacrum to the base of the skull, distributing the oil evenly along the spine. Use the pads of your fingers to lightly distribute the oils over the length of the spine.

Alternating Palm Slide: Standing at the recipient's side, place both hands next to the spine on the opposite side of the back at the base of the sacrum, with the palms down and the fingers pointing away from you. Slide one hand away from the spine toward the side using a mild pressure; then repeat using alternating hands. Continue with this sliding motion as you slowly work your hands from the base of the sacrum to the base of the skull.

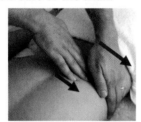

Repeat this step two more times on one side of the back; then move around the person to the opposite side, and repeat three times on that side.

5–Zone Activation: Standing at the head, place both hands together with the fingertips on either side of the spine at the base of the sacrum.

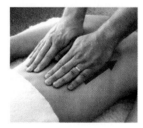

Using a medium downward pressure, pull the hands toward the head through zone 1; then continue through the neck and up to the top of the head.

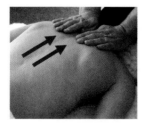

Return the hands to the base of the sacrum, and pull the hands in a similar manner through zone 2 to the shoulders.

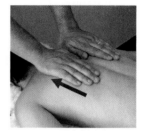

When the hands arrive at the shoulders, push the hands out to the points of the shoulders.

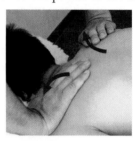

Rotate the hands around the points so that the fingers are on the underside of the shoulders.

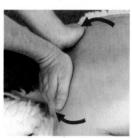

Pull the hands back to the neck, and continue up to the top of the head.

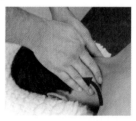

Repeat the steps for zone 2 through zones 3, 4, and 5, ending each pull at the top of the head.

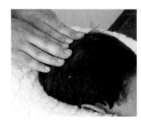

Auricular Stress Reduction: Grip each earlobe between the thumb and forefinger; using gentle pressure, work your fingers in small circles along the ear to the top.

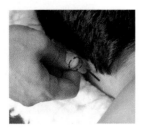

Slide your thumbs with gentle pressure along the backs of the ears returning to the lobes. Repeat this ear massage 3 times.

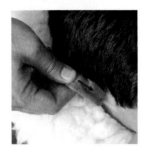

Step Two—Immune Enhancement

Melaleuca

Apply Oil: Apply melaleuca oil from the base of the sacrum to the base of the skull, distributing the oil evenly along the spine. Use the pads of your fingers to lightly distribute the oils over the length of the spine.

Alternating Palm Slide: Perform as outlined under Lavender above.

5–Zone Activation: Perform as outlined under Lavender above.

On Guard:

Apply Oil: Apply On Guard from the base of the sacrum to the base of the skull, distributing the oil evenly along the spine. Use the pads of your fingers to lightly distribute the oils over the length of the spine.

Alternating Palm Slide: Perform as outlined under Lavender above.

5–Zone Activation: Perform as outlined under Lavender above.

Thumb Walk Tissue Pull: Place the hands with palms down on either side of the spine at the base of the sacrum, with the thumbs in the small depression between the spine and the muscle tissue. Using a medium pressure, move the pads of the thumbs in small semi-circles, pulling the tissue up, away, and then down from the spine.

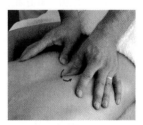

Gradually move each thumb up the spine in alternating fashion until you reach the base of the skull. Repeat this step two more times.

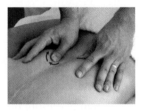

Step Three—Inflammation Reduction

AromaTouch:

Apply Oil: Apply AromaTouch from the base of the sacrum to the base of the skull, distributing the oil evenly along the spine. Use the pads of your fingers to lightly distribute the oils over the length of the spine.

Alternating Palm Slide: Perform as outlined under Lavender above.

5–Zone Activation: Perform as outlined under Lavender above.

Deep Blue:

Apply Oil: Apply Deep Blue from the base of the sacrum to the base of the skull, distributing the oil evenly along the spine. Use the pads of your fingers to lightly distribute the oils over the length of the spine.

Alternating Palm Slide: Perform as outlined under Lavender above.

5–Zone Activation: Perform as outlined under Lavender above.

Thumb Walk Tissue Pull: Perform as outlined under On Guard above.

Step Four—Autonomic Balance

Orange and Peppermint

Apply Oils to Feet: Place drops of orange oil on the palm of your hand, and apply this oil evenly over the entire bottom of the foot. Apply peppermint oil in the same manner. Hold the foot with both hands. Beginning in region 1 at the point of the heel and using a medium pressure, massage the foot using first the pad of one thumb and then the pad of the other thumb. Continue this process, alternating thumbs, back and forth through region 1 to thoroughly relax all of the tissue in that region. Repeat through regions 2 and 3.

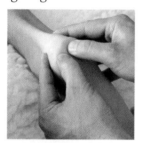

Beginning in zone 1 at the point of the heel, walk the pads of the thumbs through zone 1 using a medium pressure. Continue this process using alternating thumbs and working in a straight line through zone 1 to the tip of the big toe to thoroughly stimulate all of the tissue in that zone.

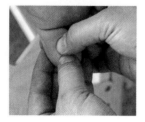

Repeat through zones 2–5.

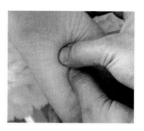

Beginning at the point of the heel and ending at the toe, use a medium pressure with the pad of your thumb to pull the tissue in zone 1. Repeat two additional times through zone 1, using alternate thumbs each time. Repeat this tissue pull process in zones 2–5 on the same foot.

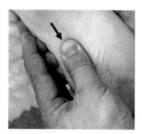

Repeat this entire process, beginning with the application of orange oil, on the opposite foot.

Apply Oils to Back: Apply first orange and then peppermint oils from the base of the sacrum to the base of the skull, distributing the oils evenly along the spine. Use the pads of your fingers to lightly distribute the oils over the length of the spine.

Alternating Palm Slide: Perform as outlined under Lavender above.

Lymphatic Stimulation:

Gentle Body Motion: Standing at the feet, grasp the feet so that the palms of your hands are against the soles of the recipient's feet and your arms are in a straight line with the recipient's legs. Use a repeated, gentle pressure on the feet that allows the recipient's body to translate (move) back and forth naturally on the table. Repeat this process for two or three 15–30 second intervals.

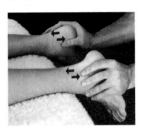

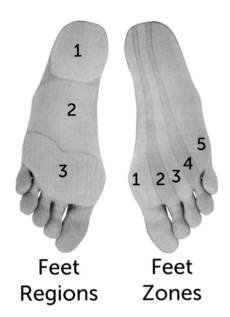

Feet Regions

Feet Zones

Zones of the Back and Head

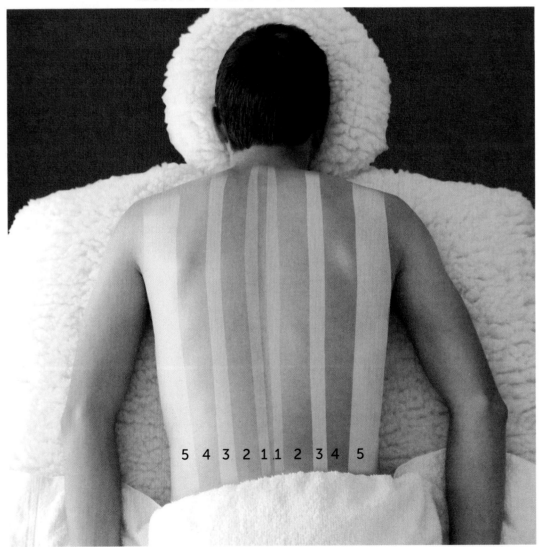

Autonomic Nervous System

Sympathetic Nervous System

Parasympathetic Nervous System

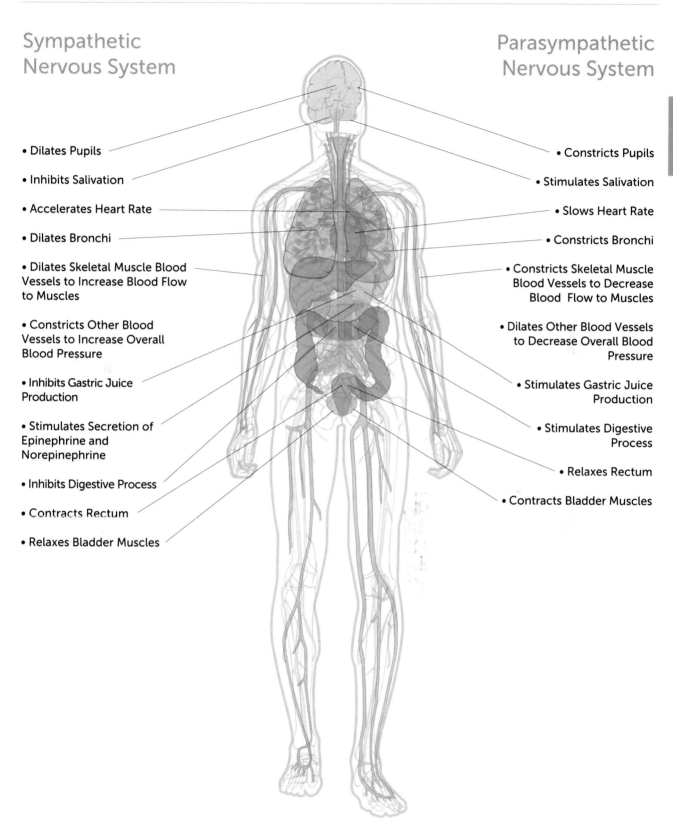

- Dilates Pupils
- Inhibits Salivation
- Accelerates Heart Rate
- Dilates Bronchi
- Dilates Skeletal Muscle Blood Vessels to Increase Blood Flow to Muscles
- Constricts Other Blood Vessels to Increase Overall Blood Pressure
- Inhibits Gastric Juice Production
- Stimulates Secretion of Epinephrine and Norepinephrine
- Inhibits Digestive Process
- Contracts Rectum
- Relaxes Bladder Muscles

- Constricts Pupils
- Stimulates Salivation
- Slows Heart Rate
- Constricts Bronchi
- Constricts Skeletal Muscle Blood Vessels to Decrease Blood Flow to Muscles
- Dilates Other Blood Vessels to Decrease Overall Blood Pressure
- Stimulates Gastric Juice Production
- Stimulates Digestive Process
- Relaxes Rectum
- Contracts Bladder Muscles

Essential Oil Application Methods: Aromatic

Aromatic application involves inhaling either a fine mist of the oil or a vapor of volatile aromatic components that have evaporated from the oil. Inhalation of the oil, or the aroma from the oil, can be a powerful way to affect memory, hormones, and emotions through the olfactory system (see the following page for further discussion on this topic). Inhalation of oils can also be a quick and effective way to affect the sinuses, larynx, bronchial tubes, and lungs.

Diffusion:

The easiest and simplest way of putting a fine mist of the whole oil into the air for inhalation is to use a nebulizing diffuser. A cool-air nebulizing diffuser uses room-temperature air to break the oils into a microfine mist that is then dispersed into the air, covering hundreds of square feet in seconds. An ultrasonic nebulizer uses ultrasonic vibrations to convert oil mixed with water into a fine water vapor. When diffused in this manner, the oils, with their oxygenating molecules, will then remain suspended for several hours to freshen and improve the quality of the air. The antiviral, antibacterial, and antiseptic properties of the oils kill bacteria and help to reduce fungus and mold.

Other diffusers may use either cool air blown through a pad containing the oil or a low level of heat to quickly evaporate the volatile oil molecules into the air. This type of diffusion is beneficial but may not be as effective for some therapeutic uses as nebulizing the whole oil can be.

Diffusers that use an intense heat source (such as a light bulb ring or candle) may alter the chemical makeup of the oil and its therapeutic qualities and are typically not recommended.

When diffused, essential oils reduce airborne chemicals and create greater physical and emotional harmony. To maximize therapeutic benefits, diffuse oils for 15 minutes every hour so that the olfactory system has time to recover before receiving more oils. The easiest way to do this is by using a timer that can be set to turn the diffuser on in 15-minute increments over a 24-hour period.

Direct Inhalation:

Direct inhalation is the simplest way to inhale the aroma of an essential oil in order to affect moods and emotions. Simply hold an opened essential oil vial close to the face, and inhale. You may also apply 1–2 drops of oil on your hands, cup your hands over your mouth and nose, and inhale.

Cloth or Tissue:

Put 1–3 drops of an essential oil on a paper towel, tissue, cotton ball, handkerchief, towel, or pillow case; hold it close to your face, and inhale.

Hot Water Vapor:

Put 1–3 drops of an essential oil into hot water, and inhale. Again, heat may reduce some of the benefits.

Vaporizer or Humidifier:

Put oil in a vaporizer or a humidifier. The cool mist types are best, since heat reduces some of the benefits. There are some commercially available diffusers that utilize ultrasonic vibration to vaporize water into a cool mist. These work well with essential oils since they produce a very fine mist that helps suspend the oil particles in the air for extended periods of time.

Fan or Vent:

Put oil on a cotton ball, and attach it to ceiling fans or air vents. This can also work well in a vehicle since the area is so small.

Perfume or Cologne:

Wearing the oils as a perfume or cologne can provide some wonderful emotional support and physical support as well—not just a beautiful fragrance. Apply 1–2 drops of oil to the wrists or neck, or create a simple perfume or cologne by dissolving 10–15 drops essential oil in 20 drops alcohol (such as vodka, or a perfumer's alcohol) and combining this mixture with 1 tsp. (5 ml) distilled water. Apply or mist on wrists or neck.

Nose and Olfactory System

When an odor molecule is inhaled into the nasal cavity, it is first sensed by the olfactory cells that are part of the olfactory epithelium. The olfactory epithelium is comprised of two small patches of olfactory nerves (each about 1 cm square) that lie on the roof of the nasal cavity. The olfactory cells within the olfactory epithelium are specialized nerve cells that extend cilia (small hair-like structures) from their dendrites into the nasal cavity. Each of these cilia have receptors that bind to a specific type of odor molecule. When an odor molecule binds to a receptor on the cilia of an olfactory cell, the olfactory cell passes the signal through the cribriform plate (the bone at the roof of the nasal cavity) to the olfactory bulb. The olfactory bulb, in turn, sends those impulses along the lateral olfactory tract to five different structures in the brain, including the amygdala (which is responsible for storing and releasing emotional trauma), the anterior olfactory nucleus (which helps process smells), the olfactory tubercle, the piriform cortex (which passes the signal on to other structures that create a conscious perception of the odor), and the entorhinal cortex (which processes stimuli before sending them on to the hippocampus, the long-term memory center of the brain). Anatomically, the olfactory system is closely connected to the limbic system of the brain. The limbic system includes structures such as the hippocampus (long-term memory), the amygdala (emotions), the hypothalamus (autonomic nervous system and hormones), and the cingulate gyrus (regulates blood pressure, heart rate, and attention). It is due to the fact that the olfactory system is so closely connected to the limbic system that essential oils have such profound physiological and psychological effects.

Olfactory System

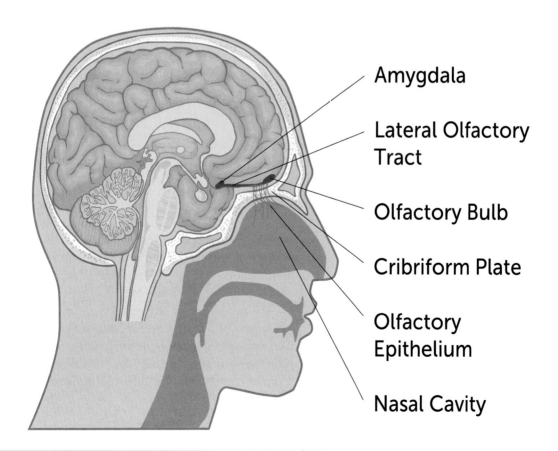

Amygdala

Lateral Olfactory Tract

Olfactory Bulb

Cribriform Plate

Olfactory Epithelium

Nasal Cavity

The Art of Blending

Blending essential oils is an art and usually requires a little bit of training and experimentation. If you choose to create your own blends, it is important to understand that the order in which the oils are blended is key to maintaining the desired therapeutic properties in a synergistic blend. An alteration in the sequence of adding selected oils to a blend may change the chemical properties, the fragrance, and, thus, the desired results. The "Blend Classification" and "Blends With" listings under each oil in the Single Oils section of this book should assist one in the blending process. In general, oils that are from the same botanical family usually blend well together. In addition, oils with similar constituents also mix well.

Four Blending Classifications

Another method utilizes four blending classifications. The following information explains the characteristics of each classification, the order in which they should be added to the blend (i.e., Personifiers first, Enhancers second, Equalizers third, and Modifiers fourth), and the amount of each type of oil as a percentage of the blend.

1st—Personifier (1–5% of blend) oils have sharp, strong, and long-lasting fragrances. They also have dominant properties with strong therapeutic action.

Oils in this classification may include birch, cinnamon, clary sage, clove, coriander, ginger, helichrysum, orange, peppermint, rose, wintergreen, and ylang ylang.

2nd—Enhancer (50–80% of blend) oils should be the predominant oil as it serves to enhance the properties of the other oils in the blend. Its fragrance is not as sharp as the personifier's and is usually of a shorter duration.

Oils in this classification may include basil, bergamot, birch, eucalyptus, frankincense, geranium, grapefruit, lavender, lemon, lemongrass, marjoram, melaleuca, orange, oregano, rose, rosemary, thyme, and wintergreen.

3rd—Equalizer (10–15% of blend) oils create balance and synergy among the oils contained in the blend. Their fragrance is also not as sharp as the personifier's and is of a shorter duration.

Oils in this classification may include basil, bergamot, cypress, fennel, white fir, frankincense, geranium, ginger, lavender, lemongrass, marjoram, melaleuca, myrrh, oregano, rose, sandalwood, and thyme.

4th—Modifier (5–8% of blend) oils have a mild and short fragrance. These oils add harmony to the blend.

Oils in this classification may include bergamot, coriander, eucalyptus, fennel, grapefruit, lavender, lemon, myrrh, rose, sandalwood, and ylang ylang.

Adding Carrier Oils

Depending upon the topical application of your blend, you will want to add some carrier/base oil. When creating a therapeutic essential oil blend, you may want to use about 28 drops of essential oil to 1 Tbs. (15 ml) of fractionated coconut oil. When creating a body massage blend, you will want to use a total of about 50 drops of essential oils to ½ cup (125 ml) of fractionated coconut oil. Remember to store your fragrant creations in dark-colored glass bottles to protect the oils from UV light and oxidation damage.

Measurement Conversion Chart

As essential oils can vary in thickness, the following are approximate measurements:

25–30 drops	= 1/4 tsp.	= 1–2 ml	= 5/8 dram
45–50 drops	= 1/2 tsp.	= 2–3 ml	= 1 dram
75–80 drops	= 3/4 tsp.	= 3–4 ml	= 1/8 oz.
100–120 drops	= 1 tsp.	= 5 ml	= 1/6 oz.
160 drops	= 1½ tsp.	= 6–8 ml	= 1/4 oz.
320–400 drops	= 3 tsp.	= 13–15 ml	= 1/2 oz.
600–650 drops	= 6 tsp.	= 25–30 ml	= 1 oz.

Learn to trust your nose, as it can help you decide which classification an oil should be in. More detailed information about these methods of blending is beyond the scope of this revision of the book. For additional information on using these classifications in your blending, we highly recommend Marcel Lavabre's *Aromatherapy Workbook*. Another very simple book about blending, with recipes and easy-to-follow guidelines, is Mindy Green's *Natural Perfumes*, which uses perfume notes (top, middle, base), odor, and odor intensity to help guide you in making your own fragrant blend creations (refer to the chart on the following page).

Natural Perfume Mixing Guide

Perfume mixing, like music, is made from notes. When used in harmony, these notes complement and accent each other to create an enjoyable aroma.

Top Notes: These are the fastest evaporating oils and the most immediately noticeable scents in a perfume. They diffuse quickly and tend to be light, crisp, and penetrating.

Middle Notes: Also called heart notes, these should make up the main body of the blend. They soften and round out the fragrance to harmonize the mixture.

Base Notes: The scents from these oils are usually not recognized until several minutes after application. Base note fragrances tend to become more pleasant over time and, when used in proper proportion, can give depth to the blend.

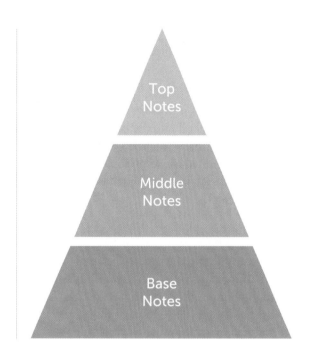

Essential Oil	Scent	Intensity
Top Notes	(5–20% of the blend)	
Orange	Fresh, citrusy, fruity, sweet, light	1
Bergamot	Sweet, lively, citrusy, fruity	2
Grapefruit	Clean, fresh, bitter, citrusy	2
Lemon	Sweet, sharp, clear, citrusy	3
Lemongrass	Grassy, lemony, pungent, earthy	4
Top to Middle Notes	(20–80% of the blend)	
Basil	Spicy, anise-like, camphorous, lively	4
Fennel	Sweet, somewhat spicy, licorice-like	4
Middle Notes	(50–80% of the blend)	
Lavender	Floral, sweet, balsamic, slightly woody	2
Cypress	Fresh, herbaceous, slightly woody	3
Eucalyptus	Slightly camphorous, sweet, fruity	3
Fir	Fresh, woody, earthy, sweet	3
Geranium	Sweet, green, citrus-rosy, fresh	3
Helichrysum	Rich, sweet, fruity, slightly honey-like	3
Marjoram	Herbaceous, green, spicy	3

Essential Oil	Scent	Intensity
Middle Notes (continued)	(50–80% of the blend)	
Melaleuca	Medicinal, fresh, woody, earthy	3
Rosemary	Strong, camphorous, slightly woody	3
Ginger	Sweet, spicy-woody, warm, fresh, sharp	4
Thyme	Fresh, medicinal, herbaceous	4
Oregano	Herbaceous, sharp	5
Peppermint	Minty, sharp, intense	5
Middle to Base Notes	(20–80% of the blend)	
Clary Sage	Spicy, hay-like, sharp, fixative	3
Rose	Floral, spicy, rich, deep, sensual, green	3
Ylang Ylang	Sweet, heavy, narcotic, tropical, floral	5
Base Notes	(5–20% of the blend)	
Frankincense	Rich, deep, warm, balsamic, sweet	3
Sandalwood	Soft, woody, sweet, earthy, balsamic	3
Myrrh	Warm, earthy, woody, balsamic	4
Vanilla	Sweet, balsamic, heavy, warm	4
Vetiver	Heavy, earthy, balsamic, smoky	5

This chart was compiled from the book *Natural Perfumes* by Mindy Green and from various other sources. It lists essential oils by note types in order of odor intensity—1 being the lightest and 5 being the strongest. Please see the previous page for more information on this blending system.

Essential Oil Application Methods: Internal

Internal use is the process of consuming or otherwise internalizing an essential oil into the body. Only pure, therapeutic-grade essential oils labeled for internal use should be used for internal consumption, as other essential oils on the market may be diluted or processed using harmful chemicals.

Sublingual

One of the most effective ways to take essential oils internally is sublingually, or by placing a drop or two of an essential oil under the tongue. Because the blood capillaries are so close to the surface of the tissue under the tongue, many essential oil constituents are able to pass directly into the bloodstream, from which they can then quickly travel to the different areas of the body where they are needed. This method provides a faster therapeutic effect than oral administration (Turley, 2009). The sublingual method enables rapid absorption and bypasses the first-pass drug metabolism in the liver, meaning that a higher dosage of chemical constituents is delivered to the body than by most other internal routes (Brenner et al., 2009). Low dosages should be given to avoid irritation to the tissue and to ensure that the essential oil is not washed away by saliva or swallowed before absorption (Brenner et al., 2009).

Capsules

One common way to take essential oils internally is by placing 1–10 drops of essential oil inside an empty capsule, closing the capsule, and then swallowing it. It is also common to dilute the pure essential oil by filling the remainder of the capsule with olive oil before closing and swallowing. This can be an effective way to take oils internally that have a less desirable taste.

Beverage

An easy way to take essential oils internally is by adding them to a beverage. This is done by placing 1 drop of essential oil in 1–4 cups (250 ml–1 L) of rice milk, almond milk, water, or another beverage before drinking.

Cooking

Essential oils can easily be incorporated into your cooking, as long as you remember that they are very concentrated. Usually only 1 drop is necessary, and sometimes even less. Use a toothpick to help control the addition of smaller amounts of oil by dipping the toothpick into the oil (more oil on the toothpick = stronger flavor, etc.) and then stirring it into the food. For more information on cooking with essential oils, see the section on cooking on page 402.

Vaginal Insertion

There are three main ways to insert essential oils vaginally. First, the oils can be diluted in 2–3 tsp. (10–15 ml) of a carrier oil, inserted using a vaginal syringe, and then held in place using a tampon. Alternately, the oils can be diluted in 1–2 tsp. (5–10 ml) of carrier oil, and then a tampon can be used to soak up the mixture. This is then inserted and retained, typically all day or overnight. The third method is to add a few drops of oil to warm water and then to use a vaginal syringe to irrigate and rinse internally using the oil and water mixture. In each case it is important to ensure that the oil is evenly dispersed to avoid irritation (Tisserand et al., 2014).

Rectal Insertion

Rectal oil insertion is often recommended to aid various respiratory problems and other internal conditions. Two ways are often recommended for implanting the oils rectally. First, a rectal syringe can be used to deposit the oils into the rectum. Second, the oils can be placed in capsules and the capsules be inserted into the rectum. The oils are typically retained inside the rectum for several hours or overnight. Ensure that the oil is evenly dispersed to avoid irritation. Rectal insertion is an important method that can produce systemic effects at a slow rate of absorption (Schellack, 2011). Rectal insertion should be used when a higher systemic concentration is needed. This higher concentration is possible because rectal insertion avoids the first-pass metabolism in the liver (Brenner et al., 2009). Diarrhea causes the rectal route to be a less effective route of administration (Schellack, 2011).

GRAS & FA Status

The U.S. Food and Drug Administration (FDA) has approved some essential oils generically for internal use and given them the following designations: GRAS (generally recognized as safe for human consumption), FA (food additive), or FL (flavoring agent). These designations are listed for each oil that is safe for human consumption in the Single Essential Oils section of this book under Oral Use as Dietary Supplement. Oils without this designation should never be used internally without first consulting a certified healthcare professional.

—Understanding GRAS, FA, and FL Status

In 1938, the United States Congress passed the Federal Food, Drug, and Cosmetic Act (FFDCA), giving authority to the FDA to regulate the food, drug, and cosmetic industries. To increase the FDA's regulatory authority, the Food Additives Amendment to the FFDCA was added in 1958. This amendment requires all food additives to be approved by the FDA. To eliminate unneeded and duplicate testing, the FDA also released a list of substances considered generally recognized as safe (GRAS) for human consumption. The designation of a substance as GRAS means that the substance, when intentionally added to food under the conditions of its intended use, is recognized by competent experts as being safe. Substances obtain GRAS status through scientific procedures or through experience based on common use in food before 1958.

Substances designated as GRAS are listed in the U.S Code of Federal Regulations (CFR). Most essential oils that are considered GRAS can be found under 21 CFR § 182.20. This section of the CFR was completed shortly after the passing of the 1958 Food Additives Amendment. Additionally, some GRAS substances are listed under section 184, including clove oil (found under 21 CFR § 184.1257) and dill oil (found under 21 CFR § 184.1282). Section 184 was added in the 1970s as part of the FDA's comprehensive review of GRAS substances.

Not all essential oils are GRAS substances. Some essential oils, like birch oil and cedarwood oil, are not recommended for internal use. Other essential oils, including frankincense oil and melaleuca oil, have been granted Food Additive (FA) or Flavoring Agent (FL) status. Food additives are used to maintain food safety, freshness, and nutritional value. Ingredients added to foods to improve the aroma or quality of taste are considered flavoring agents. A list of substances, including essential oils, that maintain Food Additive and Flavoring Agent status can be found under 21 CFR § 172.510.

Essential oils with GRAS, FA, or FL status are considered by the FDA as safe to consume and can be used internally via several routes of administration.

Common Essential Oils Designated at GRAS:	Angelica, Anise, Basil, Bay, Bergamot, Black Pepper, Chamomile, Cardamom, Cassia, Celery, Cinnamon, Citronella, Citrus (all), Clary Sage, Coriander, Cumin, Fennel, Geranium, Ginger, Grapefruit, Helichrysum, Jasmine, Juniper Berry, Lavender, Lemon, Lemongrass, Lime, Mandarin, Marjoram, Melissa, Neroli, Orange, Oregano, Palmarosa, Peppermint, Rose, Rosemary, Sage, Spearmint, Tangerine, Thyme, Vanilla, Ylang Ylang
Common Essential Oils Designated at FA/FL:	Dill, Frankincense, Melaleuca, Myrrh, Patchouli, Sandalwood, Vetiver, White Fir

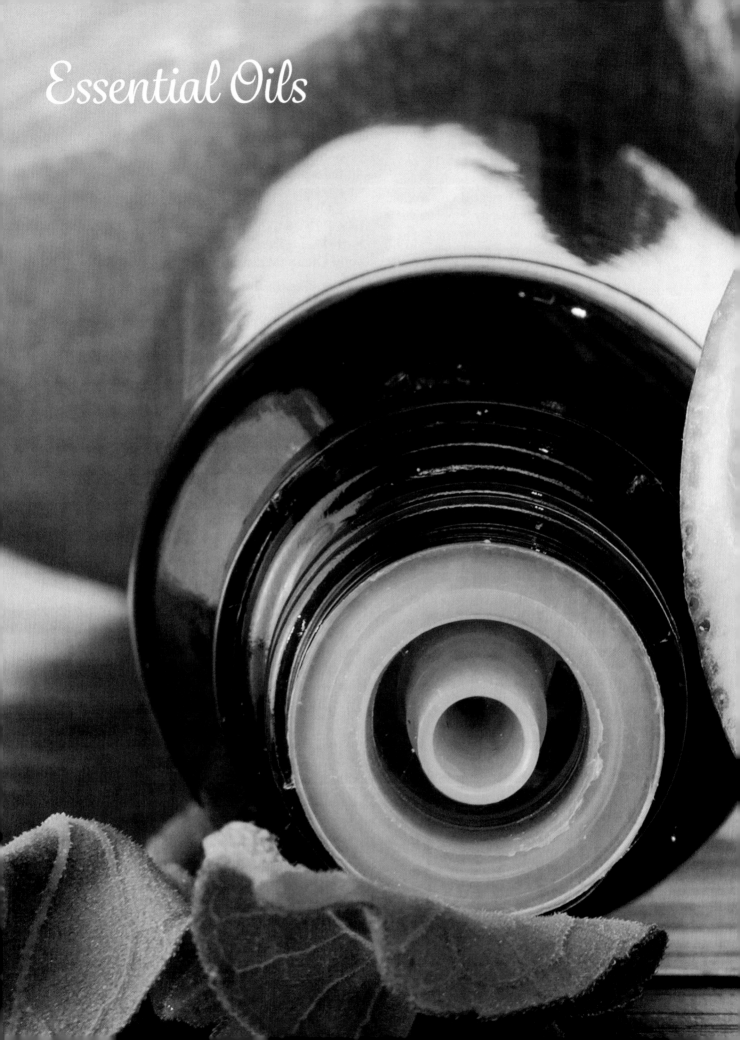

Essential Oils

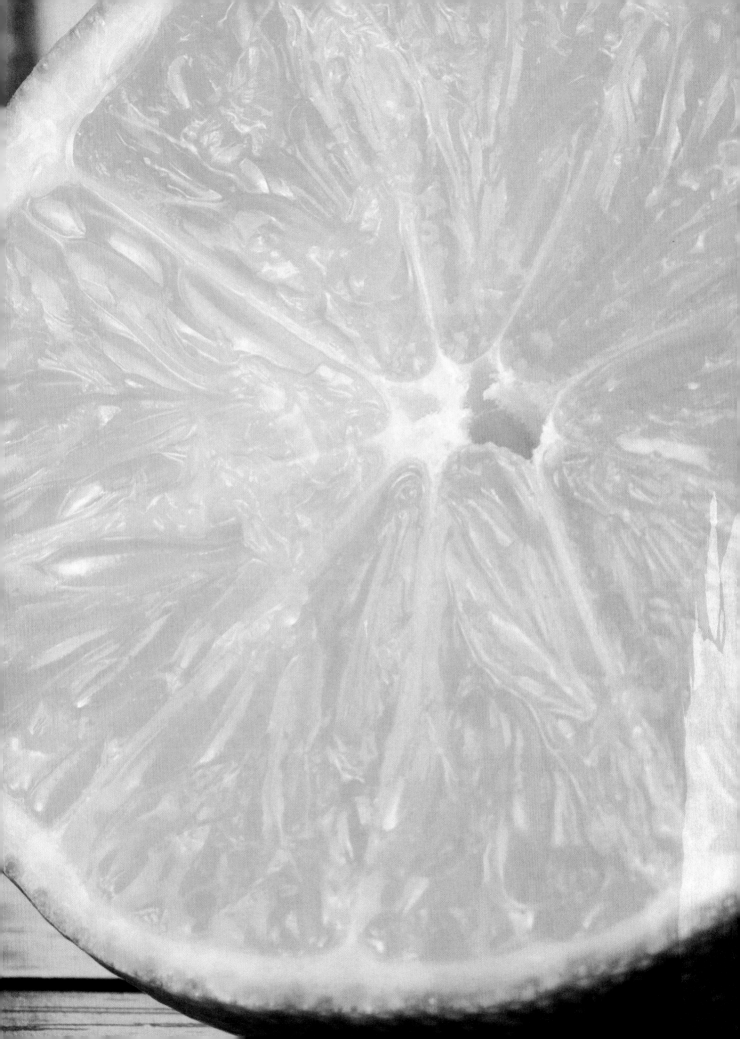

Single Essential Oils

Note: This section provides concise information about many of the pure essential oils that are available for use by the general public. The listings of possible uses are meant for external application unless otherwise directed. The included safety data is also based on the external use of the oils and may differ from other published information that is based on oral application. Any internal use indicated for these oils is based on the use of pure, therapeutic-grade essential oils only.

Since pure essential oils are powerful healing agents, please remember to check the safety data before using an oil. Because there are several different oils that can help the same health condition, it should not be difficult to find one that will work for any particular situation.

Symbols and Colors Used in This Section

 Topical

 Aromatic

 Internal

 Cleaning/Disinfecting

 Avoid sunlight for up to 12 hours after use

 Avoid sunlight for up to 72 hours after use

 Neat (can be used without dilution)

 Dilute for children and those with sensitive skin

 Dilute

 Body System(s) Affected

 See Additional Research

Arborvitae *Thuja plicata*

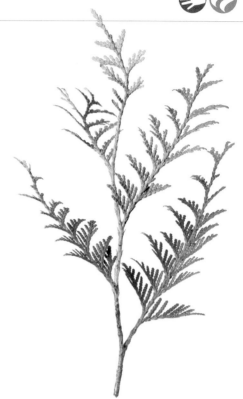

Quick Facts

Botanical Family: Cupressaceae (conifer: cypress)

Extraction Method: Steam distillation from heart-wood

Common Primary Uses*: ⚫⊘Antibacterial⊕, ⚫⊘Antifungal⊕, ⊘Calming, ⚫⊘Cancer⊕, ⊘Repellent

Common Application Methods‡:

⬤: Dilute, and apply to reflex points or to area of concern.

⊘: Diffuse into the air.

Chemical Constituents: Tropolones: α-thujaplicin, β-thujaplicin (hinokitiol), & γ-thujaplicin; methyl thujate, thujic acid, β-thujaplicinol.

Properties: Antibacterial, antifungal, antiseptic, anticancer⊕, antitumor, astringent, expectorant, insect repellent, and stimulant (nerves, immune system, uterus, and heart muscles).

Historical Uses: The arborvitae, or western red cedar, has been referred to as the "Tree of Life." It has been used by ancient civilizations to enhance their potential for spiritual communication during rituals and other ceremonies. It has also been used for coughs, fevers, intestinal parasites, cystitis, and venereal diseases.

Other Possible Uses: This oil may help with hair loss, inflammation⊕, skin (nourishing), rheumatism, sun protection⊕, warts, and psoriasis. It has powerful effects on the subconscious and unconscious mind.

✚ Body System(s) Affected: Emotional Balance, Respiratory System, Skin.

Aromatic Influence: It is calming and may help enhance spiritual awareness or meditation.

Oral Use As Dietary Supplement: None.

Safety Data: Use with caution during pregnancy. For topical and aromatic use only. Use sparingly and dilute.

Blend Classification: Enhancer and Equalizer.

Blends With: Birch, cedarwood, cassia, eucalyptus.

Odor: Type: Top to Middle Notes (10–20% of the blend); Scent: Intense, medicinal, woody, earthy; Intensity: 5.

⊕ **Additional Research:**

Anticancer Properties: Hinokitiol was found to induce autophagic signaling in murine breast and colorectal tumor cells in vitro (Wang et al., 2014).

Anticancer Properties: Mice implanted with human colon cancer tumor cells saw a decrease in tumor size and weight when treated with β-thujaplicin (hinokitiol) (Lee et al., 2013).

Anticancer Properties: Hinokitiol demonstrated inhibition of cell growth and DNA synthesis in human melanoma cells in vitro (Liu et al., 2009).

Antibacterial: *Thuja plicata* displayed antibacterial activity against two Gram-positive (*Staphylococcus aureus* and *S. epidermidis*) and four Gram-negative bacteria (*Escherichia coli*, *Enterobacter cloacae*, *Klebsiella pneumonia*, and *Pseudomonas aeruginosa*) in vitro (Tsiri et al., 2009).

Antibacterial: Arborvitae essential oil vapor and liquid displayed bactericidal activity against seven bacteria (including three Gram-positive organisms, *Bacillus subtilis*, *Streptococcus pyogenes*, and *Enterococcus fecalis*, and four Gram-negative organisms, *Acinetobacter baumannii*, *Hemophilus influenzae*, *Salmonella enteritidis*, and *Escherichia coli*) as well as the bacterial spores of *Bacillus subtilis* (Hudson et al., 2011).

Antifungal: *Thuja plicata* displayed antifungal activity against three pathogenic fungi (*Candida albicans*, *C. tropicalis*, and *C. glabrata*) in vitro (Tsiri et al., 2009).

Antifungal: Arborvitae essential oil vapor and liquid displayed antifungal activity against two commonly encountered fungi (the medically important yeast *Candida albicans* and the filamentous mold *Aspergillus niger*) (Hudson et al., 2011).

Inflammation: In a human dermal fibroblast culture model, arborvitae showed anti-inflammatory properties (Han et al., 2017).

Sunscreen: Application of β-thujaplicin on mouse ear skin decreased sunburn cell formation by 40% as compared to untreated skin, suggesting that β-thujaplicin can inhibit ultraviolet B-induced apoptosis and skin damage (Baba et al., 1998).

‡*See Application section beginning on page 16 for more details on applying essential oils.*   ⬤=Topical, ⊘=Aromatic, ◯=Internal

37

Basil *Ocimum basilicum CT linalool*

Quick Facts

Botanical Family: Lamiaceae or Labiatae (mint)

Extraction Method: Steam distillation of leaves, stems, and flowers

Common Primary Uses*: Amenorrhea, Autism, Bee/Hornet Stings, Bites/Stings, Bronchitis, Bursitis, Carpal Tunnel Syndrome, Chronic Fatigue, Cramps (Abdominal), Cuts, Earache, Frozen Shoulder, Greasy/Oily Hair, Healing, Hiatal Hernia, Incisional Hernia, Induce Sweating, Infertility, Lactation (Increase Milk Production), Mental Fatigue, Migraines, Mouth Ulcers, Muscle Spasms, Muscular Dystrophy, Olfactory Loss (Sense of Smell), Ovarian Cyst, Schmidt's Syndrome, Snake Bites, Spider Bites, Transition (Labor), Viral Hepatitis, Wounds

Common Application Methods‡:

: Can be applied neat (with no dilution) when used topically. Dilute with carrier oil for sensitive skin and for children over 6. Apply to temples, tip of nose, reflex points, and/or directly on area of concern.

: Diffuse, or inhale the aroma directly.

: Take in capsules, or use as a flavoring in cooking.

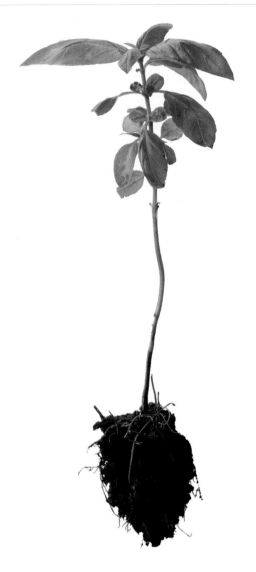

Chemical Constituents: Alcohols (up to 65%): linalool (>55%), fenchol (>10%), cis-3-hexenol; Phenolic Ethers: methyl chavicol (or estragole—up to 47%), methyl eugenol; Oxides (up to 6%): 1,8 cineol; Esters (<7%); Monoterpenes (<2%) α & β-pinenes.

Properties: Antibacterial, antifungal, anti-infectious, anti-inflammatory, antioxidant, antispasmodic (powerful), antiviral, decongestant (veins, arteries of the lungs, prostate), diuretic, disinfectant (urinary/pulmonary), stimulant (nerves, adrenal cortex), and uplifting. Basil is also anticatarrhal, antidepressant, energizing, and restorative.

Historical Uses: Basil was used anciently for respiratory problems, digestive and kidney ailments, epilepsy, poisonous insect or snake bites, fevers, epidemics, and malaria.

French Medicinal Uses: Migraines (especially from liver and gallbladder problems), mental fatigue, menstrual periods (scanty).

Other Possible Uses: This oil may be used for alertness, anxiety, chills, chronic colds, concentration, nervous depression, digestion, fainting, headaches, hiccups, insect bites (soothing), insect repellent, insomnia (from nervous tension), intestinal problems, poor memory, chronic mucus, prostate problems, rhinitis (inflammation of nasal mucous membranes), vomiting, wasp stings, and whooping cough.

---

*See Personal Usage Guide chapter for more details on these primary uses. ●=Neat, ●=Dilute for Children/Sensitive Skin, ●=Dilute

⊕ **Body System(s) Affected:** Cardiovascular System, Muscles and Bones.

Aromatic Influence: Helps one maintain an open mind and increases clarity of thought.

Oral Use As Dietary Supplement: Basil oil is generally recognized as safe (GRAS) for human consumption by the FDA (21CFR182.20). Dilute 1 drop oil in 1 tsp. (5 ml) honey or in ½ cup (125 ml) of beverage (e.g., soy/rice milk). Not for children under 6 years old; use with caution and in greater dilution for children 6 years old and over.

Safety Data: Avoid during pregnancy. Not for use by people with epilepsy. It may also irritate sensitive skin (test a small area first).

Blend Classification: Enhancer and Equalizer.

Blends With: Bergamot, cypress, white fir, geranium, helichrysum, lavender, lemongrass, marjoram, peppermint, and wintergreen.

Odor: Type: Top to Middle Notes (20–80% of the blend); Scent: Herbaceous, spicy, anise-like, camphorous, lively; Intensity: 4.

⊞ **Additional Research:**

Bronchitis: In patients with chronic bronchitis, rosemary, basil, fir, and eucalyptus oils were found to demonstrate an antioxidant effect (Siurin, 1997).

Antibacterial Properties: Basil oil was found to strongly inhibit several multidrug resistant bacteria (Opalchenova et al., 2003).

Antifungal Properties: *Ocimum basilicum* CT linalool demonstrated an ability to inhibit *Aspergillus flavus* growth (El-Soud et al., 2015).

Antioxidant Properties: Basil and its component, linalool, were found to reduce spontaneous mutagenesis in bacteria cells (Berić et al., 2008).

Insect Repellent: Two basil oils (*Ocimum basilicum* and *O. gratissimum*) were found to be insecticidal against the cowpea weevil (an agricultural pest) beetle and eggs in both a diffused and aromatized powder form (Kéita et al., 2001).

Memory: A study evaluating memory retention and retrieval of mice revealed that the hydroalcoholic extract of *Ocimum basilicum* significantly increased memory retention and retrieval. The memory enhancing effects were attributed to the antioxidant activity of flavonoids, tannins and terpenoids in the basil extract (Sarahroodi et al., 2012).

Breast Cancer: Basil extract was found to inhibit the growth of MCF-7 breast cancer cells, possess antioxidant activity, and protect against DNA damage (Al-Ali et al., 2013).

Cardiovascular System—Heart: Short-term oral administration of the hydroalcoholic extract of basil leaves to rats was found to protect the muscular tissue of the heart against a chemically induced heart attack (Fathiazad et al., 2012).

Diabetes: Results from a clinical trial showed that basil (*Ocimum sactum*) leaf extract decreased fasting and postprandial blood glucose in diabetes mellitus patients, suggesting that basil could be used as a dietary therapy in mild to moderate cases of type 2 diabetes mellitus (Agrawal et al., 1996).

Stroke: Oral pretreatment of basil extract was found to protect against brain damage induced by bilateral carotid artery occlusion in mice by reducing tissue death size and the oxidative degradation of lipids and restoring antioxidant content and motor functions. The researchers state that these results suggest that basil could be useful clinically in the prevention of stroke (Bora et al., 2011).

‡See Application section beginning on page 16 for more details on applying essential oils.   ◐=Topical, ◒=Aromatic, ◯=Internal

Bergamot *Citrus bergamia*

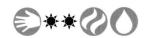

Quick Facts

Botanical Family: Rutaceae (citrus)

Extraction Method: Pressed from rind or peel; rectified and void of terpenes

Common Primary Uses*: Agitation (Calms), Brain Injury, Colic, Depression, Emotional Stress, Environmental Stress, Infection, Mental Stress, Performance Stress, Physical Energy, Physical Stress, PMS, Rheumatoid Arthritis, Sedative, Stress

Common Application Methods‡:

: Can be applied neat (with no dilution) when used topically. Apply to forehead, temples, reflex points, and/or directly on area of concern. May also be applied as a deodorant. Avoid direct sunlight or UV light for 72 hours after use.

: Diffuse, or inhale the aroma directly.

: Use as a flavoring in food and beverages.

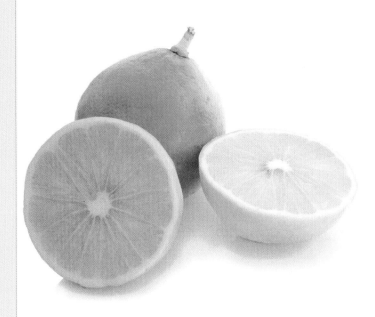

Chemical Constituents: Monoterpenes: d-Limonene (>30%), γ-terpinene, α & β-pinenes; Esters: linalyl acetate (usually around 20%); Alcohols: linalool, geraniol, nerol, α-terpineol; Sesquiterpenes: β-caryophyllene, β-bisabolene; Furanocoumarins; Aldehydes.

Properties: Analgesic, antibacterial (strep and staph infection), antifungal, anti-infectious, anti-inflammatory, antiparasitic, antiseptic, antispasmodic, digestive, neuroprotective, sedative, and uplifting.

Historical Uses: Bergamot was used by the Italians to cool and relieve fevers, protect against malaria, and expel intestinal worms.

French Medicinal Uses: Agitation, appetite (loss of), colic, depression, indigestion, infection, inflammation, insect repellent, insomnia, intestinal parasites, rheumatism, stress, and vaginal candida.

Other Possible Uses: This oil may help acne, anxiety, appetite regulation, boils, bronchitis, carbuncles, cold sores, oily complexion, coughs, cystitis, digestion, eczema, emotions, endocrine system, fever, gallstones, gonorrhea, infectious disease, insect bites, soothe lungs, psoriasis, respiratory infection, scabies, sore throat, nervous tension, thrush, acute tonsillitis, ulcers, urinary tract infection, spot varicose veins, and wounds.

Body System(s) Affected: Digestive System, Emotional Balance, Skin.

Aromatic Influence: It may help to relieve anxiety, depression, stress, and tension. It is uplifting and refreshing.

Oral Use As Dietary Supplement: Bergamot oil is generally recognized as safe (GRAS) for human consumption by the FDA (21CFR182.20). Dilute 1 drop oil in 1 tsp. (5 ml) honey or in ½ cup (125 ml) of beverage (e.g., soy/rice milk). Not for children under 6 years old; use with caution and in greater dilution for children 6 years old and over.

Safety Data: Repeated use may result in extreme contact sensitization. Avoid direct sunlight or ultraviolet light for up to 72 hours after use.

Blend Classification: Equalizer, Modifier, and Enhancer.

Blends With: Cypress, eucalyptus, geranium, lavender, lemon, and ylang ylang.

---

*See Personal Usage Guide chapter for more details on these primary uses.   ●=Neat, ●=Dilute for Children/Sensitive Skin, ●=Dilute

Odor: Type: Top Note (5–20% of the blend); Scent: Sweet, lively, citrusy, fruity; Intensity: 2.

Additional Research:

Calming: A study using 114 subjects found that listening to soft music and/or inhaling Citrus bergamia essential oil were effective methods of relaxation, as indicated by a shift of the autonomic balance toward parasympathetic (Peng et al., 2009).

Neuroprotective Properties: Bergamot essential oil demonstrated neuroprotective effects against brain injury in rats with induced cerebral ischemia (Amantea et al., 2009).

Brain—Injury: Bergamot essential oil was found to reduce excitotoxic neuronal damage caused by exposure of human neuroblastoma cells to NMDA in vitro, displaying the neuroprotection capabilities of bergamot oil (Corasaniti et al., 2007).

Antifungal: Bergamot essential oil was found to be active in vitro against several common species of ringworm (Sanguinetti et al., 2007).

Antiviral: Bergamot extract was found to have potent antiretroviral activity towards HTLV-1 (a human retrovirus that causes T-cell leukemia and lymphoma) and HIV-1 expression in infected cells (Balestrieri et al., 2011).

Anxiety: Inhalation of bergamot essential oil produced similar anxiolytic results as acute injection of an antianxiety drug, diazepam, administered to mice subjected to two behavioral measurements of anxiety (the elevated plus maze test and the hole-board test) (Saiyudthong et al., 2011).

Anxiety: Bergamot essential oil also reduced the corticosterone response to stress exposure of the mice (Saiyudthong et al., 2011).

Anxiety: In an animal model, bergamot demonstrated relaxant and anxiolytic effects (Robola et al., 2017).

Inflammation: Bergamot extract was found to display inhibitory activity on IL-8 gene expression (IL-8 is involved in the inflammatory processes associated with cystic fibrosis), indicating that bergamot may possess possible anti-inflammatory properties to reduce lung inflammation in cystic fibrosis patients (Borgatti et al., 2011).

‡See Application section beginning on page 16 for more details on applying essential oils.   ◔=Topical, ◑=Aromatic, ◯=Internal

Birch *Betula lenta*

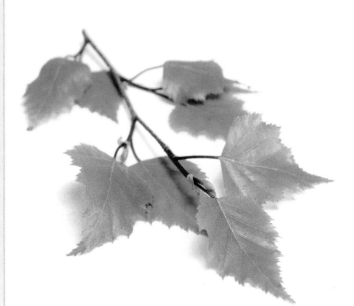

Quick Facts

Botanical Family: Betulaceae

Extraction Method: Steam distillation from wood

Common Primary Uses*: ⬤Cartilage Injury, ⬤Muscle Aches, ⬤Muscle Development, ⬤Muscle Tone, ⬤Whiplash

Common Application Methods‡:

⬤: Can be applied neat (with no dilution), or dilute 1:1 (1 drop essential oil to 1 drop carrier oil) for children and for those with sensitive skin when using topically. Apply to reflex points and/or directly on area of concern. Apply topically on location, and use only small amounts (dilute with fractionated coconut oil for application on larger areas).

⬤: Diffuse, or inhale the aroma directly.

Chemical Constituents: Esters (99%): methyl salicylate; betulene, betulinol.

Properties: Analgesic, anti-inflammatory, antirheumatic, antiseptic◔, antispasmodic, disinfectant, diuretic, stimulant (bone, liver), and warming.

Historical Uses: Birch oil has a strong, penetrating aroma that most people recognize as wintergreen. Although birch (*Betula lenta*) is completely unrelated to wintergreen (*Gaultheria procumbens*), the two oils are almost identical in chemical constituents. The American Indians and early European settlers enjoyed a tea that was flavored with birch bark or wintergreen. According to Julia Lawless, "this has been translated into a preference for 'root beer' flavourings [*sic*]." A synthetic methyl salicylate is now widely used as a flavoring agent, especially in root beer, chewing gum, toothpaste, etc.

French Medicinal Uses: Rheumatism, muscular pain, cramps, arthritis, tendinitis, hypertension, inflammation.

Other Possible Uses: This oil may be beneficial for acne, bladder infection, cystitis, dropsy, eczema, edema, reducing fever, gallstones, gout, infection, reducing discomfort in joints, kidney stones, draining and cleansing the lymphatic system, obesity, osteoporosis, skin diseases, ulcers, and urinary tract disorders. It is known for its ability to alleviate bone pain. It has a cortisone-like action due to the high content of methyl salicylate.

🜨 **Body System(s) Affected:** Muscles and Bones.

Aromatic Influence: It influences, elevates, opens, and increases awareness in the sensory system (senses or sensations).

Oral Use as a Dietary Supplement: None.

Safety Data: Avoid during pregnancy. Not for use by people with epilepsy. Some people are very allergic to methyl salicylate. Test a small area of skin first.

Blend Classification: Personifier and Enhancer.

Blends With: Basil, bergamot, cypress, geranium, lavender, lemongrass, marjoram, and peppermint.

◔ **Additional Research:**

Antiseptic Properties: Subjects using a mouthwash containing thymol, menthol, methyl salicylate, and eucalyptol for 6 months were found to not have any oral bacteria that developed a resistance to the oils (Charles et al., 2000).

---

*See Personal Usage Guide chapter for more details on these primary uses.   ⬤=Neat, ⬤=Dilute for Children/Sensitive Skin, ⬤=Dilute

Black Pepper *Piper nigrum*

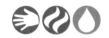

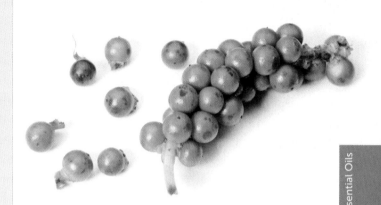

Quick Facts

Botanical Family: Piperaceae

Extraction Method: Steam distillation from berries

Common Primary Uses*: ❷Addictions (Tobacco)⬭

Common Application Methods‡:

🖐: Dilute with a carrier oil for children and for those with sensitive skin. Apply to reflex points and/or directly on area of concern. Mix very sparingly with juniper and lavender in a bath to help with chills or to warm one up in the winter.

❷: Diffuse, or inhale the aroma directly.

◍: Use as a flavoring in cooking.

Chemical Constituents: Monoterpenes (up to 70%): l-limonene (<15%), δ-3-carene (<15%), β-pinene (<14%), sabinene (<10%), α-phellandrene (<9%), α-pinene (<9%), α-thujene (<4%), γ- & α-terpinene (<7%), p-cymene (<3%), myrcene (<3%), terpinolene (<2%); Sesquiterpenes (up to 60%): β-caryophyllene (up to 35%), β-selinene (<8%), β-bisabolene (<5%), α-, α-, & δ-elemenes, β-farnesene, humulene, α-copaene, α-guaiene, α- & β-cubebenes; Oxides: caryophyllene oxide (<8%); Ketones (<2%): acetophenone, hydrocarvone, piperitone; Aldehydes: piperonal; Carboxylic Acids: piperonylic acid; Furanocoumarin: α-bergamotene.

Properties: Analgesic, anticatarrhal, anti-inflammatory, antiseptic, antispasmodic, antitoxic, aphrodisiac, expectorant, laxative, rubefacient, and stimulant (nervous, circulatory, digestive)⬭.

Historical Uses: Pepper has been used for thousands of years for malaria, cholera, and several digestive problems.

Other Possible Uses: This oil may increase cellular oxygenation, support digestive glands, stimulate the endocrine system, increase energy, and help rheumatoid arthritis. It may also help with loss of appetite, catarrh, chills, cholera, colds, colic, constipation, coughs, diarrhea, dysentery, dyspepsia, dysuria, flatulence (combine with fennel), flu, heartburn, influenza, nausea, neuralgia, poor circulation, poor muscle tone, quinsy, sprains, toothache, vertigo, viruses, and vomiting.

✛ Body System(s) Affected: Digestive and Nervous Systems.

Aromatic Influence: Pepper is comforting and stimulating.

Oral Use As Dietary Supplement: Black pepper oil is generally regarded as safe (GRAS) for human consumption by the FDA. Dilute 1 drop oil in 1 tsp. (5 ml) honey or in ½ cup (125 ml) of beverage (e.g., soy/rice milk). Not for children under 6 years old; use with caution and in greater dilution for children 6 years old and over.

Safety Data: Can cause extreme skin irritation.

Blend Classification: Enhancer.

Blends With: Fennel, frankincense, lavender, marjoram, rosemary, sandalwood, and other spice oils.

Odor: Type: Middle Note (50–80% of the blend); Scent: Spicy, peppery, musky, warm, with herbaceous undertones; Intensity: 3.

⬭ **Additional Research:**

Addiction: Inhaled vapor of black pepper oil was found to reduce cravings for cigarettes and symptoms of anxiety in smokers deprived from smoking, compared to a control (Rose et al., 1994).

Stimulant Properties: Inhalation of black pepper oil was found to increase cerebral blood flow and to improve the swallowing reflex in elderly patients who had suffered a stroke (Ebihara et al., 2006).

‡See Application section beginning on page 16 for more details on applying essential oils.   🖐=Topical, ❷=Aromatic, ◍=Internal

43

Blue Tansy *Tanacetum annuum*

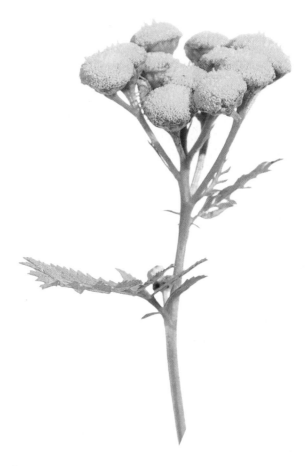

Quick Facts

Botanical Family: Compositae (daisy)

Extraction Method: Steam distillation from leaves and flowers

Common Primary Uses*: Anxiety, Calming, Wounds

Common Application Methods‡:

: Apply to reflex points and/or directly on area of concern.

: Diffuse, or inhale the aroma directly.

Chemical Constituents: Monoterpenes (up to 55%): sabinene (<17%), myrcene (<13%), d-limonene (<10%), β-pinene (<10%), α-phellandrene (<10%), p-cymene (<8%); Ketones: camphor (<17%); Sesquiterpenes: chamazulene (up to 35%).

Properties: Analgesic, antibacterial, antifungal, anti-inflammatory, antihistamine, hypotensive, hormone-like, nervine.

Historical Uses: Anciently, tansy was used to help heal wounds, as a diuretic, and for dealing with kidney issues.

Other Possible Uses: Blue tansy may help raise blood pressure, relieve itching, reduce pain, and sedate the nerves.

Body System(s) Affected: Nervous System.

Aromatic Influence: Blue tansy is uplifting, refreshing, and calming to a troubled mind. It may also help instill confidence and enthusiasm.

Oral Use As Dietary Supplement: None.

Safety Data: Consult a physician before using if taking medications.

Blend Classification: Personifier and Modifier.

Blends With: Most oils; perfumers in France have found that wild tansy has a greater fixative capability than any other oil.

Odor: Type: Middle Note (50–80% of the blend); Scent: Camphoraceous, sweet, herbaceous; Intensity: 4.

Additional Research:

Antifungal: Blue tansy oil was found to inhibit mycelial growth in several types of fungi (Greche et al., 2000).

Insecticidal: Blue tansy oil was found to have insecticidal properties against grasshoppers of the species *Paraeumigus parvulus* (Lawrence et al., 2009).

See Personal Usage Guide chapter for more details on these primary uses.   =Neat, =Dilute for Children/Sensitive Skin, =Dilute

44
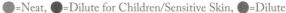

Cardamom *Elettaria cardamomum*

Essential Oils

Quick Facts

Botanical Family: Zingiberaceae (ginger)

Extraction Method: Steam distillation from seeds

Common Primary Uses*: Coughs, Digestive Support, Headaches, Inflammation, Muscle Aches, Nausea, Respiratory Ailments

Common Application Methods‡:

: Apply to reflex points and/or directly on area of concern. Dilute with base oil, and massage over the stomach, solar plexus, and thighs. This oil is excellent as a bath oil.

: Diffuse, or inhale the aroma directly.

: Place 1 drop under the tongue, or take oil in capsules. Use as a flavoring in cooking or in beverages.

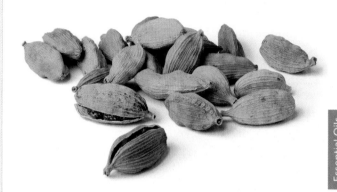

Chemical Constituents: Esters (>40%): α-terpenyl acetate (30–45%), linalyl acetate (3%); Oxides: 1,8 cineol (up to 35%); Alcohols (7%): linalool, terpinen-4-ol, α-terpineol; Monoterpenes (6%): sabinene, myrcene, l-limonene; Aldehyde: geranial.

Properties: Antibacterial, anti-infectious, anti-inflammatory, antiseptic, antispasmodic, aphrodisiac, decongestant, diuretic, expectorant, stomachic, and tonic.

Historical Uses: Anciently, cardamom was used for epilepsy, spasms, paralysis, rheumatism, cardiac disorders, all intestinal illnesses, pulmonary disease, fever, and digestive and urinary complaints. It is said to be able to neutralize the lingering odor of garlic.

Other Possible Uses: Cardamom may help with appetite (loss of), bronchitis, colic, debility, dyspepsia, flatulence, halitosis, mental fatigue, pyrosis (or heartburn), sciatica, ulcers, and vomiting. It may also help with menstrual periods, menopause, and nervous indigestion.

Body System(s) Affected: Digestive and Respiratory Systems.

Aromatic Influence: Cardamom is uplifting, refreshing, and invigorating. It may be beneficial for clearing confusion.

Oral Use As Dietary Supplement: Generally regarded as safe (GRAS) for human consumption by the FDA. Dilute 1 drop oil in 1 tsp. (5 ml) honey or in ½ cup (125 ml) of beverage (e.g., soy/rice milk). Not for children under 6 years old; use with caution and in greater dilution for children 6 years old and over.

Blend Classification: Personifier and Modifier.

Blends With: Bergamot, cedarwood, cinnamon, clove, orange, rose, and ylang ylang.

Odor: Type: Middle Note (50–80% of the blend); Scent: Sweet, spicy, balsamic, with floral undertones; Intensity: 4.

Additional Research:

Respiratory System—Lungs: Administration of cardamom to mice was found to have a protective effect against pan masala– (an herbal and tobacco blend sold in India) induced damage in the lungs of mice (Kumari et al., 2013)

Antibacterial: Cardamom essential oil was found to have powerful antibacterial activity against *Bacillus subtilis* spores when compared to 12 other essential oils and the isolated constituents of cardamom essential oil (Lawrence et al., 2009).

Inflammation: Cardamom essential oil reduced rat paw edema by 76% of the control value, illustrating significant anti-inflammatory activity (al-Zuhair et al., 1996).

Ulcers: Cardamom essential oil was found to inhibit gastric lesions induced by asprin and ethanol ligature in rats, illustrating cardamom's gastroprotective action (Jamal et al., 2006).

‡*See Application section beginning on page 16 for more details on applying essential oils.*   =Topical,   =Aromatic,   =Internal

45

Cassia *Cinnamomum cassia*

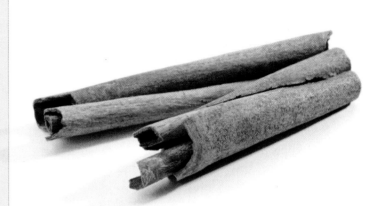

Quick Facts

Botanical Family: Lauraceae (laurel)

Extraction Method: Steam distillation from bark

Common Primary Uses*: ⬥Antiseptic[ⓘ], ⬥Cooking

Common Application Methods‡:

🖐: Dilute heavily with a carrier oil or blend with milder essential oils before applying on the skin. Apply to forehead, muscles, reflex points, and/or directly on area of concern.

🌀: Diffuse with caution: it will irritate the nasal membranes if it is inhaled directly from the diffuser.

💧: Use as a flavoring in cooking (similar to cinnamon but has a stronger, more intense flavor).

Chemical Constituents: Aldehydes: trans-cinnamaldehyde (up to 85%), benzaldehyde; Phenols (>7%): eugenol, chavicol, phenol, 2-vinylphenol; Esters: cinnamyl acetate, benzyl acetate.

Properties: Antibacterial[ⓘ], antifungal[ⓘ], anti-inflammatory[ⓘ], and antiviral.

Historical Uses: Has been used extensively as a domestic spice. Medicinally, it has been used for colds, colic, flatulent dyspepsia, diarrhea, nausea, rheumatism, and kidney and reproductive complaints.

Other Possible Uses: This oil can be extremely sensitizing to the dermal tissues. Can provide some powerful support to blends when used in very small quantities.

Oral Use As Dietary Supplement: Cassia oil is generally recognized as safe (GRAS) for human consumption by the FDA (21CFR182.20). Dilute 1 drop oil in 2 tsp. (10 ml) honey or in 1 cup (250 ml) of beverage (e.g., soy/rice milk). May need to increase dilution even more due to this oil's potential for irritating mucous membranes. Not for children under 6 years old; use with caution and in greater dilution for children 6 years old and over.

Safety Data: Repeated use can result in extreme contact sensitization. Avoid during pregnancy. Can cause extreme skin irritation. Diffuse with caution; it will irritate the nasal membranes if it is inhaled directly from the diffuser.

Blend Classification: Personifier and Enhancer.

Blends With: All citrus oils, cypress, frankincense, geranium, juniper berry, lavender, rosemary, and all spice oils.

Odor: Type: Middle Note (50–80% of the blend); Scent: Spicy, warm, sweet; Intensity: 5.

ⓘ **Additional Research:**

Antibacterial: Cinnamaldehyde, the main constituent of cassia oil, showed strong growth inhibiting activity toward five human intestinal bacteria in vitro (Lee et al., 1998).

Anxiety: A single treatment of cassia extract decreased anxiety in mice by causing a change of serotonin receptors in the dorsal raphe nucleus (Jung et al., 2012).

Antifungal: Cassia essential oil was found to have a strong inhibitory effect against Aspergillus mold in vitro and in grapes (Kocevski et al., 2013).

Anti-inflammatory: Cassia oil was found to reduce inflammation and pain perception in a mouse model (Sun et al., 2016).

Diabetes: In vitro data suggest that the constituents of cassia may be appropriate for the treatment of diabetic complications (like cataract and retinopathy) because of the constituents' ability to inhibit aldose reductase and thus prevent the conversion of glucose to corbitol (Lee, 2002).

Repellent: Cassia oil and its components were found to repel adult female mosquitoes for about 50 minutes post-application when applied to human subjects (Chang et al., 2006).

Male Impotence: Methanol extract of *Cinnamonum cassia* was found to increase the sexual function of young male rats (Goswami et al., 2014).

Male Impotence: Methanol extract of cassia was found to effectively manage sexual dysfunction in aged rats (Goswami et al., 2013).

---

*See Personal Usage Guide chapter for more details on these primary uses.   ⬤=Neat, ⬤=Dilute for Children/Sensitive Skin, ⬤=Dilute

Cedarwood *Juniperus virginiana*

Quick Facts

Botanical Family: Cupressaceae (conifer: cypress)

Extraction Method: Steam distillation from wood

Common Primary Uses*: Calming, Tension, Tuberculosis, Urinary Infection, Yoga

Common Application Methods‡:

: Dilute with a carrier oil for children and for those with sensitive skin. Apply to reflex points and/or directly on area of concern.

: Diffuse, or inhale the aroma directly.

Chemical Constituents: Sesquiterpenes: α- & β-cedrenes (up to 36%), thujopsene (up to 42%), cuparene, trans-caryophyllene; Sesquiterpene Alcohols: cedrol (up to 15%), pseudocedrol, prim-cedrol, widdrol, γ-eudesmol.

Properties: Antifungal, anti-infectious, antiseptic (urinary and pulmonary), astringent, diuretic, insect repellent, and sedative.

Historical Uses: This variety of cedarwood (also known as red or Virginian cedarwood) has been used for its strong antiseptic, diuretic, calming, and insect-repelling properties.

Other Possible Uses: This oil may help acne, anxiety, arthritis, congestion, coughs, cystitis, dandruff, inflammation, psoriasis, purification, sinusitis, skin diseases, stroke, and water retention. It may also help to reduce oily secretions.

Body System(s) Affected: Nervous and Respiratory Systems.

Oral Use As Dietary Supplement: None.

Safety Data: Use with caution during pregnancy.

Blend Classification: Enhancer and Equalizer.

Blends With: Bergamot, clary sage, cypress, eucalyptus, floral oils, juniper, resinous oils, rosemary.

Odor: Type: Base Note (5–20% of the blend); Scent: Warm, soft, woody; Intensity: 3.

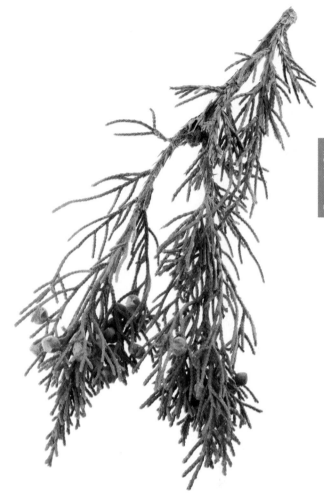

Additional Research:

Repellent: Cedarwood was found to possess highly insecticidal activity against adult mosquitoes and other household insects (Singh et al., 1984).

Inflammation: Juniperus virginiana oil was found to have anti-inflammatory activity in mice (Tumen et al., 2013).

Stroke: A chemical constituent, α-eudesmol, found in cedarwood oil demonstrated the ability to protect against brain injury after cerebral ischemia (stroke) in rats. Specifically, α-eudesmol was found to attenuate cerebral edema formation, reduce cerebral infarct size, and inhibit calcium-dependent glutamate release from synaptosomes (Asakura et al., 2000).

‡See Application section beginning on page 16 for more details on applying essential oils.   =Topical, =Aromatic, =Internal

47

Chamomile, Roman *(see Roman Chamomile)*

Cilantro *Coriandrum sativum L.*

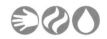

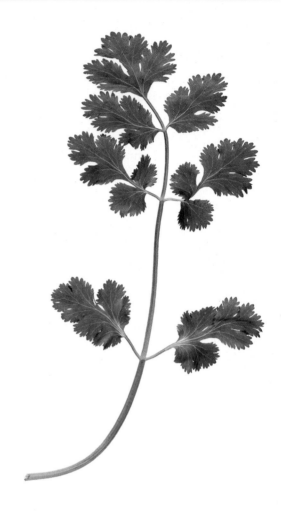

Quick Facts

Botanical Family: Umbelliferae (parsley)

Extraction Method: Steam distillation from leaves (same plant as coriander oil, which is distilled from the seeds)

Common Primary Uses*: ⵁAnxiety, ⵔCooking

Common Application Methods‡:

⊜: Can be applied neat (with no dilution) when used topically. Apply to reflex points and directly on area of concern.

ⵁ: Diffuse, or inhale the aroma directly.

◖: Use as a flavoring in cooking.

Chemical Constituents: Aldehydes (40–50%): tetra-decanal, 2-dodecenal, 13-tetradecenal, dodecanal, decanal; Alcohols (up to 40%): cyclododecanol, 1-decanol, 1-dodecanol, 1-undecanol; Phenols: eugenol; Ketones: β-ionone.

Properties: Antibacterial, antifungal⊕.

Historical Uses: Cilantro leaves have been used since the times of ancient Greece as an herb for flavoring. Its aroma has also been used for anxiety and insomnia.

Other Possible Uses: Mainly used as a flavoring in cooking. May also help with liver conditions⊕, and with protecting the skin⊕.

Oral Use As Dietary Supplement: Cilantro oil is generally recognized as safe (GRAS) for human consumption by the FDA (21CFR182.20). Dilute 1 drop oil in 1 tsp. (5 ml) honey or in ½ cup (125 ml) of beverage (e.g., soy/rice milk). Not for children under 6 years old; use with caution and in greater dilution for children 6 years old and over.

Safety Data: May cause irritation on sensitive or damaged skin.

Blend Classification: Personifier and Modifier.

Blends With: Lime, lemon.

Odor: Scent: Herbaceous, citrusy, fresh.

⊕ **Additional Research:**

Antifungal: Cilantro essential oil was found to have fungicidal effect against Candida albicans and other yeasts. The oil appeared to act by binding to membrane ergosterol, rendering the cell membrane more permeable and ultimately causing cell death (Freires Ide et al., 2014).

Liver—Cirrohsis: In rat livers, the antioxidant activity of cilantro leaves improved the adverse effect of the repeated administration of a potent liver toxin (Moustafa et al., 2012).

Liver: Ethanolic extract of the cilantro leaf was found to protect against carbon tetrachloride induced liver injury in rats, validating its use as a liver protective agent (Pandey et al., 2011).

Skin: Cilantro extract was found to protect human keratinocytes (epidermis cells) against H2O2-induced oxidative stress, suggesting that cilantro may be useful at protecting skin cells from oxidative damage (Park et al., 2012).

---

*See Personal Usage Guide chapter for more details on these primary uses.   ⬤=Neat, ⬤=Dilute for Children/Sensitive Skin, ⬤=Dilute

Cinnamon *Cinnamomum zeylanicum*

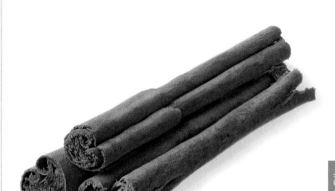

Quick Facts

Botanical Family: Lauraceae (laurel)

Extraction Method: Steam distillation from bark

Common Primary Uses*: ⊘Airborne Bacteria, ⊜⊘Bacterial Infections, ⊜Bites/Stings, ⊘⊘Breathing, ○⊜Diabetes⊕, ⊜Diverticulitis, ⊜⊘Fungal Infections, ⊜⊘General Tonic, ⊘Immune System (Stimulates), ⊜⊘Infection, ⊜⊘Libido (Low), ⊘⊘Mold, ⊜⊘Pancreas Support, ⊘Physical Fatigue, ⊘Pneumonia, ⊜⊘Typhoid, ⊜Vaginal Infection, ⊜Vaginitis, ⊜Viral Infections, ⊜Warming (Body)

Common Application Methods‡:

⊜: Dilute 1:3 (1 drop essential oil to at least 3 drops carrier oil) before using topically. Apply directly on area of concern or on reflex points.

⊘: Diffuse with caution; it may irritate the nasal membranes if it is inhaled directly from a diffuser.

○: Use as a flavoring in cooking.

Chemical Constituents: Aldehydes: trans-cinnamaldehyde (<50%), hydroxycinnamaldehyde, benzaldehyde, cuminal; Phenols (up to 30%): eugenol (<30%), phenol, 2-vinylphenol; Alcohols: linalool, cinnamic alcohol, benzyl alcohol, α-terpineol, borneol; Sesquiterpenes: β-caryophyllene; Carboxylic Acids: cinnamic acid.

Properties: Antibacterial⊕, antidepressant, antifungal⊕, anti-infectious (intestinal, urinary), anti-inflammatory⊕, antimicrobial, antioxidant, antiparasitic, antiseptic, antispasmodic (light), antiviral, astringent, immune stimulant, purifier, sexual stimulant, and warming. It also enhances the action and activity of other oils.

Historical Uses: This most ancient of spices was included in just about every prescription issued in ancient China. It was regarded as a tranquilizer, tonic, and stomachic and as being good for depression and a weak heart.

French Medicinal Uses: Sexual stimulant, topical infection, typhoid, vaginitis.

Other Possible Uses: This oil may be beneficial for circulation, colds, coughs, digestion, exhaustion, flu, infections, rheumatism⊕, and warts. This oil fights viral and infectious diseases, and testing has yet to find a virus, bacteria, or fungus that can survive in its presence.

⊕ **Body System(s) Affected:** Immune System.

Oral Use As Dietary Supplement: Cinnamon oil is generally recognized as safe (GRAS) for human consumption by the FDA (21CFR182.20). Dilute 1 drop oil in 2 tsp. (10 ml) honey or in 1 cup (250 ml) of beverage (e.g., soy/rice milk). May need to increase dilution even more due to this oil's potential for irritating mucous membranes. Not for children under 6 years old; use with caution and in greater dilution for children 6 years old and over.

Safety Data: Repeated use can result in extreme contact sensitization. Avoid during pregnancy.

Blend Classification: Personifier and Enhancer.

Blends With: All citrus oils, cypress, frankincense, geranium, juniper berry, lavender, rosemary, and all spice oils.

Odor: Type: Middle Note (50–80% of the blend); Scent: Spicy, warm, sweet; Intensity: 5.

⊕ **Additional Research:**

Diabetes: Cinnamon bark extract supplementation for three months was found to significantly improve blood glucose control in Chinese patients with type 2 diabetes taking gliclazide (a prescribed antidiabetic medication) (Lu, T. et al., 2012).

‡*See Application section beginning on page 16 for more details on applying essential oils.* ⊜=Topical, ⊘=Aromatic, ○=Internal

49

Diabetes: Cinnamaldehyde (the major constituent of cinnamon oil) produced protective action against alloxan-induced diabetic nephropathy in rats (Mishra et al., 2010).

Diabetes—Pancreas Support: Cinnamon polyphenols were found to restore pancreatic function and exert hypoglycemic and hypolipidemic effects in a diabetic mouse model (Li, R. et al., 2013).

Diabetes: Cinnamaldehyde (found in cinnamon oil) was found to significantly reduce blood glucose levels in diabetic wistar rats (Subash et al., 2007).

Diabetes: Oral administration of cinnamon oil was found to significantly reduce blood glucose levels in diabetic KK-Ay mice (Ping et al., 2010).

Antibacterial Properties: Cinnamon, thyme, and clove essential oils demonstrated an antibacterial effect on several respiratory tract pathogens (Fabio et al., 2007).

Antibacterial Properties: Cinnamon oil exhibited strong antimicrobial activity against two detrimental oral bacteria. (Filoche et al., 2005).

Antibacterial Properties: Cinnamon bark, lemongrass, and thyme oils were found to have the highest level of activity against common respiratory pathogens among 14 essential oils tested (Inouye et al., 2001).

Antibacterial Properties: Bay, cinnamon, and clove oils reduced production of alpha-toxin and enterotoxin A by *Staphylococcus aureus* bacteria (Smith-Palmer et al., 2004).

Antifungal Properties: In a test of nine oils, clove, followed by cinnamon, oregano, and mace oils, was found to be inhibitory to two toxin-producing fungi (Juglal et al., 2002).

Antifungal Properties: Cinnamon, thyme, oregano, and cumin oils inhibited the production of aflatoxin by aspergillus fungus (Tantaoui-Elaraki et al., 1994).

Antifungal Properties: Vapor of cinnamon bark oil and cinnamic aldehyde was found to be effective against fungi involved in respiratory tract mycoses (fungal infections) (Singh et al., 1995).

Anti-inflammatory: Cinnamon bark essential oil was found to demonstrate anti-inflammatory effects in a human dermal fibroblast model (Han et al., 2017).

Arthritis: The polyphenol fraction from cinnamon bark was found to improve inflammation and pain in animal models of inflammation and rheumatoid arthritis (Rathi et al., 2013).

Alzheimer's Disease: An aqueous cinnamon extract was found to inhibit beta-amyloid oligomer and fibril formation and alleviate Alzheimer's disease symptoms in the Drosophila and mouse models of Alzheimer's disease (Frydman-Marom et al., 2011).

Wound: A topically applied cinnamon oil based microemulsion showed increased wound healing ability in rats by preventing sepsis of the excised wound (Ghosh et al., 2013).

High Blood Pressure: Cinnamon bark methanol extract showed an acute antihypertensive effect on induced hypertensive rats (Nyadjeu et al., 2013).

Male Infertility: Cinnamon bark essential oil was found to have a protective effect against damages in male rat reproductive organs and cells induced by carbon tetrachloride (a common toxic substance) (Yüce et al., 2014).

Parkinson's Disease: The process of α-syn protein aggregation is a major component of Parkinson's disease. Preventing α-syn aggregation may help in the treatment of Parkinson's disease. Researchers have discovered that an aqueous cinnamon extract precipitation has a curative effect on α-syn aggregation in a Drosophila model of Parkinson's disease. Furthermore, in vitro tests have revealed that the cinnamon extract has an inhibitory effect on the process of α-syn fibrillation (Shaltiel-Karyo et al., 2012).

See Personal Usage Guide chapter for more details on these primary uses.   ●=Neat, ●=Dilute for Children/Sensitive Skin, ●=Dilute

Clary Sage *Salvia sclarea*

Quick Facts

Botanical Family: Labiatae (mint)

Extraction Method: Steam distillation from flowering plant

Common Primary Uses*: ⬤⬤Aneurysm, ⬤Breast Enlargement, ⬤Cholesterol, ⬤Convulsions, ⬤Cramps (Abdominal), ⬤Dysmenorrhea⬤, ⬤⬤Emotional Stress, ⬤Endometriosis, ⬤Epilepsy, ⬤Estrogen Balance, ⬤⬤Frigidity, ⬤Hair (Fragile), ⬤⬤Hormonal Balance, ⬤Hot Flashes, ⬤⬤Impotence, ⬤⬤Infection, ⬤⬤Infertility, ⬤⬤Insomnia (Older Children), ⬤Lactation (Start Milk Production), ⬤Mood Swings, ⬤Muscle Fatigue, ⬤Parkinson's Disease, ⬤⬤PMS⬤, ⬤⬤Postpartum Depression, ⬤Premenopause, ⬤Seizure

Common Application Methods‡:

⬤: Can be applied neat (with no dilution) when used topically. Apply to reflex points and/or directly on area of concern.

⬤: Diffuse, or inhale the aroma directly.

⬤: Take in capsules, or use as a flavoring in cooking.

Chemical Constituents: Esters (up to 75%): linalyl acetate (20–75%); Alcohols (20%): linalool (10–20%), geraniol, α-terpineol; Sesquiterpenes (<14%): germacrene-D (up to 12%), -caryophyllene; Diterpene alcohols: sclareol (1–7%); Monoterpenes: myrcene, α- and β-pinenes, l-limonene, ocimene, terpinolene; Oxides: 1,8 cineol, linalool oxide, sclareol oxide; Ketones: α- and β-thujone; Sesquiterpene alcohols; Aldehydes; Coumarins. (More than 250 constituents.)

Properties: Anticonvulsant, antifungal, antiseptic⬤, antispasmodic, astringent, nerve tonic, sedative, soothing⬤, tonic, and warming.

Historical Uses: Nicknamed "clear eyes," it was famous during the Middle Ages for its ability to

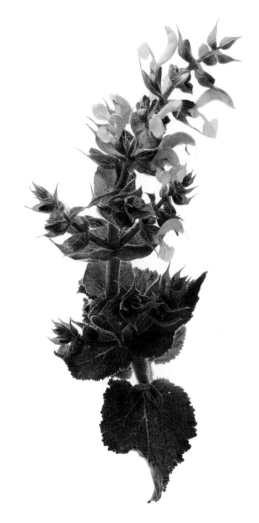

clear eye problems. During that same time, it was widely used for female complaints, kidney/digestive/skin disorders, inflammation, sore throats, and wounds.

French Medicinal Uses: Bronchitis, cholesterol, frigidity, genitalia, hemorrhoids, hormonal imbalance, impotence, infections, intestinal cramps, menstrual cramps ⬤, PMS, premenopause, weak digestion.

Other Possible Uses: This oil may be used for amenorrhea, cell regulation, circulatory problems,

---

‡*See Application section beginning on page 16 for more details on applying essential oils.*   ⬤=Topical, ⬤=Aromatic, ⬤=Internal

51

depression, insect bites, kidney disorders, dry skin, throat infection, ulcers, and whooping cough.

Body System(s) Affected: Hormonal System.

Oral Use As Dietary Supplement: Clary sage oil is generally recognized as safe (GRAS) for human consumption by the FDA (21CFR182.20). Dilute 1 drop oil in 1 tsp. (5 ml) honey or in ½ cup (125 ml) of beverage (e.g., soy/rice milk). Not for children under 6 years old; use with caution and in greater dilution for children 6 years old and over.

Safety Data: Use with caution during pregnancy. Not for babies. Avoid during and after consumption of alcohol.

Blend Classification: Personifier.

Blends With: Bergamot, citrus oils, cypress, geranium, and sandalwood.

Odor: Type: Middle to Base Notes (5–60% of the blend); Scent: Herbaceous, spicy, hay-like, sharp, fixative; Intensity: 3.

Additional Research:

Antiseptic: Clary sage oil was found to inhibit several Staphylococcus strains isolated from wound infections (Sienkiewicz et al., 2015).

Soothing Properties: Nurses working in an ICU setting demonstrated decreased perception of stress when receiving a topical application of *Lavandula angustifolia* and *Salvia sclarea* essential oils (Pemberton et al., 2008).

Anxiety: Dietary administration of clary sage oil (from conception) was found to have an anti-anxiety and submissive effect on mice, when compared to administration of sunflower oil (from conception and weaning) and clary sage (from weaning) (Gross et al., 2013).

Breast Cancer: Sclareol, a chemical constituent found in clary sage essential oil, was found to reduce regulatory T cells frequency and also tumor size in a mouse model of breast cancer, suggesting that sclareol can enhance the effect of cancer therapy as an immunostiumlant (Noori et al., 2013).

Female-Specific Conditions—Dysmenorrhea: In an experiment with 67 female college students, an aromatherapy massage with lavender, clary sage, and rose essential oils proved to be more effective at treating dysmenorrhea than a placebo treatment of almond oil or the control (Han et al., 2006).

Female-Specific Conditions—Dysmenorrhea: Compared to a synthetic fragrance, dysmenorrhea pain decreased and shortened in duration when subjects massaged a blend of lavender, marjoram, and clary sage essential oils (in a ratio of 2:1:1) daily on the abdomen between menstruations (Ou et al., 2012).

Depression: Clary sage essential oil displayed antidepressant-like effects via the dopaminergic pathway in rats submitted to the forced swim test (a common stress test) (Seol et al., 2010).

See Personal Usage Guide chapter for more details on these primary uses.   ●=Neat, ●=Dilute for Children/Sensitive Skin, ●=Dilute

52

Clove *Eugenia caryophyllata*

Essential Oils

Quick Facts

Botanical Family: Myrtaceae (shrubs and trees)

Extraction Method: Steam distillation from bud and stem

Common Primary Uses*: ⃝Addictions (Tobacco), ⃝Antioxidant, ⃝⃝Blood Clots⊕, ⃝⃝Candida, ⃝Cataracts, ⃝Corns, ⃝Disinfectant, ⃝Fever, ⃝⃝Fungal Infections, ⃝Herpes Simplex, ⃝Hodgkin's Disease, ⃝Hormonal Balance, ⃝⃝Hypothyroidism, ⃝⃝Liver Cleansing, ⃝Lupus, ⃝Macular Degeneration, ⃝⃝Memory, ⃝Metabolism Balance, ⃝⃝Mold, ⃝Muscle Aches, ⃝Muscle Pain, ⃝Osteoporosis, ⃝⃝Plague, ⃝Rheumatoid Arthritis, ⃝⃝Termites, ⃝⃝Thyroid Dysfunction, ⃝Toothache (Pain), ⃝⃝Tumor (Lipoma), ⃝⃝Viral Infections, ⃝Warts, ⃝Wounds

Common Application Methods‡:

⊗: Dilute 1:1 (1 drop essential oil to 1 drop carrier oil) before topical use. Apply to reflex points and/ or directly on area of concern. Rub directly on the gums surrounding an infected tooth. Place on tongue with finger to remove desire to smoke, or place on back of tongue to fight against tickling cough.

⊘: Diffuse with caution; it may irritate the nasal membranes if it is inhaled directly from a diffuser.

⃝: Place 1 drop under the tongue, or take in capsules. Use as a flavoring in cooking.

Chemical Constituents: Phenols: eugenol (up to 85%), chavicol, 4-allylphenol; Esters: eugenyl acetate (up to 15%), styrallyl, benzyl, terpenyl, ethyl phenyl acetates, methyl salicylate (tr.); Sesquiterpenes (up to 14%): β-caryophyllene (<12%), humulene, α-amorphene, α-muurolene, calamenene; Oxides (<3%): caryophyllene oxide, humulene oxide; Carboxylic Acids; Ketones.

Properties: Analgesic, antibacterial⊕, antifungal⊕, anti-infectious, anti-inflammatory⊕, antiparasitic, strong antiseptic, antitumor⊕, antiviral⊕, disinfectant, antioxidant, and immune stimulant.

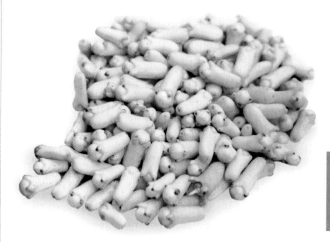

Historical Uses: Cloves were historically used for skin infections, digestive upsets, intestinal parasites, childbirth, and most notably for toothache. The Chinese also used cloves for diarrhea, hernia, bad breath, and bronchitis.

French Medicinal Uses: Impotence, intestinal parasites, memory deficiency, pain, plague, toothache, wounds (infected).

Other Possible Uses: Clove is valuable as a drawing salve—it helps pull infection from tissues. It may also help amebic dysentery, arthritis⊕, bacterial colitis, bones, bronchitis, cholera, cystitis, dental infection, diarrhea, infectious acne, fatigue, flatulence (gas), flu, halitosis (bad breath), tension headaches, hypertension, infection (wounds and more), insect bites and stings, insect control (insecticidal)⊕, multiple sclerosis, nausea, neuritis, nettles and poison oak (takes out sting), rheumatism, sinusitis, skin cancer, chronic skin disease, smoking (removes desire), sores (speeds healing of mouth and skin sores), tuberculosis, leg ulcers, viral hepatitis, and vomiting.

✛ **Body System(s) Affected:** Cardiovascular, Digestive, Immune, and Respiratory Systems.

Aromatic Influence: It may influence healing, improve memory (mental stimulant), and create a feeling of protection and courage.

‡See Application section beginning on page 16 for more details on applying essential oils.   ⃝=Topical, ⊘=Aromatic, ⃝=Internal

53

Oral Use As Dietary Supplement: Clove oil is generally recognized as safe (GRAS) for human consumption by the FDA (21CFR182.20). Dilute 1 drop oil in 1 tsp. (5 ml) honey or in ½ cup (125 ml) of beverage (e.g., soy/rice milk). Not for children under 6 years old; use with caution and in greater dilution for children 6 years old and over.

Safety Data: Repeated use can result in extreme contact sensitization. Use with caution during pregnancy. Can irritate sensitive skin.

Blend Classification: Personifier.

Blends With: Basil, bergamot, cinnamon, clary sage, grapefruit, lavender, lemon, orange, peppermint, rose, rosemary, and ylang ylang.

Odor: Type: Middle to Base Notes (20–80% of the blend); Scent: Spicy, warming, slightly bitter, woody, reminiscent of true clove buds but richer; Intensity: 5.

Additional Research:

Blood Clots: Clove oil demonstrated an ability to prevent the aggregation of platelets that can lead to blood clots and thrombosis both in vivo and in vitro (Saeed et al., 1994).

Antibacterial Properties: Cinnamon, thyme, and clove essential oils demonstrated an antibacterial effect on several respiratory tract pathogens (Fabio et al., 2007).

Antibacterial Properties: Bay, cinnamon, and clove oils reduced production of alpha-toxin and enterotoxin A by *Staphylococcus aureus* bacteria (Smith-Palmer et al., 2004).

Antifungal Properties: Clove oil was found to have very strong radical scavenging activity (antioxidant). It was also found to display an antifungal effect against tested Candida strains (Chaieb et al., 2007).

Antifungal Properties: Eugenol from clove and thymol from thyme were found to inhibit the growth of *Aspergillus flavus* and *Aspergillus versicolor* at concentrations of .4mg/ml or less. (Hitokoto et al., 1980).

Anti-inflammatory Properties: Eugenol (found in clove EO) was found to increase the anti-inflammatory activity of cod liver oil (lowered inflammation by 30%) (Reddy et al., 1994).

Inflammation: Clove oil was found to increase humoral immunity and decrease cell-mediated immunity in rats, illustrating that clove oil can modulate the immune response and overall acts as an anti-inflammatory agent (Halder et al., 2011).

Antiviral Properties: Eugenol was found to be virucidal to *Herpes simplex* and to delay the development of herpes-induced keratitis (inflammation of the cornea) in mice (Benencia et al., 2000).

Insect Control: A blend of eugenol, alpha-terpineol, and cinnamic alcohol was found to be insecticidal against American cockroaches, carpenter ants, and German cockroaches (Enan, 2001).

Insect Control: Clove oil was found to be highly termiticidal (Zhu et al., 2001).

Leukemia: Eugenol, a major chemical constituent of clove essential oil, was found to induce apoptosis in human leukemia cells via reactive oxygen species generation (Yoo et al., 2005).

Memory: Administration of clove essential oil for three weeks before treatment with scopolamine (a known agent causing memory impairment) was shown to significantly reverse the scopolamine-induced memory deficit, when compared to pretreatment with saline only (Halder et al., 2011).

Seizure: The aqueous and ethanolic extracts of clove were found to induce an anticonvulsive effect by increasing seizure latency in drug-induced seizure model mice, when compared to control (Hosseini et al., 2012).

Arthritis: Eugenol was found to ameliorate experimental arthritis in mice by inhibiting mononuclear cell infiltration into the knee joints and lowering cytokine levels (Grespan et al., 2012).

Parkinson's Disease: Eugenol administration was found to prevent induced dopamine depression and lipid peroxidation inductivity in the mouse striatum model, suggesting that eugenol may be useful in the treatment of Parkinson's disease (Kabuto et al., 2007).

Multiple Sclerosis: Beta caryophyllene (found in clove oil) was found to help protect against neuroinflammation and the demyelinating processes in the central nervous system in a murine model of multiple sclerosis (Alberti et al., 2017).

See Personal Usage Guide chapter for more details on these primary uses.   ●=Neat, ●=Dilute for Children/Sensitive Skin, ●=Dilute

Copaiba *Copaifera officinalis, C. reticulata, C. coriacea, C. langsdorffii*

Quick Facts

Botanical Family: Leguminosae (flowering plants)

Extraction Method: Steam distillation from resin

Common Primary Uses*: ⬢Acne①, ⬢⬡Antioxidant①, ⬡⬢Anxiety①, ⬢Inflammation①, ⬢Muscle Aches, ⬢Pain①

Common Application Methods‡:

⬢: Can be applied neat (with no dilution) when used topically. Apply directly on area of concern or to reflex points.

⬡: Diffuse, or inhale the aroma directly.

⬤: Take 1 drop in a beverage or in a capsule.

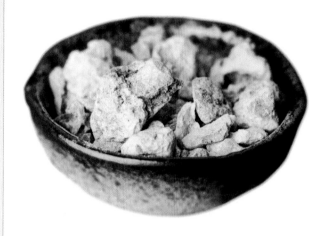

Chemical Constituents: Sesquiterpenes (up to 90%): β-caryophyllene (up to 52%), α- & β-copaene (>15%), trans-α-bergamotene (>8%), α-cubebene, α-humulene, γ- & β-elemene, β-cubebene.

Properties: Analgesic①, powerful anti-inflammatory①, antibacterial①, antiseptic, antioxidant① and stimulant (circulatory, pulmonary systems).

Historical Uses: The oleoresin has traditionally been used for inflammation (internal and external), skin disorders①, respiratory problems including bronchitis and sinusitis, and urinary tract problems including cystitis and bladder/kidney infections. It has also been used for bleeding, gonorrhea, hemorrhages, herpes, incontinence, insect bites, pain, pleurisy, sore throats, stomach ulcers, syphilis, tetanus, tonsillitis, tuberculosis, and tumors①.

Other Possible Uses: Copaiba may also help with colds, constipation, diarrhea, dyspepsia, edema, flatulence, flu, hemorrhoids, muscular aches and pains, nervous exhaustion, piles, poor circulation, stiffness, and wounds.

✛ **Body System(s) Affected:** Cardiovascular, Respiratory, and Nervous Systems, Muscles and Bones, Emotional Balance, and Skin.

Aromatic Influence: Copaiba helps to elevate the mood and lift depression. It also helps to combat nervous tension, stress problems, and anxiety①.

Oral Use As Dietary Supplement: Copaiba oil is generally recognized as safe (GRAS) for human consumption by the FDA (21CFR182.20). Dilute 1 drop oil in 1 tsp. (5 ml) honey or in ½ cup (125 ml) of beverage (e.g., soy/rice milk). Not for children under 6 years old; use with caution and in greater dilution for children 6 years old and over.

Safety Data: Repeated use may result in contact sensitization. May irritate sensitive skin in some individuals.

Blends With: Cedarwood, cinnamon, citrus oils, clary sage, jasmine, rose, ylang ylang.

Odor: Type: Base Note (5–20% of the blend); Scent: Soft, sweet, balsamic; Intensity: 3.

① **Additional Research:**

Acne: A gel containing copaiba oil was found to significantly improve acne in those suffering from acne vulgaris (da Silva et al., 2012).

Antioxidant: The overproduction of oxygen radicals, specifically NO and H2O2, and cytokines (both involved in the etiology of MS) by mouse splenocytes was significantly inhibited by copaiba oil (Dias et al., 2014).

Anxiety: In the elevated plus maze, copaiba oil was found to demonstrate anxiolitic effects on rats comparable to the antianxiety drug diazepam (Curio et al., 2009).

Pain: Oral administration of copaiba oil was found to have antinociceptive activity (blocked transmission of pain-causing stimuli) in rodents (Gomes et al., 2007).

Anti-inflammatory: beta-Caryophyllene, found in copaiba oil, was found to reduce inflammatory pain responses in an animal model (Klauke et al., 2013).

Antibacterial: Copaiba oil demonstrated inhibitory activities on several species of bacteria (Santos et al., May 2008).

Antibacterial: Copaiba oil was found to inhibit *Staphylococcus aureus* bacteria in vitro (Bonan et al., 2015).

Skin: Copaiba oil was found to inhibit the parasite *Leishmania amazonensis* (a protozoon that causes skin lesions) (Santos et al., Nov. 2008).

Anti-cancer: Beta-caryophyllene (found in copaiba oil) was found to increase the anticancer activities of paclitaxel (a chemotherapy drug derived from the yew tree) (Legault et al., 2007).

---

‡*See Application section beginning on page 16 for more details on applying essential oils.*   ⬢=Topical, ⬡=Aromatic, ⬤=Internal

Essential Oils

Coriander *Coriandrum sativum L.*

Quick Facts

Botanical Family: Umbelliferae (parsley)

Extraction Method: Steam distillation from seeds

Common Primary Uses*: Cartilage Injury, Degenerative Disease, Muscle Aches, Muscle Development, Muscle Tone, Whiplash

Common Application Methods‡:

: Can be applied neat (with no dilution) when used topically. Apply directly on area of concern or to reflex points.

: Diffuse, or inhale the aroma directly.

: Use as a flavoring in cooking.

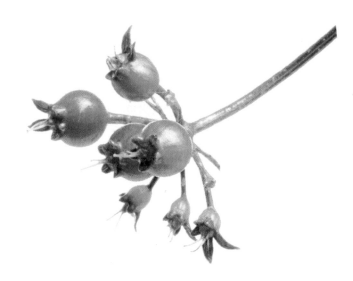

Chemical Constituents: Alcohols (up to 80%): linalool (>30%), coriandrol (<30%), geraniol, terpinen-4-ol, borneol; Monoterpenes (up to 24%): α-pinene, γ-terpinene, l-limonene, p-cymene, myrcene, camphene; Esters: geranyl acetate, linalyl acetate; Ketones: camphor, carvone; Aldehydes: decanal.

Properties: Analgesic, antibacterial, antifungal, antioxidant, antirheumatic, antispasmodic, and stimulant (cardiac, circulatory, and nervous systems). It also has anti-inflammatory and sedative properties.

Historical Uses: The Chinese have used coriander for dysentery, piles, measles, nausea, toothache, and painful hernias.

Other Possible Uses: Coriander may help with anorexia, arthritis, colds, colic, diarrhea, digestive spasms, dyspepsia, flatulence, flu, gout, infections (general), measles, migraine, nausea, nervous exhaustion, neuralgia, piles, poor circulation, rheumatism, skin (oily skin, blackheads, and other impurities), and stiffness. It may also help during convalescence and after a difficult childbirth. It may regulate and help control pain related to menstruation.

Body System(s) Affected: Digestive and Hormonal Systems.

Aromatic Influence: Coriander is a gentle stimulant for those with low physical energy. It also helps one relax during times of stress, irritability, and nervousness. It may also provide a calming influence to those suffering from shock or fear.

Oral Use As Dietary Supplement: Coriander oil is generally recognized as safe (GRAS) for human consumption by the FDA (21CFR182.20). Dilute 1 drop oil in 1 tsp. (5 ml) honey or in ½ cup (125 ml) of beverage (e.g., soy/rice milk). Not for children under 6 years old; use with caution and in greater dilution for children 6 years old and over.

Safety Data: Use sparingly, as coriander can be stupefying in large doses.

Blend Classification: Personifier and Modifier.

Blends With: Bergamot, cinnamon, clary sage, cypress, ginger, sandalwood, and other spice oils.

Odor: Type: Middle Note (50–80% of the blend); Scent: Woody, spicy, sweet; Intensity: 3.

Additional Research:

Alzheimer's Disease: Inhalation of coriander volatile oil was found to possess antianxiety, antidepressant, and antioxidant properties in Alzheimer's disease conditions in a rat model of beta-amyloid Alzheimer's disease (Cioanca et al., 2014).

Alzheimer's Disease: Repeated inhalation of coriander oil was found to prevent memory impairment and oxidative damage in a rat model of beta-amyloid Alzheimer's disease, when compared to control (Cioanca et al., 2013).

Detoxification: Coriander extract was found to have a protective role against lead toxicity in rat brain (Velaga et al., 2014).

Antispasmodic Properties: Linalool, found in several essential oils, was found to inhibit induced convulsions in rats by directly interacting with the NMDA receptor complex (Brum et al., 2001).

Arthritis: Coriander extract produced a dose dependent inhibition of joint swelling in two mice models of induced arthritis (Nair et al., 2012).

Pain: Injection of coriander extract in mice was found to have a greater analgesic effect than dexamethasone (an anti-inflammatory drug) or stress, when mice were subjected to acute and chronic pain tests (Taherian et al., 2012).

See Personal Usage Guide chapter for more details on these primary uses. =Neat, =Dilute for Children/Sensitive Skin, =Dilute

Cypress *Cupressus sempervirens*

Essential Oils

Quick Facts

Botanical Family: Cupressaceae (conifer: cypress)

Extraction Method: Steam distillation from branches

Common Primary Uses*: ☽⊘Aneurysm, ☽Bone Spurs, ☽Bunions, ☽Bursitis, ☽Carpal Tunnel Syndrome, ☽⊘Catarrh, ☽⊘Circulation, ☽Concussion, ☽Dysmenorrhea, ☽Edema, ☽Endometriosis, ☽⊘Environmental Stress, ☽⊘Flu (Influenza), ☽Greasy/Oily Hair, ☽Hemorrhoids, ☽Hernia (Hiatal), ☽Incontinence, ☽Lou Gehrig's Disease, ☽⊘Lymphatic Decongestant, ☽Menopause, ☽Menorrhagia, ☽Muscle Fatigue, ☽Muscle Tone, ☽Pain (Chronic), ☽⊘Pleurisy, ☽⊘Preeclampsia, ☽Prostatitis, ☽⊘Raynaud's Disease, ☽Retina (Strengthen), ☽Rheumatoid Arthritis, ☽Skin (Revitalizing), ☽⊘Stroke, ☽Swollen Eyes, ☽⊘Toxemia, ☽⊘Tuberculosis, ☽Varicose Veins

Common Application Methods‡:

☽: Can be applied neat (with no dilution) when used topically. Apply to reflex points and directly on area of concern.

⊘: Diffuse, or inhale the aroma directly.

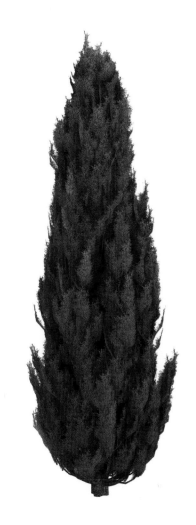

Chemical Constituents: Monoterpenes: α-pinene (>55%), δ-3-carene (<22%), l-limonene, terpinolene, sabinene, β-pinene; Sesquiterpene Alcohols: cedrol (up to 15%), cadinol; Alcohols: borneol (<9%), α-terpineol, terpinene-4-ol, linalool sabinol; Esters: α-terpinyl acetate (<5%), isovalerate, terpinen-4-yl acetate; Sesquiterpenes: δ-cadinene, α-cedrene; Diterpene Alcohols; labdanic alcohols, manool, sempervirol; Diterpene Acids; Oxides.

Properties: Antibacterial ⊕, anti-infectious, antimicrobial, mucolytic, antiseptic, astringent, deodorant, diuretic, lymphatic and prostate decongestant, refreshing, relaxing, and vasoconstricting.

Historical Uses: It was used anciently for its benefits on the urinary system and in instances where there is excessive loss of fluids, such as perspiration, diarrhea, and menstrual flow. The Chinese valued cypress for its benefits to the liver and to the respiratory system.

French Medicinal Uses: Arthritis, bronchitis, circulation, cramps, hemorrhoids, insomnia, intestinal parasites, lymphatic decongestant, menopausal problems, menstrual pain, pancreas insufficiencies, pleurisy, prostate decongestion, pulmonary tuberculosis, rheumatism, spasms, throat problems, varicose veins, water retention.

Other Possible Uses: This oil may be beneficial for asthma, strengthening blood capillary walls, reducing cellulite, improving the circulatory system, colds, strengthening connective tissue, spasmodic coughs, diarrhea, energy, fever, gallbladder, bleeding gums, hemorrhaging, influenza, laryngitis, liver disorders ⊕, lung circulation, muscular cramps, nervous tension, nose bleeds, ovarian cysts, increasing perspiration, skin care, scar tissue, whooping cough, and wounds.

---

‡*See Application section beginning on page 16 for more details on applying essential oils.*   ☽=Topical, ⊘=Aromatic, ◯=Internal

57

⊕ **Body System(s) Affected:** Cardiovascular System, Muscles and Bones.

Aromatic Influence: It influences and strengthens and helps ease the feeling of loss. It creates a feeling of security and grounding.

Oral Use As Dietary Supplement: None.

Safety Data: Use with caution during pregnancy.

Blend Classification: Equalizer.

Blends With: Bergamot, clary sage, lavender, lemon, orange, and sandalwood.

Odor: Type: Middle Note (50–80% of the blend); Scent: Fresh, herbaceous, slightly woody with evergreen undertones; Intensity: 3.

◍ **Additional Research:**

Antibacterial: Cypress essential oil was found to possess antibacterial activity against Staphlococcus aureus, *Klebsiella pneumoniae*, and Salmonella indica when tested for antimicrobial properties against 13 microorganisms (Selim et al., 2014).

Liver—Hepatitis: Oral administration of cypress methanolic extract displayed preventive action against CCl4-induced hepatotoxicity in rats. These results suggest that the antioxidant activity of the flavonoid content of cypress could have potential use as a treatment for liver diseases (Ali et al., 2010).

See Personal Usage Guide chapter for more details on these primary uses.   ●=Neat, ●=Dilute for Children/Sensitive Skin, ●=Dilute

Dill *Anethum graveolens*

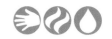

Quick Facts

Botanical Family: Umbelliferae (parsley)

Extraction Method: Steam distillation from whole plant

Common Primary Uses*: ⬡⚪Cholesterol▱, ⚪Flavoring

Common Application Methods‡:

⬡: Can be applied neat (with no dilution) when used topically. Apply to reflex points on the feet and/or directly on area of concern. A drop or two on the wrists may help remove addictions to sweets.

⚖: Diffuse, or inhale the aroma directly.

⚫: Take in a capsule. Use as a flavoring in cooking.

Chemical Constituents: Monoterpenes (up to 65%): d-limonene (up to 25%), α- & β-pinenes (<30%), α- & β-phellandrenes, p-cymene; Ketones: d-carvone (<45%); Ethers (<11%).

Properties: Antispasmodic, antibacterial, expectorant, and stimulant.

Other Possible Uses: This oil may help with bronchial catarrh, colic, constipation, dyspepsia, flatulence, headaches, indigestion, liver deficiencies, lowering glucose levels, nervousness, normalizing insulin levels, promoting milk flow in nursing mothers, supporting pancreas function, and clearing toxins▱. It may also act as an insect repellent▱.

⊕ **Body System(s) Affected:** Digestive & Cardiovascular Systems.

Aromatic Influence: It helps calm the autonomic nervous system and, when diffused with Roman chamomile, may help fidgety children.

Oral Use As Dietary Supplement: Generally regarded as safe (GRAS) for human consumption by the FDA. Dilute 1 drop oil in 1 tsp. (5 ml) honey or in ½ cup (125 ml) of beverage (e.g., soy/rice milk). Not for children under 6 years old; use with caution and in greater dilution for children 6 years old and over.

Safety Data: Use with caution if susceptible to epilepsy.

Blend Classification: Enhancer.

Blends With: Citrus oils.

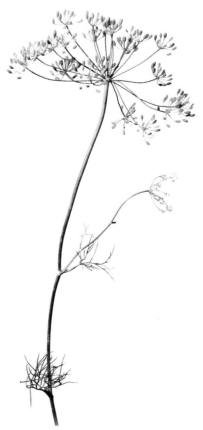

Odor: Type: Middle Note (50–80% of the blend); Scent: Fresh, sweet, herbaceous, slightly earthy; Intensity: 2

▱ **Additional Research:**

Cholesterol: Different fractions of *Anethum graveolens* extract improved hypercholesterolemia in rats fed a high fat diet. Hypercholesterolemia has been found to be a risk factor for the development of atherosclerosis (Bahramikia et al., 2009).

Clearing Toxins: Three compounds derived from dill and caraway oil—anethofuran, carvone, and limonene—were found to induce the enzyme glutathione S-transferase (involved in transforming or binding to toxins in tissues) in several mice tissues (Zheng et al., 1992).

Repellent: Dill proved to be an effective repellent against male and female adult German cockroaches (Lee et al., 2017).

Gastric Ulcers: Oral administration of dill seed extract was found to have effective antisecretory and anti-ulcer activity against HCl- and ethanol-induced stomach lesions in mice (Hosseinzadeh et al., 2002).

Inflammation: Oil-based dill extract displayed greater anti-inflammatory activity when topically applied to inflamed rat paws than the anti-inflammatory drug diclofenac (Naseri et al., 2012).

Skin: An in vitro study using human fibroblast cells from adult skin showed that dill extract was able to stimulate LOXL gene expression to induce elastogenesis in adult skin cells. These findings suggest that dill extract may be able to increase skin elasticity and firming (Cenizo et al., 2006).

Antifungal: Dill essential oil was demonstrated to induce apoptosis (cell death) in Candida albicans in a metacaspase-dependent manner (Chen et al., 2014).

Memory: A combined extract of *Cissampelos pareira* and **Anethum graveolens** was found to produce cognitive-enhancing and neuroprotective effects on spatial memory in memory deficit induced rats (Thukham-Mee et al., 2012).

Diabetes: Dill seed extract suppressed high-fat diet-induced hyperlipidemia through hepatic PPAR-α activation in diabetic obese mice (Takahashi et al., 2013).

---

‡See Application section beginning on page 16 for more details on applying essential oils.   ⬡=Topical, ⚖=Aromatic, ⚫=Internal

59

Douglas Fir *Pseudotsuga menziesii*

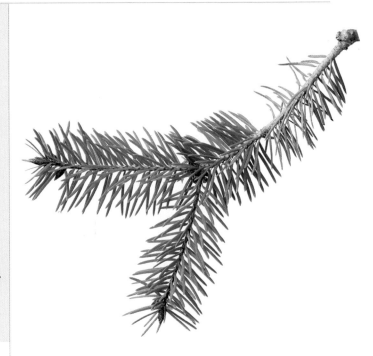

Quick Facts

Botanical Family: Pinaceae (conifer)

Extraction Method: Steam distillation from twigs and needles

Common Primary Uses*: ⊘⊝Asthma, ⊘⊝Bronchitis⊕, ⊘⊝Congestion, ⊘⊝Coughs, ⊝Disinfectant (skin), ⊘⊝Flu (Influenza), ⊘Focus, ⊘⊝Infection

Common Application Methods‡:

⊝: Can be applied neat (with no dilution) when used topically. Dilute 1:1 (1 drop essential oil to at least 1 drop carrier oil) for children and for those with sensitive skin. Apply directly on area of concern or to reflex points.

⊘: Diffuse, or inhale the aroma directly.

Chemical Constituents: Monoterpenes (up to 80%): α-pinene (10–20%), β-pinene (30–40%), l-limonene (<5%), δ-3-carene, camphene, terpinolene; Esters (up to 15%): bornyl acetate (<15%), geranyl acetate (<4%), bornyl & geranyl coproates; Alcohols (up to 10%): borneol, geraniol; Aldehydes: benzoicaldehyde, citrals; Ketones: camphor; Oxides: 1,8 cineol.

Properties: Antiseptic, astringent, diuretic, expectorant, sedative (nerves), and tonic.

Historical Uses: The Douglas fir is highly regarded for its fragrant scent. Douglas fir has also been valued through the ages for its ability to help support the body with respiratory complaints, fever, and muscular and rheumatic pain.

Other Possible Uses: Douglas fir may be beneficial for anxiety, catarrh, colds, respiratory weakness, rheumatism, tension (nervous), and wounds. It is soothing to sore muscles and can help soothe overworked or tired muscles and joints.

⊕ **Body System(s) Affected:** Respiratory System, Muscles and Bones.

Aromatic Influence: This beautiful aroma can help create a feeling of grounding and anchoring and promotes a sense of focus. It can help balance the emotions and stimulate the mind while allowing the body to relax.

Oral Use As Dietary Supplement: None.

Safety Data: Can irritate sensitive skin.

Blend Classification: Equalizer.

Blends With: Cedarwood, eucalyptus, frankincense, juniper, lavender, lemon, orange, and sandalwood.

Odor: Type: Middle Notes (50–80% of the blend); Scent: Fresh, woody, earthy, sweet; Intensity: 3.

⊡ **Additional Research:**

Bronchitis: In patients with chronic bronchitis, rosemary, basil, fir, and eucalyptus oils were found to demonstrate an antioxidant effect (Siurin et al., 1997).

*See Personal Usage Guide chapter for more details on these primary uses.   ●=Neat, ●=Dilute for Children/Sensitive Skin, ●=Dilute

Eucalyptus *Eucalyptus radiata*

Quick Facts

Botanical Family: Myrtaceae (Myrtle shrubs and trees)

Extraction Method: Steam distillation from leaves

Common Primary Uses*: ⚬Arterial Vasodilator, ⚬Asthma, ⚬Brain Blood Flow, ⚬Bronchitis⊕, ⚬Congestion, ⚬Cooling (Body), ⚬Coughs, ⚬Diabetes, ⚬Disinfectant, ⚬Dysentery, ⚬Ear Inflammation, ⚬Emphysema, ⚬Expectorant, ⚬Fever, ⚬Flu (Influenza), ⚬Hypoglycemia, ⚬Inflammation, ⚬Iris Inflammation, ⚬Jet Lag, ⚬Kidney Stones, ⚬Lice⊕, ⚬Measles, ⚬Neuralgia, ⚬Neuritis, ⚬Overexercised Muscles, ⚬Pain, ⚬Pneumonia, ⚬Respiratory Viruses, ⚬Rhinitis, ⚬Shingles, ⚬Sinusitis, ⚬Tennis Elbow, ⚬Tuberculosis

Common Application Methods‡:

🖐: Can be applied neat (with no dilution), or dilute 1:1 (1 drop essential oil to at least 1 drop carrier oil) for children and for those with sensitive skin when using topically. Apply to reflex points and/or directly on area of concern.

🌀: Diffuse, or inhale the aroma directly.

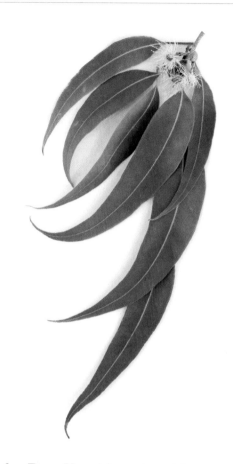

Chemical Constituents: Oxides: 1,8 cineol (62–72%), caryophyllene oxide; Monoterpenes (up to 24%): α- & β-pinenes (<12%), l-limonene (<8%), myrcene, p-cymene; Alcohols (<19%): α-terpineol (14%), geraniol, borneol, linalool; Aldehydes (8%): myrtenal, citronellal, geranial, neral.

Properties: Analgesic⊕, antibacterial⊕, anticatarrhal, anti-infectious, anti-inflammatory⊕, antiviral⊕, insecticidal⊕, and expectorant.

Other Possible Uses: This oil, when combined with bergamot, has been used effectively on herpes simplex. It may also help with acne, endometriosis, hay fever, high blood pressure⊕, nasal mucous membrane inflammation, and vaginitis.

✛ Body System(s) Affected: Respiratory System, Skin.

Oral Use As Dietary Supplement: None.

Safety Data: Use with caution with very small children.

Blend Classification: Enhancer.

Blends With: Geranium, lavender, lemon, sandalwood, juniper berry, lemongrass, melissa, thyme.

Odor: Type: Middle Note (50–80% of the blend); Scent: Slightly camphorous, sweet, fruity; Intensity: 3.

⊕ Additional Research:

Analgesic Properties: 1,8 cineole (eucalyptol) was found to have antinociceptive (pain-reducing) properties similar to morphine (Liapi et al., 2007).

Analgesic Properties: 1,8 cineole (eucalyptol) was found to display an anti-inflammatory effect on rats in several tests and was found to exhibit antinociceptive (pain-reducing) effects in mice, possibly by depressing the central nervous system (Santos et al., 2000).

Bronchitis: Therapy with 1.8 cineole (eucalyptol) in both healthy and bronchitis-afflicted humans was shown to reduce production of LTB4 and PGE2 (both metabolites of arachidonic acid, a known chemical messenger involved in inflammation) in white blood cells (Juergens et al., 1998).

Bronchitis: In patients with chronic bronchitis, rosemary, basil, fir, and eucalyptus oils were found to demonstrate an antioxidant effect. Lavender was found to promote normalization of lipid levels (Siurin et al., 1997).

Antibacterial Properties: Subjects using a mouthwash containing thymol, menthol, methyl salicylate, and eucalyptol for 6 months were found to not have developed oral bacteria that were resistant to the oils (Charles et al., 2000).

Anti-inflammatory Properties: 1,8 cineole (eucalyptol) was found to display an anti-inflammatory effect on rats in several tests and was found to exhibit anti-

‡*See Application section beginning on page 16 for more details on applying essential oils.*   🖐=Topical, 🌀=Aromatic, O=Internal

61

nociceptive (pain-reducing) effects in mice, possibly by depressing the central nervous system (Santos et al., 2000).

Anti-inflammatory Properties: Eucalyptus oil was shown to ameliorate inflammatory processes by interacting with oxygen radicals and interfering with leukocyte activation (Grassmann et al., 2000).

Antiviral Properties: Tea tree and eucalyptus oil demonstrated ability to inhibit the Herpes simplex virus (Schnitzler et al., 2001).

Insecticidal Properties: A blend of eugenol, alpha-terpineol, and cinnamic alcohol was found to be insecticidal against American cockroaches, carpenter ants, and German cockroaches (Enean, 2001).

High Blood Pressure: Treatment of rats with 1,8-cineole (or eucalyptol, found in eucalyptus and rosemary) demonstrated an ability to lower mean aortic pressure (blood pressure), without decreasing heart rate, through vascular wall relaxation (Lahlou et al., 2002).

Lice: Researchers found that an 8% eucalyptus oil spray was the most effective treatment (when compared against other concentrations of eucalyptus and clove oil sprays) against lice and insecticide-resistant head lice (Choi et al., 2010).

Lice: Researchers found that eucalyptus oil was an effective treatment for head lice in school-aged children (Greive et al., 2017).

Bones—Osteoporosis: Oral intake of rosemary or eucalyptus essential oil (as well as several monoterpenes found in other essential oils) was shown to inhibit bone resorption in rats (Mühlbauer et al., 2003).

Childhood Diseases—Mumps: A plaque reduction assay showed that eucalyptus essential oil possessed a mild antiviral activity against mumps virus (Cermelli et al., 2008).

See Personal Usage Guide chapter for more details on these primary uses.   ●=Neat, ●=Dilute for Children/Sensitive Skin, ●=Dilute

Fennel (Sweet) *Foeniculum vulgare*

Quick Facts

Botanical Family: Umbelliferae (parsley)

Extraction Method: Steam distillation from the crushed seeds

Common Primary Uses*: ⬢Benign Prostatic Hyperplasia, ⬢⬢⬢Blood Clots, ⬢Bruises, ⬢⬢⬢Digestive System Support, ⬢⬢Gastritis, ⬢IBS⬤, ⬢Kidney Stones, ⬢Lactation (Increase Milk Production), ⬢⬢Pancreas Support, ⬢⬢Parasites, ⬢Skin (Revitalizing), ⬢Tissue (Toxin Cleansing), ⬢Wrinkles

Common Application Methods‡:

⬢: Can be applied neat (with no dilution), or dilute 1:1 (1 drop essential oil to at least 1 drop carrier oil) for children and for those with sensitive skin when using topically. Apply directly on area of concern or to reflex points.

⬢: Diffuse, or inhale the aroma directly.

⬢: Place 1–2 drops under the tongue, or take in a capsule. Use as a flavoring in cooking.

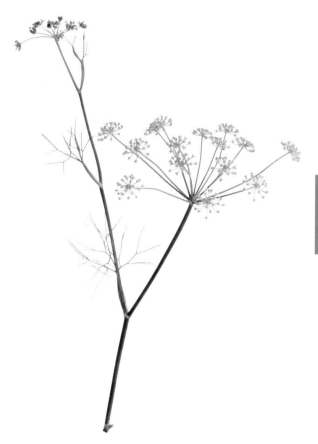

Chemical Constituents: Phenolic Ethers (up to 80%): trans-anethole (70%), methyl chavicol (or estragole) (>3%); Monoterpenes (up to 50%): trans-ocimene (<12%), l-limonene (<12%), γ-terpinene (<11%), α- & β-pinenes (<10%), p-cymene, α- & β-phellandrenes, terpiolene, myrcene, sabinene; Alcohols (up to 16%): linalool (<12%), α-fenchol (<4%); Ketones (<15%): fenchone (12%), camphor; Oxides; Phenols.

Properties: Antiparasitic, antiseptic, antispasmodic⬤, antitoxic, diuretic, and expectorant.

Historical Uses: The ancient Egyptians and Romans awarded garlands of fennel as praise to victorious warriors because fennel was believed to bestow strength, courage, and longevity. It has been used for thousands of years for snakebites, to stave off hunger pains, to tone the female reproductive system, for earaches, eye problems, insect bites, kidney complaints, lung infections, and to expel worms.

French Medicinal Uses: Cystitis, sluggish digestion, flatulence, gout, intestinal parasites, intestinal spasms, increase lactation, menopause problems⬤, premenopause, urinary stones, vomiting.

Other Possible Uses: Fennel oil may be used for colic⬤, stimulating the cardiovascular system, constipation, digestion (supports the liver), balancing hormones, nausea, obesity, PMS⬤, and stimulating the sympathetic nervous system⬤.

⬢ **Body System(s) Affected:** Digestive and Hormonal Systems.

Aromatic Influence: It increases and influences longevity, courage, and purification.

Oral Use As Dietary Supplement: Fennel oil is generally recognized as safe (GRAS) for human consumption by the FDA (21CFR182.20). Dilute 1 drop oil in 1 tsp. (5 ml) honey or in ½ cup (125 ml) of beverage (e.g., soy/rice milk). Not for children under 6 years old; use with caution and in greater dilution for children 6 years old and over.

Safety Data: Repeated use can possibly result in contact sensitization. Use with caution if susceptible to epilepsy. Use with caution during pregnancy.

‡*See Application section beginning on page 16 for more details on applying essential oils.*   ⬢=Topical, ⬢=Aromatic, ⬢=Internal

63

Essential Oils

Blend Classification: Equalizer and Modifier.

Blends With: Basil, geranium, lavender, lemon, rosemary, and sandalwood.

Odor: Type: Top to Middle Notes (20–80% of the blend); Scent: Sweet, somewhat spicy, licorice-like; Intensity: 4.

Additional Research:

IBS: Patients with moderate IBS symptoms who took a pill with curcumin and fennel essential oils had significantly improved symptoms and quality of life compared to those who took a placebo (Portincasa et al., 2016).

Antispasmodic Properties: Fennel oil was found to reduce contraction frequency and intensity in rat uterus induced to contract (Ostad et al., 2001).

Menopause: Using a mouse model of postmenopausal bone loss researchers found that oral administration of fennel oil for six weeks had an intermediate effect on the prevention of femoral bone mineral density and bone mineral content when compared to controls. These findings suggest that fennel oil has potential in preventing bone loss in postmenopausal osteoporosis (Kim et al., 2012).

Menopause: In a triple-blind, placebo-controlled trial with 90 postmenopausal women aged 45 to 60 years, fennel demonstrated an ability to reduce menopausal symptoms in postmenopausal women (Rahimikian et al., 2017).

Colic: Fennel seed oil was found to be superior to a placebo in decreasing intensity of infantile colic in a randomized placebo-controlled trial including 121 infants. The oil was administered four times a day and consumption was limited to a maximum of 12 mg/kg/day of fennel seed oil (Alexandrovich et al., 2003).

Colic: Colic improved in breastfed infants within 1 week of administering a phytotherapeutic agent containing *Matricariae recutita, Foeniculum vulgare,* and *Melissa officinalis* when compared to a placebo containing vitamins (Savino et al., 2005).

PMS: Fennel oil was found to reduce contraction frequency and intensity in rat uterus induced to contract (Ostad et al., 2001).

Stimulating the Sympathetic Nervous System: Inhalation of essential oils such as pepper, estragon, fennel, and grapefruit was found to have a stimulating effect on sympathetic activity in healthy adults (Haze et al., 2002).

Cells: Oral pretreatment with fennel essential oil was found to inhibit in vivo genotoxicity of cyclophosphamide (an important chemotherapy medication with adverse effects) in mouse bone marrow and sperm. These findings suggest that fennel could be used as an adjuvant in chemotherapeutic applications to help diminish adverse effects (Tripathi et al., 2013).

Hair: Fennel extract gel, when compared to a placebo, was effective in decreasing hair thickness in women suffering from mild to moderate idiopathic hirsutism (Akha et al., 2014).

See Personal Usage Guide chapter for more details on these primary uses.   ●=Neat, ●=Dilute for Children/Sensitive Skin, ●=Dilute

Fir, Douglas *(see Douglas Fir)*   Fir, White *(see White Fir)*

Frankincense *Boswellia frereana, Boswellia carteri, Boswellia sacra*

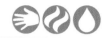

Quick Facts

Botanical Family: Burseraceae (resinous trees and shrubs)

Extraction Method: Steam distillation from gum/resin

Common Primary Uses*: Alzheimer's Disease, Aneurysm, Arthritis, Asthma, Balance, Brain (Aging), Brain Injury, Breathing, Cancer, Coma, Concussion, Confusion, Coughs, Depression, Fibroids, Genital Warts, Hepatitis, Immune System Support, Improve Vision, Infected Wounds, Inflammation, Liver Cirrhosis, Lou Gehrig's Disease, Memory, Mental Fatigue, Miscarriage (After), Moles, MRSA, Multiple Sclerosis, Nasal Polyp, Parkinson's Disease, Plague, Postpartum Depression, Scarring (Prevention), Tumor (Lipoma), Ulcers, Uterus Tissue Regeneration, Virus of Nerves, Warts, Wrinkles

Common Application Methods‡:

🖐: Can be applied neat (with no dilution) when used topically. Apply directly on area of concern or to reflex points.

🌀: Diffuse, or inhale the aroma directly.

💧: Place 1–2 drops under the tongue, or take in a capsule.

Chemical Constituents: Monoterpenes: α-phellandrenes (up to 25%), α- & β-pinenes (up to 15%), α-thujene (<15%), l-limonene (<5%), sabinene (<7%), p-cymene (<10%), α-terpinene, camphene, myrcene; Sesquiterpenes (<10%): β-elemene (<5%), α-copaene; Alcohols (<10%): cis-verbenol (<5%), 4-terpineol, α-terpineol, borneol, cis-sabinol, olibanol, trans-pinocarveol, farnesol; Ketones: verbenone.

Properties: Anticatarrhal, anticancer, antidepressant, anti-infectious, anti-inflammatory, antiseptic, antitumor, expectorant, immune stimulant, and sedative.

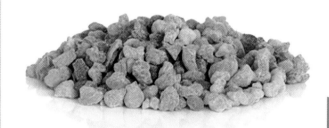

Historical Uses: Frankincense is a holy oil in the Middle East. As an ingredient in the holy incense, it was used anciently during sacrificial ceremonies to help improve communication with the creator.

French Medicinal Uses: Asthma, depression, ulcers.

Other Possible Uses: This oil may help with aging, allergies, bites (insect and snake), bronchitis, carbuncles, catarrh, colds, diarrhea, diphtheria, gonorrhea, headaches, healing, hemorrhaging, herpes, high blood pressure, jaundice, laryngitis, meningitis, nervous conditions, prostate problems, pneumonia, respiratory problems, sciatic pain, sores, spiritual awareness, staph, strep, stress, syphilis, T.B., tension, tonsillitis, typhoid, and wounds. It contains sesquiterpenes, enabling it to go beyond the blood-brain barrier. It may also help oxygenate the pineal and pituitary glands. It increases the activity of leukocytes, defending the body against infection. Frankincense may also help a person have a better attitude, which may help to strengthen the immune system.

Body System(s) Affected: Emotional Balance, Immune and Nervous Systems, Skin.

Aromatic Influence: This oil helps to focus energy, minimize distractions, and improve concentration. It eases hyperactivity, impatience, irritability, and restlessness and can help enhance spiritual awareness and meditation.

Oral Use As Dietary Supplement: Frankincense oil in general is approved by the FDA (21CFR172.510) for use as a Food Additive (FA) and Flavoring

‡*See Application section beginning on page 16 for more details on applying essential oils.*   🖐=Topical, 🌀=Aromatic, 💧=Internal

65

Agent (FL). Dilute 1 drop oil in 1 tsp. (5 ml) honey or in ½ cup (125 ml) of beverage (e.g., soy/rice milk). Not for children under 6 years old; use with caution and in greater dilution for children 6 years old and over.

Blend Classification: Enhancer and Equalizer.

Blends With: All oils.

Odor: Type: Base Note (5–20% of the blend); Scent: Rich, deep, warm, balsamic, sweet, with incense-like overtones; Intensity: 3.

Additional Research:

Arthritis: Alpha-phellandrene (found in frankincense oil) was found to have antinociceptive (pain sensation–blocking) properties in animal models (Lima et al., 2012).

Anticancer Properties: An extract from frankincense was found to produce apoptosis in human leukemia cells (Bhushan et al., 2007).

Anticancer Properties: β-elemene—a sesquiterpene found in curcumin and *Boswellia frereana* and black pepper essential oils—is currently being studied for its promising potential to induce apoptosis and inhibit cancer cell proliferation in ovarian (Zou et al., 2013), liver (Dai et al., 2013), breast (Zhang et al., 2013, Ding et al., 2013), bladder (Li et al., 2013), lung (Li et al., 2013, Chen et al., 2012), and brain (Li et al., 2013) cancer cell lines, both on its own and in combination with cisplatin chemotherapy.

Antidepressant Properties: Incensole acetate (found in frankincense) was found to open TRPV receptors in mice brain, a possible channel for emotional regulation (Moussaieff et al., 2008).

Anti-inflammatory Properties: Alpha-pinene was found to block proinflammatory responses in THP-1 cells (Zhou et al., 2004).

Anti-inflammatory Properties: *Boswellia frereana* extracts were found to inhibit proinflammatory molecules involved in joint cartilage degradation (Blain et al., 2009).

See Personal Usage Guide chapter for more details on these primary uses.   ●=Neat, ●=Dilute for Children/Sensitive Skin, ●=Dilute

66

Geranium *Pelargonium graveolens*

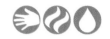

Quick Facts

Botanical Family: Geraniaceae

Extraction Method: Steam distillation from leaves

Common Primary Uses*: ⊘⊜Agitation (Calms), ⊘Airborne Bacteria, ⊜Autism, ⊜Bleeding, ⊜Breasts (Soothes), ⊜Bruises, ⊜Calcified Spine, ⊜⊘Cancer, ⊜Capillaries (Broken), ⊜⊘Diabetes, ⊜Diarrhea, ⊜Dysmenorrhea, ⊜Endometriosis, ⊘⊜Environmental Stress, ⊜Gallbladder Stones, ⊜Hair (Dry), ⊜Hernia (Incisional), ⊜Impetigo, ⊘⊜Insomnia (Older Children), ⊜⊘Jaundice, ⊜Jet Lag, ⊜Libido (Low), ⊜Menorrhagia, ⊜Miscarriage (After), ⊜MRSA, ⊜Osteoarthritis, ⊜Osteoporosis, ⊜⊘Pancreas Support, ⊜⊘Paralysis, ⊜Pelvic Pain Syndrome, ⊘⊜Physical Stress, ⊜⊘PMS, ⊜Post Labor, ⊜Rheumatoid Arthritis, ⊜Skin (Dry), ⊜Skin (Sensitive), ◐⊜Ulcer (Gastric), ⊜Varicose Ulcer, ⊜Vertigo, ⊜Wrinkles

Common Application Methods‡:

⊜: Can be applied neat (with no dilution) when used topically. Apply directly on area of concern or to reflex points.

⊘: Diffuse, or inhale the aroma directly.

◐: Take in capsules.

Chemical Constituents: Alcohols (up to 70%): citronellol (>32%), geraniol (<23%), linalool (<14%), nerol, γ-eudesmol, α-terpineol, menthol; Esters (up to 30%): citronellyl formate (14%), geranyl formate & acetate (<12%), other propionates, butyrates, & tiglates; Ketones: isomenthone (<8%), menthone, piperitone; Sesquiterpenes: 4-guaiadiene-6,9, α-copaene, δ- & γ-cadinenes, δ-guaiazulene, β-farnesene; Aldehydes: geranial (<6%), neral, citronellal; Monoterpenes (<5%): α- & β-pinenes, l-limonene, myrcene, ocimene; Sesquiterpene Alcohols: farnesol (<3%).

Properties: Antibacterial⊕, anticonvulsant⊕, antidepressant, anti-inflammatory⊕, antiseptic, astringent, diuretic, insect repellent⊕, refreshing, relaxing, sedative, and tonic.

Historical Uses: Geranium oil has been used for dysentery, hemorrhoids, inflammations, heavy menstrual flow, and possibly even cancer (if the folktale is correct). It has also been said to be a remedy for bone fractures, tumors, and wounds.

French Medicinal Uses: Diabetes, diarrhea, gallbladder, gastric ulcer, jaundice, liver, sterility, urinary stones.

Other Possible Uses: This oil may be used for acne, bleeding (increases to eliminate toxins, then stops), burns, circulatory problems (improves blood flow), depression, digestion, eczema, hormonal imbalance⊕, insomnia, kidney stones, dilating biliary ducts for liver detoxification, menstrual problems, neuralgia (severe pain along the nerve), regenerating tissue and nerves, pancreas (balances), ringworm, shingles, skin (may balance the sebum, which is the fatty secretion in the sebaceous glands of the skin that keeps the skin

Essential Oils

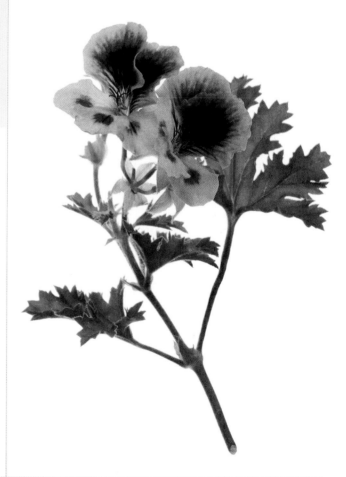

‡*See Application section beginning on page 16 for more details on applying essential oils.*   ⊜=Topical, ⊘=Aromatic, ◐=Internal

67

supple. It is good for expectant mothers. It works as a cleanser for oily skin and may even liven up pale skin), sores, sore throats, and wounds.

Body System(s) Affected: Emotional Balance, Skin.

Aromatic Influence: It may help to release negative memories and take a person back to peaceful, joyful moments. It may also help ease nervous tension and stress, balance the emotions, lift the spirit, and foster peace, well-being, and hope.

Oral Use As Dietary Supplement: Geranium oil is generally recognized as safe (GRAS) for human consumption by the FDA (21CFR182.20). Dilute 1 drop oil in 1 tsp. (5 ml) honey or in ½ cup (125 ml) of beverage (e.g., soy/rice milk). Not for children under 6 years old; use with caution and in greater dilution for children 6 years old and over.

Safety Data: Repeated use can possibly result in some contact sensitization.

Blend Classification: Enhancer and Equalizer.

Blends With: All oils.

Odor: Type: Middle Note (50–80% of the blend); Scent: Sweet, green, citrus-rosy, fresh; Intensity: 3.

Additional Research:

Antibacterial Properties: A combination of Citricidal and geranium oil demonstrated strong antibacterial effects on MRSA. Geranium and tea tree demonstrated strong antibacterial effects on *Staphylococcus aureus* (Edwards-Jones et al., 2004).

Antibacterial Properties: A formulation of lemongrass and geranium oil was found to reduce airborne bacteria by 89% in an office environment after diffusion for 15 hours (Doran et al., 2009).

Anticonvulsant Properties: Linalool, found in several essential oils, was found to inhibit induced convulsions in rats by directly interacting with the NMDA receptor complex (Brum et al., 2001).

Anti-inflammatory Properties: Topical application of geranium oil was found to reduce the inflammatory response of neutrophil (white blood cell) accumulation in mice (Maruyama et al., 2005).

Insect Repellent—Ticks: A sesquiterpene alcohol from geranium essential oil proved to be an effective repellent of the lone star tick (*Amblyomma americanum*) and at concentrations greater than 0.052 mg the oil was comparable to the repellant capability of DEET (Tabanca et al., 2013).

Male Infertility: Male mice exposed to a harmful insecticide, known to cause sperm damage, were successfully treated with geranium essential oil through its antioxidant effects. Compared to the control group, the oral administration of geranium oil prevented testicular oxidative damage, reduced lipid peroxidation, and improved total sperm motility, viability, and morphology in mice spermatozoa (Slima et al., 2013).

Hormonal Balance: Perimenopausal women exposed to geranium and rose otto oils were found to have increased salivary estrogen concentration compared to those exposed to a control odor (Shinohara et al., 2017).

See Personal Usage Guide chapter for more details on these primary uses.   ●=Neat, ●=Dilute for Children/Sensitive Skin, ●=Dilute

68

Ginger *Zingiber officinale*

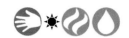

Quick Facts

Botanical Family: Zingiberaceae (ginger)

Extraction Method: Steam distillation from rhizomes

Common Primary Uses*: ◑⊘Angina, ◐Club Foot, ⚪◐Diarrhea, ◑◐Gas/Flatulence, ◑⊘Indigestion, ⊘◐Libido (Low), ⚪◑⊘Morning Sickness, ◑⊘Nausea◒, ◐Pelvic Pain Syndrome, ◐Rheumatic Fever (Pain), ◐Rheumatoid Arthritis◒, ◑◐Scurvy, ◑⊘Vertigo, ◑⊘Vomiting

Common Application Methods‡:

◑: Can be applied neat (with no dilution), or dilute 1:1 (1 drop essential oil to 1 drop carrier oil) for children and for those with sensitive skin when using topically. Apply directly on area of concern or to reflex points.

⊘: Diffuse, or inhale the aroma directly.

◐: Take in capsules. Use as a flavoring in cooking.

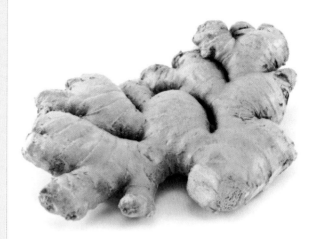

Chemical Constituents: Sesquiterpenes (up to 90%): zingiberene (up to 50%), α- & β-curcumene (<33%), β-farnesene (<20%), β-sesquiphellandrene (<9%), β- & γ-bisabolene (<7%), β-ylangene, β-elemene, α-selinene, germacrene-D; Monoterpenes: camphene (8%), β-phellandrene, l-limonene, p-cymene, α and β-pinenes, myrcene; Alcohols: nonanol (<8%), citronellol (<6%), linalool (<5%), borneol, butanol, heptanol; Sesquiterpene Alcohols: nerolidol (<9%), zingeberol, elemol; Ketones (<6%): heptanone, acetone, 2 hexanone; Aldehydes: butanal, citronellal, geranial; Sesquiterpene Ketones: gingerone.

Properties: Antiseptic, laxative, stimulant, tonic, and warming.

Historical Uses: Anciently esteemed as a spice and recognized for its affinity for the digestive system, it has been used in gingerbread (up to 4,000 years ago in Greece), in Egyptian cuisine (to ward off epidemics), in Roman wine (for its aphrodisiac powers), in Indian tea (to soothe upset stomachs), and in Chinese tonics (to strengthen the heart and to relieve head congestion). It was also used in Hawaii to scent clothing, to cook with, and to cure indigestion. The Hawaiians also added it to their shampoos and massage oils.

French Medicinal Uses: Angina, prevention of contagious diseases, cooking, diarrhea, flatulence, impotence, rheumatic pain, scurvy, and tonsillitis.

Other Possible Uses: Ginger may be used for alcoholism, loss of appetite, arthritis◒, broken bones, catarrh (mucus), chills, colds, colic, congestion, coughs, cramps, digestive disorders, fevers, flu, impotence, indigestion, infectious diseases, memory, motion sickness, muscular aches/pains, rheumatism, sinusitis, sore throats, and sprains. Ginger may also be used in cooking.

✚ **Body System(s) Affected:** Digestive and Nervous Systems.

Aromatic Influence: The aroma may help influence physical energy, love, money, and courage.

Oral Use As Dietary Supplement: Ginger oil is generally recognized as safe (GRAS) for human consumption by the FDA (21CFR182.20). Dilute 1 drop oil in 1 tsp. (5 ml) honey or in ½ cup (125 ml) of beverage (e.g., soy/rice milk). Not for children under 6 years old; use with caution and in greater dilution for children 6 years old and over.

Safety Data: Repeated use can possibly result in contact sensitization. Avoid direct sunlight for 3 to 6 hours after use.

Blend Classification: Personifier and Equalizer.

‡*See Application section beginning on page 16 for more details on applying essential oils.*   ◑=Topical, ⊘=Aromatic, ◐=Internal

69

Blends With: All spice oils, all citrus oils, eucalyptus, frankincense, geranium, and rosemary.

Odor: Type: Middle Note (50–80% of the blend); Scent: Sweet, spicy-woody, warm, tenacious, fresh, sharp; Intensity: 4.

Additional Research:

Nausea: Ginger root given one hour before major gynecological surgery resulted in lower nausea and fewer incidences of vomiting compared to a control (Nanthakomon et al., 2006).

Nausea: Ginger root given orally to pregnant women was found to decrease the severity of nausea and the frequency of vomiting compared to a control (Vutyavanich et al., 2001).

Nausea: In a trial of women receiving gynecological surgery, women receiving ginger root had less incidences of nausea compared to a placebo. Ginger root demonstrates results similar to the antiemetic drug (a drug effective against vomiting and nausea) metoclopramide (Bone et al., 1990).

Arthritis: Powdered ginger supplementation was found to lower pain and swelling in arthritic patients and to relieve pain from muscle discomfort (Srivastava et al., 1992).

Arthritis: Eugenol and ginger oil taken orally were found to reduce paw and joint swelling in rats with induced severe arthritis (Sharma et al., 1994).

Liver: Daily oral administration of ginger (*Z. officinale R.*) essential oil and isolated citral (a constituent of ginger essential oil) displayed preventative effects on the formation of alcohol fatty liver disease in mice administered an alcoholic liquid diet for four weeks (Liu et al., 2013).

Pain: A double-blind, placebo-controlled study demonstrated that aroma massage with ginger and orange essential oils relieved knee joint pain in elderly subjects more than the placebo (massage with olive oil) or the control (conventional treatment without massage) (Yip et al., 2008).

See Personal Usage Guide chapter for more details on these primary uses.   ●=Neat, ●=Dilute for Children/Sensitive Skin, ●=Dilute

Grapefruit *Citrus x paradisi*

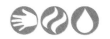

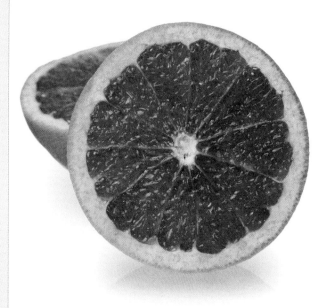

Quick Facts

Botanical Family: Rutaceae (hybrid between *Citrus maxima* and *Citrus sinensis*)

Extraction Method: Cold expressed from rind

Common Primary Uses*: Addictions (Drugs), Anorexia, Appetite Suppressant, Bulimia, Cellulite, Dry Throat, Edema, Gallbladder Stones, Hangovers, Lymphatic Decongestant, Mental Stress, Miscarriage (After), Obesity, Overeating, Performance Stress, PMS, Slimming/Toning, Stress, Withdrawal

Common Application Methods‡:

: Can be applied neat (with no dilution) when used topically. Apply directly on area of concern or to reflex points. Because grapefruit oil has many of the same uses as other citrus oils, it can be used in their place when immediate exposure to the sun is unavoidable. This is because grapefruit oil does not cause as much photosensitivity as the other citrus oils.

: Diffuse, or inhale the aroma directly.

: Take 1–2 drops in a beverage or in capsules. Use as a flavoring in cooking.

Chemical Constituents: Monoterpenes (up to 95%): d-Limonene (<92%), myrcene, α-pinene, sabinene, β-phellandrene; Tetraterpenes: β-carotene, lycopene; Aldehydes (>2%): nonanal, decanal, citral, citronellal; Furanocoumarins: aesculetin, auraptene, bergaptol; Sesquiterpene Ketones (<2%): nootketone (used to determine harvest time); Alcohols: octanol.

Properties: Antidepressant, antiseptic, disinfectant, diuretic, stimulant, and tonic.

French Medicinal Uses: Cellulite, digestion, dyspepsia, lymphatic decongestant, water retention.

Other Possible Uses: Grapefruit oil may help with cancer, depression, eating disorders, fatigue, jet lag, liver disorders, migraine headaches, premenstrual tension, stress, and sympathetic nervous system stimulation. It may also have a cleansing effect on the kidneys, the lymphatic system, and the vascular system.

Body System(s) Affected: Cardiovascular System.

Aromatic Influence: It is balancing and uplifting to the mind and may help to relieve anxiety.

Oral Use As Dietary Supplement: Grapefruit oil is generally recognized as safe (GRAS) for human consumption by the FDA (21CFR182.20). Dilute 1 drop oil in 1 tsp. (5 ml) honey or in ½ cup (125 ml) of beverage (e.g., soy/rice milk). Not for children under 6 years old; use with caution and in greater dilution for children 6 years old and over.

Blend Classification: Modifier and Enhancer.

Blends With: Basil, bergamot, cypress, frankincense, geranium, lavender, peppermint, rosemary, and ylang ylang.

Odor: Type: Top Note (5–20% of the blend); Scent: Clean, fresh, bitter, citrusy; Intensity: 2.

Additional Research:

Obesity: The scent of grapefruit oil and its component, limonene, was found to affect the autonomic nerves and to reduce appetite and body weight in rats exposed to the oil for 15 minutes three times per week (Shen et al., 2005).

Obesity: Grapefruit essential oil was found to directly inhibit adipogenesis of adipocytes, indicating that grapefruit has an antiobesity effect (Haze et al., 2010).

Cancer: In a study of older individuals, it was found that there was a dose-dependent relationship between citrus peel consumption (which is high in d-Limonene) and a lower degree of squamous cell carcinoma (SCC) of the skin (Hakim et al., 2000).

Cancer: In clinical trials, d-Limonene (found in most citrus oils) was found to elicit a response (kept patients stable) in some patients in advanced stages of cancer (1 breast and 3 colorectal carcinoma of 32 total patients). A secondary trial with just breast-cancer patients did not elicit any responses (Vigushin et al., 1998).

Sympathetic Nervous System Stimulation: Inhalation of essential oils such as pepper, estragon, fennel, and grapefruit was found to have a stimulating effect on sympathetic activity in healthy adults (Haze et al., 2002).

Diabetes: Helichrysum and grapefruit extracts were found to improve post-prandial glycemic control in a dietary model of insulin resistance in rats (da la Garza et al., 2013).

Addiction: Injection of limonene, a common terpene found in many citrus essential oils, inhibited behavioral manifestations of drug use on rats administered methamphetamine (METH). Examination of the nucleus accumbens of the rats revealed that limonene may produce its effects by regulating dopamine levels and serotonin receptor function (Yun, 2014).

Ticks: Nootkatone, found in grapefruit essential oil, was found to be toxic to four tick species (Flor-Weiler et al., 2011).

Anxiety: Inhalation of grapefruit oil was found to help alleviate abdominal pain associated with anxiety in colonoscopy patients (Hozumi et al., 2017).

See Personal Usage Guide chapter for more details on these primary uses.   ●=Neat, ●=Dilute for Children/Sensitive Skin, ●=Dilute

Green Mandarin *Citrus nobilis*

Essential Oils

Quick Facts

Botanical Family: Rutaceae (citrus)

Extraction Method: Cold pressed from peel

Common Primary Uses*: Nausea, Calming, GERD, Skin (Toning), Soothing

Common Application Methods‡:

: Can be applied neat (with no dilution) when used topically. Apply directly on area of concern or to reflex points. Avoid UV light for up to 12 hours after using on skin.

: Diffuse, or inhale the aroma directly.

: Take in capsules or in a beverage (add 1 drop to 1 cup (250 ml). Use as a flavoring in cooking.

Chemical Constituents: Monoterpenes (up to 97%): limonene (<75%), γ-terpinene (<18%); α- & β-pinenes, β-myrcene, terpinolene, p-cymene; Aldehydes: decanal, octanal; Esters: methyl n-methyl anthranilate; Alcohols: linalool, citronellol, nerol.

Properties: Anticoagulant, anti-inflammatory, anti-microbial, antispasmodic, antitumor, antiviral, expectorant, laxative, and sedative.

Historical Uses: Green mandarin essential oil is distilled from the green, unripened fruit of the mandarin tree. Distilling at this time gives the oil a brighter, fresher aroma. Mandarin trees are native to Asia, but they are now cultivated around the world.

Other Possible Uses: This oil may help wth cellulite, circulation, constipation, diarrhea, digestive system disorders, dizziness, fat digestion, fear, flatulence, gallbladder (gallstones), heartburn, insomnia, intestinal spasms, irritability, limbs (tired and aching), liver problems, lymphatic system congestion (helps stimulate drainage), obesity, parasites, sadness, stomach (tonic), stress, stretch marks (smooths when blended with lavender), swelling, and water retention (alleviates edema).

Body System(s) Affected: Emotional Balance, Digestive System, Immune System, Skin.

Aromatic Influence: The bright, fresh aroma of green mandarin is effective for soothing strong emotions such as anger, grief, and shock. It can also be sedating and calming to the nervous system while promoting courage and quiet strength.

Oral Use As Dietary Supplement: Green mandarin oil is generally regarded as safe (GRAS) for human consumption by the FDA. Dilute 1 drop oil in 1 tsp. (5 ml) honey or in ½ cup (125 ml) of beverage (e.g., soy/rice milk). Not for children under 6 years old; use with caution and in greater dilution for children 6 years old and over.

Safety Data: Old or oxidized oil may irritate highly sensitive skin. Consult with a physician before use if taking medications, pregnant, or nursing.

Blend Classification: Personifier and Enhancer.

Blends With: Basil, bergamot, clary sage, frankincense, grapefruit, lavender, lemon, marjoram, orange, Roman chamomile, sandalwood, spearmint.

Odor: Type: Top Note (5–20% of the blend); Scent: Bright, citrusy, fresh, sweet, herbal; Intensity: 3.

Additional Research:

GERD: Oral administration of d-limonene over several days was found to significantly reduce symptoms of gastroesophageal reflux compared to a placebo in a limited human trial (Sun, 2007).

Skin: Limonene and its metabolite perillyl alcohol were found in animal tests to aid in tissue regeneration and reduced inflammation in animal models (d'Alessio et al., 2014).

Anti-inflammatory: Limonene was found to demonstrate anti-inflammatory activity in laboratory tests (Kummer et al., 2013).

Antitumor: In several animal and laboratory studies, d-limonene was found to inhibit cancer cell growth of several cancer types (Elegbede et al., 1984; Maltzman et al., 1989; Uedo et al., 1999).

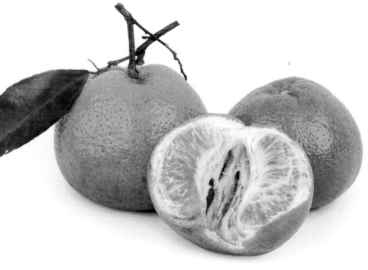

‡See Application section beginning on page 16 for more details on applying essential oils.   =Topical, =Aromatic, =Internal

73

Hawaiian Sandalwood *Santalum paniculatum*

Quick Facts

Botanical Family: Santalaceae (sandalwood)

Extraction Method: Steam distillation from heartwood

Common Primary Uses*: Alzheimer's Disease, Aphrodisiac, Back Pain, Cancer, Cartilage Repair, Confusion, Exhaustion, Fear, Hair (Dry), Hiccups, Laryngitis, Lou Gehrig's Disease, Meditation, Moles, Multiple Sclerosis, Rashes, Skin (Dry), Ultraviolet Radiation, Vitiligo, Yoga

Common Application Methods‡:

: Can be applied neat (with no dilution) when used topically. Apply directly on area of concern or to reflex points.

: Diffuse, or inhale the aroma directly.

: Take in capsules.

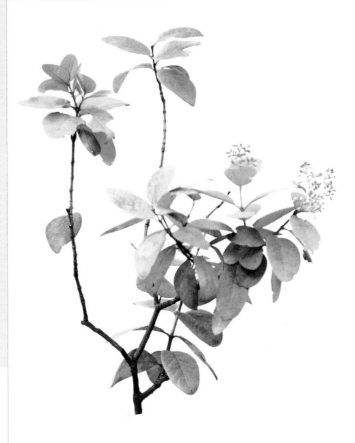

Chemical Constituents: Sesquiterpene Alcohols (up to 98%): α- & β-santalols (up to 70%), α-bergamotol (up to 5%), cis-nuciferol, lanceol; Sesquiterpenes: α- & β-santalenes; Sesquiterpene Aldehydes: teresantalal; Carboxylic Acids: nortricycloekasantalic acid.

Properties: Antidepressant, antiseptic, antitumor, aphrodisiac, astringent, calming, sedative, and tonic.

Historical Uses: Hawaiian sandalwood was traditionally used to help clear dandruff, repel insects, and to help heal diseases of the reproductive organs.

Other Possible Uses: Sandalwood may support the cardiovascular system and relieve symptoms associated with lumbago and the sciatic nerves. It may also be beneficial for acne, regenerating bone cartilage, catarrh, circulation (similar in action to frankincense), coughs, cystitis, depression, hiccups, lymphatic system, menstrual problems, nerves (similar in action to frankincense), nervous tension, increasing oxygen around the pineal and pituitary glands, skin infection and regeneration, and tuberculosis.

Body System(s) Affected: Emotional Balance, Muscles and Bones, Nervous System, Skin.

Aromatic Influence: Calms, harmonizes, and balances the emotions. It may help enhance meditation.

Oral Use As Dietary Supplement: While this specific species of sandalwood has not yet been approved for oral use by the FDA, regular *Santalum album* oil is approved by the FDA (21CFR172.510) for use as a Food Additive (FA) and Flavoring Agent (FL) and possesses a similar chemical profile. Dilute 1 drop oil in 1 tsp. (5 ml) honey or in ½ cup (125 ml) of beverage (e.g., soy/rice milk). Not for children under 6 years old; use with caution and in greater dilution for children 6 years old and over.

Blend Classification: Modifier and Equalizer.

Blends With: Cypress, frankincense, lemon, myrrh, and ylang ylang.

Odor: Type: Base Note (5–20% of the blend); Scent: Soft, woody, spicy, sweet, earthy, balsamic, tenacious; Intensity: 3.

See Personal Usage Guide chapter for more details on these primary uses.   ●=Neat, ●=Dilute for Children/Sensitive Skin, ●=Dilute

Additional Research:

Antitumor Properties: Alpha-santalol, derived from sandalwood EO, was found to delay and decrease the incidence and multiplicity of skin tumor (papilloma) development in mice (Dwivedi et al., 2003).

Antitumor Properties: Various concentrations of alpha-santalol (from sandalwood) were tested against skin cancer in mice. All concentrations were found to inhibit skin cancer development (Dwivedi et al., 2005).

Antitumor Properties: Alpha-santalol was found to induce apoptosis in human skin cancer cells (Kaur et al., 2005).

‡*See Application section beginning on page 16 for more details on applying essential oils.*   ◐=Topical, ◑=Aromatic, ○=Internal

75

Helichrysum *Helichrysum italicum*

Quick Facts

Botanical Family: Compositae

Extraction Method: Steam distillation from flowers

Common Primary Uses*: Abscess (Tooth), AIDS/HIV, Aneurysm, Bleeding, Bone Bruise, Broken Blood Vessels, Bruises, Catarrh, Cholesterol, Cleansing, Colitis, Cuts, Dermatitis/Eczema, Detoxification, Earache, Fibroids, Gallbladder Infection, Hematoma, Hemorrhaging, Herpes Simplex, Incisional Hernia, Liver Stimulant, Lymphatic Drainage, Nose Bleed, Pancreas Stimulant, Phlebitis, Psoriasis, Sciatica, Shock, Staph Infection, Stroke, Sunscreen, Swollen Eyes, Taste (Impaired), Tennis Elbow, Tinnitus, Tissue Pain, Tissue Repair, Vertigo, Viral Infections, Wounds

Common Application Methods‡:

: Can be applied neat (with no dilution) when used topically. Apply directly on area of concern or to reflex points.

: Diffuse, or inhale the aroma directly.

: Take in capsules.

Chemical Constituents: Esters (up to 60%): neryl acetate (up to 50%), neryl propionate & butyrate (<10%); Ketones: italidione (<20%), β-diketone; Sesquiterpenes: γ-curcumene (<15%), β-caryophyllene (<5%); Monoterpenes: l-limonene (<13%), α-pinene; Alcohols: nerol (<5%), linalool (<4%), geraniol; Oxides: 1,8 cineol; Phenols: eugenol.

Properties: Antibacterial, anticatarrhal, anticoagulant, antioxidant, antispasmodic, antiviral, expectorant, and mucolytic.

Historical Uses: Helichrysum has been used for asthma, bronchitis, whooping cough, headaches, liver ailments, and skin disorders.

French Medicinal Uses: Blood cleansing, chelating agent for metallics, chemicals, and toxins, viral colitis, detoxification, gallbladder infection, hematoma, hypo-cholesterol, liver cell function stimulant, lymph drainage, pain reduction, pancreas stimulant, phlebitis, sciatica, sinus infection, skin conditions (eczema, dermatitis, psoriasis), stomach cramps, sunscreen.

Other Possible Uses: This oil may help with anger management, bleeding, circulatory functions, hearing, detoxifying and stimulating the liver cell function, pain (acute), relieving respiratory conditions, reducing scarring, scar tissue, regenerating tissue, and varicose veins.

Body System(s) Affected: Cardiovascular System, Muscles and Bones.

Aromatic Influence: It is uplifting to the subconscious and may help calm feelings of anger.

Oral Use As Dietary Supplement: Helichrysum oil is generally recognized as safe (GRAS) for human consumption by the FDA (21CFR182.20). Dilute 1 drop oil in 1 tsp. (5 ml) honey or in ½ cup (125 ml) of beverage (e.g., soy/rice milk). Not for children under 6 years old; use with caution and in greater dilution for children 6 years old and over.

Blend Classification: Personifier.

Blends With: Geranium, clary sage, rose, lavender, spice oils, and citrus oils.

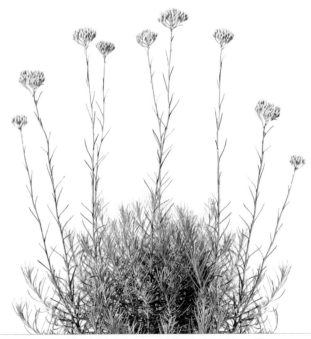

Odor: Type: Middle Note (50–80% of the blend); Scent: Rich, sweet, fruity, with tea and honey undertones; Intensity: 3.

Additional Research:

Antibacterial Properties: Helichrysum oil exhibited definite antibacterial activity against six tested Gram (+/-) bacteria (Chinou et al., 1996).

Antibacterial Properties: Helichrysum was found to inhibit both the growth and the formation of some enzymes of *Staphylococcus aureus* (staph) bacteria (Nostro et al., 2001).

Antioxidant Properties: Arzanol (extracted from helichrysum) at non-cytotoxic concentrations showed a strong inhibition of TBH-induced oxidative stress in VERO cells (Rosa et al., 2007)

Antiviral Properties: Arzanol, extracted from helichrysum, inhibited HIV-1 replication in T-cells and also inhibited the release of pro-inflammatory cytokines (chemical messengers) in monocytes (Appendino et al., 2007).

Antiviral Properties: Helichrysum showed significant antiviral activity against the herpes virus at non-cytotoxic concentrations (Nostro et al., 2003).

Diabetes: Helichrysum and grapefruit extracts were found to improve postprandial glycemic control in a dietary model of insulin resistance in rats (da la Garza et al., 2013).

‡*See Application section beginning on page 16 for more details on applying essential oils.*   =Topical, =Aromatic, =Internal

77

Hinoki *Chamaecyparis obtusa*

Quick Facts

Botanical Family: Cupressaceae (conifer: cypress)

Extraction Method: Steam distillation from wood

Common Primary Uses*: ⊘⊙Calming, ⊙Cleaning, ⊘⊙Colds, ⊙Cuts/Scrapes, ⊙Rashes

Common Application Methods‡:

⊙: Can be applied neat (with no dilution) when used topically. Apply directly on area of concern or to reflex points. Add 1–2 drops to bathwater before bathing. Use in massage oil.

⊘: Diffuse, or inhale the aroma directly.

Chemical Constituents: Sesquiterpene Alcohols (up to 60%): α-cadinol, T-muurolol, T-cadinol, cadin-1(10)-en-4,β-ol, β-caryophyllene alcohol; Sesquiterpenes (up to 30%): γ-cadinene, δ-cadinene, α-muurolene, β-caryophyllene, α-elemene; Mono-terpenes: α-pinene, limonene.

Properties: Antibacterial, antifungal, anti-infectious, anti-inflammatory, antiseptic, antiviral, disinfec-tant, and insecticidal.

Historical Uses: Hinoki wood has long been used in Japan for building royal palaces and sacred baths because of its beautiful look, wonderful smell, and natural properties for resisting insects, bacteria, and fungi—allowing the wood to last for hundreds of years.

Other Possible Uses: Hinoki may be beneficial for respiratory conditions such as colds, coughs, and bronchitis. It is also often used as an antiseptic to help clean and aid in tissue healing from abrasions, cuts, scrapes, and rashes. It may also be an effective insect repellent. It can be used to clean and polish wood.

Body System(s) Affected: Emotional Balance, Immune System, Respiratory System, Skin.

Aromatic Influence: Hinoki oil is believed to impart a calming influence, helping to alleviate stress and anxiety. It also uplifts the mind and increases spiritual awareness.

Oral Use As Dietary Supplement: None.

Safety Data: Consult with a physician before use if taking medications, pregnant, or nursing.

Blend Classification: Enhancer.

Blends With: Bergamot, clary sage, cypress, eucalyptus, floral oils, frankincense, juniper berry, resinous oils, and rosemary.

Odor: Type: Top Note (5–20% of the blend); Scent: Clean, woody, citrusy, spicy; Intensity: 2.

Additional Research:

Antibacterial: Hinoki essential oil was found to demonstrate antibacterial activity and to inhibit biofilm formation of methicillin-resistant Staphylococcus aureus in vitro (Kim et al., 2015).

Anti-inflammatory: *Chamaecyparis obtusa* essential oil displayed anti-inflammatory activity in rats by regulating the production of prostaglandin E2 and transforming growth factor alpha gene expression (An et al., 2013).

Insecticidal: Hinoki essential oil demonstrated repellent properties and inhibited the activities of flies and mites in experimental models (Ando, 1994; Lee et al., 2015).

Calming: Inhaling hinoki oil was found to decrease heart rate and blood pressure and to affect the autonomic nervous system and stimulate a positive mood state in a limited human trial (Chen et al., 2015).

Anxiety: Inhalation treatment with *Chamaecyparis obtusa* essential oil reduced anxiety-related behavior shown in maternal separation rats. This behavioral activity was further emphasized by altered expression of cytokine genes in the hippocampus of maternal separation rats treated with essential oil (Park et al., 2014).

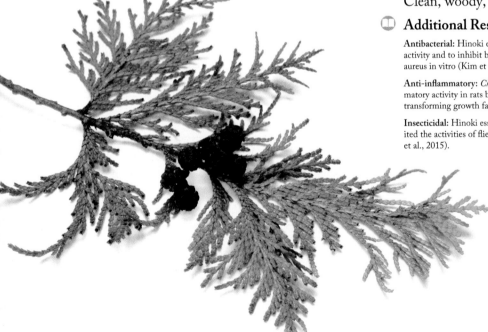

See Personal Usage Guide chapter for more details on these primary uses.　　●=Neat, ●=Dilute for Children/Sensitive Skin, ●=Dilute

78

Jasmine *Jasminum officinale*

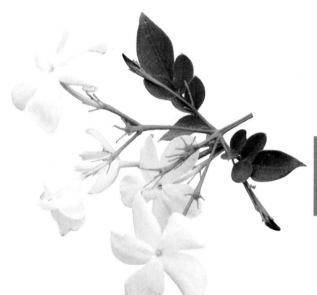

Quick Facts

Botanical Family: Oleaceae (olive)

Extraction Method: Absolute extraction from flowers

Common Primary Uses*: ⬤Hoarse Voice, ⬤Pink Eye, ⬤Sensitive Skin

Common Application Methods‡:

⬤: Can be applied neat (with no dilution) when used topically. Apply directly on area of concern or to reflex points.

⬤: Diffuse, or inhale the aroma directly.

⬤: Take in capsules.

Chemical Constituents: Esters (up to 50%): benzyl acetate (<28%), benzyl benzoate (<21%), methyl anthranilate, methyl jasmonate; Diterpene Alcohols: phytol (<12%), isophytol (<7%); Alcohols: linalool (<8%), benzyl alcohol, farnesol; Triterpenes: squalene (<7%); Pyrroles: indole, scatole; Ketone: cis-jasmone.

Properties: Anticatarrhal, antidepressant, and antispasmodic⬤.

Historical Uses: Known in India as the "queen of the night" and "moonlight of the grove," women have treasured jasmine for centuries for its beautiful, aphrodisiac-like fragrance. According to Roberta Wilson, "In many religious traditions, the jasmine flower symbolizes hope, happiness, and love." Jasmine has been used for hepatitis, cirrhosis of the liver, dysentery, depression, nervousness, coughs, respiratory congestion, reproductive problems, and "to stimulate uterine contractions in pregnant women as childbirth approached." It was also used in teas, perfumes, and incense.

Other Possible Uses: This oil may help with catarrh (mucus), conjunctivitis, coughs, dysentery, eczema (when caused by emotions), frigidity, hepatitis (cirrhosis of the liver), hoarseness, labor pains, laryngitis, lethargy (abnormal drowsiness), menstrual pain and problems, muscle spasms, nervous exhaustion and tension, pain relief, respiratory conditions, sex, skin care (dry, greasy, irritated, and sensitive), sprains, and uterine disorders. Jasmine is an oil that affects the emotions; it penetrates the deepest layers of the soul, opening doors to our emotions. It produces a feeling of confidence, energy, euphoria, and optimism. It helps to reduce anxiety, apathy, depression, indifference, listlessness, and relationship dilemmas. As a cologne, it increases feelings of attractiveness.

⬤ Body System(s) Affected: Emotional Balance, Hormonal System⬤.

Aromatic Influence: It is very uplifting to the emotions and may help increase intuitive powers and wisdom. It may also help to promote powerful, inspirational relationships.

Oral Use As Dietary Supplement: Jasmine oil is generally regarded as safe (GRAS) for human consumption by the FDA. Dilute 1 drop oil in 1 tsp. (5 ml) honey or in ½ cup (125 ml) of beverage (e.g., soy/rice milk). Not for children under 6 years old; use with caution and in greater dilution for children 6 years old and over.

Blend Classification: Equalizer, Modifier, and Enhancer.

‡*See Application section beginning on page 16 for more details on applying essential oils.*   ⬤=Topical, ⬤=Aromatic, ⬤=Internal

79

Blends With: Bergamot, frankincense, geranium, helichrysum, lemongrass, melissa, orange, rose, sandalwood, spearmint.

Odor: Type: Base Note (5–20% of the blend); Scent: Powerful, sweet, tenacious, floral with fruity-herbaceous undertones; Intensity: 4.

Additional Research:

Antispasmodic Properties: While inhaled jasmine has been shown to stimulate in vivo, jasmine applied to guinea pig and rat tissue was shown to be spasmolytic (anti-spasm) (Lis-Balchin et al., 2002).

Hormonal System: Jasmine flowers applied to the breast were found to be as effective as the anti-lactation drug bromocriptine at reducing breast engorgement, milk production, and analgesic (pain-relieving drug) intake in women after giving birth (Shrivastav et al., 1988).

See Personal Usage Guide chapter for more details on these primary uses.   ●=Neat, ●=Dilute for Children/Sensitive Skin, ●=Dilute

80

Juniper Berry *Juniperus communis*

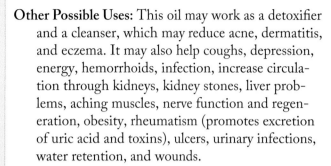

Quick Facts

Botanical Family: Cupressaceae (conifer: cypress)

Extraction Method: Steam distillation from berries and needles

Common Primary Uses*: ⬤Acne, ⬤Alcoholism, ⬤Dermatitis/Eczema, ⬤Kidney Stones, ⬤Tinnitus

Common Application Methods‡:

⬤: Can be applied neat (with no dilution) when used topically. Apply directly on area of concern or to reflex points.

⬤: Diffuse, or inhale the aroma directly.

⬤: Place 1 drop under the tongue, or take in capsules. Use with caution if pregnant or nursing.

Chemical Constituents: Monoterpenes (>50%): α-pinene (up to 40%), sabinene (<18%), β-myrcene (<8%), l-limonene (<6%); Sesquiterpenes (up to 30%): β-caryophyllene, α-humulene, germacrene; Esters: bornyl acetate, terpinyl acetate; Ketones: camphor, junionone, pinocamphone, thujone.

Properties: Antiseptic, antispasmodic, astringent, cleanser, detoxifier, diuretic, stimulant, and tonic.

Historical Uses: Over the centuries, juniper has been used for physical and spiritual purification, for cleansing infections and healing wounds, for liver complaints, for embalming, for relieving arthritis and urinary tract infections, for warding off plagues, epidemics, and contagious diseases, and for headaches, kidney and bladder problems, pulmonary infections, and fevers.

French Medicinal Uses: Acne, dermatitis, eczema.

Other Possible Uses: This oil may work as a detoxifier and a cleanser, which may reduce acne, dermatitis, and eczema. It may also help coughs, depression, energy, hemorrhoids, infection, increase circulation through kidneys, kidney stones, liver problems, aching muscles, nerve function and regeneration, obesity, rheumatism (promotes excretion of uric acid and toxins), ulcers, urinary infections, water retention, and wounds.

⬤ **Body System(s) Affected:** Digestive System, Emotional Balance, Nervous System, Skin.

Aromatic Influence: Juniper evokes feelings of health, love, and peace and may help to elevate one's spiritual awareness.

Oral Use As Dietary Supplement: Juniper berry oil is generally recognized as safe (GRAS) for human consumption by the FDA (21CFR182.20). Dilute 1 drop oil in 1 tsp. (5 ml) honey or in ½ cup (125 ml) of beverage (e.g., soy/rice milk). Not for children under 6 years old; use with caution and in greater dilution for children 6 years old and over. Use with caution during pregnancy or while nursing.

Blend Classification: Equalizer.

Blends With: Bergamot, all citrus oils, cypress, geranium, lavender, melaleuca, and rosemary.

Odor: Type: Middle Note (50–80% of the blend); Scent: Sweet, balsamic, tenacious; Intensity: 3.

⬤ **Additional Research:**

Cholesterol: Oral administration of juniper berry essential oil to rats fed a high cholesterol diet resulted in increased antioxidant enzyme activities in the rat heart tissue (Gumral et al., 2013).

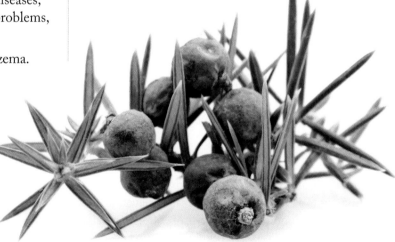

‡*See Application section beginning on page 16 for more details on applying essential oils.*   ⬤=Topical, ⬤=Aromatic, ⬤=Internal

81

Lavender *Lavandula angustifolia*

Quick Facts

Botanical Family: Labiatae (mint)

Extraction Method: Steam distillation from flowering top

Common Primary Uses*: ⬡Abuse (Healing From), ⬡⬡Agitation (Calms), ⬡Allergies, ⬡⬡Anxiety⊕, ⬡Appetite Loss, ⬡⬡Arrhythmia, ⬡Atherosclerosis, ⬡Bites/Stings, ⬡Blisters, ⬡Boils, ⬡Breasts (Soothes), ⬡Burns, ⬡⬡Calming, ⬡⬡Cancer, ⬡Chicken Pox, ⬡Club Foot, ⬡Concentration, ⬡Convulsions, ⬡⬡Crying, ⬡Cuts, ⬡Dandruff, ⬡⬡ODepression, ⬡Diabetic Sores, ⬡Diaper Rash, ⬡Diuretic, ⬡Dysmenorrhea, ⬡Exhaustion, ⬡Fever, ⬡Gangrene, O⬡Gas/Flatulence, O⬡Giardia, ⬡Gnats and Midges (Repellent), ⬡⬡Grief/Sorrow, ⬡Hair (Dry), ⬡Hair (Fragile), ⬡Hair (Loss), ⬡Hay Fever, ⬡Hernia (Inguinal), ⬡Herpes Simplex, ⬡⬡Hyperactivity, ⬡Impetigo, ⬡Inflammation, ⬡⬡Insomnia, ⬡Itching, ⬡Jet Lag, ⬡Lips (Dry), ⬡Mastitis, ⬡Menopause, ⬡⬡Mental Stress, ⬡Mood Swings, ⬡Mosquito Repellent, ⬡Muscular Paralysis, ⬡⬡Pain, ⬡⬡Parasympathetic Nervous System Stimulation, ⬡Parkinson's Disease, ⬡⬡Phlebitis, ⬡⬡Physical Stress, ⬡Poison Ivy/Oak, ⬡Post Labor, ⬡⬡Postpartum Depression, ⬡Rashes, ⬡⬡Relaxation, ⬡Rheumatoid Arthritis, ⬡⬡Sedative, ⬡Seizure, ⬡Skin (Dry), ⬡Skin (Sensitive), ⬡Skin Ulcers, ⬡⬡Sleep, ⬡⬡Stress⊕, ⬡Stretch Marks, ⬡Sunburn, ⬡⬡Tachycardia, ⬡Teeth Grinding, ⬡Teething Pain, ⬡⬡Tension, ⬡Thrush, ⬡Ticks, ⬡Ulcers (Leg), ⬡Varicose Ulcer, ⬡Vertigo, ⬡⬡Withdrawal, O⬡Worms, ⬡Wounds, ⬡Wrinkles

Common Application Methods‡:

🖐: Can be applied neat (with no dilution) when used topically. Apply directly on area of concern or to reflex points.

🌀: Diffuse, or inhale the aroma directly.

💧: Place 1–2 drops under the tongue, or take in capsules. Can also be used in beverages or as a flavoring in cooking.

Chemical Constituents: Alcohols (up to 58%): linalool (>41%), α-terpineol, borneol, lavendulol, geraniol, nerol; Esters (approx. 50%): linalyl acetate (up to 45%), lavendulyl & geranyl acetates, α-terpenyl acetate; Monoterpenes (up to 24%): β-ocimene (<16%), d-Limonene (<5%), α- & β-pinenes, camphene, δ-3-carene; Sesquiterpenes: β-caryophyllene (<7%), χ-farnesene; Phenols: terpinen-4-ol (<6%); Aldehydes: benzaldehyde, cuminal, geranial, hexanal, myrtenal, neral; Oxides: 1,8 cineol, caryophyllene oxide, linalool oxide; Coumarins (<4%); Ketones: octanone (<3%), camphor; Lactones.

Properties: Analgesic⊕, anticoagulant, anticonvulsant⊕, antidepressant, antifungal⊕, antihistamine, anti-infectious, anti-inflammatory⊕, antimicrobial⊕, antimutagenic⊕, antiseptic, antispasmodic, antitoxic, antitumor⊕, cardiotonic, regenerative, and sedative⊕.

Historical Uses: During Medieval times, people were obviously divided on the properties of lavender

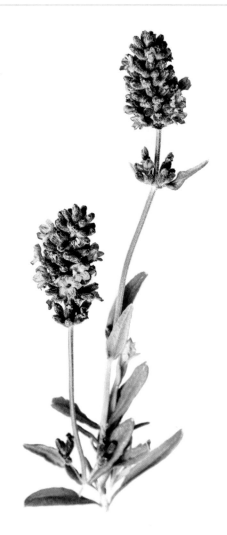

---

*See Personal Usage Guide chapter for more details on these primary uses.   ⬤=Neat, ⬤=Dilute for Children/Sensitive Skin, ⬤=Dilute

82

regarding love. Some would claim that it could keep the wearer chaste, while others claimed just the opposite—touting its aphrodisiac qualities. Its list of uses is long.

French Medicinal Uses: Acne, allergies⊕, burns (cell renewal), cramps (leg), dandruff, diaper rash, flatulence, hair loss, herpes, indigestion, insomnia⊕, lowering blood pressure⊕, lymphatic system drainage, menopausal conditions⊕, mouth abscess, nausea, phlebitis, premenstrual conditions, scarring (minimizes), stretch marks, tachycardia, thrush, water retention.

Other Possible Uses: Lavender is a universal oil that has traditionally been known to balance the body and to work wherever there is a need. If in doubt, use lavender. It may help anxiety, arthritis, asthma⊕, body systems balance, bronchitis⊕, bruises, carbuncles, cold sores, earaches, fainting, gallstones, relieve headaches⊕, heart irregularity, reduce high blood pressure⊕, hives (urticaria), hysteria, insect bites and bee stings, infection, influenza, injuries, repel insects⊕, laryngitis, migraine headaches, mental clarity⊕, mouth abscess, reduce mucus, nervous tension, pineal gland (activates), respiratory function, rheumatism, skin conditions (eczema, psoriasis, rashes), sprains, sunstroke, throat infections, tuberculosis, typhoid fever, and whooping cough.

Body System(s) Affected: Cardiovascular System, Emotional Balance, Nervous System, Skin.

Aromatic Influence: It promotes consciousness, health, love, peace, and a general sense of well-being. It also nurtures creativity.

Oral Use As Dietary Supplement: Lavender oil is generally recognized as safe (GRAS) for human consumption by the FDA (21CFR182.20). Dilute 1 drop oil in 1 tsp. (5 ml) honey or in ½ cup (125 ml) of beverage (e.g., soy/rice milk). Not for children under 6 years old; use with caution and in greater dilution for children 6 years old and over.

Blend Classification: Enhancer, Modifier, and Equalizer.

Blends With: Most oils (especially citrus oils), clary sage, and geranium.

Odor: Type: Middle Note (50–80% of the blend); Scent: Floral, sweet, herbaceous, balsamic, woody undertones; Intensity: 2.

Additional Research:

Anxiety: Patients waiting for dental treatment were found to be less anxious and have a better mood when exposed to the odor of lavender or orange oil compared to control (Lehrner et al., 2005).

Anxiety and Sleep: A study with 56 percutaneous coronary intervention patients in an intensive care unit found that an aromatherapy blend of lavender, Roman chamomile, and neroli decreased anxiety and improved sleep quality when compared to conventional nursing intervention (Cho et al., 2013).

Anxiety: Lavender essential oil was found to bind to and supress several receptors believed to play a role in anxiety and depression (Lopez et al., 2017).

Stress: Lavender odor was found to reduce mental stress while increasing arousal (Motomura et al., 2001).

Stress: Nurses working in an ICU setting demonstrated decreased perception of stress when receiving a topical application of *Lavandula angustifolia* and *Salvia sclarea* essential oils (Pemberton et al., 2008).

Analgesic Properties: Lavender oil was found to work as an anaesthetic (reducing pain) in rabbit reflex tests (Ghelardini et al., 1999).

Analgesic Properties: A triple blind randomized placebo-controlled trial, consisting of 60 subjects and evaluating the use of lavender oil for Cesarean post-operative pain management, found that inhalation of lavender (when compared to inhalation of a placebo) decreased postoperative pain and increased patient satisfaction. Furthermore, patients inhaling lavender oil required significantly lower dosages of Diclofenac suppository as a supplemental analgesic drug than the placebo group. The researchers state that lavender essential oil is not recommended as the sole analgesic treatment (Olapour et al., 2013).

Analgesic Properties: Inhaling lavender oil was found to decrease the severity of labor pains in a small study of women giving birth for the first time (Yazdkhasti et al., 2016).

Anticonvulsant Properties: Linalool, found in several essential oils, was shown to inhibit induced convulsions in rats by directly interacting with the NMDA receptor complex (Brum et al., 2001).

Antifungal Properties: Lavender oil demonstrated both fungistatic (stopped growth) and fungicidal (killed) activity against *Candida albicans* (D'Auria et al., 2005).

Anti-inflammatory Properties: Oil from *Lavandula angustifolia* was found to reduce writhing in induced writhing in rats and to reduce edema (swelling) in carrageenan-induced paw edema, indicating an anti-inflammatory effect (Hajhashemi et al., 2003).

Anti-inflammatory Properties: Linalool and linalyl acetate (from lavender and other essential oils) were found to exhibit anti-inflammatory activity in rats subjected to carrageenin-induced edema (inflammation) (Peana et al., 2002).

Antimicrobial Properties: Essential oil from *Lavandula angustifolia* demonstrated ability to eliminate protozoal pathogens *Giardia duodenalis*, *Thrichomonas vaginalis*, and *Hexamita inflata* at concentrations of 1% or less (Moon et al., 2006).

Antibacterial: Scanning electron microscopy analysis and zeta potential measurement revealed that lavender essential oil's antibacterial action against multi-drug-resistant *Escherichia coli* occurs via two mechanisms: alteration of outer membrane permeability and possible inhibition of bacterial quorum sensing (Yap et al., 2014).

Antimutigenic Properties: In tests for mutagenicity, both melaleuca (tea tree) and lavender oils were found to not be mutagenic. Lavender oil was also found to demonstrate a strong antimutagenic activity, reducing mutations of cells exposed to a known mutagen (Evandri et al., 2005).

Antitumor Properties: Mice treated with perillyl alcohol (found in lavender and mint plants) had a 22% reduction in tumor incidence and a 58% reduction in tumor multiplicity during a mouse lung tumor bioassay (Lantry et al., 1997).

Antitumor Properties: Rats with liver tumors that were treated with perillyl alcohol had smaller tumor sizes than untreated rats due to apoptosis in cancer cells in treated rats (Mills et al., 1995).

Antitumor Properties: Rats fed diets containing perillyl alcohol (derived from lavender plants) were found to have less incidence of colon tumors and less multiplicity of tumors in the colon compared to a control. Colon tumors of animals fed perillyl alcohol were found to exhibit increased apoptosis of cells compared to control (Reddy et al., 1997).

Sedative Properties: Exposure to lavender odor was found to decrease anxiety in gerbils in the elevated plus maze. A further decrease in anxiety was found in females after prolonged (2 week) exposure (Bradley et al., 2007).

‡*See Application section beginning on page 16 for more details on applying essential oils.*   ◐=Topical, ◉=Aromatic, ◯=Internal

83

Sedative Properties: Exposure to lavender oil and to its constituents, linalool and linalyl acetate, was found to decrease normal movement in mice and was also found to return mice to normal movement rates after caffeine-induced hyperactivity (Buchbauer et al., 1991).

Sedative Properties: In patients admitted to an intensive care unit, those receiving lavender aromatherapy reported a greater improvement in mood and in perceived levels of anxiety compared to those receiving just massage or a period of rest (Dunn et al., 1995).

Sedative Properties: Swiss mice fed lavender oil diluted in olive oil were found to be more sedate in several common tests (Guillemain et al., 1989).

Sedative Properties: Patients being treated with chronic hemodialysis demonstrated less anxiety when exposed to lavender aroma (Itai et al., 2000).

Sedative Properties: Inhaling lavender oil was found to lower agitation in older adults suffering from dementia (Lin et al., 2007).

Sedative Properties: Lavender oil was found to inhibit sympathetic nerve activity in rats while exciting parasympathetic nerve activity. Linalool, a component of lavender, was shown to have similar effects (Shen et al., 2005).

Sedative Properties: Lavender oil demonstrated anticonflict effects in mice similar to the anxiolytic (antianxiety) drug diazepam (Umezu et al., 2000).

Allergies: Lavender oil was found to inhibit immediate-type allergic reactions in mice and rats by inhibiting mast cell degranulation (Kim et al., 1999).

Insomnia: Female students suffering from insomnia were found to sleep better and to have lower levels of depression during weeks they used a lavender fragrance when compared to weeks they did not use a lavender fragrance (Lee et al., 2006).

Insomnia: Twenty-four sessions of lavender essential oil aromatherapy was found to improve sleep quality in midlife women with insomnia up to one week after the end of the intervention when compared to the control group (Chien et al., 2012).

Sleep: Sixty nurses with shifting sleep schedules were found to have better quality sleep after inhaling lavender essential oil (Kim et al., 2016).

Lowering Blood Pressure: Lavender oil scent was found to lower sympathetic nerve activity and blood pressure in rats while elevating parasympathetic nerve activity. It was further found that applying an anosmia-inducing agent (something that causes a loss of smell) eliminated the effects of the lavender oil scent (Tanida et al., 2006).

Menopause: Inhalation of linalool or *Lavandula burnatii* super-derived essential oil (composed from the five main lavender oils and containing a high level of linalool) was found to aid in the recovery of ether-inhalation induced decrease in adrenaline, noradrenaline, and dopamine levels in female menopausal model rats. The researchers stated that these results suggest that lavender or linalool may contribute to relieving tension and may be applicable to the treatment of menopausal disorders (Yamada et al., 2005).

Asthma: Long-term inhalation of lavender oil was found to suppress allergic airway inflammation and mucous cell hyperplasia in a mouse model of acute asthma (Ueno-Iio et al., 2014).

Headaches: Inhalation of lavender essential oil was found to be more effective than inhalation of a placebo for reducing the severity of headaches in subjects diagnosed with migraine headaches (Sasannejad et al., 2012).

Bronchitis: In patients with chronic bronchitis, lavender was found to promote normalization of lipid levels (Siurin et al., 1997).

High Blood Pressure: Eighty-three hypertensive or prehypertensive subjects were divided into the following three groups: a study group (exposed to an essential oil blend containing lavender, ylang ylang, marjoram, and neroli), a placebo group (exposed to artificial fragrance), and a control group (no interventions). The study group was found to have an immediate and long-term decrease in home blood pressure (Kim et al., 2012).

Insect Repellent: Lavender oil was found to be comparable to DEET in its ability to repel ticks (*Hyalomma marginatum*) (Mkolo et al., 2007).

Insect Repellent: An infestation of the red bud borer pest was reduced by more than 95% in the grafted buds of apple trees by application of the essential oil of *Lavandula angustifolia* (van Tol et al., 2007).

Mental Clarity: Subjects exposed to 3 minutes of lavender aroma were more relaxed and were able to perform math computations faster and more accurately (Diego et al., 1998).

Mental Clarity: Subjects who smelled a cleansing gel with lavender aroma were more relaxed and were able to complete math computations faster (Field et al., 2005).

Dysmenorrhea: Compared to a synthetic fragrance, dysmenorrhea pain decreased and shortened in duration when subjects massaged a blend of lavender, marjoram, and clary sage essential oils (in a ratio of 2:1:1) daily on the abdomen between menstruations (Ou et al., 2012).

Alzheimer's Disease: Lavender and its main component, linolool, were found to relieve oxidative stress in certain brain pathways related to cognitive function in a mouse model of Alzheimer's disease (Xu et al., 2017).

---

*See Personal Usage Guide chapter for more details on these primary uses.   ●=Neat, ●=Dilute for Children/Sensitive Skin, ●=Dilute

Lemon *Citrus limon*

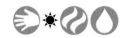

Quick Facts

Botanical Family: Rutaceae (citrus)

Extraction Method: Cold expressed from rind (requires 3,000 lemons to produce a kilo of oil)

Common Primary Uses*: ⊘Air Pollution, ⊘Anxiety⊕, ⊘⊜Atherosclerosis, ⊜Bites/Stings, OBlood Pressure (Regulation), ⊘⊜Brain Injury, ⊜Cold Sores, ⊘⊜Colds (Common), ⊘Concentration⊕, ⊜Constipation, ⊘⊜ODepression, ⊜Digestion (Sluggish), ⊜⊘Disinfectant, O⊜Dry Throat, ⊜Dysentery, ⊜Energizing, ⊜Exhaustion, O⊜Fever, ⊜⊘Flu (Influenza), ⊜Furniture Polish, O⊜Gout, ⊜Greasy/Oily Hair, ⊘⊜Grief/Sorrow, ⊜Gum/Grease Removal, ⊜⊘Hangovers, ⊜Heartburn, O⊜Intestinal Parasites, OKidney Stones, ⊘⊜Lymphatic Cleansing, ⊜MRSA, ⊘Overeating, ⊜⊘Pancreatitis, ⊘Physical Energy, ⊘⊜Postpartum Depression, ⊘Purification, ⊘Relaxation, ⊜Skin (Tones), ⊘⊜Stress⊕, ⊜⊘OThroat Infection, ⊜Tonsillitis, ⊘Uplifting, ⊜Varicose Veins, O⊜Water Purification

Common Application Methods‡:

⊜: Can be applied neat (with no dilution) when used topically. Apply directly on area of concern or to reflex points. Avoid direct sunlight or UV light for up to 12 hours after using on the skin.

⊘: Diffuse, or inhale the aroma directly.

O: Place 1–2 drops under the tongue, or drink with a beverage. Take in capsules. Use as a flavoring in cooking.

Chemical Constituents: Monoterpenes (up to 90%): d-Limonene (up to 72%), α- & β-pinenes (<30%), α- & γ-terpinenes (7–14%), sabinene, p-cymene, terpinolene, α- & β-phellandrenes; Aldehydes (up to 12%): citral, citronellal, neral, geranial, heptanal, hexanal, nonanal, octanal, undecanal; Alcohols: hexanol, octanol, nonanol, decanol, linalool, α-terpineol; Esters (<5%): geranyl acetate, neryl acetate, methyl anthranilate; Sesquiterpenes (<5%): β-bisabolene, β-caryophyllene; Tetraterpenes (<4%): β-carotene, lycopene; Phenols: terpinen-4-ol; Coumarins and Furocoumarins (<3%): umberlliferone, bergaptene,

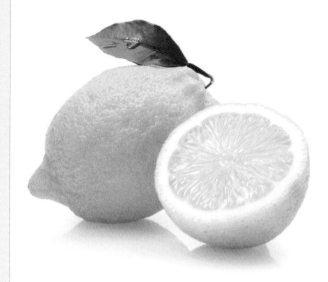

α-bergamotene, limettine, psoralen, bergamottin, bergaptol, citroptene scopoletin.

Properties: Anticancer⊕, antidepressant⊕, antiseptic, antifungal⊕, antioxidant⊕, antiviral, astringent, invigorating, refreshing, and tonic.

Historical Uses: Lemon has been used to fight food poisoning, malaria and typhoid epidemics, and scurvy. (In fact, sources say that Christopher Columbus carried lemon seeds to America—probably just the leftovers from the fruit that was eaten during the trip.) Lemon has also been used to lower blood pressure and to help with liver problems, arthritis, and muscular aches and pains.

French Medicinal Uses: Air disinfectant, anemia, asthma, cold, fever (reduces), germicide, gout, heartburn, intestinal parasites, red blood cell formation, rheumatism, throat infection, ureter infections, varicose veins, water purification, white blood cell formation.

Other Possible Uses: This oil may be beneficial for aging⊕, soothing broken capillaries, dissolving cellulite, clarity of thought, debility, digestive problems⊕, energy, gallstones, hair (cleansing), promoting leukocyte formation, liver deficiencies in children, memory improvement, nails (strengthening and hardening), nerves⊕, nervous conditions, respiratory problems, cleaning children's skin, sore throats, and promoting a sense of well-being. It works extremely well in removing gum, wood stain, oil, and grease spots. It may

‡*See Application section beginning on page 16 for more details on applying essential oils.* ⊜=Topical, ⊘=Aromatic, O=Internal

85

also brighten a pale, dull complexion by removing dead skin cells.

🜨 **Body System(s) Affected:** Digestive, Immune, and Respiratory Systems.

Aromatic Influence: It promotes health, healing, physical energy, and purification. Its fragrance is invigorating, enhancing, and warming.

Oral Use As Dietary Supplement: Lemon oil is generally recognized as safe (GRAS) for human consumption by the FDA (21CFR182.20). Dilute 1 drop oil in 1 tsp. (5 ml) honey or in ½ cup (125 ml) of beverage (e.g., soy/rice milk). Not for children under 6 years old; use with caution and in greater dilution for children 6 years old and over.

Safety Data: Avoid direct sunlight for up to 12 hours after use. Can cause extreme skin irritation.

Blend Classification: Modifier and Enhancer.

Blends With: Eucalyptus, fennel, frankincense, geranium, peppermint, sandalwood, and ylang ylang.

Odor: Type: Top Note (5–20% of the blend); Scent: Sweet, sharp, clear, citrusy; Intensity: 3.

📖 **Additional Research:**

Anxiety: Rats exposed long-term to lemon essential oil were found to demonstrate different anxiety and pain threshold levels than untreated rats. It was also found that exposure to lemon oil induced chemical changes in the neuronal circuits involved in anxiety and pain (Ceccarelli et al., 2004).

Concentration: Daily inhalation of lemon essential oil aroma for five minutes was found to have a positive effect on learning in mice (Ogeturk et al., 2010).

Stress: Lemon odor was found to enhance the positive mood of volunteers exposed to a stressor (Kiecolt-Glaser et al., 2008).

Stress: Lemon oil vapor was found to have strong antistress and antidepressant effects on mice subjected to several common stress tests (Komiya et al., 2006).

Anticancer Properties: In a study of older individuals, it was found that there was a dose-dependent relationship between citrus peel consumption (which are high in d-Limonene) and a lower degree of squamous cell carcinoma (SCC) of the skin (Hakim et al., 2000).

Anticancer Properties: In clinical trials, d-Limonene (found in most citrus oils and in dill, caraway, citronella, and nutmeg) was found to elicit a response (kept patients stable) in some patients in advanced stages of cancer (1 breast and 3 colorectal carcinoma of 32 total patients). A secondary trial with just breast cancer patients did not elicit any responses (Vigushin et al., 1998).

Antidepressant Properties: Lemon oil and its component, citral, were found to decrease depressed behavior in rats involved in several stress tests in a manner similar to antidepressant drugs (Komori et al., 1995).

Antifungal Properties: Lemon oil was found to be an effective antifungal agent against two bread-mold species (Caccioni et al., 1998).

Antioxidant Properties: Lemon oil and one of its components, gamma-terpinene, were found to inhibit oxidation of low-density lipoprotein (LDL). Oxidation of LDL has been found to increase the risk of atherosclerosis and cardiac disease (Grassmann et al., 2001).

Aging: Based on lemon essential oil's acetylcholinesterase inhibitory activity, butyrylcholinesterase inhibitiory activity, and antioxidant power, this essential oil could be used in the management and/or prevention of neurodegenerative conditions like Alzheimer's disease (Oboh et al., 2014).

Aging: A study using mice demonstrated that pretreatment with lemon essential oil causes an increase in antioxidant enzymatic activities and decreased lipid degradation in the hippocampus (Campelo et al., 2011). Antioxidant and bioprotective activities, like that of lemon essential oil, can reduce damage to neurons produced by neurodegenerative disease (Campelo et al., 2011).

Digestive Problems: The use of rosemary, lemon, and peppermint oils in massage demonstrated an ability to reduce constipation and to increase bowel movements in elderly subjects, compared to massage without the oils (Kime et al., 2005).

Gastric Ulcer: Lemon essential oil and its majority compound (limonene) exhibited a gastroprotective effect against induced gastric ulcers in rats (Rozza et al., 2011).

Nerves: Pretreatment of human and rat astrocyte cells (cells found in the nerve and brain that support the blood-brain barrier and help repair the brain and spinal cord following injuries) with lemon oil was found to inhibit heat-shock induced apoptosis of these cells (Koo et al., 2002).

Nose—Rhinitis: A study including 100 patients (ages 3 to 79) suffering from vasomotor allergic rhinopathy, showed that topical application of a citrus lemon based spray resulted in a total reduction of eosinophils granulocytes and mast cells. These results suggest that the lemon-based nasal spray is a good alternative to conventional medicine for the treatment of perennial and seasonal allergic and vasomotor rhinopathy (Ferrara et al., 2012).

Morning Sickness: A randomized clinical trial carried out on 100 pregnant women suffering from mild to moderate nausea found inhalation of lemon essential oil to be more effective at preventing nausea than inhalation of a carrier oil on days two and four of a four day trial (Yavari kia et al., 2014).

See Personal Usage Guide chapter for more details on these primary uses.   ●=Neat, ●=Dilute for Children/Sensitive Skin, ●=Dilute

Lemon Myrtle *Backhousia citriodora*

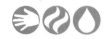

Quick Facts

Botanical Family: Myrtaceae (myrtle: shrubs and trees)

Extraction Method: Steam distillation from leaves

Common Primary Uses*: Antibacterial, Antifungal, Candida, Staph/MRSA

Common Application Methods‡:

: Dilute 1:3 (1 drop essential oil to at least 3 drops carrier oil) before applying topically. Apply directly on area of concern or to reflex points.

: Diffuse, or inhale the aroma directly.

: Add 1 drop to 1 cup (250 ml) of water or other beverage.

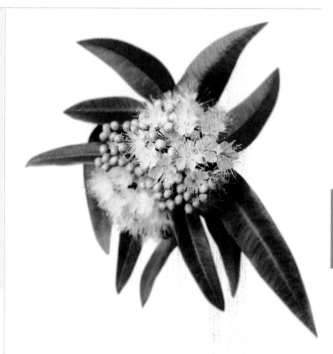

Chemical Constituents: Aldehydes (>90%): geranial (57%), neral (37%), citronellal; Alcohols (<4%): cis- & trans-verbenol (<3%), linalool, nerol. Other trace elements include linalyl acetate, myrcene, methylheptenone, and geranic acid.

Properties: Analgesic, anxiolytic, antibacterial, antifungal, anti-inflammatory, antimicrobial, antitumor, and sedative.

Historical Uses: Dried leaves from the lemon myrtle tree have been used as food flavoring for poultry and seafood. They have also served as air fresheners in wardrobes, shoe cabinets, and vehicles. Lemon myrtle is said to smell more "lemony" than lemon. Research indicates that lemon myrtle oil has very good antibacterial activity and excellent antifungal activity, perhaps even more than Melaleuca alternifolia. Tests have also shown lemon myrtle to possess strong germicidal powers, twice that of Eucalyptus citriodora and 19.5 times that of citral alone.

Other Possible Uses: Lemon myrtle may help with viral, bacterial, and fungal infections. It has also been reported to help with sprained or torn ligaments and tendons. Due to antibacterial, antifungal, and antimicrobial actions, lemon myrtle works well as an additive to any natural cleaning product. What more agreeable way to clean than with the strong lemon scent from this oil!

Body System(s) Affected: Immune System, Respiratory System, Muscles and Bones.

Aromatic Influence: Lemon myrtle is elevating and refreshing.

Oral Use As Dietary Supplement: While the FDA has given no guidance on this oil, leaves from the lemon myrtle are commonly used as a spice or flavoring in Australia. Use in cooking or in beverages in small amounts (1 drop or less). Dilute 1 drop oil in 1 tsp. (5 ml) honey or in 1 cup (250 ml) of beverage (e.g., soy/rice milk). Not for children under 6 years old; use with caution and in greater dilution for children 6 years old and over.

Safety Data: Oils may irritate sensitive or damaged skin. Dilute before applying on the skin. Consult with a physician before use if taking medications (especially for diabetes), pregnant, or nursing.

Blend Classification: Enhancer and Equalizer.

Blends With: Basil, clary sage, citrus oils, eucalyptus, geranium, lavender, melaleuca, and rosemary.

Odor: Type: Top (5–20% of the blend); Scent: Lemony, crisp, sweet, slightly herbal; Intensity: 5.

‡*See Application section beginning on page 16 for more details on applying essential oils.*   =Topical, =Aromatic, =Internal

87

Lemongrass *Cymbopogon flexuosus*

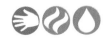

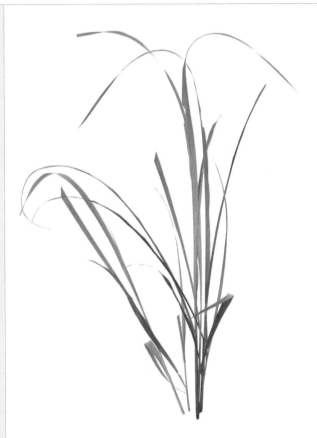

Quick Facts

Botanical Family: Gramineae (grasses)

Extraction Method: Steam distillation from leaves

Common Primary Uses*: ⊘Air Pollution, ⊘Airborne Bacteria, ⊜Carpal Tunnel Syndrome, ○Cholesterol⊕, ⊜Cramps/Charley Horses, ⊜Cystitis/Bladder Infection, ⊜Diuretic, ⊜Edema, ⊜Fleas, ⊜Frozen Shoulder, ○Gastritis, ⊜⊘Grave's Disease, ⊜⊘Hashimoto's Disease, ⊜Hernia (Incisional), ⊜Hernia (Inguinal), ⊜Improve Vision, ○⊜Lactose Intolerance, ⊜⊘Lymphatic Drainage, ⊘⊜Mental Fatigue, ⊜Muscular Dystrophy, ⊜⊘Paralysis, ⊘Purification, ⊜Retina (Strengthen), ⊜Sprains, ⊜Strain (Muscle), ⊜Tissue Repair, ⊜⊘Urinary Tract Infection, ⊜Varicose Veins, ⊜Whiplash (Ligaments), ⊜Wounds

Common Application Methods‡:

◐: Can be applied neat (with no dilution), or dilute 1:1 (1 drop essential oil to 1 drop carrier oil) for children and for those with sensitive skin when using topically. Apply directly on area of concern or to reflex points.

⊘: Diffuse, or inhale the aroma directly.

○: Take in capsules. Use as a flavoring in cooking.

Chemical Constituents: Aldehydes (up to 80%): geranial (<42%), neral (<38%), farnesal (<3%), decanal; Alcohols (<15%): geraniol (<10%), α-terpineol (<3%), borneol (<2%), nerol, linalool, citronellol; Sesquiterpene Alcohols: farnesol (<13%); Esters (<11%): geranyl & linalyl acetates; Monoterpenes (<9%): myrcene (<5%), d-Limonene (<3%), β-ocimene; Sesquiterpenes: β-caryophyllene (<6%); Oxides: caryophyllene oxide (<4%); Ketones: methyl heptanone (<3%).

Properties: Analgesic, antibacterial⊕, anticancer⊕, anti-inflammatory⊕, antiseptic, insect repellent, revitalizer, sedative, tonic, and vasodilator.

Historical Uses: Lemongrass has been used for infectious illnesses and fever, as an insecticide, and as a sedative to the central nervous system.

French Medicinal Uses: Bladder infection (cystitis), connective tissue (regenerates), digestive system, edema, fluid retention, kidney disorders, lymphatic drainage, parasympathetic nervous system (regulates), varicose veins, vascular walls (strengthens).

Other Possible Uses: This oil may help with circulation, improving digestion, improving eyesight, fevers, flatulence, headaches, clearing infections, repairing ligaments, waking up the lymphatic system, getting the oxygen flowing, respiratory problems⊕, sore throats, tissue regeneration, and water retention.

⊕ Body System(s) Affected: Immune System, Muscles and Bones.

Aromatic Influence: It promotes awareness and purification.

Oral Use As Dietary Supplement: Lemongrass oil is generally recognized as safe (GRAS) for human consumption by the FDA (21CFR182.20). Dilute 1 drop oil in 1 tsp. (5 ml) honey or in ½ cup (125 ml) of beverage (e.g., soy/rice milk). Not for children

See Personal Usage Guide chapter for more details on these primary uses.   ●=Neat, ●=Dilute for Children/Sensitive Skin, ●=Dilute

88

under 6 years old; use with caution and in greater dilution for children 6 years old and over.

Safety Data: Can cause extreme skin irritation.

Blend Classification: Enhancer and Equalizer.

Blends With: Basil, clary sage, eucalyptus, geranium, lavender, melaleuca, and rosemary.

Odor: Type: Top Note (5–20% of the blend); Scent: Grassy, lemony, pungent, earthy, slightly bitter; Intensity: 4.

Additional Research:

Cholesterol: Internal use of lemongrass capsules was found to reduce cholesterol in some subjects (Elson et al., 1989).

Antibacterial Properties: A formulation of lemongrass and geranium oil was found to reduce airborne bacteria by 89% in an office environment after diffusion for 15 hours (Doran et al., 2009).

Antibacterial Properties: Lemongrass and lemon verbena oil were found to be bactericidal to *Helicobacter pylori* at very low concentrations. Additionally, it was found that this bacteria did not develop a resistance to lemongrass oil after 10 passages; while this bacteria did develop resistance to clarithromycin (an antibiotic) under the same conditions (Ohno et al., 2003).

Antibacterial Properties: Two components of lemongrass demonstrated antibacterial properties, while the addition of a third component, myrcene, enhanced the antibacterial activities (Onawunmi et al., 1984).

Anticancer Properties: Geraniol, found in lemongrass oil (among others), was found to inhibit colon cancer cell growth while inhibiting DNA synthesis in these cells (Carnesecchi et al., 2001).

Anticancer Properties: Lemongrass oil and its constituent, isointermedeol, were found to induce apoptosis in human leukemia cells (Kumar et al., 2008).

Anticancer Properties: An extract from lemongrass was found to inhibit hepatocarcinogenesis (liver cancer genesis) in rats (Puatanachokchai et al., 2002).

Anticancer Properties: Lemongrass oil was found to inhibit multiple cancer cell lines, both in vitro and in vivo in mice (Sharma et al., 2009).

Anti-inflammatory Properties: Lemongrass was found to demonstrate anti-inflammatory activity in human skin cells (Han et al., 2017).

Respiratory Problems: Cinnamon bark, lemongrass, and thyme oils were found to have the highest level of activity against common respiratory pathogens among 14 essential oils tested (Inouye et al., 2001).

‡*See Application section beginning on page 16 for more details on applying essential oils.*   ◐=Topical, ◑=Aromatic, ○=Internal

89

Lime *Citrus aurantifolia*

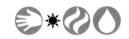

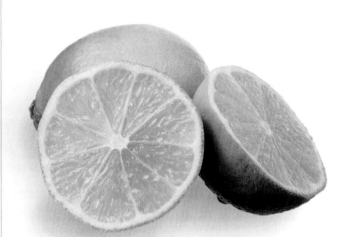

Quick Facts

Botanical Family: Rutaceae (citrus)

Extraction Method: Cold expressed from peel

Common Primary Uses*: Bacterial Infections, Fever, Gum/Grease Removal, Skin (Revitalizing)

Common Application Methods‡:

: Can be applied neat (with no dilution) when used topically. Apply directly on area of concern or to reflex points. It makes an excellent addition to bath and shower gels, body lotions, and deodorants.

: Diffuse, or inhale the aroma directly.

: Place 1–2 drops under the tongue, or drink with a beverage. Take in capsules. Use as a flavoring in cooking.

Chemical Constituents: Monoterpenes (up to 80%): d-Limonene (<65%), α- & β-pinenes (<17%), camphene, sabinene, p-cymene, myrcene, bisabolene, dipentene, phellandrene, cadinene; Oxides (<22%): 1,8 cineol (<20%), 1,4 cineol; Aldehydes (<20%): geranial (<8%), neral (<5%), citral, citronellal, octanal, nonanal, decanal, lauric aldehyde; Alcohols (4%): α-terpineol (<2%), borneol, α-fenchol, linalool; Coumarins: limettine; Furanoids: furfural, garanoxycoumarin.

Properties: Antibacterial, antiseptic, antiviral, restorative, and tonic.

Historical Uses: For some time, lime was used as a remedy for dyspepsia with glycerin of pepsin. It was often used in place of lemon for fevers, infections, sore throats, colds, etc.

Other Possible Uses: This oil may be beneficial for anxiety, blood pressure, soothing broken capillaries, dissolving cellulite, improving clarity of thought, debility, energy, gallstones, hair (cleansing), promoting leukocyte formation, liver deficiencies in children, lymphatic system cleansing, memory improvement, nails (strengthening), nervous conditions, cleaning children's skin, sore throats, water and air purification, and promoting a sense of well-being. It works extremely well in removing gum, wood stain, oil, and grease spots.

It may also help brighten a pale, dull complexion by removing the dead skin cells. Lime oil is capable of tightening skin and connective tissue.

Body System(s) Affected: Digestive, Immune, and Respiratory Systems.

Aromatic Influence: Lime oil has a fresh, lively fragrance that is stimulating and refreshing. It helps one overcome exhaustion, depression, and listlessness. Although unverifiable, some sources claim that inhaling the oil may stimulate the muscles around the eyes.

Oral Use As Dietary Supplement: Lime oil is generally regarded as safe (GRAS) for human consumption by the FDA. Dilute 1 drop oil in 1 tsp. (5 ml) honey or in ½ cup (125 ml) of beverage (e.g., soy/rice milk). Not for children under 6 years old; use with caution and in greater dilution for children 6 years old and over.

Safety Data: Avoid direct sunlight 12 hours after use.

Blend Classification: Enhancer and Equalizer.

Blends With: Citronella, clary sage, lavender, rosemary, other citrus oils.

Odor: Type: Top Note (5–20% of the blend); Scent: Sweet, tart, intense, lively; Intensity: 3

Additional Research:

Weight—Obesity: Injection of lime essential oil prevented weight gain by suppressing the appetite of mice even when administered ketotifen, an antihistamine with the undesirable side effects of decreased metabolism and increased appetite (Asnaashari et al., 2010).

*See Personal Usage Guide chapter for more details on these primary uses.   =Neat, =Dilute for Children/Sensitive Skin, =Dilute

Litsea *Litsea cubeba*

Essential Oils

Quick Facts

Botanical Family: Lauraceae (laurel)

Extraction Method: Steam distillation from fruit

Common Primary Uses*: ⚌⚌Bacterial Infections◻, ⚌⚌Cleaning, ⚌⚌Energizing, ◖Flavoring, ⚌⚌Meditation, ⚌⚌Yoga

Common Application Methods‡:

⚌: Can be applied neat (with no dilution) when used topically. Apply directly on area of concern or to reflex points. Use in massage oil.

⚌: Diffuse, or inhale the aroma directly.

◖: Place 1–2 drops in liquid, and drink as a beverage. Use as a flavoring in cooking.

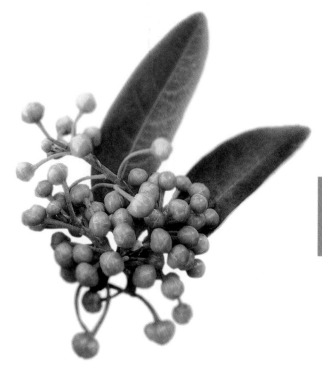

Chemical Constituents: Aldehydes (up to 75%): geranial (<42%), neral (<35%), citronellal; Monoterpenes (up to 25%): limonene (<23%), myrcene (<3%), sabinene, β-ocimene, α- & β-pinenes, camphene; Alcohols: geraniol, nerol, α-terpineol, linalool, citronellol; Esters: terpinyl acetate; Sesquiterpenes: β-caryophyllene; Ketones: 6-methyl-5-hepten-2-one.

Properties: Antibacterial◻, antifungal, antiseptic, antiviral.

Historical Uses: Litsea (also known as mei (may) chang) has been used medicinally in Taiwan and China for centuries to treat pain, asthma, and digestive issues.

Other Possible Uses: This oil may also be beneficial for allergies, asthma, throat congestion, and heart arrhythmia.

✛ **Body System(s) Affected:** Digestive, Immune, and Respiratory Systems.

Aromatic Influence: Litsea oil has a sweet, citrusy, floral aroma that is uplifting and energizing and may help promote feelings of balance.

Oral Use As Dietary Supplement: There is no FDA designation for *Litsea cubeba* oil at this time, but it is commonly used as a flavoring in cooking. Dilute 1 drop oil in 1 tsp. (5 ml) honey or in ½ cup (125 ml) of beverage (e.g., soy/rice milk). Not for

children under 6 years old; use with caution and in greater dilution for children 6 years old and over.

Safety Data: May cause skin sensitivity. Consult with a physician before using if pregnant, nursing, or being treated for diabetes or other medical conditions.

Blend Classification: Enhancer and Equalizer.

Blends With: Lavender, rosemary, rose, petitgrain, citrus oils, ylang ylang, sandalwood, frankincense, fennel, geranium, vetiver.

Odor: Type: Middle Note (50–80% of the blend); Scent: Citrusy, floral, fresh, sweet; Intensity: 3

◻ **Additional Research:**

Antibacterial: Essential oil from the fruit of *Litsea cubeba* demonstrated an excellent antibacterial property (Su et al., 2016).

‡*See Application section beginning on page 16 for more details on applying essential oils.*   ⚌=Topical, ⚌=Aromatic, ◖=Internal

91

Magnolia *Michelia alba (Magnolia alba)*

Quick Facts

Botanical Family: Magnoliaceae

Extraction Method: Steam distillation from flowers

Common Primary Uses*: Anxiety, Calming, Soothing (skin)

Common Application Methods‡:

: Can be applied neat (with no dilution) when used topically. Apply directly on area of concern or to reflex points.

: Diffuse, or inhale the aroma directly.

Chemical Constituents: Alcohols: linalool (up to 80%); Sesquiterpenes (up to 10%): β-caryophyllene, selinine, β-elemene; Monoterpenes: β-ocimene.

Properties: Analgesic, anxiolytic, antibacterial, anti-inflammatory, antimicrobial, antitumor, sedative.

Historical Uses: Magnolia trees are native to Southeast Asia, and the bark of one magnolia species (*Magnolia officinalis*) is used in traditional Chinese medicine to help with digestive and respiratory issues. This variety of magnolia (*M. alba*) is believed to be a hybrid of *M. champaca* and *M. montana*.

Other Possible Uses: This oil may also be beneficial for calming, depression, and skin (cleansing and soothing).

Body System(s) Affected: Hormonal System, Immune System, Skin.

Aromatic Influence: benefitIt also has calming and sedating properties when inhaled.

Oral Use As Dietary Supplement: None.

Safety Data: Old or oxidized oil may irritate sensitive skin. Consult with a physician before use if taking medications, pregnant, or nursing.

Blend Classification: Enhancer and Equalizer.

Blends With: Bergamot, geranium, grapefruit, lime, marjoram, rose, sandalwood, vetiver, ylang ylang.

Odor: Type: Top to Middle (50–80% of the blend); Scent: Sweet, floral, fruity, herbal; Intensity: 2.

Additional Research:

Pain: Linalool was found to demonstrate an antinociceptive effect (blocked pain perception) due to its ability to inhibit the production and release of nitric oxide (Peana et al., 2006).

Sedative: In a mouse model, inhaled linalool was found to demonstrate sedative properties (Linck et al., 2009).

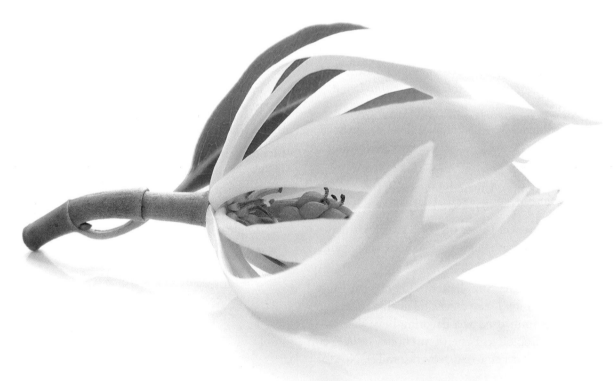

*See Personal Usage Guide chapter for more details on these primary uses.   ●=Neat, ●=Dilute for Children/Sensitive Skin, ●=Dilute

92

Manuka *Leptospermum scoparium*

Quick Facts

Botanical Family: Myrtaceae (myrtle)

Extraction Method: Steam distillation from leaves, flowers, and branches

Common Primary Uses*: ⚗⚗Respiratory Infections, ⚗⚗Arthritis, ⚗Rheumatism, ⚗Skin

Common Application Methods‡:

⚗: Can be applied neat (with no dilution) when used topically. Apply directly on area of concern or to reflex points. Use in baths.

⚗: Diffuse, or inhale the aroma directly.

Chemical Constituents: Sesquiterpenes (up to 50%): trans-calamenene (<15%), Cadina-3,5-diene (<10%>, δ-cadinene (<7%), α-copaene (<7%), α- & β-selinene, α-cubebene, δ-amorphene, β-caryophyllene, aromadendrene, humulene; Cyclic Triketones (20–30%): leptospermone (<17%), iso-leptospermone (<5%), flavesone (<5%); Alcohols: linalool, geraniol; Monoterpenes: α- & β-pinenes.

Properties: Analgesic, antibacterial⚬, antifungal, anti-infectious, antiviral, antihistamine, antiseptic, decongestant, and insecticidal.

Historical Uses: This oil has a long history of use by the Maori people for bronchitis, rheumatism, and similar conditions. Also, manuka oil has been used to treat a range of skin problems including chronic sores, ringworm, eczema, fungal infections (athlete foot and fungal nail infections), scalp itch, and dandruff. A decoction of leaves was used for urinary complaints and to reduce fever. The leaves were boiled in water and inhaled for head colds, blocked sinuses, hay fever, and even bronchitis and asthma. Leaves and bark were boiled together, and the warm liquid was rubbed on stiff backs and rheumatic joints. The leaves and young branches were put into vapor baths. The crushed leaves were applied as a poultice for many skin diseases and were directly applied to wounds and deep gashes to enhance healing and to reduce the risk of infection. The young shoots were chewed and swallowed for dysentery.

Other Possible Uses: This oil may be beneficial for abrasions, acne, bronchitis, catarrh, chafing, colds, cuts, dandruff, fungal infections, infections, insect bites and stings, muscle and joint pains, odor, rashes, scratches, skin irritations, sinusitis, sunburn, and ulcers.

✛ **Body System(s) Affected:** Muscles and Bones, Respiratory System, and Skin.

Aromatic Influence: Manuka oil helps to calm sensitive nerves and to produce a feeling of well-being. Its calming aroma helps to combat stress and irritability.

Oral Use As Dietary Supplement: None.

Safety Data: Use with caution when pregnant or nursing.

Blend Classification: Enhancer and Equalizer.

Blends With: All citrus oils, cypress, eucalyptus, lavender, rosemary, and thyme.

Odor: Type: Middle Note (50–80% of the blend); Scent: Rich, fresh, woody, earthy, herbaceous; Intensity: 3.

⊞ **Additional Research:**

Antibacteial: Manuka oil demonstrated strong antibacterial activity against detrimental oral bacteria (Takarada et al., 2004).

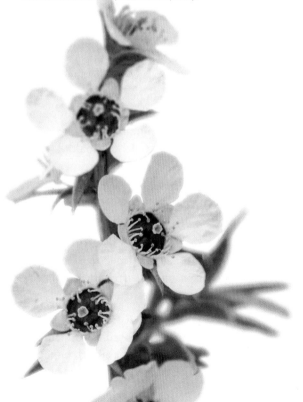

‡See Application section beginning on page 16 for more details on applying essential oils.   ⚗=Topical, ⚗=Aromatic, O=Internal

93

Marjoram *Origanum majorana*

Quick Facts

Botanical Family: Labiatae (mint)

Extraction Method: Steam distillation from leaves

Common Primary Uses*: Arterial Vasodilator, Arthritis, Bone Spurs, Carpal Tunnel Syndrome, Cartilage Injury, Colic, Constipation, Cramps/Charley Horses, Croup, Expectorant, High Blood Pressure, Muscle Aches, Muscle Fatigue, Muscle Spasms, Muscle Tone, Muscular Dystrophy, Neuralgia, Osteoarthritis, Pancreatitis, Parkinson's Disease, Physical Stress, Prolapsed Mitral Valve, Rheumatoid Arthritis, Sprains, Stiffness, Tendinitis, Tension (Muscle), Whiplash (Muscles)

Common Application Methods‡:

: Can be applied neat (with no dilution) when used topically. Apply directly on area of concern or to reflex points. Use with caution during pregnancy.

: Diffuse, or inhale the aroma directly.

: Place 1–2 drops under the tongue, or take in a capsule. Use as a flavoring in cooking.

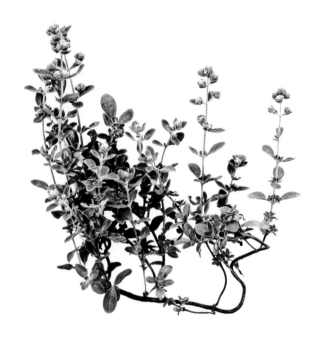

Chemical Constituents: Monoterpenes (up to 60%): α- & γ-terpinenes (<30%), sabinene (<8%), myrcene (<7%), terpinolene, ocimene, δ-3-carene, p-cymene, α- and β-pinenes, δ-cadinene, α- & β-phellandrenes, l-limonene; Alcohols (<30%): α-terpineol (<15%), cis- & trans-thujanol-4 (<12%), linalool (<8%); Phenols: terpinen-4-ol (>21%), terpinen-1-ol-3; Esters: geranyl acetate (<7%), linalyl acetate, α-terpenyl acetate; Aldehydes: citral (<6%); Sesquiterpenes (<5%): β-caryophyllene, humulene; Phenolic Ethers: trans-anethole.

Properties: Antibacterial, anti-infectious, antiseptic, antisexual, antispasmodic, arterial vasodilator, digestive stimulant, diuretic, expectorant, sedative, and tonic.

Historical Uses: Marjoram was used to combat poisoning, fluid retention, muscle spasms, rheumatism, sprains, stiff joints, bruises, obstructions of the liver and spleen, and respiratory congestions. According to Roberta Wilson, "Those curious about their futures anointed themselves with marjoram at bedtime so that they might dream of their future mates."

French Medicinal Uses: Aches, arthritis, asthma, bronchitis, colic, constipation, cramps, insomnia, intestinal peristalsis, migraine headaches, muscles, neuralgia, pains, parasympathetic nervous system (tones), blood pressure (regulates), rheumatism, sprains.

Other Possible Uses: It may be relaxing and calming to the muscles that constrict and sometimes contribute to headaches. It may help anxiety, boils, bruises, burns, carbuncles, celibacy (vow not to marry), colds, cold sores, cuts, fungus and viral infections, hysteria, menstrual problems, calm the respiratory system, ringworm, shingles, shock, sores, relieve spasms, sunburns, and water retention.

Body System(s) Affected: Cardiovascular System, Muscles and Bones.

Aromatic Influence: It promotes peace and sleep.

Oral Use As Dietary Supplement: Marjoram oil is generally recognized as safe (GRAS) for human consumption by the FDA (21CFR182.20). Dilute 1 drop oil in 1 tsp. (5 ml) honey or in ½ cup (125 ml) of beverage (e.g., soy/rice milk). Not for

---

*See Personal Usage Guide chapter for more details on these primary uses.   ●=Neat, ●=Dilute for Children/Sensitive Skin, ●=Dilute

children under 6 years old; use with caution and in greater dilution for children 6 years old and over.

Safety Data: Use with caution during pregnancy.

Blend Classification: Enhancer and Equalizer.

Blends With: Bergamot, cypress, lavender, orange, rosemary, and ylang ylang.

Odor: Type: Middle Note (50–80% of the blend); Scent: Herbaceous, green, spicy; Intensity: 3.

Additional Research:

High Blood Pressure: Eighty-three hypertensive or prehypertensive subjects were divided into the following three groups: a study group (exposed to an essential oil blend containing lavender, ylang ylang, marjoram, and neroli), a placebo group (exposed to artificial fragrance), and a control group (no interventions). The study group was found to have an immediate and long-term decrease in home blood pressure (Kim et al., 2012).

Arthritis: In patients suffering from arthritis, it was found that a blend of lavender, marjoram, eucalyptus, rosemary, and peppermint blended with carrier oils reduced perceived pain and depression compared to control (Kim et al., 2005).

Dysmenorrhea: Compared to a synthetic fragrance, dysmenorrhea pain decreased and shortened in duration when subjects massaged a blend of lavender, marjoram, and clary sage essential oils (in a ratio of 2:1:1) daily on the abdomen between menstruations (Ou et al., 2012).

Ulcers: Oral administration of marjoram extract was shown to significantly decrease the incidence of ulcers, basal gastric secretion, and acid output in rats (Al-Howiriny et al., 2009).

‡*See Application section beginning on page 16 for more details on applying essential oils.*   ◗=Topical, ◗=Aromatic, ◗=Internal

95

Melaleuca (Tea Tree) *Melaleuca alternifolia*

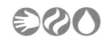

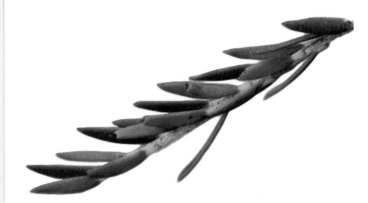

Quick Facts

Botanical Family: Myrtaceae (Myrtle: shrubs and trees)

Extraction Method: Steam distillation from leaves

Common Primary Uses*: Acne, Allergies, Aneurysm, Athlete's Foot, Bacterial Infections, Boils, Bronchitis, Candida, Canker Sores, Cavities, Chicken Pox, Cleansing, Cold Sores, Colds (Common), Coughs, Cuts, Dermatitis/Eczema, Dry/Itchy Eyes, Ear Infection, Earache, Flu (Influenza), Fungal Infections, Gum Disease, Hepatitis, Herpes Simplex, Hives, Immune System (Stimulates), Infected Wounds, Infection, Inflammation, Jock Itch, Lice, MRSA, Mumps, Nail Infection, Pink Eye, Rashes, Ringworm, Rubella, Scabies, Shingles, Shock, Sore Throat, Staph Infection, Sunburn, Thrush, Tonsillitis, Vaginal Infection, Varicose Ulcer, Viral Infections, Warts, Wounds

Common Application Methods‡:

🖐: Can be applied neat (with no dilution) when used topically. Apply directly on area of concern or to reflex points.

🌀: Diffuse, or inhale the aroma directly.

⭘: Take in capsules.

Chemical Constituents: Monoterpenes (up to 70%): α- & γ-terpinenes (<40%), p-cymene (<12%), α- and β-pinenes (<8%), terpinolene, l-limonene, sabinene, myrcene, α-thujene; Phenols: terpinen-4-ol (<40%); Sesquiterpenes (up to 20%): α- & δ-cadinenes (<8%), aromadendrene (<7%), viridiflorene (<5%), β-caryophyllene, α-phellandrene; Oxides: 1,8 cineol (<14%), 1,4 cineol (<3%), caryophyllene oxide; Alcohols: α- & β-terpineols (<8%); Sesquiterpene Alcohols (<5%): globulol, viridiflorol.

Properties: Analgesic, antibacterial, antifungal, anti-infectious, anti-inflammatory, antioxidant, antiparasitic, a strong antiseptic, antiviral, decongestant, digestive, expectorant, immune stimulant, insecticidal, neurotonic, stimulant, and tissue regenerative.

Historical Uses: The leaves of the melaleuca tree (or tea tree) have been used for centuries by the Aboriginal people of Australia to heal cuts, wounds, and skin infections. With 12 times the antiseptic power of phenol, it has some strong immune-building properties.

French Medicinal Uses: Athlete's foot, bronchitis, colds, coughs, diarrhea, flu, periodontal (gum) disease, rash, skin healing, sore throat, sunburn, tonsillitis, vaginal thrush.

Other Possible Uses: This oil may help burns, digestion, hysteria, infectious diseases, mites, and ticks.

✛ **Body System(s) Affected:** Immune and Respiratory Systems, Muscles and Bones, Skin.

Aromatic Influence: It promotes cleansing and purity.

Oral Use As Dietary Supplement: Melaleuca oil in general is approved by the FDA (21CFR172.510) for use as a Food Additive (FA) or Flavoring Agent (FL). Dilute 1 drop oil in 1 tsp. (5 ml) honey or in ½ cup (125 ml) of beverage (e.g., soy/rice milk). Not for children under 6 years old; use with caution and in greater dilution for children 6 years old and over.

Safety Data: Repeated use can possibly result in contact sensitization.

Blend Classification: Enhancer and Equalizer.

Blends With: All citrus oils, cypress, eucalyptus, lavender, rosemary, and thyme.

---

*See Personal Usage Guide chapter for more details on these primary uses.   ●=Neat, ●=Dilute for Children/Sensitive Skin, ●=Dilute

Odor: Type: Middle Note (50–80% of the blend); Scent: Medicinal, fresh, woody, earthy, herbaceous; Intensity: 3.

Additional Research:

Acne: A gel with 5% tea tree oil was found to be as effective as a 5% benzoyl peroxide (a common chemical used to treat acne) lotion at treating acne, with fewer side effects (Bassett et al., 1990).

Acne: A topical gel containing 5% tea tree oil was found to be more effective than a placebo at preventing acne vulgaris lesions and at decreasing severity in patients suffering from acne vulgaris (Enshaieh et al., 2007).

Acne: Tea tree oil and several of its main components were found to be active against *Propionibacterium acnes*, a bacteria involved in the formation of acne. This oil was also found to be active against two types of Staphylococcus bacteria (Raman et al., 1995).

Boils: In a human trial, most patients receiving treatment with *Melaleuca alternifolia* oil placed topically on boils experienced healing or reduction of symptoms; while of those receiving no treatment (control), half required surgical intervention, and all still demonstrated signs of the infection (Feinblatt et al., 1960).

Influenza: In vitro research has found that *Melaleuca alternifolia* concentrate can disturb the normal viral membrane fusion of the influenza virus and inhibit entry of influenza virus into the host cell (Li et al., 2013).

Antibacterial Properties: MRSA (methicillin-resistant staph) and MSSA (methicillin-sensitive staph) in biofilms (plaque/microcolonies) were eradicated by a 5% solution of tea tree oil as well as 5 of 9 CoNS (coagulase-negative staph) (Brady et al., 2006).

Antibacterial Properties: 66 isolates of *Staphylococcus aureus* (Staph), including 64 methicillin-resistant (MRSA) strains and 33 mupirocin-resistant strains, were inhibited by tea tree essential oil (Carson et al., 1995).

Antibacterial Properties: Tea tree oil was found to disrupt the cellular membrane and to inhibit respiration in *Candida albicans,* Gram-negative *E. coli*, and Gram-positive *Staphylococcus aureus* (Staph) (Cox et al., 2000).

Antibacterial Properties: Geranium and tea tree demonstrated strong antibacterial effects on *Staphylococcus aureus* (Edwards-Jones et al., 2004).

Antibacterial Properties: Tea tree oil and its component terpinen-4-ol demonstrated an effective antibacterial activity against *Staphylococcus aureus* (Staph) bacteria, superior to the activity of several antibiotic drugs—even against antibiotic-resistant strains (Ferrini et al., 2006).

Antibacterial Properties: Tea tree oil was found to kill transient skin flora at lower concentrations than it killed resident skin flora (Hammer et al., 1996).

Antibacterial Properties: Gram-positive strains of *Staphylococcus aureus* and *Enterococcus faecalis* were shown to have very low frequencies of resistance to tea tree oil (Hammer et al., 2008).

Antibacterial Properties: Tea tree oil demonstrated ability to kill *Staphylococcus aureus* (Staph) bacteria both within biofilms and in the stationary growth phase at concentrations below 1% (Kwieciński et al., 2009).

Antifungal Properties: Tea tree oil was found to inhibit 301 different types of yeasts isolated from the mouths of cancer patients suffering from advanced cancer, including 41 strains that are known to be resistant to antifungal drugs (Bagg et al., 2006).

Antifungal Properties: Eleven types of Candida were found to be highly inhibited by tea tree oil (Banes-Marshall et al., 2001).

Antifungal Properties: Topical application of 100% tea tree oil was found to have results similar to topical application of 1% clotrimazole (antifungal drug) solution on onychomycosis (also known as tinea, or fungal nail infection) (Buck et al., 1994).

Antifungal Properties: Tea tree oil was found to alter the membrane properties and functions of *Candida albicans* cells, leading to cell inhibition or death (Hammer et al., 2004).

Antifungal Properties: Terpinen-4-ol, a constituent of tea tree oil, and tea tree oil were found to be effective against several forms of vaginal candida infections in rats, including azole-resistant forms (Mondello et al., 2006).

Antifungal Properties: Patients with tinea pedis (athlete's foot) were found to have a higher rate of cure and a higher clinical response when treated topically with 25% or 50% tea tree oil solution compared to control (Satchell et al., 2002).

Antifungal: When applied as a coating to protect oranges after harvest, a mixture containing chitosan and melaleuca essential oil was found to reduce fungal growth by 50% (Cháfer et al., 2012).

Anti-inflammatory Properties: Tea tree oil was found to reduce swelling during a contact hypersensitivity response in the skin of mice sensitized to the chemical hapten (Brand et al., 2002).

Anti-inflammatory Properties: *Melaleuca alternifolia* oil was found to reduce reactive oxygen species (ROS) production in neutrophils (a type of white blood cell), indicating an antioxidant effect and decreased Interleukin 2 (a chemical messenger that helps trigger an inflammatory response) secretion, while increasing the secretion of Interleukin 4 (a chemical messenger involved in turning off the inflammatory response) (Caldefie-Chézet et al., 2006).

Anti-inflammatory Properties: Inhaled tea tree oil was found to have anti-inflammatory influences on male rats with induced peritoneal inflammation (Golab et al., 2007).

Anti-inflammatory Properties: The water soluble terpinen-4-ol component of tea tree was found to suppress the production of pro-inflammatory mediators in human monocytes (a type of white blood cell that is part of the human immune system) (Hart et al., 2000).

Anti-inflammatory Properties: Tea tree oil applied to histamine-induced weal and flare in human volunteers was found to decrease the mean weal volume when compared to a control (Koh et al., 2002).

Antiviral Properties: Tea tree and eucalyptus oil demonstrated ability to inhibit the *Herpes simplex* virus (Schnitzler et al., 2001).

Mites: Tea tree oil scrub and shampoo were found to reduce demodex mite infestation on the eyelids of patients suffering from ocular irritation and inflammation who used this treatment daily for six weeks. It also dramatically decreased ocular irritation and inflammation (Kheirkhah et al., 2007).

Mites: Tea tree oil was found to be effective against both lice and dust mites in a mite chamber assay (Williamson et al., 2007).

Ticks: Essential oil of *Melaleuca alternifolia* was found to be lethal for more than 80% of Ixodes ricinus tick nymphs (a carrier or Lyme disease) when they inhaled a 10 microl dose of the oil for 90 minutes or more (Iori et al., 2005).

Oral Conditions: In 34 patients with fixed orthodontic appliances, a dental gel containing 5% melaleuca essential oil performed better than Colgate Total gel when comparing microbial biofilm and quantification of Streptococcus mutans in the patients' saliva (Santamaria et al., 2014).

Parasites: Melaleuca oil was effective at killing *Anisakis simplex* larva in vitro. Data suggests that the mechanism of action against anisakis involves inhibition of acetylcholinesterase (Gómez-Rincón et al., 2014).

‡See Application section beginning on page 16 for more details on applying essential oils.   =Topical,   =Aromatic,   =Internal

97

Melissa (Lemon Balm) *Melissa officinalis*

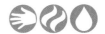

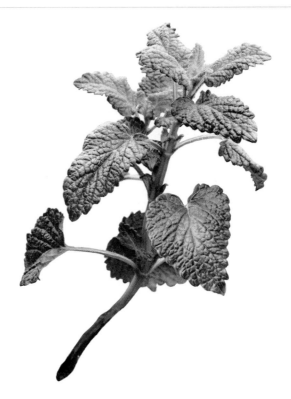

Quick Facts

Botanical Family: Labiatae (mint)

Extraction Method: Steam distillation from leaves and flowers

Common Primary Uses*: Calming, Cold Sores, Viral Infections

Common Application Methods‡:

: Can be applied neat (with no dilution) when used topically. Apply directly on area of concern or to reflex points.

: Diffuse, or inhale the aroma directly.

: Take in capsules. Use as a flavoring in cooking.

Chemical Constituents: Aldehydes (up to 65%): geranial (<35%), neral (<28%), citronellal (<3%), α-cyclocitral; Sesquiterpenes (<35%): β-caryophyllene (<19%), α-copaene (<5%), germacrene-D (<4%), β-bourbonene, δ- & γ-cadinenes, humulene, β-elemene; Oxides (<11%): caryophyllene oxide (<7%), 1,8 cineol (<4%); Alcohols (<7%): linalool, octen-3ol, nerol, geraniol, citronellol, isopulegol, caryophyllenol, farnesol; Esters (<7%): methyl citronellate (<5%), citronellyl, geranyl, neryl, & linalyl acetates; Ketones (<7%): methyl heptanone (<5%), farnesylacetone, octanone; Monoterpenes (<3%): cis- & trans-ocimenes, l-limonene; Sesquiterpene Alcohols: elemol, α-cadinol; Furanocoumarins: aesculetin.

Properties: Antibacterial, antidepressant, antihistamine, antimicrobial, antispasmodic, antiviral, hypotensive, nervine, sedative, tonic, and uterine.

Historical Uses: Anciently, melissa was used for nervous disorders and many different ailments dealing with the heart or the emotions. It was also used to promote fertility. Melissa was the main ingredient in Carmelite water, distilled in France since 1611 by the Carmelite monks.

Other Possible Uses: Allergies, anxiety, asthma, bronchitis, chronic coughs, colds, cold-sore blisters (apply directly three times per day), colic, depression, dysentery, eczema, erysipelas, fevers, heart conditions (where there is over-stimulation or heat), hypertension, indigestion, inflammation, insect bites, insomnia, menstrual problems, migraine, nausea, nervous tension, palpitations, shock, sterility (in women), throat infections, vertigo, and vomiting. Dr. Dietrich Wabner, a professor at the Technical University of Munich, reported that a one-time application of true melissa oil led to complete remission of herpes simplex lesions. According to Robert Tisserand, "Melissa is the nearest one can find to a rejuvenator—not something which will make us young again, but which helps to cushion the effect of our mind and the world outside on our body."

Body System(s) Affected: Emotional Balance, Skin.

Aromatic Influence: Melissa has a delicate, delightful, lemony scent that is unique among essential oils, providing a wonderful support to both body and mind. It is calming and uplifting and may help to balance the emotions.

Oral Use As Dietary Supplement: Melissa oil is generally recognized as safe (GRAS) for human consumption by the FDA (21CFR182.20). Dilute 1 drop oil in 1 tsp. (5 ml) honey or in ½ cup (125 ml) of beverage (e.g., soy/rice milk). Not for children

*See Personal Usage Guide chapter for more details on these primary uses.   ●=Neat, ●=Dilute for Children/Sensitive Skin, ●=Dilute

98

under 6 years old; use with caution and in greater dilution for children 6 years old and over.

Safety Data: Use with caution when pregnant or nursing.

Blend Classification: Enhancer, Equalizer, and Modifier.

Blends With: Geranium, lavender, and other floral and citrus oils.

Odor: Type: Middle Note (50–80% of the blend); Scent: Delicate, lemony; Intensity: 2.

Additional Research:

Antiviral Properties: Melissa oil demonstrated inhibition of *Herpes simplex* type 1 and 2 viruses. (Schnitzler et al., 2008).

Cold-sore Blisters: Melissa oil demonstrated inhibition of *Herpes simplex* type 1 and 2 viruses. (Schnitzler et al., 2008).

Sedative Properties: Results of a clinical trial indicate that a combination of melissa and valerian oils may have anxiety-reducing properties at some doses (Kennedy et al., 2006).

Sedative Properties: Melissa (lemon balm) oil applied topically in a lotion was found to reduce agitation and to improve quality of life factors in patients suffering severe dementia compared to those receiving a placebo lotion (Ballard et al., 2002).

Colic: Colic improved in breastfed infants within 1 week of administering a phytotherapeutic agent containing *Matricariae recutita*, *Foeniculum vulgare*, and *Melissa officinalis* when compared to a placebo containing vitamins (Savino et al., 2005).

Inflammation: Melissa oil was found to help reduce inflammation in an animal model (Bounihi 2013).

Atherosclerosis: Melissa essential oil was found to have hypolipidemic effects in transgenic mice. Mice orally administered Melissa essential oil for two weeks had lower plasma triglyceride concentrations and altered metabolic pathways. These results indicate that melissa oil could be beneficial in preventing hypertriglyceridemia, one of the main contributors to the development of cardiovascular disease (Jun et al., 2012).

Diabetes: Oral supplementation of melissa essential oil significantly reduced plasma glucose levels compared with the control group, and increased glucose tolerance in a type 2 diabetic mouse model (Chung et al., 2010).

‡See Application section beginning on page 16 for more details on applying essential oils.   ◔=Topical, ◑=Aromatic, ●=Internal

99

Myrrh *Commiphora myrrha*

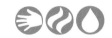

Quick Facts

Botanical Family: Burseraceae (resinous trees and shrubs)

Extraction Method: Steam distillation from gum/resin

Common Primary Uses*: Cancer, Chapped/Cracked Skin, Congestion, Dysentery, Gum Disease, Hashimoto's Disease, Hepatitis, Hyperthyroidism, Infection, Liver Cirrhosis, Skin Ulcers, Stretch Marks, Ulcers (Duodenal), Weeping Wounds

Common Application Methods‡:

: Can be applied neat (with no dilution) when used topically. Apply directly on area of concern or to reflex points.

: Diffuse, or inhale the aroma directly.

: Place 1–2 drops under the tongue, or take in capsules.

Chemical Constituents: Sesquiterpenes (up to 75%): lindestrene (up to 30%), β-, γ-, & δ-elemenes (<40%), α-copaene (<12%), β-bourbonene (<5%), muurolene, δ-cadinene, humulene, curzerene; Furanoids (<27%): methoxyfurogermacrene (<9%), furoendesmadiene (<8%), α-bergamotene (<5%), methylisopropenylfurone (<5%), furfural (<3%), furanodione (<2%), rosefuran; Ketones: (<20%): curzenone (<11%), methylisobutyl ketone (<6%), germacrone (<4%); Triterpenes (<7%): α-amyrin (<4%), α-amyrenone (<3%); Monoterpenes (<6%): ocimene, p-cymene, α-thujene, l-limonene, myrcene; Aldehydes: methylbutynal (<3%), cinnamaldehyde, cuminal; Arenes: xylene; Carboxylic Acids: acetic acid, formic acid, palmitic acid; Phenols: eugenol, cresol.

Properties: Anti-infectious, anti-inflammatory ⊕, antiseptic, antitumor ⊕, astringent, and tonic.

Historical Uses: Myrrh was used as incense in religious rituals, in embalming, and as a cure for cancer, leprosy, and syphilis. Myrrh, mixed with coriander and honey, was used to treat herpes.

French Medicinal Uses: Bronchitis, diarrhea, dysentery, hyperthyroidism, stretch marks, thrush, ulcers, vaginal thrush, viral hepatitis.

Other Possible Uses: This oil may help with appetite (increase), asthma, athlete's foot, candida, catarrh (mucus), coughs, eczema, digestion, dyspepsia (impaired digestion), flatulence (gas), fungal infection, gingivitis, hemorrhoids, mouth ulcers, decongesting the prostate gland, ringworm, sore throats, skin conditions (chapped, cracked, and inflamed)⊕, wounds, and wrinkles.

Body System(s) Affected: Hormonal, Immune, and Nervous Systems; Skin.

Aromatic Influence: It promotes awareness and is uplifting.

Oral Use As Dietary Supplement: Myrrh oil in general is approved by the FDA (21CFR172.510) for use as a Food Additive (FA) and Flavoring Agent (FL). Dilute 1 drop oil in 1 tsp. (5 ml) honey or in ½ cup (125 ml) of beverage (e.g., soy/rice milk). Not for children under 6 years old; use with caution and in greater dilution for children 6 years old and over.

Safety Data: Use with caution during pregnancy.

Blend Classification: Modifier and Equalizer.

Blends With: Frankincense, lavender, sandalwood, and all spice oils.

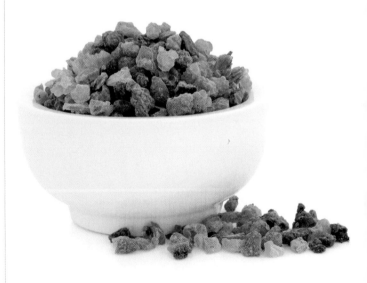

See Personal Usage Guide chapter for more details on these primary uses.   ●=Neat, ●=Dilute for Children/Sensitive Skin, ●=Dilute

100

Odor: Type: Base Note (5–20% of the blend); Scent: Warm, earthy, woody, balsamic; Intensity: 4.

Additional Research:

Anti-inflammatory Properties: At subtoxic levels, myrrh oil was found to reduce interleukin (chemical signals believed to play a role in the inflammation response) by fibroblast cells in the gums (Tipton et al., 2003).

Antitumor Properties: Treatment with elemene (found in myrrh oil) was found to increase survival time and to reduce tumor size in patients with malignant brain tumor, as compared to chemotherapy (Tan et al., 2000).

Skin: Myrrh essential oil was shown to be an efficient quencher of singlet oxygen (a type of antioxidant action) by its ability to decrease formation of squalene peroxide in UV irradiated sebum on the facial skin of human subjects. These findings suggest that topical application of myrrh essential oil can help decrease sebum damage and in turn protect skin from aging (Auffray 2007).

Brain—Aging: Three new cadinane sesquiterpenes isolated from myrrh resin were found to have neuroprotective activities against 1-methyl-4-phenylpyridinium induced neuronal cell death in a human derived cell line cells (Xu et al., 2011).

‡See Application section beginning on page 16 for more details on applying essential oils.   =Topical, =Aromatic, =Internal

101

Neroli (Orange Blossom) *Citrus aurantium*

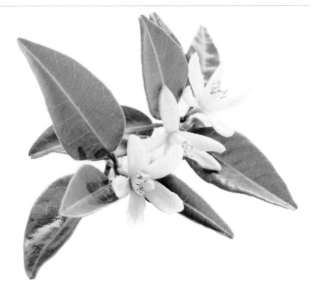

Quick Facts

Botanical Family: Rutaceae (citrus)

Extraction Method: Extracted from flowers of the bitter orange tree

Common Primary Uses*: Anxiety, Emotional Balance, Relaxing, Sensitive Skin, Stress.

Common Application Methods‡:

: Can be applied neat (with no dilution) when used topically. Apply directly on area of concern or to reflex points.

: Diffuse, or inhale the aroma directly.

Chemical Constituents: Alcohols (up to 53%): linalool (<44%), α-terpineol (<6%), geraniol (<3%), nerol; Sesquiterpene Alcohols (<7%): trans-nerolidol (<5%), farnesol (<2%); Monoterpenes (up to 40%): d-limonene (<18%), β-pinene (<17%), ocimene (<8%), myrcene (<4%), α-pinene, neptadecene, sabinene, camphene; Esters (>25%): linalyl acetate (<15%), methyl anthranilate (<10%), neryl & geranyl acetates; Aldehydes: decanal, benzaldehyde, vinylhexanal; Phenols: phenylethanol, benzyl alcohol; Pyrroles: indole, scatole.

Properties: Antibacterial⌑, antidepressant, anti-infectious, antiparasitic, antiseptic, antispasmodic, antiviral, aphrodisiac, deodorant, sedative, and tonic.

Historical Uses: Neroli has been regarded traditionally by the Egyptian people for its great attributes for healing the mind, body, and spirit. It brings everything into the focus of one and at the moment.

Other Possible Uses: This oil may help support the digestive system and may help inhibit bacteria, infections, parasites, and viruses. It may also help with anxiety, chronic diarrhea, colic, convulsions⌑, depression, digestive spasms, fear, flatulence, headaches, heart (regulates rhythm), hysteria, insomnia, mature and sensitive skin, menopause⌑, nervous dyspepsia, nervous tension, palpitations, PMS, poor circulation, scars, shock, stress-related conditions, stretch marks, tachycardia, thread veins, and wrinkles. In support of the skin, it works at the cell level to help shed the old skin cells and stimulate new cell growth.

 Body System(s) Affected: Digestive System, Skin.

Aromatic Influence: Neroli has some powerfully soothing psychological effects. It is calming and relaxing to the body and spirit. It may also help to strengthen and stabilize the emotions and bring relief to seemingly hopeless situations. It encourages confidence, courage, joy, peace, and sensuality.

Oral Use As Dietary Supplement: Neroli oil is generally recognized as safe (GRAS) for human consumption by the FDA (21CFR182.20). Dilute 1 drop oil in 1 tsp. (5 ml) honey or in ½ cup (125 ml) of beverage (e.g., soy/rice milk). Not for children under 6 years old; use with caution and in greater dilution for children 6 years old and over. Follow label instructions, and use orally only if recommended.

Safety Data: Consult with a physician before using if pregnant or being treated for a medical condition.

Blend Classification: Equalizer, Modifier, and Personifier.

Blends With: Rose, lavender, sandalwood, jasmine, cedarwood, geranium, lemon.

Odor: Type: Middle Note (50–80% of the blend); Scent: Floral, citrusy, sweet, delicate, slightly bitter; Intensity: 3.

 Additional Research:

Antibacterial: Neroli essential oil demonstrated antibacterial, antifungal, and antioxidant activity when tested in vitro (Ammar et al., 2012).

Menopause: Post menopausal women who inhaled neroli oil were found to have improved scores on a menopausal symptom questionnaire compared to a control group (Choi et al., 2014).

Anticonvulsant: Neroli oil demonstrated an anticonvulsant ability on mice (Azanchi et al., 2014).

---

*See Personal Usage Guide chapter for more details on these primary uses.   =Neat, =Dilute for Children/Sensitive Skin, =Dilute

Orange (or Wild Orange) *Citrus sinensis*

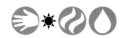

Quick Facts

Botanical Family: Rutaceae (citrus)

Extraction Method: Cold expressed from rind

Common Primary Uses*: Anxiety, Digestion (Sluggish), Fear, Heart Palpitations, Insomnia, Menopause, Nervousness, Uplifting, Withdrawal

Common Application Methods‡:

: Can be applied neat (with no dilution) when used topically. Apply directly on area of concern or to reflex points. Avoid direct sunlight for up to 12 hours after using on skin.

: Diffuse, or inhale the aroma directly.

: Place 1–2 drops under the tongue, or take in a beverage. Take in capsules. Use as a flavoring in cooking.

Chemical Constituents: Monoterpenes (up to 95%): d-Limonene (<90%), terpinolene, myrcene, α-pinene; Tetraterpenes (<8%): β-carotene (<6%), lycopene; Aldehydes (<8%): citral, decanal, citronellal, dodecanal, nonanal, octanal, α-sinensal; Alcohols (<6%): linalool, cis & trans-carveol, α-terpineol, geraniol; Ketones (<4%): 1- & d-carvone (<3%), α-ionone; Esters (<3%): citronellyl acetate, geranyl acetate, linalyl acetate, methyl anthranilate; Furanoids: auraptene, bergaptol, imperatarine; Sesquiterpene Ketones: nootkatone.

Properties: Anticancer, antidepressant, antiseptic, antispasmodic, digestive, sedative, and tonic.

Historical Uses: Oranges, particularly the bitter oranges, have been used for palpitation, scurvy, jaundice, bleeding, heartburn, relaxed throat, prolapse of the uterus and the anus, diarrhea, and blood in the feces.

French Medicinal Uses: Angina (false), cardiac spasm, constipation, diarrhea (chronic), dyspepsia (nervous), insomnia, menopause, palpitation.

Other Possible Uses: This oil may help appetite, bones (rickety), bronchitis, colds, colic (dilute for infants; helps them sleep), complexion (dull and oily), dermatitis, digestive system, fever, flu, lower high cholesterol, mouth ulcers, muscle soreness,

obesity, sedation, tissue repair, water retention, and wrinkles.

Body System(s) Affected: Digestive and Immune Systems, Emotional Balance, Skin.

Aromatic Influence: Orange is calming and uplifting to the mind and body.

Oral Use As Dietary Supplement: Orange oil is generally recognized as safe (GRAS) for human consumption by the FDA (21CFR182.20). Dilute 1 drop oil in 1 tsp. (5 ml) honey or in ½ cup (125 ml) of beverage (e.g., soy/rice milk). Not for children under 6 years old; use with caution and in greater dilution for children 6 years old and over.

Safety Data: Avoid direct sunlight for up to 12 hours after use.

Blend Classification: Enhancer and Personifier.

Blends With: Cinnamon, frankincense, geranium, and lavender.

Odor: Type: Top Note (5–20% of the blend); Scent: Fresh, citrusy, fruity, sweet; Intensity: 1.

Additional Research:

Anxiety: Healthy male subjects displayed reduced anxiety after five minutes of inhalation of orange essential oil compared to the inhalation of melaleuca essential oil or distilled water when submitted to an anxiety inducing situation (Goes et al., 2012).

Anxiety: Rats subjected to the elevated plus-maze following exposure to the aroma of orange essential oil for five minutes displayed reduced anxiety as compared to exposure to melaleuca essential oil (Faturi et al., 2010).

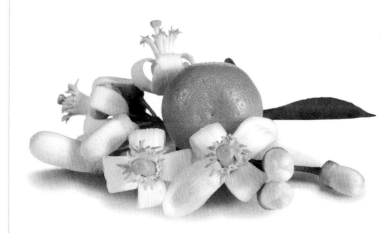

‡See Application section beginning on page 16 for more details on applying essential oils.   =Topical, =Aromatic, =Internal

103

Anxiety: Dental patients (aged 6–9 years) displayed reduce salivary cortisol, pulse rate, and anxiety while undergoing dental treatments when inhaling wild orange essential oil, compared to no aroma (Jafarzadeh et al., 2013).

Anticancer Properties: In a study of older individuals, it was found that there was a dose-dependent relationship between citrus peel consumption (which is high in d-Limonene) and a lower degree of squamous cell carcinoma (SCC) of the skin (Hakim et al., 2000).

Anticancer Properties: In clinical trials, d-Limonene (found in most citrus oils, dill, caraway, citronella, and nutmeg) was found to elicit a response (kept patients stable) in some patients in advanced stages of cancer (1 breast and 3 colorectal carcinoma of 32 total patients). A secondary trial with just breast cancer patients did not elicit any responses (Vigushin et al., 1998).

Sedative Properties: Female patients waiting for dental treatment were found to be less anxious, more positive, and more calm when exposed to orange oil odor than patients who were not exposed to the orange oil odor (Lehrner et al., 2000).

Sedative Properties: Patients waiting for dental treatment were found to be less anxious and to have a better mood when exposed to the odor of lavender or orange oil compared to control (Lehrner et al., 2005).

Addiction: Injection of limonene, a common terpene found in many citrus essential oils, inhibited behavioral manifestations of drug use on rats administered methamphetamine (METH). Examination of the nucleus accumbens of the rats revealed that limonene may produce its effects by regulating dopamine levels and serotonin receptor function (Yun, 2014).

See Personal Usage Guide chapter for more details on these primary uses.   ●=Neat, ●=Dilute for Children/Sensitive Skin, ●=Dilute

Oregano *Origanum vulgare*

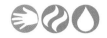

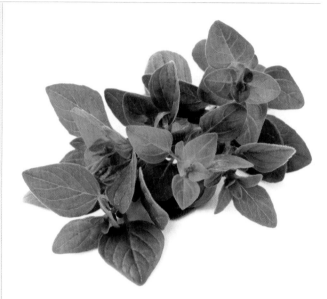

Quick Facts

Botanical Family: Labiatae

Extraction Method: Steam distillation from herb

Common Primary Uses*: Athlete's Foot, Calluses, Candida, Canker Sores, Carpal Tunnel Syndrome, Ebola Virus, Fungal Infections, Immune System (Stimulates), Inflammation⊕, Intestinal Parasites, MRSA, Muscle Aches, Nasal Polyp, Parasites, Plague, Pneumonia, Ringworm, Staph Infection, Vaginal Candida, Viral Infections, Warming (Body), Warts, Whooping Cough

Common Application Methods‡:

🖐: Dilute 1:3 (1 drop essential oil to at least 3 drops carrier oil) when used topically. Dilute more heavily for children over 6 or for those with sensitive skin. Apply directly on area of concern or to reflex points.

🌀: Diffuse, or inhale the aroma directly.

⚪: Dilute and take in capsules. Use as a flavoring in cooking.

Chemical Constituents: Phenols (up to 80%): carvacrol (<75%), thymol (<5%), terpinen-4-ol; Monoterpenes (<25%): p-cymene (<10%), γ-terpinene (<9%), myrcene (<3%), α- and β-pinenes, camphene, l-limonene, α-terpinene; Sesquiterpenes (<6%): β-caryophyllene (<5%), β-bisabolene; Carboxylic Acids: rosmaric acid (<5%); Esters: linalyl acetate (<4%); Ketones: camphor, d-carvone; Alcohols: borneol, linalool, α-terpineol.

Properties: Antibacterial⊕, antifungal⊕, antiparasitic⊕, antiseptic to the respiratory system, antiviral, and immune stimulant⊕.

French Medicinal Uses: Asthma, bronchitis (chronic), mental disease, pulmonary tuberculosis, and rheumatism (chronic).

Other Possible Uses: This oil may help colds, digestive problems, metabolic balance, obesity⊕, viral and bacterial pneumonia, and strengthen vital centers.

🜨 Body System(s) Affected: Immune and Respiratory Systems, Muscles and Bones.

Aromatic Influence: Strengthens one's feeling of security.

Oral Use As Dietary Supplement: Oregano oil is generally recognized as safe (GRAS) for human consumption by the FDA (21CFR182.20). Dilute 1 drop oil in 1 tsp. (5 ml) honey or in ½ cup (125 ml) of beverage (e.g., soy/rice milk). Not for children under 6 years old; use with caution and in greater dilution for children 6 years old and over.

Safety Data: Can cause extreme skin irritation.

Blend Classification: Enhancer and Equalizer.

Blends With: Basil, fennel, geranium, lemongrass, thyme, and rosemary.

Odor: Type: Middle Note (50–80% of the blend); Scent: Herbaceous, sharp; Intensity: 5.

ⓘ **Additional Research:**

Inflammation: Oregano oil was found to alter signal pathways involved in inflammation in a human skin model (Han et al., 2017).

Antibacterial Properties: Oregano oil was found to inhibit MRSA (Nostro et al., 2004).

Antibacterial Properties: Oregano oil was found to kill antibiotic-resistant strains of *Staph, E. coli, Klebsiella pneumoniae, Helicobacter pylori,* and *Mycobacterium terrae* (Preuss et al., 2005).

Antifungal Properties: The vapor of oregano oil was found to be fungicidal against the *Trichophyton mentagrophytes* fungus (a fungus that causes a skin infection known as Malabar itch) (Inouye et al., 2006).

Antifungal Properties: In a test of nine oils, clove (followed by cinnamon, oregano, and mace oils) was found to be inhibitory to two toxin-producing fungi (Juglal et al., 2002).

‡*See Application section beginning on page 16 for more details on applying essential oils.*   🜔=Topical, 🌀=Aromatic, ⚪=Internal

105

Antifungal Properties: Mice infected with *Candida albicans* who were fed origanum oil or carvacrol diluted in olive oil had an 80% survival rate after 30 days, while infected mice fed olive oil alone all died after 10 days (Manohar et al., 2001).

Antifungal Properties: Cinnamon, thyme, oregano, and cumin oils inhibited the production of aflatoxin by aspergillus fungus (Tantaoui-Elaraki et al., 1994).

Antiparasitic Properties: Oregano oil administered orally was found to improve gastrointestinal symptoms in 7 of 11 patients who had tested positive for the parasite *Blastocystis hominis* and caused the disappearance of this parasite in 8 cases (Force et al., 2000).

Immune Stimulant Properties: Growth-retarded pigs receiving a supplementation of oregano leaves and flowers enriched with cold-pressed oregano oil were found to have increased growth, decreased mortality, and higher numbers of immune-system cells and compounds when compared to control pigs who did not receive supplementation (Walter et al., 2004).

Weight—obesity: After 10 weeks of feeding, the body weight gain, visceral fat-pad weights, and final body weights of mice fed a high-fat diet and carvacrol were significantly lower than that of mice fed a high-fat diet without carvacrol (specifically a 24% decrease in final body weight, a 43% decrease in body weight gain, and a 36% decrease in total visceral fat-pad weight was observed when carvacrol was ingested)(Cho et al., 2012). Interestingly, the food intake during the 10-week feeding period did not differ among the groups and mRNA expressions were different between the two groups (Cho et al., 2012).

Antioxidant: The antioxidant activity of oregano essential oil added to extra virgin olive oil at 0.05% was found to retard the lipid oxidation process in olive oil and prolong the olive oil's shelf life (Asensio et al., 2011).

Cats—Antifungal: Four out of seven cats with the fungus mycoses (*Microsporum canis*) recovered both clinically and culturally with topical application of diluted oregano oil for a month (Mugnaini et al., 2012).

Anxiety: Carvacrol is a monoterpenic phenol found in thyme and oregano. Oral administration of carvacrol produced antianxiety-like effects in mice (Melo et al., 2010).

Colon—Colitis: Oral administration of thyme and oregano oil at a dose of 0.2% thyme and 0.1% oregano was found to be effective in decreasing the mortality rate, accelerating body weight gain recovery, and significantly reducing the macroscopic damage of colonic tissue of mice with induced colitis (Bukovska et al., 2007).

*See Personal Usage Guide chapter for more details on these primary uses.   ●=Neat, ●=Dilute for Children/Sensitive Skin, ●=Dilute

Patchouli (or Patchouly) *Pogostemon cablin*

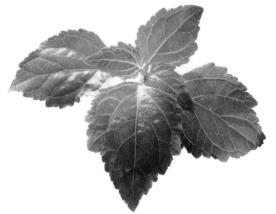

Quick Facts

Botanical Family: Labiatae (mint)

Extraction Method: Steam-distilled from leaves

Common Primary Uses*: ⬤Diuretic, ⬤⬤⬤Fever, ⬤⬤Mosquito Repellent, ⬤⬤Termite Repellent

Common Application Methods‡:

⬤: Can be applied neat (with no dilution) when used topically. Apply directly on area of concern or to reflex points.

⬤: Diffuse, or inhale the aroma directly.

⬤: Take in capsules.

Chemical Constituents: Sesquiterpenes (up to 63%): α-bulnesene (<20%), β-bulnesene (<16%), aromadendrene (<15%), α-gaiene (>12%), seychellene (6%), α-, β- & γ-patchoulenes (<12%), β-caryophyllene (<4%), δ-cadinene (<3%), β-gaiene, β-elemene, humulene; Sesquiterpene Alcohols (<38%): patchoulol (up to 35%), pogostol, bulnesol, guaiol, patchoulenol; Oxides (<5%): bulnesene oxide, caryophyllene oxide, guaiene oxide; Ketones: patchoulenone (<3%); Monoterpenes: α- & β-pinenes, l-limonene.

Properties: Anti-infectious, anti-inflammatory, antifungal, antiseptic, antitoxic, astringent, decongestant, deodorant, diuretic, insecticidal⬤, stimulant (digestive), and tonic.

Historical Uses: For centuries, the Asian people used patchouli to fight infection, cool fevers, tone the skin (and entire body), and to act as an antidote for insect and snake bites. It was also used to treat colds, headaches, nausea, vomiting, diarrhea, abdominal pain, and halitosis (bad breath).

French Medicinal Uses: Allergies, dermatitis, eczema, hemorrhoids, tissue regeneration.

Other Possible Uses: This oil is a digester of toxic material in the body. It may also help acne, appetite (curbs), bites (insect and snake), cellulite, congestion, dandruff, depression, digestive system, relieve itching from hives, mastitis⬤, skin conditions (chapped and tightens loose skin), UV radiation (protects against)⬤, water retention, weeping wounds, weight reduction, and wrinkles prevention.

⬤ **Body System(s) Affected:** Skin.

Aromatic Influence: It is sedating, calming⬤, and relaxing—allowing it to reduce anxiety. It may have some particular influence on sex, physical energy, and money.

Oral Use As Dietary Supplement: Patchouli oil in general is approved by the FDA for use as a Food Additive (FA) and Flavoring Agent (FL). Dilute 1 drop oil in 1 tsp. (5 ml) honey or in ½ cup (125 ml) of beverage (e.g., soy/rice milk). Not for children under 6 years old; use with caution and in greater dilution for children 6 years old and over.

Blend Classification: Enhancer

Blends With: Bergamot, clary sage, frankincense, geranium, ginger, lavender, lemongrass, myrrh, pine, rosewood, sandalwood.

Odor: Type: Base Note (5–20% of the blend); Scent: Earthy, herbaceous, sweet-balsamic, rich, with woody undertones; Intensity: 4.

⬤ **Additional Research:**

Insecticidal Properties: In a test of 34 different essential oils, patchouli (*Pogostemon cablin*) oil proved to be the most effective insecticide against the common house fly (Pavela, 2008).

Insecticidal Properties: Both patchouli oil and its constituent, patchouli alcohol (patchoulol), were found to be repellent and insecticidal to Formosan termites when applied topically (Zhu et al., 2003).

Insecticidal Properties: Clove, citronella, and patchouli oils were found to effectively repel 3 species of mosquitoes (Trongtokit et al., 2005).

Pregnancy/Motherhood—Mastitis: Patchouli alcohol (a tricyclic sesquiterpene and an essential oil of *Pogostemon cablin*) was found to inhibit chemically induced mastitis in a mouse model by inhibiting inflammation, suggesting patchouli may prevent mastitis (Li et al., 2014).

UV Radiation: Patchouli was found to protect the skin's structure and prevent photoaging effects caused by UV radiation in an animal model (Lin et al., 2014).

Calming Aromatic Influence: Inhalation of essential oils such as pepper, estragon, fennel, and grapefruit was found to have a stimulating effect on sympathetic activity, while inhalation of essential oils of rose or patchouli caused a decrease in sympathetic activity in healthy adults (Haze et al., 2002).'

‡*See Application section beginning on page 16 for more details on applying essential oils.*   ⬤=Topical, ⬤=Aromatic, ⬤=Internal

107

Peppermint *Mentha piperita*

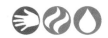

Quick Facts

Botanical Family: Labiatae (mint)

Extraction Method: Steam distillation from leaves

Common Primary Uses*: ◐◖Alertness, ○◐◖Antioxidant, ◐◖Asthma, ◖Autism, ◖Bacterial Infections, ◐◖Bell's Palsy, ◐◖Brain Injury, ◐◖Chronic Fatigue, ○◖Cold Sores, ○◖Colon Polyps, ◐◖Congestion, ◖Constipation, ◐◖Cooling (Body), ◖Cramps/Charley Horses, ◐○Crohn's Disease, ○◖Diarrhea, ◖Dysmenorrhea, ◖Endurance⊕, ◖Fainting, ○◐◖Fever, ◐◖○Flu (Influenza), ○◖Gamma Radiation Exposure⊕, ◐○Gastritis, ◖Halitosis, ◐◖Headaches⊕, ◖Heartburn, ◖Heatstroke, ◖Hernia (Hiatal), ◖Herpes Simplex, ◖Hives, ◖Hot Flashes, ◐◖Huntington's Disease, ◐◖Hypothyroidism, ○◐◖Indigestion, ○◖Irritable Bowel Syndrome⊕, ◖Itching, ◖Jet Lag, ◖Lactation (Decrease Milk Production), ◐◖Memory⊕, ◐◖Migraines, ◖Motion Sickness, ◖MRSA, ◐◖Multiple Sclerosis, ◖Muscle Aches, ◖Muscle Fatigue, ◐◖Myelin Sheath, ◖Nausea⊕, ◐◖Olfactory Loss (Sense of Smell), ◖Osteoporosis, ◐◖Paralysis, ◐◖Rhinitis, ◖Scabies, ◖Sciatica, ◐◖Shock, ◐◖Sinusitis, ◖Surgical Wounds, ◖Swollen Eyes, ◖Tennis Elbow, ◐◖○Throat Infection, ◐◖Typhoid, ○◖Ulcer (Gastric), ◖Varicose Veins, ○◐◖Vomiting

Common Application Methods‡:

◖: Can be applied neat (with no dilution), or dilute 1:1 (1 drop essential oil to 1 drop carrier oil) for children and for those with sensitive skin when using topically. Apply directly on area of concern or to reflex points.

◔: Diffuse, or inhale the aroma directly.

○: Place 1–2 drops under the tongue or in a beverage. Take in capsules. Use as a flavoring in cooking.

Chemical Constituents: Phenolic Alcohols (up to 44%): menthol (<44%), piperitols; Ketones (<25%): menthone (20–30% and up to 65% if distilled in September when flowering), pulegone (<5%), piperitone (<2%), carvone, jasmone; Monoterpenes (< 15%): α and β-pinenes (<6%), l-limonene (<6%), ocimene, myrcene, p-cymene,

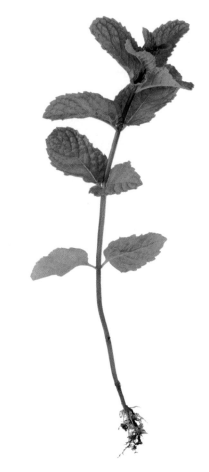

β-phellandrene, sabinene, α-terpinene, terpinolene, camphene; Sesquiterpenes (<10%): germacrene-D (<5%), β-bourbonene, ζ-bulgarene, γ-cadinene, β-caryophyllene, β-elemene, β-farnesene, muurolene; Esters (<9%): menthyl acetate (<9%), also menthyl butyrate & isovalerate; Oxides (<9%): 1,8 cineol (<5%), piperitone oxide, caryophyllene oxide; Furanoids: menthofuran (<8%); Phenols: terpinen-4-ol (<3%); Alcohols (<3%): α-terpineol, linalool; Sesquiterpene Alcohols: viridiflorol; Furanocoumarins: aesculetin; Sulphides: mint sulfide, dimenthyl sulfide.

Properties: Analgesic, antibacterial⊕, anticarcinogenic, anti-inflammatory⊕, antiseptic, antispasmodic⊕, antiviral⊕, and invigorating.

Historical Uses: For centuries, peppermint has been used to soothe digestive difficulties, freshen breath, and to relieve colic, gas, headaches, heartburn, and indigestion.

---

*See Personal Usage Guide chapter for more details on these primary uses.   ●=Neat, ●=Dilute for Children/Sensitive Skin, ●=Dilute

French Medicinal Uses: Asthma, bronchitis, candida, diarrhea, digestion (aids)⊕, fever (reduces), flu, halitosis, heartburn, hemorrhoids, hot flashes, indigestion⊕, menstrual irregularity, migraine headache, motion sickness, nausea, respiratory function (aids), shock, skin (itchy), throat infection, varicose veins, vomiting.

Other Possible Uses: This oil may help anger, arthritis, colic, depression, fatigue, food poisoning, hysteria, inflammation, liver problems, nerves⊕ (regenerate and support), rheumatism, seizures⊕, elevate and open sensory system, soothe and cool skin (may help keep body cooler on hot days), toothaches, tuberculosis, and add flavor to water.

Body System(s) Affected: Digestive System, Muscles and Bones, Nervous and Respiratory Systems, Skin.

Aromatic Influence: It is purifying and stimulating to the conscious mind and may aid with memory and mental performance. It is cooling and may help reduce fevers.

Oral Use As Dietary Supplement: Peppermint oil is generally recognized as safe (GRAS) for human consumption by the FDA (21CFR182.20). Dilute 1 drop oil in 1 tsp. (5 ml) honey or in ½ cup (125 ml) of beverage (e.g., soy/rice milk). Not for children under 6 years old; use with caution and in greater dilution for children 6 years old and over.

Safety Data: Repeated use can possibly result in contact sensitization. Use with caution if dealing with high blood pressure. Use with caution during pregnancy.

Blend Classification: Personifier

Blends With: Basil, black pepper, cinnamon, cypress, dill, grapefruit, juniper berry, lavender, lemon, rosemary, spearmint, tea tree.

Odor: Type: Middle Note (50–80% of the blend); Scent: Minty, sharp, intense; Intensity: 5.

⊕ **Additional Research:**

Endurance: A quasi experiment comparing exercise performance before and after consumption of mineral water containing peppermint essential oil for 10 days found that exercise performance improved after consumption of peppermint oil (including increases in respiratory efficiency, energy expenditure, time to exhaustion, and distance during exercise and decreases in resting and exercise heart rates) (Meamarbashi et al., 2013).

Gamma Radiation Exposure: In mice exposed to whole-body gamma irradiation, only 17% of mice who had been fed peppermint oil died, while 100% of mice who did not receive peppermint oil died. It was also found that mice pre-fed peppermint oil were able to return blood cell levels to normal after 30 days, while control mice were not (and consequently died), suggesting a protective or stimulating effect of the oil on blood stem cells (Samarth et al., 2004).

Gamma Radiation Exposure: Peppermint extract fed orally to mice demonstrated the ability to protect the testis from gamma radiation damage (Samarth et al., 2009).

Gamma Radiation Exposure: Mice pretreated with peppermint leaf extract demonstrated less bone marrow cell loss than mice not pretreated with peppermint when exposed to gamma radiation (Samarth et al., 2007).

Headaches: A combination of peppermint oil and ethanol was found to have a significant analgesic effect with a reduction in sensitivity to headache; while a combination of peppermint, eucalyptus, and ethanol was found to relax muscles and to increase cognitive performance in humans (Göbel et al., 1994).

Irritable Bowel Syndrome: In irritable bowel syndrome patients without bacterial overgrowth, lactose intolerance, or celiac disease, peppermint oil was found to reduce IBS symptoms significantly more than a placebo over 8 weeks (Cappello et al., 2007).

Irritable Bowel Syndrome: Children suffering from irritable bowel syndrome (IBS) who received peppermint oil in enteric-coated capsules (encapsulated so the capsules wouldn't open until they reached the intestines) reported a reduced severity of pain associated with IBS (Kline et al., 2001).

Irritable Bowel Syndrome: Patients with IBS symptoms who took a peppermint-oil formulation in an enteric-coated capsule were found to have a significantly higher reduction of symptoms compared to patients taking a placebo (Liu et al., 1997).

Irritable Bowel Syndrome: Peppermint oil in enteric-coated capsules was found to relieve symptoms of irritable bowel syndrome better than a placebo in patients suffering from IBS (Rees et al., 1979).

Memory: In human trials, the aroma of peppermint was found to enhance memory and to increase alertness (Moss et al., 2008).

Nausea: Oral administration of capsules containing two drops of either spearmint or peppermint oil to cancer patients during chemotherapy cycles was found to reduce the intensity of nausea when compared to the control (Tayarani-Najaran et al., 2013).

Antibacterial Properties: Subjects using a mouthwash containing thymol, menthol, methyl salicylate, and eucalyptol for 6 months were found to not have developed oral bacteria that were resistant to the oils (Charles et al., 2000).

Antibacterial Properties: Peppermint and spearmint oil inhibited resistant strains of *Staphylococcus, E. Coli, Salmonella,* and *Helicobacter pylori* (Imai et al., 2001).

Antibacterial Properties: Peppermint and rosemary oils were each found to be more effective at preventing dental biofilm (plaque) formation than chlorhexidine (an antiseptic) (Rasooli et al., 2008).

Antibacterial Properties: Peppermint oil blended with toothpaste was found to be more effective at lower concentrations in inhibiting the formation of dental plaque than chlorhexidine (an antiseptic) in human volunteers (Shayegh et al., 2008).

Anti-inflammatory Properties: A combination of peppermint and caraway oil was found to reduce visceral hyperalgesia (pain hypersensitivity in the gastrointestinal tract) after induced inflammation in rats (Adam et al., 2006).

Anti-inflammatory Properties: L-menthol was found to inhibit production of inflammation mediators in human monocytes (a type of white blood cell involved in the immune response) (Juergens et al., 1998).

Antispasmodic Properties: Peppermint oil was found to be as effective as Buscopan (an antispasmodic drug) at preventing spasms during a barium enema (a type of enema used to place barium in the colon for X-ray imaging purposes) (Asao et al., 2003).

Antiviral Properties: Peppermint oil demonstrated a direct virucidal activity against Herpes type 1 and 2 viruses (Schuhmacher et al., 2003).

Digestion (aid): The use of rosemary, lemon, and peppermint oils in massage demonstrated an ability to reduce constipation and to increase bowel movements in elderly subjects compared to massage without the oils (Kim et al., 2005).

Indigestion: In patients with dyspepsia (indigestion), treatments with capsules containing peppermint and caraway oil were found to decrease pain and pain frequency (Freise et al., 1999).

Indigestion: An enteric-coated capsule with peppermint and caraway oil was found to reduce pain and symptoms in patients with non-ulcer dyspepsia (indigestion) compared to a control (May et al., 1996).

Nerves: Pretreatment of human and rat astrocyte cells (cells found in the nerve and brain that support the blood-brain barrier and help repair the brain and spinal cord following injuries) with peppermint oil was found to inhibit heat-shock-induced apoptosis of these cells (Koo et al., 2001).

Seizure: Mice pretreated with an injection of peppermint essential oil demonstrated no seizures and 100% post-treatment survival after being injected with a lethal dose of pentylenetetrazol (PTZ) to cause seizures (Koutroumanidou et al., 2013).

‡See Application section beginning on page 16 for more details on applying essential oils. ❂=Topical, ❂=Aromatic, ○=Internal

Essential Oils

Petitgrain *Citrus aurantium*

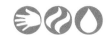

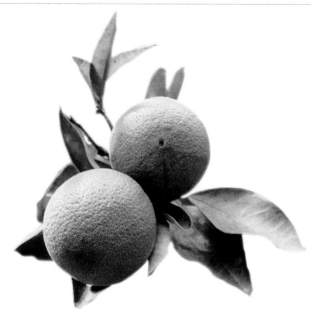

Quick Facts

Botanical Family: Rutaceae (citrus)

Extraction Method: Steam distillation from leaves

Common Primary Uses*: Depression, Focus, Greasy/Oily Hair, Stress, Uplifting

Common Application Methods‡:

: Can be applied neat (with no dilution) when used topically. Apply directly on area of concern or to reflex points.

: Diffuse, or inhale the aroma directly.

: Take a small amount in capsules.

Chemical Constituents: Esters (up to 65%): linalyl acetate (<55%), geranyl acetate (<5%), neryl & α-terpenyl acetates, methyl anthranilate; Alcohols (40%): linalool (<28%), α-terpineol (<8%), geraniol (<5%), nerol, citronellol; Monoterpenes (<28%): myrcene (<6%), β-cymene (<5%), cis- & trans-ocimenes (<5%), p-cymene (<3%), β-pinene, γ-terpinene, d-limonene, phellandrene, sabinene, terpinolene; Aldehydes: decanal, geranial, neral; Phenols: thymol, terpinen-4-ol; Furanocoumarins: bergaptene, citroptene.

Properties: Antibacterial, anti-infectious, anti-inflammatory, antioxidant, antiseptic, antispasmodic, deodorant, and stimulant (digestive, nervous).

Historical Uses: Petitgrain (from the French term *petit grain*, meaning "small grain") derives its name from the extraction of the oil, which at one time was from the green unripe oranges when they were still about the size of a cherry. This oil is now derived from the plant's leaves. Because of its very pleasing scent, petitgrain has been used extensively in high-quality perfumes and cosmetics.

Other Possible Uses: This oil may help with acne, dyspepsia, fatigue, flatulence, greasy hair, insomnia, and excessive perspiration.

Body System(s) Affected: Emotional Balance.

Aromatic Influence: Petitgrain is uplifting and refreshing and helps to refresh the senses, clear confusion, reduce mental fatigue, and reduce depression. It may also help stimulate the mind, support memory, and gladden the heart.

Oral Use As Dietary Supplement: Petitgrain is generally regarded as safe (GRAS) for use in small amounts as a flavoring or additive in foods by the FDA. Dilute 1 drop oil in 1 tsp. (5 ml) honey or in ½ cup (125 ml) of beverage (e.g., soy/rice milk). Not for children under 6 years old; use with caution and in greater dilution for children 6 years old and over.

Safety Data: May cause slight skin irritation in some individuals.

Blend Classification: Enhancer, Modifier, and Personifier.

Blends With: Bergamot, clary sage, clove, geranium, jasmine, lavender, orange, and rosemary.

Odor: Type: Top Note (5–20% of the blend); Scent: Fresh, floral, citrusy, lighter in fragrance than neroli and slightly woody; Intensity: 3.

Additional Research:

Antibacterial: *Citrus aurantium* leaf essential oils were found to have antibacterial effects on *Escherichia coli*, *Bacillus subtilis*, and *Staphylococcus aureus* in vitro (Ellouze et al., 2012).

Antioxidant: Petitgrain oil was found to demonstrate free radical–scavenging activity in a DPPH test, with oil from older leaves demonstrating the greatest activity (Sarrou et al., 2013).

Sedative: Extracts from *Citrus aurantium* leaf were found to have sedating properties in animal models of sedation (Carvalho-Freitas et al., 2002).

---

*See Personal Usage Guide chapter for more details on these primary uses.   ●=Neat, ●=Dilute for Children/Sensitive Skin, ●=Dilute

Pink Pepper *Schinus molle*

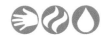

Quick Facts

Botanical Family: Anacardiaceae

Extraction Method: Steam distillation from fruit

Common Primary Uses*: Alertness, Antibacterial, Cleaning

Common Application Methods‡:

: Can be applied neat (with no dilution) when used topically. Apply directly on area of concern or to reflex points.

: Diffuse, or inhale the aroma directly.

: Add 1 drop to 1 cup (250 ml) of water, tea, or other beverage.

Chemical Constituents: Monoterpenes (up to 80%): α- & β-phellandrene, limonene, myrcene, α-pinene, p-cymene; Sesquiterpenes (up to 15%): α- & β-caryophyllene, α-humulene, others; Sesquiterpinols (up to 10%): viridiflorol, spathulenol, t-cadinol, t-muurolol, elemol.

Properties: Antibacterial, antifungal, anti-inflammatory, antitumor, antiviral, antimicrobial, antispasmodic, astringent, diuretic, stimulant (digestive), and wound healing.

Historical Uses: According to Leslie Taylor, ND, "Virtually all parts of this tropical tree, including its leaves, bark, fruit, seeds, resin, and oleoresin (or balsam), have been used medicinally by indigenous peoples throughout the tropics."

Other Possible Uses: This oil may help with bronchitis, cancer, diabetes (high blood sugar), gingivitis, gonorrhea, gout, heart problems (hypertension and irregular heart beat), inflammation (general), insects (repellent), menstrual disorders (excessive bleeding), pain relief, rheumatism, sores, swelling, tuberculosis, tumors, ulcers, urethritis, urogenital disorders, venereal diseases, warts, and wounds.

Body System(s) Affected: Immune System, Respiratory System, Skin.

Aromatic Influence: Pink pepper has a warm, spicy aroma that can help increase alertness.

Oral Use As Dietary Supplement: Pink pepper oil is generally regarded as safe (GRAS) for human consumption by the FDA. Dilute 1 drop oil in 1

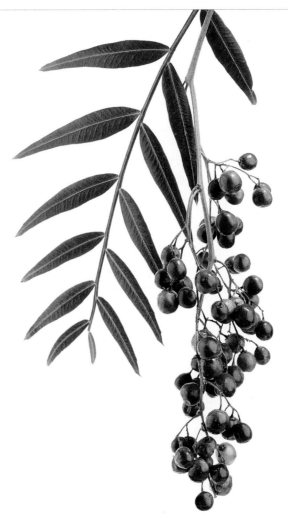

tsp. (5 ml) honey or in 1 cup (250 ml) of beverage (e.g., soy/rice milk). Not for children under 6 years old; use with caution and in greater dilution for children 6 years old and over.

Safety Data: May irritate highly sensitive skin. Consult with a physician before using if taking medications, pregnant, or nursing.

Blends With: Fennel, frankincense, lavender, marjoram, rosemary, sandalwood, and other spice oils.

Odor: Type: Middle Note (50–80% of the blend); Scent: spicy, fruity, with slight woody undertone; Intensity: 3.

Additional Research:

Antibacterial: Schinus molle essential oil was found to demonstrate antibacterial properties against several strains of gram-positive and gram-negative bacteria (Martins et al., 2014; Guerra-Boone et al., 2013; Gundidza, 1993).

Cancer: Oil from Schinus molle was found to inhibit leukemia and breast cancer cell lines in laboratory tests (Lin et al., 2015, Diaz et al., 2008).

Insects: Pink pepper essential oil was found to be insecticidal and repellant to several varieties of beetles and fleas (Benzi et al., 2009; Abdel-Sattar et al., 2010; Batista et al., 2016).

‡See Application section beginning on page 16 for more details on applying essential oils.   =Topical, =Aromatic, =Internal

111

Roman Chamomile *Chamaemelum nobile or Anthemis nobilis*

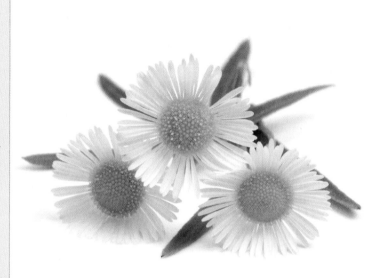

Quick Facts

Botanical Family: Compositae (daisy)

Extraction Method: Steam distillation from flowers

Common Primary Uses*: ⊖Bee/Hornet Stings, ⊘⊖Calming⊕, ⊖Club Foot, ⊖Dysentery, ⊘⊖Hyperactivity, ⊘⊖Insomnia, ⊖Menopause, ⊖Muscle Spasms, ⊖Neuralgia, ⊖Neuritis, ⊙⊖Parasites, ⊖Rashes, ⊖Sciatica, ⊖Shock, ⊖Skin (Dry), ⊖Sore Nipples

Common Application Methods‡:

⋐: Can be applied neat (with no dilution), or dilute 1:1 (1 drop essential oil to 1 drop carrier oil) for children and for those with sensitive skin when using topically.

⧀: Diffuse, or inhale the aroma directly.

◍: Take in capsules.

Chemical Constituents: Esters (up to 75%): isobutyl angelate (up to 25%), isoamyl methacylate (up to 25%), amyl butyrate (<15%), other angelate, butyrate, acetate, and tiglate esters; Monoterpenes (<35%): α- & β-pinenes (<20%), terpinenes, sabinene, camphene, d-Limonene, p-cymene, myrcene; Ketones: pinocarvone (14%); Sesquiterpenes (up to 12%): β-caryophyllene, chamazulene; Alcohols (>7%): trans-pinocarveol, farnesol, nerolidol.

Properties: Anti-infectious, anti-inflammatory⊕, antiparasitic, antispasmodic⊕, calming, and relaxing.

Historical Uses: It was traditionally used by the ancient Romans to give them a clear mind and to empower them with courage for their battles. According to Roberta Wilson, "Chamomile was nicknamed the 'plant's physician' because it supposedly cured any ailing plant placed near it."

French Medicinal Uses: Intestinal parasites, neuritis, neuralgia, shock (nervous).

Other Possible Uses: Chamomile neutralizes allergies and increases the ability of the skin to regenerate. It is a cleanser of the blood and also helps the liver to reject poisons and to discharge them. This oil may help with allergies, bruises, cuts, depression, insomnia, muscle tension, nerves (calming and promoting nerve health), restless legs, and skin conditions such as acne, boils, dermatitis, eczema, rashes, and sensitive skin. Chamomile is mild enough to use on infants and children. For centuries, mothers have used chamomile to calm crying children, ease earaches, fight fevers, soothe stomachaches and colic, and relieve toothaches and teething pain. It can safely and effectively reduce irritability and minimize nervousness in children, especially hyperactive children.

✛ **Body System(s) Affected:** Emotional Balance, Nervous System, Skin.

Aromatic Influence: Because it is calming and relaxing, it can combat depression, insomnia⊕, and stress. It eliminates some of the emotional charge of anxiety, irritability, and nervousness. It may also be used to soothe and clear the mind, creating an atmosphere of peace and patience.

Oral Use As Dietary Supplement: Roman chamomile oil is generally recognized as safe (GRAS) for human consumption by the FDA (21CFR182.20). Dilute 1 drop oil in 1 tsp. (5 ml) honey or in ½ cup (125 ml) of beverage (e.g., soy/rice milk). Not for children under 6 years old; use with caution and in greater dilution for children 6 years old and over.

---

*See Personal Usage Guide chapter for more details on these primary uses.   ●=Neat, ●=Dilute for Children/Sensitive Skin, ●=Dilute

Safety Data: Can irritate sensitive skin.

Blend Classification: Personifier

Blends With: Lavender, rose, geranium, and clary sage.

Odor: Type: Middle Note (50–80% of the blend); Scent: Fresh, sweet, fruity-herbaceous, apple-like, no tenacity; Intensity: 4.

Additional Research:

Anxiety and Sleep: A study with 56 percutaneous coronary intervention patients in an intensive care unit found that an aromatherapy blend of lavender, Roman chamomile, and neroli decreased anxiety and improved sleep quality when compared to conventional nursing intervention (Cho et al., 2013).

Anti-inflammatory Properties: Chamazulene, a chemical in chamomile oil, was found to block formation of leukotriene (a signaling chemical involved in the inflammation process) in neutrophilic (immune system) granulocytes (white blood cells containing granules). It also demonstrated an antioxidant effect (Safayhi et al., 1994).

Antispasmodic: Roman chamomile essential oil demonstrated a relaxant effect on smooth muscle cells in vitro (Sándor et al., 2018).

‡*See Application section beginning on page 16 for more details on applying essential oils.*   ⟳=Topical, ⊘=Aromatic, ◯=Internal

113

Rose *Rosa damascena*

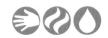

Quick Facts

Botanical Family: Rosaceae

Extraction Method: Steam distillation from flowers (a two-part process)

Common Primary Uses*: Anxiety, Aphrodisiac, Poison Ivy/Oak, Scarring (Prevention)

Common Application Methods‡:

: Can be applied neat (with no dilution) when used topically. Apply directly on area of concern or to reflex points.

: Diffuse, or inhale the aroma directly.

: Take in capsules. Use as a flavoring in cooking.

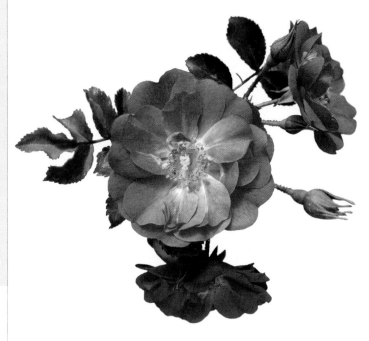

Chemical Constituents: Alcohols (up to 70%): citronellol (up to 45%), geraniol (up to 28%), nerol (<9%), linalool, borneol, α-terpineol; Monoterpenes (<25%): stearoptene (<22%), α & β-pinenes, camphene, α-terpinene, l-limonene, myrcene, p-cymene, ocimene; Alkanes (<19%): nonadecane (<15%), octadecane, eicosane, and others; Esters (<5%): geranyl, neryl, and citronellyl acetates; Phenols (<4%): eugenol, phenylethanol; Sesquiterpene Alcohols: farnesol (<2%); Oxides: rose oxide; Ketones: α- & β-damascenone, β-ionone; Furanoids: rosefuran; Many other trace elements.

Properties: Antihemorrhagic, anti-infectious, aphrodisiac, and sedative.

Historical Uses: The healing properties of the rose have been utilized in medicine throughout the ages and still play an important role in the East. Rose has been used for digestive and menstrual problems, headaches and nervous tension, liver congestion, poor circulation, fever (plague), eye infections, and skin complaints.

Other Possible Uses: This oil may help aging, asthma, chronic bronchitis, frigidity, gingivitis, hemorrhaging, herpes simplex, impotence, infections, lower-back pain (pregnancy), opioid addiction, prevent scarring, seizures, sexual debilities, skin disease, sprains, thrush, tuberculosis, ulcers, wounds, and wrinkles.

Body System(s) Affected: Emotional Balance, Skin.

Aromatic Influence: It is stimulating and elevating to the mind, creating a sense of well-being. Its beautiful fragrance is almost intoxicating and aphrodisiac-like.

Oral Use As Dietary Supplement: Rose oil is generally recognized as safe (GRAS) for human consumption by the FDA (21CFR182.20). Dilute 1 drop oil in 1 tsp. (5 ml) honey or in ½ cup (125 ml) of beverage (e.g., soy/rice milk). Not for children under 6 years old; use with caution and in greater dilution for children 6 years old and over.

Safety Data: Use with caution during pregnancy.

Blend Classification: Personifier, Enhancer, Equalizer, and Modifier

Blends With: bergamot, cedarwood, cinnamon, clary sage, clove, fennel, frankincense, geranium, jasmine, lavender, melissa, myrrh, patchouli, petitgrain, vetiver, ylang ylang.

---

*See Personal Usage Guide chapter for more details on these primary uses.   ●=Neat, ●=Dilute for Children/Sensitive Skin, ●=Dilute

Odor: Type: Middle to Base Notes (20–80% of the blend); Scent: Floral, spicy, rich, deep, sensual, green, honey-like; Intensity: 3.

Additional Research:

Anxiety: Inhalation and a warm foot bath with rose oil was found to decrease anziety levels in women during the first stage of labor (Kheirkhah et al., 2014).

Anxiety: Self-massage with rose oil was found to help decrease pain and anxiety in women experiencing menstrual pain (Kim et al., 2011).

Sedative Properties: Rose oil was found to have effects similar to the antianxiety drug diazepam (Valium) in mice but through a different cellular mechanism (Umezu, 1999).

Digestive System: Rose essential oil and its main constituents were found to inhibit rat isolated ileum (a section of the small intestine), suggesting that rose oil can be used as an antispasmodic remedy for treatment of abdominal spasm (Sadraei et al., 2013).

Female-Specific Conditions—Dysmenorrhea: A study with 92 university age female students with primary dysmenorrhea found that ingestion of a capsule containing 200 mg of Rosa damascena extract every 6 hours at the first 3 days of menstruation was as effective as administration of Mefenamic acid (a drug with possible adverse reactions and side effects) (Bani et al., 2014).

PMS: In a study with 66 female participants, aromatherapy with rose oil twice a day for a total of five days during the luteal phase proved to improve psychological, physical, and social PMS symptoms compared with baseline (Heydari et al., 2018).

Brain—Aging: The chloroform extract of *Rosa damascena* was found to cause neurite outgrowth activity in rat cortical neurons subjected to neurotic atrophy conditions. These findings suggest that *Rosa damascena* possesses neuronal protective properties that may benefit persons with dementia (Awale et al., 2011).

Aging—Memory: Oral administration of Rosa damascena extract for one month was found to enhance adult neurogenesis, hippocampal volume, and synaptic plasticity, as well as reverse the amyloid-β-associated memory abnormalities in a rat model of amyloid-β-induced Alzheimer's disease. These results indicate that rose extract may have memory-enhancing ability (Esfandiary et al., 2014).

Lower-Back Pain: Topical administration of rose oil in pregnant women with low back pain demonstrated a significant decrease in pain intensity and functional ability compared to placebo and no intervention. (Shirazi et al., 2016).

Opioid Addiction: Rose oil demonstrated an ability to reduce morphine (an opioid) withdrawal symptoms in mice. (Abbasi et al., 2013).

Seizure: Aqueous and ethanolic extracts of Rosa damascena were found to have potential anticonvulsant effect in drug-induced seizure model mice (Hosseini et al., 2011).

Seizure: Injection of rose essential oil before induction of amygdala kindling seizures in male rats significantly retarded the development of seizure stages and possessed the ability to counteract kindling stimulation when compared to the control group (Ramezani et al., 2008).

‡*See Application section beginning on page 16 for more details on applying essential oils.*   ⬢=Topical, ⬡=Aromatic, ⬤=Internal

115

Rosemary *Rosmarinus officinalis CT 1,8 Cineol*

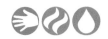

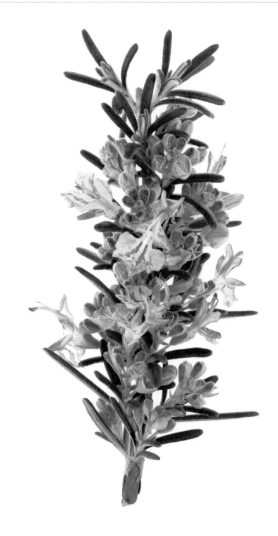

Quick Facts

Botanical Family: Labiatae (mint)

Extraction Method: Steam distillation from flowering plant

Common Primary Uses*: ⊘⊘Addictions (Alcohol), ⊘Adenitis, O⊘⊘Antioxidant, ⊘Arterial Vasodilator, ⊘⊘Arthritis, ⊘⊘Bell's Palsy, ⊘⊘Cancer, ⊘Cellulite, ⊘⊘Chemical Stress, ⊘Cholera, ⊘Club Foot, ⊘Constipation, ⊘Detoxification, ⊘⊘Diabetes, ⊘Diuretic, ⊘Fainting, ⊘⊘Fatigue, ⊘⊘Flu (Influenza), ⊘Greasy/Oily Hair, ⊘Hair (Loss), ⊘⊘Headaches, ⊘Inflammation, ⊘Kidney Infection, ⊘Lice, ⊘⊘Low Blood Pressure⊕, ⊘⊘Memory, ⊘Muscular Dystrophy, ⊘Osteoarthritis, ⊘Schmidt's Syndrome, ⊘⊘Sinusitis, ⊘Vaginal Infection, ⊘Vaginitis, ⊘⊘Viral Hepatitis, ⊘OWorms

Common Application Methods‡:

⊘: Can be applied neat (with no dilution), or dilute 1:1 (1 drop essential oil to 1 drop carrier oil) for children and for those with sensitive skin when used topically. Apply directly on area of concern or to reflex points. Avoid use during pregnancy.

⊘: Diffuse, or inhale the aroma directly.

O: Take in capsules, or place 1–2 drops under the tongue. Use as a flavoring in cooking.

Chemical Constituents: Oxides: 1,8 cineol (up to 55%), caryophyllene oxide, humulene oxide; Monoterpenes: α-pinene (<14%), β-pinene (<9%), camphene (<8%), l-limonene, myrcene, p-cymene, α- & β-phellandrenes, α- & γ-terpinenes; Ketones (<32%): camphor (<30%), β-thujone, verbenone, d-carvone, hexanone, heptanone; Alcohols (<20%): borneol (<12%), α-terpineol (<5%), linalool, verbenol; Sesquiterpenes (<3%): β-caryophyllene, humulene; Phenols: terpinen-4-ol; Esters: bornyl and fenchyl acetates; Acids: rosemaric acid.

Properties: Analgesic⊕, antibacterial⊕, anticancer⊕, anticatarrhal, antifungal⊕, anti-infectious, anti-inflammatory⊕, antioxidant⊕, and expectorant.

Historical Uses: The rosemary plant was regarded as sacred by many civilizations. It was used as a fumigant to help drive away evil spirits and to protect against plague and infectious illness.

French Medicinal Uses: Arthritis⊕, blood pressure (low), bronchitis⊕, cellulite, cholera, colds, dandruff, depression (nervous)⊕, diabetes, fatigue (nervous/mental), flu, fluid retention, hair loss⊕, headache, hepatitis (viral), menstrual periods (irregular), sinusitis, tachycardia, vaginitis.

Other Possible Uses: This oil may help arteriosclerosis, bronchitis, chills, colds, colitis, cystitis, dyspepsia, nervous exhaustion, immune system (stimulate), otitis, palpitations, prevent respiratory infections, sour stomach, stress-related illness⊕. Note: This chemotype is said to be best used for

*See Personal Usage Guide chapter for more details on these primary uses.   ●=Neat, ●=Dilute for Children/Sensitive Skin, ●=Dilute

116

pulmonary congestion, slow elimination, candida, chronic fatigue, and infections (especially staph and strep).

Body System(s) Affected: Immune, Respiratory, and Nervous Systems.

Aromatic Influence: Stimulates memory and opens the conscious mind.

Oral Use As Dietary Supplement: Rosemary oil is generally recognized as safe (GRAS) for human consumption by the FDA (21CFR182.20). Dilute 1 drop oil in 1 tsp. (5 ml) honey or in ½ cup (125 ml) of beverage (e.g., soy/rice milk). Not for children under 6 years old; use with caution and in greater dilution for children 6 years old and over.

Safety Data: Avoid during pregnancy. Not for use by people with epilepsy. Avoid if dealing with high blood pressure.

Blend Classification: Enhancer

Blends With: Basil, frankincense, lavender, peppermint, eucalyptus, and marjoram.

Odor: Type: Middle Note (50–80% of the blend); Scent: Herbaceous, strong, camphorous, with woody-balsamic and evergreen undertones; Intensity: 3.

Additional Research:

Blood Pressure—Low: Oral treatment with rosemary essential oil on primary hypotensive subjects was found to increase blood pressure values when compared to the subjects' placebo treatments before and after rosemary treatment (Fernández et al., 2014).

Analgesic Properties: An ethanol extract of rosemary was found to demonstrate antinociceptive (pain-blocking) and anti-inflammatory activity in mice and rats (González-Trujano et al., 2007).

Antibacterial Properties: Peppermint and rosemary oils were each found to be more effective at preventing dental biofilm (plaque) formation than chlorhexidine (an antiseptic) (Rasooli et al., 2008).

Anticancer Properties: An ethanol extract of rosemary was found to have an antiproliferative effect on human leukemia and breast carcinoma cells, as well as an antioxidant effect (Cheung et al., 2007).

Anticancer Properties: Rosemary extract injected in rats was found to decrease mammary adenocarcinomas in rats (Singletary et al., 1996).

Anticancer Properties: Carnosic acid (derived from rosemary) was found to inhibit the proliferation of human leukemia cells in vitro (Steiner et al., 2001).

Antifungal Properties: Rosemary oil was found to inhibit aflatoxin production by aspergillus fungi (a highly toxic and carcinogenic substance produced by these fungi (Rasooli et al., 2008).

Anti-inflammatory Properties: Rosemary oil was found to have anti-inflammatory and peripheral antinociceptive (pain-sensitivity-blocking) properties in mice (Takaki et al., 2008).

Antioxidant Properties: Extracts from rosemary were found to have high antioxidant properties. Rosmarinic acid and carnosic acid from rosemary were found to have the highest antioxidant activities of studied components of rosemary (Almela et al., 2006).

Antioxidant Properties: Extracts from rosemary were found to have high antioxidant levels (Moreno et al., 2006).

Antioxidant Properties: An ethanol extract of rosemary demonstrated a protective effect against the oxidative damage to DNA in cells exposed to H2O2 and light-excited methylene blue (Slamenova et al., 2002).

Arthritis: In patients suffering from arthritis, it was found that a blend of lavender, marjoram, eucalyptus, rosemary, peppermint, and carrier oils reduced perceived pain and depression compared to control (Kim et al., 2005).

Bronchitis: In patients with chronic bronchitis, rosemary, basil, fir, and eucalyptus oils were found to demonstrate an antioxidant effect. Lavender was found to promote normalization of lipid levels (Siurin, 1997).

Depression: Many fractions of *Rosmarinus officinalis*, including its essential oil, were found to have antidepressant-like effects on mice submitted to two stress tests after oral administration of the rosemary plant fractions (Machado et al., 2013).

Hair Loss: Patients with alopecia areata (hair loss) that massaged carrier oils containing a blend of thyme, rosemary, lavender, and cedarwood oils into their scalps were more likely to show improvement when compared to a control group that massaged carrier oils alone into their scalps (Hay et al., 1998).

Memory: Subjects exposed to rosemary aroma were more alert and completed math computations faster than subjects not exposed to the aroma (Diego et al., 1998).

Memory: Volunteers completing a battery of tests were found to be more content when exposed to lavender and rosemary aromas. Rosemary aroma also was found to enhance quality of memory compared to control (Moss et al., 2003).

Stress: Mice who inhaled rosemary oil were found to exhibit less stress-related behaviors in a tail suspension test than mice whot didn't (Villareal et al., 2017).

Stress-related Illness: Rosemary oil demonstrated a relaxant effect on smooth muscle from the trachea of rabbit and guinea pig (Aqel, 1991).

Liver—Cirrhosis: Daily administration of rosemary essential oil displayed a protective effect against chemical-induced liver injury in rats (Ra Kovi et al., 2014).

Bone: Oral intake of rosemary or eucalyptus essential oil (as well as several monoterpenes found in other essential oils) was shown to inhibit bone resorption in rats (Mühlbauer et al., 2003).

Colon—Colitis: Rosemary essential oil was found to be effective in reducing colon tissue lesions and colitis indices when administered orally or intraperitoneally to rats induced with colitis, suggesting that rosemary has anti-colitic activity (Minaiyan et al., 2011).

‡*See Application section beginning on page 16 for more details on applying essential oils.*   ◐=Topical, ◐=Aromatic, ○=Internal

117

Sandalwood *Santalum album*

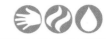

Quick Facts

Botanical Family: Santalaceae (sandalwood)

Extraction Method: Steam distillation from wood

Common Primary Uses*: Alzheimer's Disease, Aphrodisiac, Back Pain, Cancer, Cartilage Repair, Coma, Confusion, Exhaustion, Fear, Hair (Dry), Hiccups, Laryngitis, Lou Gehrig's Disease, Meditation, Moles, Multiple Sclerosis, Rashes, Skin (Dry), Ultraviolet Radiation, Vitiligo, Yoga

Common Application Methods‡:

🖐: Can be applied neat (with no dilution) when used topically. Apply directly on area of concern or to reflex points.

🌀: Diffuse, or inhale the aroma directly.

⭘: Take in capsules.

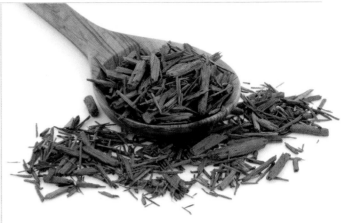

Chemical Constituents: Sesquiterpene Alcohols: α- & β-santalols (<80%); Sesquiterpenes: α- & β-santalenes (<11%); Sesquiterpene Aldehydes: teresantalal (<3%); Carboxylic Acids: nortricycloekasantalic acid (<2%).

Properties: Antidepressant, antiseptic, antitumor, aphrodisiac, astringent, calming, sedative, and tonic.

Historical Uses: Sandalwood was traditionally used as an incense during ritual work for enhancing meditation. The Egyptians also used sandalwood for embalming.

French Medicinal Uses: Bronchitis (chronic), diarrhea (obstinate), hemorrhoids, impotence.

Other Possible Uses: Sandalwood is very similar to frankincense in action. It may support the cardiovascular system and relieve symptoms associated with lumbago and the sciatic nerves. It may also be beneficial for acne, regenerating bone cartilage, catarrh, circulation (similar in action to frankincense), coughs, cystitis, depression, hiccups, lymphatic system, menstrual problems, nerves (similar in action to frankincense), nervous tension, increasing oxygen around the pineal and pituitary glands, skin infection and regeneration, and tuberculosis.

Body System(s) Affected: Emotional Balance, Muscles and Bones, Nervous System, Skin.

Aromatic Influence: Calms, harmonizes, and balances the emotions. It may help enhance meditation.

Oral Use As Dietary Supplement: Sandalwood oil is approved by the FDA (21CFR172.510) for use as a Food Additive (FA) and Flavoring Agent (FL). Dilute 1 drop oil in 1 tsp. (5 ml) honey or in ½ cup (125 ml) of beverage (e.g., soy/rice milk). Not for children under 6 years old; use with caution and in greater dilution for children 6 years old and over.

Blend Classification: Modifier and Equalizer

Blends With: Cypress, frankincense, lemon, myrrh, and ylang ylang.

Odor: Type: Base Note (5–20% of the blend); Scent: Soft, woody, sweet, earthy, balsamic, tenacious; Intensity: 3.

Additional Research:

Alzheimer's Disease: A blend of ethanol extracts from 8 herbs, including sandalwood, orally administered to a mice model of Alzheimer's disease was shown to improve amyloid β protein-induced memory impairment, suppress amyloid β protein levels, and diminish plaque deposition in the brain as much as that of donepezil treatment. (Jeon et al., 2011).

Antitumor Properties: Alpha-santalol, derived from sandalwood EO, was found to delay and decrease the incidence and multiplicity of skin tumor (papilloma) development in mice (Dwivedi et al., 2003).

Antitumor Properties: Various concentrations of alpha-santalol (from sandalwood) were tested against skin cancer in mice. All concentrations were found to inhibit skin cancer development (Dwivedi et al., 2005).

Antitumor Properties: Alpha-santalol was found to induce apoptosis in human skin cancer cells (Kaur et al., 2005).

Antiviral: Sandalwood oil was found to possess antiviral activities against herpes simplex virus 1 and 2 in a dose-dependent manner (Benencia et al., 1999).

---

*See Personal Usage Guide chapter for more details on these primary uses.   ●=Neat, ●=Dilute for Children/Sensitive Skin, ●=Dilute

Siberian Fir *Abies sibirica*

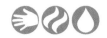

Quick Facts

Botanical Family: Pinaceae (conifer)

Extraction Method: Steam distillation from needles and twigs

Common Primary Uses*: 🌀🌑Bronchitis, 🌑Bursitis, 🌑Cartilage Inflammation, 🌑Cleaning, 🌀🌑Emotional Balance, 🌀🌑Energizing, 🌑Frozen Shoulder, 🌑Furniture Polish, 🌑Massage (soothing), 🌑Muscle Fatigue, 🌑Muscle Pain, 🌑Overexercised Muscles, 🌀🌑Relaxing, 🌑Sprains

Common Application Methods‡:

🌑: Can be applied neat (with no dilution) when used topically. Dilute 1:1 (1 drop essential oil to at least 1 drop carrier oil) for children and for those with sensitive skin. Apply directly on area of concern or to reflex points.

🌀: Diffuse, or inhale the aroma directly.

🌢: Take in capsules, or take 1 drop in a beverage.

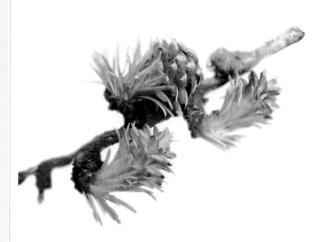

Chemical Constituents: Monoterpenes (60–70%): camphene (<30%), α- & β-pinene (<20%), δ-3-carene (up to 12%), l-limonene (<5%), santene; Esters: bornyl acetate (up to 35%); Alcohols: borneol.

Properties: Analgesic, antiarthritic, anticatarrhal, antiseptic (pulmonary), expectorant, and stimulant.

Historical Uses: Sibirian fir is found throughout the cold taiga forest in northern Eurasia and North America. Though highly regarded for its fragrant scent, the fir tree has been prized through the ages for its medicinal virtues in regards to respiratory complaints, fever, and muscular and rheumatic pain.

French Medicinal Uses: Bronchitis◷, respiratory congestion, energy.

Other Possible Uses: Fir creates the symbolic effect of an umbrella protecting the earth and bringing energy in from the universe. At night the animals in the wild lie down under the tree for the protection, recharging, and rejuvenation the trees bring them. Fir may be beneficial for reducing aches/pains from colds and the flu, fighting airborne germs/bacteria, arthritis, asthma, supporting the blood, bronchial obstructions, coughs, fevers, oxygenating the cells, rheumatism, sinusitis, and urinary tract infections.

🜨 **Body System(s) Affected:** Respiratory System.

Aromatic Influence: It creates a feeling of grounding, anchoring, and empowerment. It can stimulate the mind while allowing the body to relax.

Oral Use As Dietary Supplement: Siberian fir oil is approved by the FDA (21CFR172.510) for use as a Food Additive (FA) and Flavoring Agent (FL). Dilute 1 drop oil in 1 tsp. (5 ml) honey or in ½ cup (125 ml) of beverage (e.g., soy/rice milk). Not for children under 6 years old; use with caution and in greater dilution for children 6 years old and over.

Safety Data: Can irritate sensitive skin.

Blend Classification: Equalizer.

Blends With: Frankincense and lavender.

Odor: Type: Middle Notes (50–80% of the blend); Scent: Fresh, woody, earthy, sweet; Intensity: 3.

◷ **Additional Research:**

Bronchitis: In patients with chronic bronchitis, rosemary, basil, fir, and eucalyptus oils were found to demonstrate an antioxidant effect (Siurin et al., 1997).

‡See Application section beginning on page 16 for more details on applying essential oils.   🌑=Topical, 🌀=Aromatic, 🌢=Internal

119

Essential Oils

Spearmint *Mentha spicata*

Quick Facts

Botanical Family: Labiatae (mint)

Extraction Method: Steam distillation from leaves

Common Primary Uses*: O Cooking, O Indigestion

Common Application Methods‡:

🤚: Can be applied neat (with no dilution), or dilute 1:1 (1 drop essential oil to 1 drop carrier oil) for children and for those with sensitive skin when used topically. Use with caution during pregnancy. Avoid use on babies. Apply directly on area of concern or to reflex points.

🌀: Diffuse, or inhale the aroma directly.

💧: Take in capsules or in a beverage. Use as a flavoring in cooking.

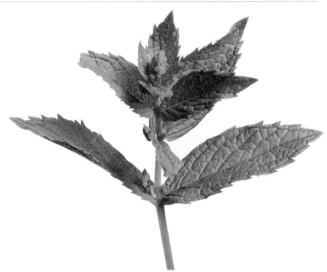

Chemical Constituents: Ketones (up to 70%): l-carvone (<58%), dihydrocarvone (<10%), menthone (<2%), pulegone; Monoterpenes (<30%): l-limonene (<25%), myrcene (<3%), camphene, α- & β-pinenes, α-phellandrene; Alcohols (<10%): carveol (<3%), linalool, trans-thujanol-4, octanol, borneol; Sesquiterpenes (<5%): β-caryophyllene, β-bourbonene, α-elemene, β-farnesene; Esters: carvyl acetates (<4%); Oxides: 1,8 cineol (<3%); Sesquiterpene Alcohols: α-cadinol, farnesol, elemol; Phenolic Alcohols: menthol.

Properties: Antibacterial⬚, anticatarrhal, antifungal, anti-inflammatory, antiseptic, antispasmodic, hormone-like, insecticidal, and stimulant.

Historical Uses: Spearmint has been used to relieve hiccough, colic, nausea, indigestion, flatulence, headaches, sores, and scabs.

French Medicinal Uses: Bronchitis, candida, cystitis, hypertension.

Other Possible Uses: This oil may help balance and increase metabolism, which may help burn up fats and toxins in the body. It may aid the glandular, nervous, and respiratory systems. It may also help with acne, appetite (stimulates), arthritis (pain)⬚, bad breath, balance, childbirth (promotes easier labor), constipation, depression, diarrhea, digestion, dry skin, eczema, fevers, headaches, intestines (soothes), kidney stones, menstrua-tion (slow, heavy periods), migraines, nausea, sore gums, stomach (relaxes muscles), urine retention, vaginitis, weight (reduces), and bring about a feeling of well-being.

Body System(s) Affected: Digestive System, Emotional Balance.

Aromatic Influence: Its hormone-like activity may help open and release emotional blocks to bring about a feeling of balance. It acts as an antidepressant by relieving mental strain and fatigue, and by lifting one's spirits.

Oral Use As Dietary Supplement: Generally regarded as safe (GRAS) for human consumption by the FDA. Dilute 1 drop oil in 1 tsp. (5 ml) honey or in ½ cup (125 ml) of beverage (e.g., soy/rice milk). Not for children under 6 years old; use with caution and in greater dilution for children 6 years old and over.

Safety Data: Use with caution during pregnancy. Not for use on babies.

Blend Classification: Personifier

Blends With: Basil, lavender, peppermint, rosemary.

Odor: Top Note (5–20% of the blend); Scent: Minty, slightly fruity, less bright than peppermint; Intensity: 3.

📖 **Additional Research:**

Antibacterial Properties: Peppermint and spearmint oil inhibited resistant strains of *Staphylococcus*, *E. Coli*, *Salmonella*, and *Helicobacter pylori* (Imai et al., 2001).

Arthritis: Spearmint oil was found to help reduce pain in patients with osteoarthritis (Mahboubi, 2017).

Anti-inflammatory: In an animal model, spearmint essential oil was found to have anti-inflammatory and antinociceptive properties (Mogosan et al., 2017).

---

*See Personal Usage Guide chapter for more details on these primary uses.   ●=Neat, ●=Dilute for Children/Sensitive Skin, ●=Dilute

Spikenard *Nardostachys jatamansi*

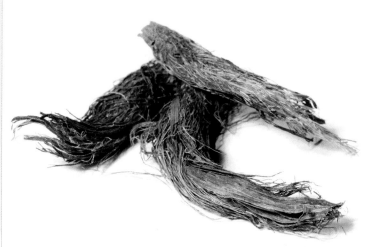

Quick Facts

Botanical Family: Valerianaceae

Extraction Method: Steam distillation from rhizomes

Common Primary Uses*: ⬢Aging Skin, ⬢⬢Insomnia, ⬢⬢Nervousness, ⬢Perfume, ⬢Rashes

Common Application Methods‡:

⬢: Can be applied neat (with no dilution) when used topically. Apply directly on area of concern or to reflex points.

⬢: Diffuse, or inhale the aroma directly.

Chemical Constituents: Sesquiterpenes (up to 50%): β-gurjunene (<30%), β-maalene (<9%), aristoladiene (<7%), aristolene (5%), seychellene, dihydroazulene, β-patchoulene; Monoterpenes (up to 45%): calarene (<35%), β-ionene (<8%), α- & β-pinenes, limonene, aristolene; Sesquiterpene Alcohols (<11%): patchoulol (<7%), nardol, calarenol, maaliol, valerianol; Ketones (<10%): aristolenone (<7%), β-ionone, nardostachone, valerianone (=jatamansone); Phenolic Aldehydes: valerianal; Coumarins; Oxides: 1,8 cineol; Carboxylic Acids: jatamanshinic acid.

Properties: Antibacterial, antifungal, anti-inflammatory, antioxidant⬡, deodorant, relaxing, and skin tonic.

Historical Uses: Spikenard gets its name from the spike-shaped rhizomes (or "spikes") of the plant that the oil is distilled from. Highly prized in the Middle East during the time of Christ, spikenard is referred to several times in the Bible. Spikenard was also used in the preparation of nardinum, a scented oil of great renown during ancient times. Prized in early Egypt, it was used in a preparation called *kyphi* with other oils like saffron, juniper, myrrh, cassia, and cinnamon.

Other Possible Uses: The oil is known for helping in the treatment of allergic skin reactions, and according to Victoria Edwards, "The oil redresses the skin's physiological balance and causes permanent regeneration." Spikenard may also help with allergies, candida, flatulent indigestion, insomnia, menstrual difficulties, migraine, nausea, neurological diseases⬡, rashes, staph infections, stress, tachycardia⬡, tension, and wounds that will not heal.

Body System(s) Affected: Emotional Balance, Skin.

Aromatic Influence: Spikenard has an earthy, animal-like fragrance. It is balancing, soothing, and harmonizing.

Oral Use As Dietary Supplement: None.

Blend Classification: Modifier and Personifier.

Blends With: lavender, patchouli, pine, and vetiver.

Odor: Base Note (5–20% of the blend); Scent: Heavy, earthy, animal-like, similar to valerian; Intensity: 5.

Additional Research:

Antioxidant: Spikenard oil and spikenard extracts have demonstrated an ability to protect neural and cardiac cells by exhibiting an antioxidant effect in vitro and in animal models (Maiwalanjiang et al., 2014; Maiwalanjiang et al., 2013; Maiwalanjiang et al., 2015).

‡*See Application section beginning on page 16 for more details on applying essential oils.*   ⬢=Topical, ⬢=Aromatic, ⬡=Internal

121

Star Anise *Illicium verum*

Quick Facts

Botanical Family: Illiciaceae

Extraction Method: Steam distillation from the fruit, seed, and leaf

Common Primary Uses*: ⚪Colic, ⚪⚫Flatulence, ⚪⚫⚭Indigestion, ⚪⚫⚭Relaxing

Common Application Methods‡:

⚫: Can be applied neat (with no dilution) when used topically. Apply directly on area of concern or to reflex points. Use in a massage oil.

⚭: Diffuse, or inhale the aroma directly.

⚪: Add 1 drop to 1 cup (250 ml) of warm water, tea, or other beverage.

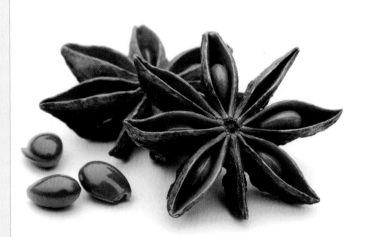

Chemical Constituents: Phenolic Ethers: (E)-anethole (up to 95%), (methyl chavicol) (1–10%); Monoterpenes: limonene; Alcohols: linalool.

Properties: Antifungal⚪, antiseptic, antispasmodic, estrogen-like, diuretic, stimulant (heart), and tonic (heart).

Historical Uses: Native to Asia, star anise has been used for centuries in Chinese medicine to help with various digestive issues such as indigestion, flatulence, colic, and cramping. It has also been used to help with back pain and rheumatism.

Other Possible Uses: This oil may be beneficial for bronchitis, colitis, constipation, digestion (accelerates), diverticulitis, estrogen (increases), fertility, flatulence, hormonal imbalance, irritable bowel syndrome, menopause, parasites, PMS, prostate cancer (blend with frankincense), and respiratory system (strengthens).

⊕ **Body System(s) Affected:** Cardiovascular System, Digestive System, Hormonal System, Respiratory System.

Aromatic Influence: The aroma of star anise is grounding and balancing to the emotions.

Oral Use As Dietary Supplement: Star anise oil is generally regarded as safe (GRAS) for human consumption by the FDA. Dilute 1 drop oil in 1 tsp. (5 ml) honey or in ½ cup (125 ml) of beverage (e.g., soy/rice milk). Not for children under 6 years old; use with caution and in greater dilution for children 6 years old and over.

Safety Data: May irritate highly sensitive skin. Consult with a physician before use if taking medications, pregnant, or nursing.

Blends With: Bergamot, black pepper, blue tansy, fennel, ginger, juniper berry, lemongrass, patchouli, peppermint, tangerine, tarragon, and ylang ylang.

Odor: Type: Top to Middle Note (20–80% of the blend); Scent: Sweet, licorice-like, spicy, warm, slightly balsamic; Intensity: 4.

⚪ **Additional Research:**

Antifungal: Anethol from star anise was found to inhibit 3 *Aspergillus* strains at concentrations of 2 mg/ml (Hitokoto et al., 1980).

Antifungal: Essential oil of anise was found to be highly antifungal against several *Candida* species at low concentrations (Kosalec et al., 2005).

See Personal Usage Guide chapter for more details on these primary uses.   ⚫=Neat, ⚫=Dilute for Children/Sensitive Skin, ⚫=Dilute

122

Tangerine *Citrus reticulata*

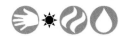

Quick Facts

Botanical Family: Rutaceae (citrus)

Extraction Method: Cold expressed from rind

Common Primary Uses*: ^OCooking, Calming, Uplifting

Common Application Methods‡:

: Can be applied neat (with no dilution) when used topically. Apply directly on area of concern or to reflex points. Avoid direct sunlight or UV light for up to 12 hours after using on the skin.

: Diffuse, or inhale the aroma directly.

: Take in capsules or in a beverage. Use as a flavoring in cooking.

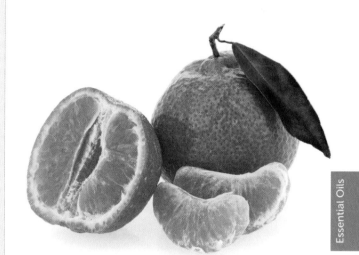

Chemical Constituents: Monoterpenes (up to 95%): d-limonene (<80%), γ-terpinene (<20%), myrcene (<4%), p-cymene, α- & β-phellandrenes, β-ocimene, α- & β-pinenes, terpinolene, cadinene; Tetraterpenes (<10%): β-carotene (<6%), lycopene (<4%); Alcohols: linalool, citronellol; Aldehydes: citral, neral.

Properties: Anticoagulant, anti-inflammatory, laxative, and sedative.

Other Possible Uses: It may help cellulite (dissolve), circulation, constipation, diarrhea, digestive system disorders, fat digestion, dizziness, fear, flatulence, gallbladder, insomnia, intestinal spasms, irritability, limbs (tired and aching), liver problems, decongest the lymphatic system (helps to stimulate draining), obesity, parasites, sadness, the stomach (tonic), stretch marks (smooths when blended with lavender), stress, swelling, and help alleviate water retention (edema).

Body System(s) Affected: Emotional Balance, Immune System, Skin.

Aromatic Influence: Tangerine oil contains esters and aldehydes, which are sedating and calming to the nervous system. When diffused together with marjoram, tangerine can soothe emotions such as grief, anger, and shock.

Oral Use As Dietary Supplement: Tangerine oil is generally regarded as safe (GRAS) for human consumption by the FDA. Dilute 1 drop oil in 1 tsp. (5 ml) honey or in ½ cup (125 ml) of beverage (e.g., soy/rice milk). Not for children under 6 years old; use with caution and in greater dilution for children 6 years old and over.

Blend Classification: Modifier and Personifier

Blends With: Basil, bergamot, clary sage, frankincense, geranium, grapefruit, lavender, lemon, orange, and Roman chamomile.

Odor: Top Note (5–20% of the blend); Scent: Fresh, sweet, citrusy; Intensity: 3.

Additional Research:

Pneumonia: In rats with induced pulmonary fibrosis oral treatment of hydrodistilled tangerine essential oil suppressed body weight loss and significantly improved scores of alveolitis and fibrosis of lung tissue. The effects of tangerine essential oil on lung fibrosis were associated with free radical scavenging and antioxidant activity (Zhou et al., 2012).

---

‡*See Application section beginning on page 16 for more details on applying essential oils.*   =Topical, =Aromatic, =Internal

123

Thyme *Thymus vulgaris CT Thymol*

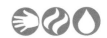

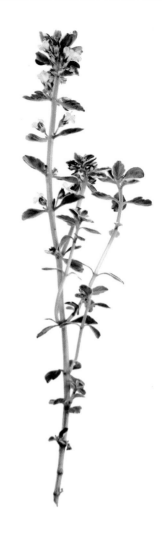

Quick Facts

Botanical Family: Labiatae (mint)

Extraction Method: Steam distillation from leaves, stems, and flowers

Common Primary Uses*: 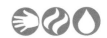Antioxidant, Asthma, Bacterial Infections, Bites/Stings, Blood Clots, Brain (Aging), Bronchitis, Colds (Common), Croup, Dermatitis/Eczema, Fatigue, Fungal Infections, Greasy/Oily Hair, Hair (Fragile), Hair (Loss), Mold, MRSA, Parasites, Pleurisy, Pneumonia, Prostatitis, Psoriasis, Radiation Wounds, Sciatica, Tuberculosis

Common Application Methods‡:

: Dilute 1:4 (1 drop essential oil to at least 4 drops carrier oil) when used topically. Dilute heavily for children and for those with sensitive skin. Apply directly on area of concern or to reflex points.

: Diffuse, or inhale the aroma directly.

: Place 1–2 drops under the tongue, or take in capsules. Use as a flavoring in cooking.

Chemical Constituents: Phenols (up to 60%): thymol (<55%), carvacrol (<10%); Monoterpenes (<54%): p-cymene (<28%), γ-terpinene (<11%), terpinolene (<6%), α-pinene (<6%), myrcene (<3%); Oxides: 1,8 cineol (<15%); Alcohols (<14%): linalool (<8%), borneol (<7%), thujanol, geraniol; Sesquiterpenes: β-caryophyllene (<8%); Carboxylic Acids: rosmaric acid (<2%), triterpenic acids (tr.); Ethers: methyl thymol (tr.), methyl carvacrol (tr.); Ketone: camphor (tr.); Also trace elements of menthone.

Properties: Highly antibacterial, antifungal, antimicrobial, antioxidant, antiviral, antiseptic.

Historical Uses: It was used by the Egyptians for embalming and by the ancient Greeks to fight against infectious illnesses. It has also been used for respiratory problems, digestive complaints, the prevention and treatment of infection, dyspepsia, chronic gastritis, bronchitis, pertussis, asthma, laryngitis, tonsillitis, and enuresis in children.

French Medicinal Uses: Anthrax, asthma, bronchitis, colitis (infectious), cystitis, dermatitis, dyspepsia, fatigue (general), pleurisy, psoriasis, sciatica, tuberculosis, vaginal candida.

Other Possible Uses: This oil is a general tonic for the nerves and stomach. It may also help with circulation, depression, digestion, dysmenorrhea, physical weakness after illness, flu, headaches, immunological functions, insomnia, rheumatism, urinary infections, viruses along the spine, and wounds.

Body System(s) Affected: Immune System, Muscles and Bones.

Aromatic Influence: It helps energize in times of physical weakness and stress. It has also been thought to aid concentration. It is uplifting and helps to relieve depression.

*See Personal Usage Guide chapter for more details on these primary uses. ●=Neat, ●=Dilute for Children/Sensitive Skin, ●=Dilute

Oral Use As Dietary Supplement: Thyme oil is generally recognized as safe (GRAS) for human consumption by the FDA (21CFR182.20). Dilute 1 drop oil in 2 tsp. (10 ml) honey or in 1 cup (250 ml) of beverage (e.g., soy/rice milk). However, more dilution may be necessary due to this oil's potential for irritating mucous membranes. Not for children under 6 years old; use with caution and in greater dilution for children 6 years old and over.

Safety Data: This type of thyme oil may be somewhat irritating to the mucous membranes and dermal tissues (skin). This type of thyme should be avoided during pregnancy. Use with caution when dealing with high blood pressure.

Blend Classification: Equalizer and Enhancer.

Blends With: Bergamot, melaleuca, oregano, and rosemary.

Odor: Type: Middle Note (50–80% of the blend); Scent: Fresh, medicinal, herbaceous; Intensity: 4.

Additional Research:

Antibacterial Properties: Subjects using a mouthwash containing thymol, menthol, methyl salicylate, and eucalyptol for 6 months did not have oral bacteria that had developed a resistance to the oils (Charles et al., 2000).

Antibacterial Properties: Cinnamon, thyme, and clove essential oils demonstrated an antibacterial effect on several respiratory tract pathogens (Fabio et al., 2007).

Antibacterial Properties: Thyme oil demonstrated a strong antibacterial effect against *Staph* and *E. Coli* bacteria (Mohsenzadeh et al., 2007).

Antifungal Properties: Thyme oil was found to inhibit Candida species by causing lesions in the cell membrane and inhibiting germ tube (an outgrowth that develops when the fungi is preparing to replicate) formation (Pina-Vaz et al., 2004).

Antifungal Properties: Cinnamon, thyme, oregano, and cumin oils inhibited the production of aflatoxin by aspergillus fungus (Tantaoui-Elaraki et al., 1994).

Antimicrobial Properties: Cinnamon bark, lemongrass, and thyme oils were found to have the highest level of activity against common respiratory pathogens among 14 essential oils tested (Inouye et al., 2001).

Antioxidant Properties: Older rats whose diets were supplemented with thyme oil were found have higher levels of the antioxidant enzymes superoxide dismutase and glutathione peroxidase in the heart, liver, and kidneys than did older rats without this supplementation (Youdim et al., 1999).

Antioxidant Properties: Aging rats fed thyme oil or the constituent thymol were found to have higher levels of the antioxidant enzymes superoxide dismutase and glutathione peroxidase in the brain than did aging rats not fed the oil or constituent (Youdim et al., 2000).

Colon—Colitis: Oral administration of thyme and oregano oil at a dose of 0.2% thyme and 0.1% oregano was found to be effective in decreasing the mortality rate, accelerating body weight gain recovery, and significantly reducing the macroscopic damage of colonic tissue of mice with induced colitis (Bukovska et al., 2007).

Dysmenorrhea: A study comparing administration of thyme essential oil, ibuprofen, and placebo treatment revealed that thyme essential oil alleviates dysmenorrhea pain as well as ibuprofen and works significantly better than the placebo treatment (Salmalian et al., 2014).

Anxiety: Carvacrol is a monoterpenic phenol found in thyme and oregano. Oral administration of carvacrol produced antianxiety-like effects in mice (Melo et al., 2010).

Weight—Obesity: After 10 weeks of feeding, the body weight gain, visceral fat-pad weights, and final body weights of mice fed a high-fat diet and carvacrol were significantly lower than that of mice fed a high-fat diet without carvacrol (specifically a 24% decrease in final body weight, a 43% decrease in body weight gain, and a 36% decrease in total visceral fat-pad weight was observed when carvacrol was ingested)(Cho et al., 2012). Interestingly, the food intake during the 10-week feeding period did not differ among the groups and mRNA expressions were different among the two groups (Cho et al., 2012).

‡See Application section beginning on page 16 for more details on applying essential oils.   🜨=Topical, ⊘=Aromatic, ◯=Internal

125

Essential Oils

Turmeric *Curcuma longa*

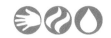

Quick Facts

Botanical Family: Zingiberaceae (ginger)

Extraction Method: Steam distillation from rhizome

Common Primary Uses*: ⬡⬢⬢Antioxidant, ⬢⬢Antibacterial, ⬡⬢⬢Indigestion, ⬡⬢⬢Neurological Diseases (Protects), ⬢Skin

Common Application Methods‡:

⬢: Can be applied neat (with no dilution) when used topically. Apply directly on area of concern or to reflex points.

⬢: Diffuse, or inhale the aroma directly.

⬢: Add 1 drop to 1 cup (250 ml) of water, tea, or other beverage.

Chemical Constituents: Ketones (up to 50%): turmerone, ar-turmerone, carlone; Sesquiterpenes (up to 35%): zingiberene, β-sesquiphellandrene, ar-curcumene, β-curcumene, α- & β-caryophyllene, β-bisabolene; Monoterpenes (up to 16%): α-phellandrene, turpinolene, p-cymene; Oxide: 1,8 cineole (up to 7%).

Properties: Analgesic, anticonvulsant, anti-inflammatory⬡, antimicrobial, antimutagenic, antioxidant, antitumor, insecticidal.

Historical Uses: Native to India, the rhizome of curcumin is a bright orange-yellow color. Turmeric's unique color makes it valuable as a dye coloring, but it is also an important spice in many dishes. The herb has been used in Ayurvedic medicine for centuries to help with gastritis, jaundice, and nausea.

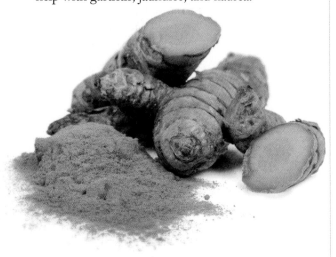

Other Possible Uses: Turmeric essential oil may also be beneficial for arthritis, blood clots⬡, cancer, depression, epilepsy⬡, joint health, neurological health⬡, skin conditions (ringworm and other fungal skin conditions)⬡, and pain. It may also have neuroprotective⬡ properties.

⬢ **Body System(s) Affected:** Digestive System, Immune System, Skin.

Aromatic Influence: The warm, earthy aroma of turmeric is grounding to the mind and emotions, and it can help promote feelings of relaxation.

Oral Use As Dietary Supplement: Turmeric oil is generally regarded as safe (GRAS) for human consumption by the FDA. Dilute 1 drop oil in 1 tsp. (5 ml) honey or in ½ cup (125 ml) of beverage (e.g., soy/rice milk). Not for children under 6 years old; use with caution and in greater dilution for children 6 years old and over.

Safety Data: May irritate highly sensitive skin. Consult with a physician before use if taking medications (especially for diabetes), pregnant, or nursing.

Blend Classification: Personifier and Equalizer.

Blends With: Citrus oils (tangerine, in particular), ginger, pink pepper, and spice oils.

Odor: Type: Middle Note (50–80% of the blend); Scent: Warm, earthy, spicy, slightly woody; Intensity: 4.

⬡ **Additional Research:**

Anti-inflammatory: In a laboratory test, aromatic termerone from turmeric oil was found to demonstrate an anti-inflammatory effect (Oh et al., 2014).

Blood Clots: *Curcuma longa* oil was found to suppress intravascular platelet aggregation in induced thrombosis models in mice (Prakash et al., 2011).

Neurological Health: Aromatic turmerone (ar-turmerone) was found to induce neural stem cell proliferation both in vitro and in mouse models.

Epilepsy: In a mouse model, aromatic turmerone (ar-turmerone) was found to reduce convulsions in an induced epileptic seizure mouse model without causing any perceived neurological side effects. Ar-turmerone was also found to cross the blood-brain barrier.

Neuroprotective: *Curcuma longa* essential oil was found to increase the survival rate of neurons in a mouse model of ischemic stroke (Preeti et al., 2008).

Neuroprotective: Aromatic turmerone (ar-turmerone) from turmeric essential oil was found to protect neurons in the brain from damage by inhibiting inflammation in a mouse model (Chen et al., 2018).

Skin: Ar-turmerone (a component of turmeric oil) was found to inhibit the growth of several fungi responsible for skin conditions such as ringworm and tinea (Mukda et al., 2013).

*See Personal Usage Guide chapter for more details on these primary uses.   ●=Neat, ●=Dilute for Children/Sensitive Skin, ●=Dilute

126

Vetiver *Vetiveria zizanioides*

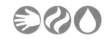

Quick Facts

Botanical Family: Gramineae (grasses)

Extraction Method: Steam distillation from roots

Common Primary Uses*: ⊘⊙ADD/ADHD, ⊘⊘Balance, ⊘⊘Termite Repellent, ⊙Vitiligo

Common Application Methods‡:

⊙: Can be applied neat (with no dilution) when used topically. Apply directly on area of concern or to reflex points. Also excellent in baths or in massage blends. A very small amount of vetiver oil is all that is needed in most applications.

⊘: Diffuse, or inhale the aroma directly.

○: Take in capsules.

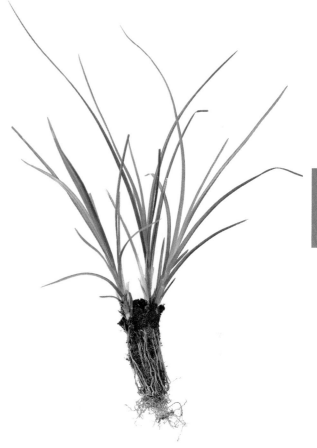

Chemical Constituents: Sesquiterpene Alcohols (up to 42%): isovalencenol (<15%), bicyclovetiverol (<13%), khusenol (<11%), tricyclovetiverol (<4%), vetiverol, zizanol, furfurol; Sesquiterpene Ketones (<22%): α- & β-vetivones (<12%), khusimone (<6%), nootkatone (<5%); Sesquiterpenes (<4%): vitivene, tricyclovetivene, vetivazulene, β- & δ-cadinenes; Sesquiterpene Esters: vetiveryl acetate; Carboxylic Acids: benzoic, palmitic, and vetivenic acids.

Properties: Antiseptic, antispasmodic, calming, grounding, immune stimulant, rubefacient (locally warming), sedative (nervous system), stimulant (circulatory, production of red corpuscles).

Historical Uses: The distillation of vetiver is a painstaking, labor-intensive activity. The roots and rootlets of vetiver have been used in India as a perfume since antiquity.

Other Possible Uses: Vetiver may help acne, anorexia, anxiety, arthritis, breasts (enlarge), cuts, depression (including postpartum), insomnia, muscular rheumatism, nervousness (extreme), skin care (oily, aging, tired, irritated), sprains, stress, and tuberculosis ⊕.

⊕ **Body System(s) Affected:** Emotional Balance, Hormonal and Nervous Systems, Skin.

Aromatic Influence: Vetiver has a heavy, smoky, earthy fragrance reminiscent of patchouli with lemon-like undertones. Vetiver has been valuable for relieving stress and helping people recover from emotional traumas and shock. As a natural tranquilizer, it may help induce a restful sleep. It is known to affect the parathyroid gland.

Oral Use As Dietary Supplement: Vetiver oil is approved by the FDA (21CFR172.510) for use as a Food Additive (FA) and Flavoring Agent (FL). Dilute 1 drop oil in 1 tsp. (5 ml) honey or in ½ cup (125 ml) of beverage (e.g., soy/rice milk). Not for children under 6 years old; use with caution and in greater dilution for children 6 years old and over.

Safety Data: Use with caution during pregnancy.

Blends With: Clary sage, lavender, rose, sandalwood, and ylang ylang.

Odor: Type: Base Note (5–20% of the blend); Scent: Heavy, earthy, balsamic, smoky, sweet undertones; Intensity: 5.

⊕ **Additional Research:**

Tuberculosis: The ethanolic extract of vetiver root was found to inhibit both virulent and avirulent strains of *M. tuberculosis*, suggesting that vetiver could be useful in treating tubercular infections (Saikia et al., 2012).

‡*See Application section beginning on page 16 for more details on applying essential oils.*   ⊙=Topical, ⊘=Aromatic, ○=Internal

127

Essential Oils

White Fir *Abies alba*

Quick Facts

Botanical Family: Pinaceae (conifer)

Extraction Method: Steam distillation from needles

Common Primary Uses*: ⊘Bronchitis, ⊘Bursitis, ⊘Cartilage Inflammation, ⊘Energizing, ⊘Frozen Shoulder, ⊘Furniture Polish, ⊘Muscle Fatigue, ⊘Muscle Pain, ⊘Overexercised Muscles, ⊘Sprains

Common Application Methods‡:

⊘: Can be applied neat (with no dilution) when used topically. Dilute 1:1 (1 drop essential oil to at least 1 drop carrier oil) for children and for those with sensitive skin. Apply directly on area of concern or to reflex points.

⊘: Diffuse, or inhale the aroma directly.

⊘: Take in capsules.

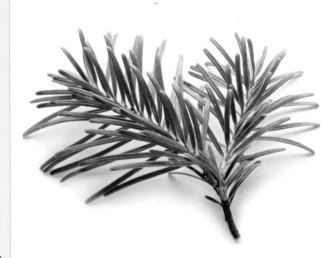

Chemical Constituents: Monoterpenes (75–95%): l-limonene (34%), α-pinene (24%), camphene (21%), santene, δ-3-carene; Esters: bornyle acetate (up to 10%).

Properties: Analgesic, antiarthritic, anticatarrhal, antiseptic (pulmonary), expectorant, and stimulant.

Historical Uses: The fir tree is the classic Christmas tree (short with the perfect pyramidal shape and silvery white bark). Though highly regarded for its fragrant scent, the fir tree has been prized through the ages for its medicinal virtues in regards to respiratory complaints, fever, and muscular and rheumatic pain.

French Medicinal Uses: Bronchitis⊕, respiratory congestion, energy.

Other Possible Uses: Fir creates the symbolic effect of an umbrella protecting the earth and bringing energy in from the universe. At night the animals in the wild lie down under the tree for the protection, recharging, and rejuvenation the trees bring them. Fir may be beneficial for reducing aches/pains from colds and the flu, fighting airborne germs/bacteria, arthritis, asthma, supporting the blood, bronchial obstructions, coughs, fevers,

oxygenating the cells, rheumatism, sinusitis, and urinary tract infections.

Body System(s) Affected: Respiratory System.

Aromatic Influence: It creates a feeling of grounding, anchoring, and empowerment. It can stimulate the mind while allowing the body to relax.

Oral Use As Dietary Supplement: White fir oil in general is approved by the FDA (21CFR172.510) for use as a Food Additive (FA) and Flavoring Agent (FL). Dilute 1 drop oil in 1 tsp. (5 ml) honey or in ½ cup (125 ml) of beverage (e.g., soy/rice milk). Not for children under 6 years old; use with caution and in greater dilution for children 6 years old and over.

Safety Data: Can irritate sensitive skin.

Blend Classification: Equalizer.

Blends With: Frankincense and lavender.

Odor: Type: Middle Notes (50–80% of the blend); Scent: Fresh, woody, earthy, sweet; Intensity: 3.

⊕ **Additional Research:**

Bronchitis: In patients with chronic bronchitis, rosemary, basil, fir, and eucalyptus oils were found to demonstrate an antioxidant effect. (Siurin et al., 1997).

See Personal Usage Guide chapter for more details on these primary uses. ●=Neat, ●=Dilute for Children/Sensitive Skin, ●=Dilute

128

Wintergreen *Gaultheria fragrantissima or G. procumbens*

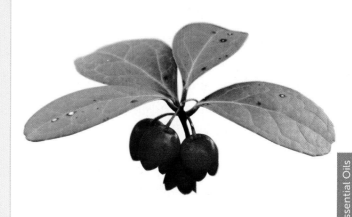

Quick Facts

Botanical Family: Ericaceae (heather)

Extraction Method: Steam distillation from leaves

Common Primary Uses*: ⊖Arthritic Pain, ⊖Bone Pain, ⊖Bone Spurs, ⊖Cartilage Injury, ⊖Dandruff, ⊖Frozen Shoulder, ⊖Joint Pain, ⊖Muscle Development, ⊖Muscle Tone, ⊖Pain, ⊖Rotator Cuff (Sore)

Common Application Methods‡:

⊖: Can be applied neat (with no dilution), or dilute 1:1 (1 drop essential oil to 1 drop carrier oil) for children and for those with sensitive skin when using topically. Apply directly on area of concern or to reflex points. Apply topically on location, and use only small amounts (dilute with fractionated coconut oil for application on larger areas).

🌀: Diffuse, or inhale the aroma directly.

Chemical Constituents: Phenolic Esters: methyl salicylate (>90%); Carboxylic Acids: salicylic acid.

Properties: Analgesic, anti-inflammatory⊕, antirheumatic, antiseptic, antispasmodic, disinfectant, diuretic, stimulant (bone), and warming.

Historical Uses: Wintergreen oil has a strong, penetrating aroma. The American Indians and early European settlers enjoyed a tea that was flavored with birch bark or wintergreen. According to Julia Lawless, "this has been translated into a preference for 'root beer' flavourings [*sic*]." A synthetic methyl salicylate is now widely used as a flavoring agent, especially in root beer, chewing gum, toothpaste, etc. In fact, the true essential oil is produced in such small quantities (compared to the very extensive uses of the synthetic methyl salicylate) that those desiring to use wintergreen essential oil for therapeutic uses should verify the source of their oil to make sure they have a true oil, not a synthetic one.

French Medicinal Uses: Rheumatism, muscular pain, cramps, arthritis, tendinitis, hypertension, inflammation.

Other Possible Uses: This oil may be beneficial for acne, bladder infection, cystitis, dropsy, eczema, edema, reducing fever, gallstones, gout, infection, reducing discomfort in joints, kidney stones, draining and cleansing the lymphatic system, obesity, osteoporosis, skin diseases, ulcers, and urinary tract disorders. It is known for its ability to alleviate bone pain. It has a cortisone-like action due to the high content of methyl salicylate.

⊕ **Body System(s) Affected:** Muscles and Bones.

Aromatic Influence: It influences, elevates, opens, and increases awareness in sensory system.

Safety Data: Avoid during pregnancy. Not for use by people with epilepsy. Some people are very allergic to methyl salicylate. Test a small area of skin first for allergies.

Blend Classification: Personifier and Enhancer.

Blends With: Basil, bergamot, cypress, geranium, lavender, lemongrass, marjoram, and peppermint.

⊕ **Additional Research:**

Anti-inflammatory Properties: Methyl salicylate (found in wintergreen or birch oils) was found to inhibit leukotriene C4 (a chemical messenger involved in the inflammatory response), while also demonstrating gastroprotective against ethanol-induced gastric injury in rats (Trautmann, et al., 1991).

‡*See Application section beginning on page 16 for more details on applying essential oils.*   ⊖=Topical, 🌀=Aromatic, ○=Internal

129

Yarrow *Achillea millefolium*

Quick Facts

Botanical Family: Compositae (daisy)

Extraction Method: Steam distillation from flowering top

Common Primary Uses*: ◐☯⊘Antioxidant[⊕], ☯Bleeding, ⊘Calming, ⊘Uplifting, ☯Wounds

Common Application Methods‡:

☯: Can be applied neat (with no dilution) when used topically. Apply directly on area of concern or to reflex points.

⊘: Diffuse, or inhale the aroma directly.

◐: Add 1 drop to 1 cup (250 ml) of water, tea, or other beverage.

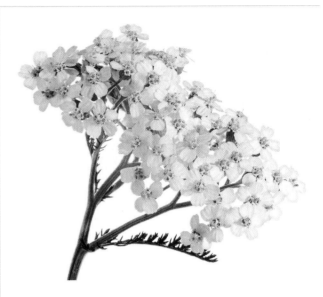

Chemical Constituents: Monoterpenes (up to 65%): sabinene (<40%), α- & β-pinenes (<16%), camphene (<6%), γ-terpinene; Sesquiterpenes (<55%): chamazulene (<30%), germacrene-D (<13%), trans-β-caryophyllene, humulene, dihydroazulenes; Ketones (<30%): camphor (<18%), isoartemisia ketone (<10%), thujone; Alcohols (<10%): borneol (<9%), terpineol; Oxides (<12%): 1,8 cineol (<10%), caryophyllene oxide; Phenols: terpinen-4-ol; Esters: bornyl acetate; Lactones: achillin; Sesquiterpene Alcohols: α-cadinol.

Properties: Anti-inflammatory, antiseptic[⊕], astringent, and styptic (stops bleeding).

Historical Uses: Yarrow was used by Germanic tribes to treat battle wounds. The Chinese also considered it sacred for the harmony of the yin and yang energies within it.

Other Possible Uses: This oil may be beneficial for prostate health and hormonal balance. It may also help with acne, amenorrhea, appetite (lack of), colds, catarrh, digestion (poor), dysmenorrhea, eczema, fevers, flatulence, gastritis, gout, hair growth, headaches, hemorrhoids, hypertension, injuries, kidney stones, liver, menopause problems, neuritis, neuralgia, open leg sores, pelvic infections, prostatitis, rheumatism, scarring, sprains, stomach issues, sunburn, ulcers, urinary infections, vaginitis, varicose veins, and wounds (promotes healing).

✚ **Body System(s) Affected:** Hormonal System, Immune System, Skin.

Aromatic Influence: Balancing highs and lows, both external and internal, yarrow may allow us to have our heads in the clouds while our feet remain firm on the ground. Its balancing properties may also make it useful during meditation.

Oral Use As Dietary Supplement: Yarrow oil is approved by the FDA (21CFR172.510) for use as a Flavoring Agent (FL) in beverages. Dilute 1 drop oil in 1 tsp. (5 ml) honey or in ½ cup (125 ml) of beverage (e.g., soy/rice milk). Not for children under 6 years old; use with caution and in greater dilution for children 6 years old and over.

Safety Data: May irritate highly sensitive skin. Consult with a physician before use if taking medications, pregnant, or nursing.

Blend Classification: Personifier and Enhancer.

Blends With: Clary sage and vetiver.

Odor: Type: Middle Note (50–80% of the blend); Scent: Sharp, woody, herbaceous, with a slight floral undertone; Intensity: 4.

⊕ **Additional Research:**

Antioxidant: Yarrow essential oil demonstrated antioxidant and antimicrobial activity against several pathogenic bacteria and fungi (Candan et al., 2003).-

*See Personal Usage Guide chapter for more details on these primary uses.   ●=Neat, ●=Dilute for Children/Sensitive Skin, ●=Dilute

130

Ylang Ylang *Cananga odorata*

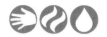

Quick Facts

Botanical Family: Annonaceae (tropical trees and shrubs—custard-apple)

Extraction Method: Steam distillation from flowers

Common Primary Uses*: Aphrodisiac, Arrhythmia, Calming, Colic, Crying, Diabetes, Exhaustion, Fear, Hair (Loss), High Blood Pressure, Hormonal Balance, Hyperpnea, Libido (Low), Palpitations, Relaxation, Sedative, Stress, Tachycardia, Tension

Common Application Methods‡:

: Can be applied neat (with no dilution) when used topically. Apply directly on area of concern or to reflex points. It may be beneficial when applied over the thymus (to help stimulate the immune system).

: Diffuse, or inhale the aroma directly.

: Take in capsules.

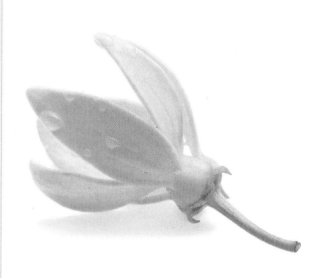

Chemical Constituents: Sesquiterpenes (up to 55%): β-caryophyllene (<22%), germacrene-D (<20%), α-farnesene (<12%), humulene (<5%); Esters (<50%): benzyl acetate & benzoate (<25%), methyl salicylate & benzoate (<17%), farnesyl acetate (<7%), geranyl acetate (<4%), linalyl acetate; Alcohols (<45%): linalool (<40%), geraniol; Ethers: paracresyl methyl ether (<15%); Phenols (<10%): methyl p-cresol (<9%), methyl chavicol (estragole), eugenol, isoeugenol; Oxides: caryophyllene oxide (<7%); Sesquiterpene Alcohols: farnesol.

Properties: Antidepressant, antiseptic, antispasmodic, sedative, and tonic.

Historical Uses: Interestingly enough, the original wild flowers had no fragrance. Through selection and cloning, we have this unique fragrance today. Ylang ylang has been used to cover the beds of newlywed couples on their wedding night, for skin treatments, to soothe insect bites, and in hair preparations to promote thick, shiny, lustrous hair (it is also reported to help control split ends). It has been used to treat colic, constipation, indigestion, stomachaches, and to regulate the heartbeat and respiration.

French Medicinal Uses: Anxiety, arterial hypertension, depression, diabetes, fatigue (mental), frigidity, hair loss, hyperpnea (reduces), insomnia, palpitations, tachycardia.

Other Possible Uses: Ylang ylang may help with rapid breathing, balancing equilibrium, frustration, balancing heart function, impotence, infection, intestinal problems, sex drive problems, shock, and skin problems.

Body System(s) Affected: Emotional Balance, Cardiovascular and Hormonal Systems.

Aromatic Influence: It influences sexual energy and enhances relationships. It may help stimulate the adrenal glands. It is calming and relaxing and may help alleviate anger.

Oral Use As Dietary Supplement: Ylang ylang oil is generally recognized as safe (GRAS) for human consumption by the FDA (21CFR182.20). Dilute 1 drop oil in 1 tsp. (5 ml) honey or in ½ cup (125 ml) of beverage (e.g., soy/rice milk). Not for children under 6 years old; use with caution and in greater dilution for children 6 years old and over.

---

‡See Application section beginning on page 16 for more details on applying essential oils.   =Topical, =Aromatic, =Internal

Safety Data: Repeated use can possibly result in contact sensitization.

Blend Classification: Personifier and Modifier.

Blends With: Bergamot, geranium, grapefruit, lemon, marjoram, sandalwood, and vetiver.

Odor: Type: Middle to Base Notes (20–80% of the blend); Scent: Sweet, heavy, narcotic, cloying, tropical floral, with spicy-balsamic undertones; Intensity: 5.

Additional Research:

Calming—Sedative: In healthy control subjects, inhalation of ylang ylang aroma significantly reduced the P300 (an event-related potential interpreted to reflect attentional allocation and working memory) amplitude when compared to inhalation without aroma. These results suggest that ylang ylang produces a relaxing effect on cognition (Watanabe et al., 2013).

Blood Pressure: Inhaled ylang ylang oil was found to decrease blood pressure and pulse rate and to enhance attentiveness and alertness in volunteers compared to an odorless control (Hongratanaworakit et al., 2004).

Blood Pressure: Subjects who had ylang ylang oil applied to their skin had decreased blood pressure, increased skin temperature, and reported feeling more calm and relaxed compared to subjects in a control group (Hongratanaworakit et al., 2006).

Sedative Properties: In human trials, ylang ylang aroma was found to increase calmness (Moss et al., 2008).

Urinary tract: Ylang ylang oil induced relaxation in rat (in vitro) and rabbit (in vivo) bladder smooth muscle, suggesting that ylang ylang may be effective at alleviating an overactive bladder (Kim et al., 2003).

See Personal Usage Guide chapter for more details on these primary uses.   ●=Neat, ●=Dilute for Children/Sensitive Skin, ●=Dilute

132

Yuzu *Citrus junos*

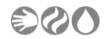

Quick Facts

Botanical Family: Rutaceae (citrus)

Extraction Method: Cold pressed from peel

Common Primary Uses*: Calming, Warming

Common Application Methods‡:

: Can be applied neat (with no dilution) when used topically. Apply directly on area of concern or to reflex points. Use in bath water.

: Diffuse, or inhale the aroma directly.

: Add 1 drop to 1 cup (250 ml) of warm water, tea, or other beverage.

Chemical Constituents: Monoterpenes (up to 95%): limonene (<80%), α- & γ-terpinenes (<10%), α- & β-pinenes (<5%), camphene, sabinene, β-myrcene, β-phellandrene; Alcohols (<4%): terpineol, linalool; Coumarins: limettin; Sesquiterpenes (<1%): β-farnesene.

Properties: Antibacterial, calming, and warming.

Historical Uses: Yuzu fruit has been used in Japan since the 18th century in a traditional bath at winter solstice to help warm the body, improve circulation, promote healthy-looking skin, and prevent illness.

Other Possible Uses: This oil may be beneficial for acne, arthritic pain, circulation, clarity, concentration, focus, moisturizing skin, neuralgia, premenstrual syndrome, skin tone, sore throat, and sore muscles.

Body System(s) Affected: Digestive System, Immune System, Skin.

Aromatic Influence: Yuzu oil has a refreshing, citrusy aroma that is often used to help improve focus and concentration. It can also help purify the air.

Oral Use As Dietary Supplement: Citrus peel oils are generally regarded as safe (GRAS) for human consumption by the FDA. Dilute 1 drop oil in 1 tsp. (5 ml) honey or in 1 cup (250 ml) of beverage (e.g., soy/rice milk). Not for children under 6 years old; use with caution and in greater dilution for children 6 years old and over.

Safety Data: Old or oxidized oils may irritate sensitive skin. Consult with a physician before using if taking medications.

Blend Classification: Enhancer and Equalizer.

Blends With: Clary sage, lavender, neroli, rosemary, and citrus oils.

Odor: Type: Top Note (5–20% of the blend); Scent: Sweet, citrusy; Intensity: 3.

Additional Research:

Calming: In a limited trial, the aroma of yuzu essential oil was found to affect parasympathetic nervous system activity and to have a mood-balancing effect on women experiencing premenstrual emotional symptoms (Matsumoto et al., 2016; Matsumoto et al., 2017).

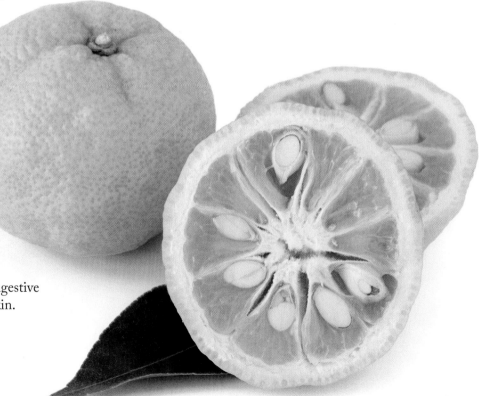

‡See Application section beginning on page 16 for more details on applying essential oils. =Topical, =Aromatic, =Internal

133

Essential Oil Blends

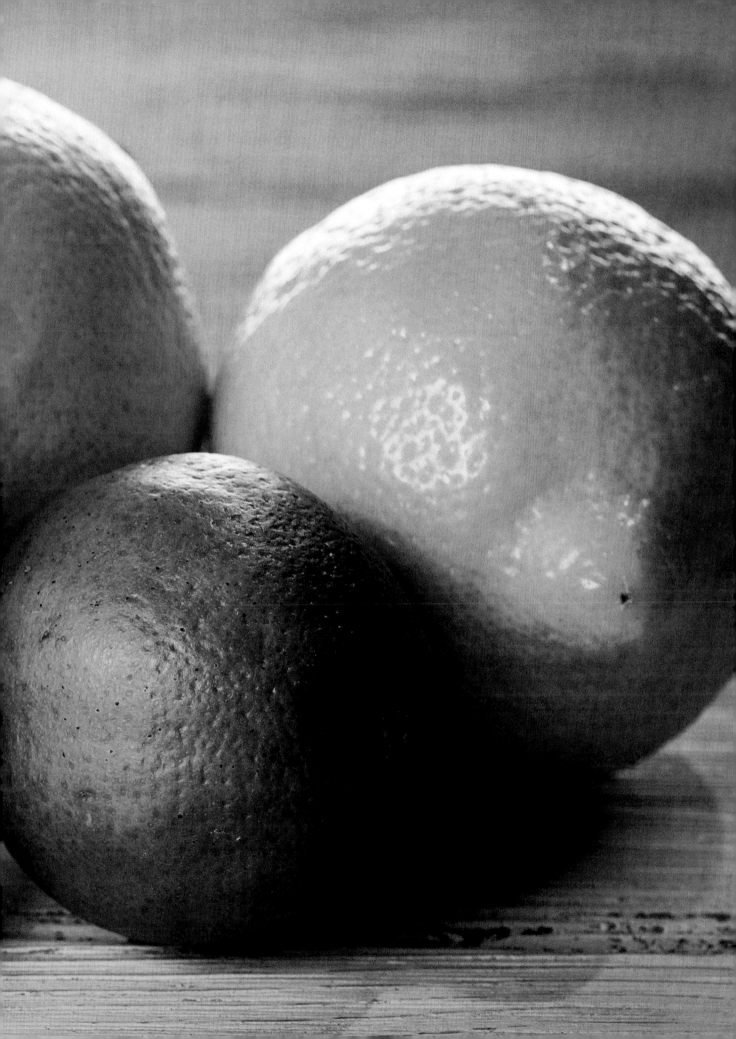

Essential Oil Blends

Note: This section contains examples of various essential oil blends that may be available commercially as well as examples of essential oils that each blend may contain.

For further information and research on many of the single oils contained in these blends, see the Single Essential Oils section of this book. Any internal use indicated for these blends is based on the use of pure, therapeutic-grade essential oils only.

Symbols and Colors Used in This Section

 Topical

 Aromatic

 Internal

 Cleaning/Disinfecting

 Avoid sunlight for up to 12 hours after use

 Avoid sunlight for up to 72 hours after use

 Neat (can be used without dilution)

 Dilute for children and those with sensitive skin

 Dilute

 Body System(s) Affected

 See Additional Research

AromaTouch® *(Massage Blend)*

Quick Facts

The oils in this blend were selected specifically for their abilities to relax, calm, and relieve the tension of muscles, to soothe irritated tissue, and to increase circulation. AromaTouch may help promote an anti-inflammatory effect on soft tissue and enhance all aspects of massage.

Common Primary Uses*: Anxiety, Massage, Muscle Aches/Pain, Muscular Dystrophy, Relaxation, Tension.

Application:

: Best if applied on location for all muscles. It may also be applied over the heart or diluted with fractionated coconut oil for a full body massage. It is also beneficial when placed in bathwater.

Single Oils in This Blend:

Basil: has anti-inflammatory and antispasmodic properties. It is relaxing to spastic muscles, including those that contribute to headaches and migraines.

Grapefruit: has calming and sedative properties. It may help with fatigue and stress.

Cypress: is anti-infectious, mucolytic, antiseptic, lymphatic-decongestive, refreshing, and relaxing. It may help improve lung circulation as well as help relieve other respiratory problems. It may also help relieve muscle cramps and improve overall circulation.

Marjoram: is an antispasmodic and is relaxing, calming, and appeasing to the muscles that constrict and sometimes contribute to headaches. It may be useful for muscle spasms, sprains, bruises, migraines, and sore muscles.

Lavender: is an oil that has traditionally been known to balance the body and to work wherever there is a need. It has antispasmodic and analgesic properties. It may help with sprains, sore muscles, headaches, and general healing.

Peppermint: is an anti-inflammatory to the nerves and helps reduce inflammation in damaged tissue. It is soothing, cooling, and dilating to the systems of the body. It may help to reduce fevers, candida, nausea, vomiting, and also help to strengthen the respiratory system.

Body System(s) Affected: The oils in this blend may help it be effective for dealing with various problems related to the Respiratory System, Cardiovascular System, and to Muscles and Bones.

Companion Oils: Basil, helichrysum, marjoram, and wintergreen.

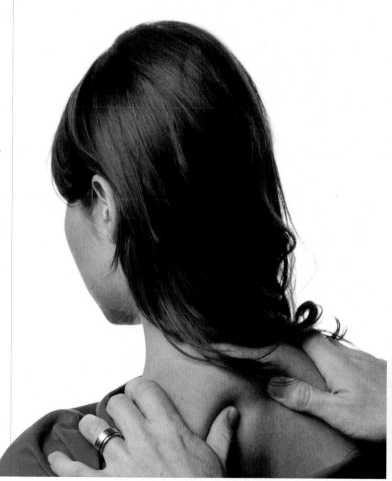

Essential Oil Blends

=Topical, =Aromatic, =Internal

Balance® *(Grounding Blend)*

Quick Facts

The oils in this blend may help establish a feeling of calmness, peace, and relaxation. It may aid in harmonizing the various physiological systems of the body and promote tranquility and a sense of balance.

Common Primary Uses*: Anxiety, Back Pain, Balance, Brain Integration, Bursitis, Coma, Confusion, Convulsions, Depression, Diabetic Sores, Energy, Fear, Grand Mal Seizure, Grief/Sorrow, Herniated Discs, Hot Flashes, Hyperactivity, Jet Lag, Lou Gehrig's Disease, Lupus, Metabolism (Balance), Mood Swings, Parkinson's Disease, Seizure

Application:

: This blend works best on the bottoms of the feet. Put six drops on bottoms of feet. Put on heart, wrists, and solar plexus from neck to thymus. To balance left and right brain, put on left fingers, and rub on right temple; or put on right fingers, and rub on left temple; or cross arms, and rub reflex points on bottoms of feet. To relieve pain along the spine, apply to reflex points on feet and on spine.

: Wear as perfume or cologne. Diffuse or inhale the aroma directly.

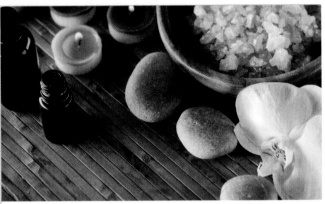

Single Oils in This Blend:

Spruce: grounds the body, creating the balance and the opening necessary to receive and to give. It may help dilate the bronchial tract to improve the oxygen exchange. It may also help a person to release emotional blocks.

Ho Wood: is soothing to the skin, appeasing to the mind, relaxing to the body, and creates a feeling of peace and gentleness.

Blue Tansy: may help cleanse the liver and calm the lymphatic system to help rid oneself of anger and promote a feeling of self-control.

Frankincense: contains sesquiterpenes, which may help oxygenate the pineal and pituitary glands. As one of the ingredients for the holy incense, frankincense was used anciently to help enhance one's communication with the Creator. It may help promote a positive attitude.

German (Blue) Chamomile: is soothing to the muscles and joints. It may help ease nervous tension and eliminate emotional tension.

Osmanthus: is one of the 10 famous traditional flowers of China. The blossoms are highly aromatic and are used in the world's rarest and most expensive perfumes. Its warm, floral aroma helps with concentration and focus while meditating, helping to relieve stress and clutter in the mind.

Carrier Oil in This Blend: Fractionated coconut oil.

Body System(s) Affected: The oils in this blend may help it be effective for dealing with various problems related to Muscles and Bones, Skin, the Nervous System, and Emotional Balance.

Aromatic Influence: This blend of oils may help balance the body and mind. Diffuse wherever and whenever possible.

---

*See Personal Usage Guide chapter for more details on these primary uses.   ●=Neat, ●=Dilute for Children/Sensitive Skin, ●=Dilute

Breathe® *(Respiratory Blend)*

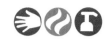

Essential Oil Blends

Quick Facts

Many of the oils in this blend have been studied for their abilities to open and soothe the tissues of the respiratory system and also for their abilities to combat airborne bacteria and viruses that could be harmful to the system.

Common Primary Uses*: ⊘Antiviral, ⊘Anxiety, ⊘⊘Asthma, ⊘⊘Bronchitis, ⊘⊘Congestion, ⊘⊘Cough, ⊘⊘Emphysema, ⊘⊘Influenza, ⊘⊘Mono, ⊘⊘Nasal Polyp, ⊘⊘Pneumonia, ⊘⊘Respiratory System, ⊘⊘Sinusitis, ⊘⊘Tuberculosis

Application:

⊘: May be applied on the chest, the back, or the bottoms of the feet.

⊘: Diffuse into the air. Apply to palms of hands: cup hands over nose and mouth, and breathe deeply, or inhale the aroma of the oil directly.

Single Oils in This Blend:

Laurel Leaf (Bay): has antiseptic and antifungal properties. It may also help with asthma, bronchitis, and viral infections.

Peppermint: is antiseptic, antispasmodic, and anti-inflammatory. It is soothing, cooling, and dilating to the system.

Eucalyptus radiata: may have a profound antiviral effect upon the respiratory system. It may also help reduce inflammation of the nasal mucous membrane.

Melaleuca alternifolia: has antibacterial, antifungal, antiviral, and expectorant properties. It may also help with bronchitis, coughs, and inflammation.

Lemon: promotes health, healing, physical energy, and purification. Its fragrance is invigorating, enhancing, and warming. It is an antiseptic and is great for the respiratory system.

Ravintsara: has antiviral properties and is often used for colds, bronchitis, mononeucleosis, and sinusitis.

Ravensara: is a powerful antiviral, antibacterial, antifungal, and anti-infectious oil. It may help dilate, open, and strengthen the respiratory system. As a cross between clove and nutmeg, it may also help support the adrenal glands.

Cardamom: has antiseptic and anti-inflammatory properties. It may also help with congestion and other respiratory problems.

⊕ **Body System(s) Affected:** The oils in this blend may help it be effective for dealing with various problems related to the Respiratory System and to the Skin.

Aromatic Influence: This blend of oils is excellent for opening the respiratory system when the blend is diffused or inhaled and is perfect for nighttime diffusion, allowing for restful sleep.

Application: Apply topically to the chest, the back, or the bottoms of the feet. Diffuse.

Safety Data: Can be irritating to sensitive skin. Dilute for young or sensitive skin.

Companion Oils: Run hot steaming water in sink; put Breathe and wintergreen in water; put towel over head; and inhale to open sinuses that have been blocked by flu, colds, or pneumonia. Also try On Guard.

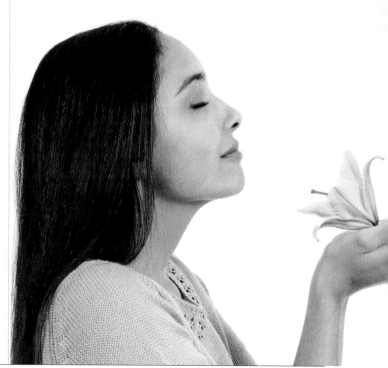

Cheer® *(Uplifting Blend)*

Quick Facts

This blend contains citrus and spice oils that are known to help combat feelings of gloom, distress, and disinterest, helping to cheer and uplift the mind, body, and spirit.

Common Primary Uses*: 🜓Coldness, 🜓Creativity, 🜓Depression, 🜓Grief, 🜓Joy, 🜓Positive (Feeling), 🜓Uplifting

Application:

🜋: Diffuse or inhale the aroma directly.

🜊: Apply on wrists, back of neck, over the heart area, or on the bottoms of the feet.

Single Oils in This Blend:

Orange: has calming properties that help ease feelings of anxiousness. Its aroma is uplifting to the mind and body.

Clove: has an energizing aroma that helps create a feeling of protection and courage.

Star Anise: from China has a licorice-like aroma that is believed to be energizing and to promote feelings of euphoria.

Lemon Myrtle: has calming, sedative properties and has an elevating, refreshing aroma.

Nutmeg: is often used to help increase energy and to support the nervous system from feelings of fatigue.

Vanilla: is calming and balancing and may help ease tension.

Ginger: is often used for its stimulating, warming influence. The aroma may help influence physical energy and love.

Cinnamon: has warming, stimulating properties and is often used to help relieve feelings of depression.

Zdravetz: is a variety of geranium found in Bulgaria. This oil has calming and relaxing properties.

❂ **Body System(s) Affected:** Hormonal System, Emotional Balance.

Safety Data: Repeated use can result in contact sensitization. Consult your doctor before using if you are pregnant, epileptic, or have a medical condition.

Companion Blends: Console, Motivate, Passion, Peace, Forgive.

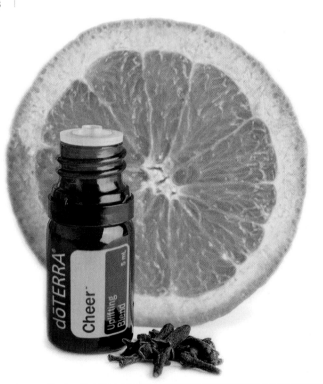

---

*See Personal Usage Guide chapter for more details on these primary uses.   ●=Neat, ●=Dilute for Children/Sensitive Skin, ●=Dilute

Citrus Bliss® *(Invigorating Blend)*

Quick Facts

This uniquely exhilarating blend brings together all of the uplifting and stress-reducing benefits of citrus essential oils in a sweetly satisfying way. In addition to their elevating properties, many of the citrus oils in this blend have been studied for their ability to cleanse and to disinfect.

Common Primary Uses*: 🌿Calming, 🌿🍃Depression, 🌿Eating Disorders, 🍃Mastitis, 🌿Sedative

Application:

🖐: May be applied on the ears, heart, and wrists or may be worn as a perfume or cologne. It may be diluted with fractionated coconut oil for a full-body massage. It may also be added to water for a relaxing bath.

🌀: Diffuse or inhale the aroma directly.

🧴: Mixed with water, this blend can also be used to disinfect countertops and other surfaces.

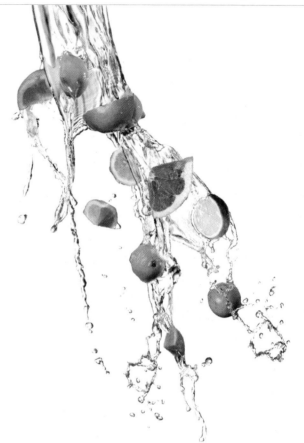

Single Oils in This Blend:

Orange: brings peace and happiness to the mind and body and joy to the heart, which feelings provide emotional support to help one overcome depression.

Lemon: promotes health, healing, physical energy, and purification. Its fragrance is invigorating, enhancing, and warming.

Grapefruit: is an antidepressant, an antiseptic, and a diuretic. It is balancing and uplifting to the mind and may help to relieve anxiety.

Mandarin: is appeasing, gentle, and promotes happiness. It is also refreshing, uplifting, and revitalizing. Because of its sedative properties, it is very good for combating stress and irritability.

Bergamot: has uplifting properties. It may also help with depression and agitation.

Tangerine: contains esters and aldehydes, which are sedating and calming to the nervous system. It is also a diuretic and a decongestant of the lymphatic system.

Clementine: is soothing and sedating and may help ease tension.

Vanilla Bean Extract: is calming and may help ease tension.

⊕ **Body System(s) Affected:** The oils in this blend may help it be effective for dealing with various problems related to the Immune System and to Emotional Balance.

Aromatic Influence: This blend of oils may create an enjoyable aromatic fragrance in the home or workplace. Simple diffusion can be achieved by applying a few drops of this blend on a cotton ball and placing it on a desk at work or placing it in an air vent.

Safety Data: May cause skin irritation. Avoid exposure to direct sunlight for up to 12 hours after use.

🖐=Topical, 🌀=Aromatic, ◯=Internal

ClaryCalm® *(Women's Monthly Blend)*

Quick Facts

This blend combines many different oils often used to help alleviate symptoms often associated with PMS, menopause, and aging.

Common Primary Uses*: ⊙⊘Hot Flashes, ⊙⊘Hormones (Balancing), ⊙⊘Menopause, ⊙Menstruation, ⊙⊘PMS

Application:

⊖: Apply to the chest, abdomen, or back of neck as needed.

⊘: Diffuse or inhale from the hands.

Single Oils in This Blend:

Clary Sage: is often used to help balance estrogen and other hormones associated with PMS and menopause symptoms.

Lavender: has soothing properties and is often used to help balance and calm emotions associated with PMS.

Bergamot: helps relieve feelings of stress and agitation, relieves tension, and helps balance emotions.

Roman Chamomile: is antispasmodic and has calming and relaxing properties. It is often used to help balance emotions and relieve symptoms related to menopause.

Cedarwood: is calming and soothes nervous tension.

Ylang Ylang: has calming and sedative properties. It brings a feeling of self-love, confidence, joy, and peace, and is often used to help balance hormones.

Geranium: may help with hormonal balance, and is often used to combat bone problems such as osteoporosis. It has a calming influence and is used in treating symptoms associated with PMS.

Fennel: is often used to help alleviate issues associated with menopause and premenopause. It has hormone balancing properties, and may be helpful in soothing symptoms related to PMS. It is also often used to help alleviate skin issues related to aging.

Carrot Seed: is often used to help regulate menstruation and soothe symptoms related to PMS.

Palmarosa: helps reduce stress and tension, and uplifts the emotions. It is often used to help alleviate many different skin problems.

Vitex: has been studied for its abilities to regulate estrogen levels, and to alleviate symptoms associated with PMS and menopause (Meier et al., 2000).

✚ **Body System(s) Affected:** Hormonal System, Emotional Balance, Skin.

Aromatic Influence: Helps to balance mood and calm stress and tension.

Safety Data: Repeated use may result in contact sensitization—dilute with fractionated coconut oil if this occurs. Consult your doctor before using if you are pregnant or have a medical condition.

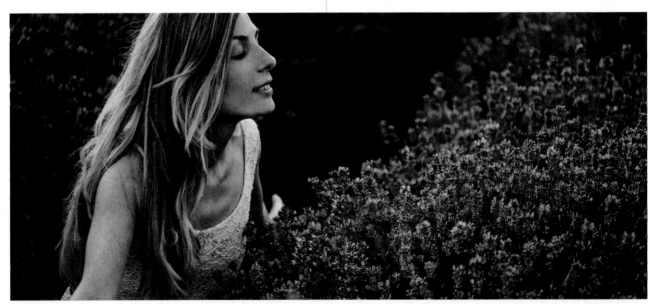

*See Personal Usage Guide chapter for more details on these primary uses. ●=Neat, ●=Dilute for Children/Sensitive Skin, ●=Dilute

Console® *(Comforting Blend)*

Quick Facts

This blend contains floral and tree oils that can help soothe feelings of sorrow and grief and promote uplifting feelings of peace and hope.

Common Primary Uses*: ⊘⊜Anger, ⊘⊜Depression, ⊘⊜Grief/Sorrow, ⊘⊜Happiness, ⊘⊜Uplifting

Application:

⊘: Diffuse or inhale the aroma directly.

⊜: Apply on wrists, back of neck, over the heart area, or on the bottoms of the feet.

Single Oils in This Blend:

Frankincense: is often used to help promote feelings of balance, to help with focus and meditation, and to help ease impatience and restlessness.

Patchouli: has sedating, calming, and relaxing properties and is often used to help reduce anxious feelings.

Ylang Ylang: has antidepressant and sedative properties. It is often used to help calm and relax.

Labdanum: or cistus, was one of the first aromatic substances used anciently. It is stimulating to the senses and is often used to help elevate the emotions and soothe the nerves.

Amyris: is similar to sandalwood in nature and is often called East Indies sandalwood. It is often used for its sedative properties and to help relieve tension and stress.

Sandalwood: is often used to help soothe feelings of sadness and depression. It has calming and sedative properties and helps harmonize and balance the emotions.

Rose: is stimulating and elevating to the mind, creating a sense of well-being.

Osmanthus: is one of the 10 famous traditional flowers of China. The blossoms are highly aromatic and are used in the world's rarest and most expensive perfumes. It is used in Chinese medicine to "reduce phlegm and remove blood stasis."

⊕ **Body System(s) Affected:** Hormonal System, Emotional Balance.

Safety Data: Repeated use can result in contact sensitization. Consult your doctor before using if you are pregnant, epileptic, or have a medical condition.

Companion Blends: Motivate, Passion, Peace, Forgive, Cheer.

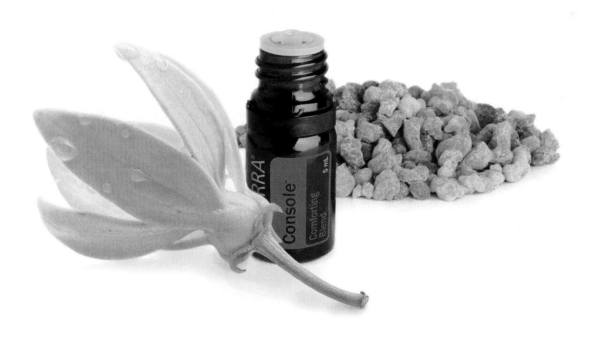

⊜=Topical, ⊘=Aromatic, ◯=Internal

DDR Prime® *(Cellular Complex)*

Quick Facts

The oils in this blend have been chosen for their abilities to provide antioxidant support for the cells and to promote a healthy cellular life cycle.

Common Primary Uses*: ^OAging, ^OAntioxidant, ^OAtherosclerosis, ^OCancer, ^OCellular Health, ^OTumors

Application:

⊘: Dilute as needed, and apply on area of concern.

⊘: Diffuse or inhale the aroma directly.

○: Adults can take up to 8 drops internally, twice a day with food.

Single Oils in This Blend:

Frankincense: has anti-inflammatory and immune-stimulant properties. It is often used to help support the body's response to cancer and other cellular diseases.

Orange: contains high levels of d-limonene, which has demonstrated potential in inhibiting cancer tumor growth (Chidambara et al., 2012) and has also been shown to reduce cholesterol levels in animal studies (Sorentino et al., 2005).

Litsea: has antibacterial properties, and is energizing and uplifting. It is used traditionally to help with pain and digestive issues.

Lemongrass: has anti-inflammatory and antiseptic properties. Constituents found in this oil have demonstrated an ability to inhibit cancer cell growth (Carnesecchi et al., 2001) and to induce apoptosis (cellular death) in human leukemia cells (Kumar et al., 2008).

Thyme: has strong antioxidant and antiseptic properties. It is often used to help support the brain as it ages.

Summer Savory (*Satureja hortensis*): has demonstrated antifungal (Sabzghabaee et al., 2012) and anti-inflammatory (Hajhashemi et al., 2012) properties. Studies have also demonstrated the ability of summer savory oil to decrease lipid peroxidation associated with aging in mice (Misharina et al., 2011) and to reduce DNA damage caused by oxidative stress in rat lymphocytes (Mosaffa et al., 2006). Additionally, a methanol extract of Satureja hortensis was found to reduce blood platelet adhesion (a risk factor in cardiovascular disease) in vitro (Yazdanparast et al., 2008).

Clove: has high antioxidant properties and is anti-infectious and helps support healthy liver and thyroid function.

Niaouli (*Melaleuca quinquenervia*): has powerful antifungal properties and is anti-inflammatory. It is often used to help protect against radiation and also to help regenerate damaged tissue.

✛ **Body System(s) Affected:** The oils in this blend may help it be effective for dealing with various problems related to the Cardiovascular System, Immune System, Nervous System, Muscles and Bones, and Skin and Hair.

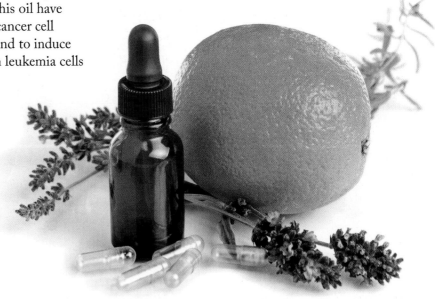

*See Personal Usage Guide chapter for more details on these primary uses.   ●=Neat, ●=Dilute for Children/Sensitive Skin, ●=Dilute

144

Deep Blue® *(Soothing Blend)*

Quick Facts

This blend contains oils that are well-known and are frequently studied for their abilities to soothe inflammation, alleviate pain, and reduce soreness.

Common Primary Uses*: ⬤Arthritis, ⬤Back Pain, ⬤Bone Pain, ⬤Bruises, ⬤Bursitis, ⬤Fibromyalgia, ⬤Inflammation, ⬤Joint Pain, ⬤Muscle Aches/Pain, ⬤Muscle Tension, ⬤Pain, ⬤Tension Headaches, ⬤Whiplash

Application:

⬤: Apply as a compress on spine and on reflex points on feet. Apply on location for muscle cramps, bruises, or any other pain.

Single Oils in This Blend:

Wintergreen: contains 99% methyl salicylate, which gives it cortisone-like properties. It may be beneficial for arthritis, rheumatism, tendinitis, and any other discomfort that is related to the inflammation of bones, muscles, and joints.

Camphor: is analgesic (pain-relieving) and anti-inflammatory. It may be beneficial for arthritis, rheumatism, muscle aches and pains, sprains, and bruises.

Peppermint: is anti-inflammatory to the prostate and to damaged tissues. It has a soothing and cooling effect that may help with arthritis and rheumatism.

Ylang Ylang: is often used to help calm and relax from exhaustion. It can help relieve anxious feelings, and soothe skin irritations.

Blue Tansy: is analgesic and anti-inflammatory. It may also help with low blood pressure, arthritis, and rheumatism.

German (Blue) Chamomile: is antioxidant, anti-inflammatory, and analgesic. It may also help relieve congestion and arthritis.

Helichrysum: may help cleanse the blood and improve circulatory functions. It is anticatarrhal in structure and nature. As a powerful anti-inflammatory, it may even help reduce inflammation in the meninges of the brain. On a spiritual level, it may help one let go of angry feelings that prevent one from forgiving and moving forward.

Osmanthus: is one of the 10 famous traditional flowers of China. The blossoms are highly aromatic and are used in the world's rarest and most expensive perfumes. It is used in Chinese medicine to "reduce phlegm and remove blood stasis."

⬤ **Body System(s) Affected:** The oils in this blend may help it be effective for dealing with various problems related to the Nervous System and to Muscles and Bones.

Safety Data: Repeated use may possibly result in contact sensitization. Use with caution during pregnancy.

Companion Oils: Add frankincense (to enhance) or wintergreen (for bone pain).

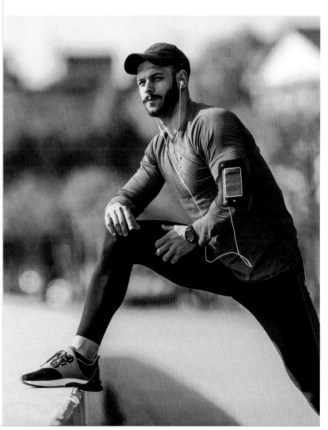

Essential Oil Blends

⬤=Topical, ⬤=Aromatic, ⬤=Internal

DigestZen® *(Digestive Blend)*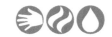

Quick Facts

This blend may be useful for improving digestive function. The oils in this blend have been studied for their abilities in balancing the digestive system and in soothing many of that system's ailments.

Common Primary Uses*: ⚬⚭Bloating, ⚭⚬Colitis, ⚬⚭Constipation, ⚬⚭Cramps (Abdominal), ⚬⚭Crohn's Disease, ⚬⚭Diarrhea, ⚬Food Poisoning, ⚬⚭Gastritis, ⚭⚬Heartburn, ⚭⚬Nausea, ⚬⚭Parasites, ⚭Sinusitis

Application:

⚭: May be applied to reflex points on the feet and on the ankles. It may also be applied topically over the stomach, as a compress on the abdomen, and at the bottom of the throat (for gagging). Apply to animal paws for parasites.

⚋: Diffuse or inhale the aroma directly.

⚬: As a dietary supplement, dilute 1 drop in ½ cup (125 ml) of water or soy/rice milk, and sip slowly. May also be used in a retention enema for ridding the colon of parasites and for combating digestive candida.

Single Oils in This Blend:

Ginger: is warming, uplifting, and empowering. Emotionally, it may help influence physical energy, love, and courage. Because of its calming influence on the digestive system, it may help reduce feelings of nausea and motion sickness.

Peppermint: is an anti-inflammatory to the prostate and nerves. It is soothing, cooling, and dilating to the system. It may also be beneficial for counteracting food poisoning, vomiting, diarrhea, constipation, flatulence, halitosis, colic, nausea, and motion sickness.

Tarragon: may help to reduce anorexia, dyspepsia, flatulence, intestinal spasms, nervous and sluggish digestion, and genital urinary tract infection.

Fennel: may help improve digestive function by supporting the liver. It may also help balance the hormones.

Caraway: is antiparasitic and antispasmodic. It may also help with indigestion, gas, and colic.

Coriander: is antispasmodic and has anti-inflammatory properties. It may also help with indigestion, flatulence, diarrhea, and other spasms of the digestive tract.

Anise: may help calm and strengthen the digestive system.

⊕ Body System(s) Affected: The oils in this blend may help it be effective for dealing with various problems related to the Digestive System.

Safety Data: Use with caution during pregnancy (only a drop massaged on the outer ear for morning sickness). Not for use by people with epilepsy.

Companion Oils: Peppermint.

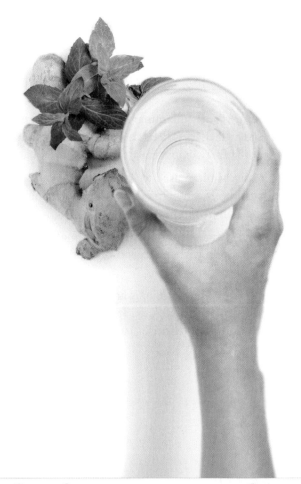

See Personal Usage Guide chapter for more details on these primary uses.   ●=Neat, ●=Dilute for Children/Sensitive Skin, ●=Dilute

146

Elevation *(Joyful Blend)*

Essential Oil Blends

Quick Facts

This uplifting combination of essential oils creates an energetic aroma that can help stimulate the body's chemistry when a person is feeling lethargic or sad.

Common Primary Uses*: ⚬Abuse, ⚬Anxiety, ⚬Cushing's Syndrome, ⚬⚬Depression, ⚬⚬Energy, ⚬⚬Grief/Sorrow, ⚬⚬Lupus, ⚬Poison Oak/Ivy, ⚬⚬Postpartum Depression, ⚬Shock, ⚬⚬Stimulating, ⚬⚬Stress, ⚬Uplifting, ⚬Weight Loss

Application:

⚬: Rub over heart, ears, neck, thymus, temples, across brow, and on wrists. Apply on heart reflex points. Put in bathwater. Use as compress; dilute with fractionated coconut oil for a full-body massage. Place on areas of poor circulation.

⚬: Wear as perfume or cologne, especially over the heart. Put two drops on a wet cloth, and put the cloth in the dryer with washed laundry for great-smelling clothes. Diffuse or inhale the aroma directly.

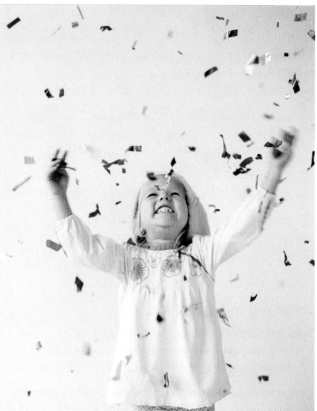

Single Oils in This Blend:

Lavandin: may help dispel feelings of depression or anxiety.

Lavender: is a universal oil that is traditionally used to balance the body, relieve depression, and increase relaxation.

Amyris (West Indian Sandalwood): contains a high level of sesquiterpenes and may help promote calmness and relief from stress and tension.

Clary Sage: has sedative and soothing properties and is often used to help with hormonal balance.

Tangerine: is sedative in nature. It may help calm and relieve feelings of stress while enhancing energy.

Lemon Myrtle: has a strong lemony aroma that is elevating and refreshing.

Melissa: may help with depression and anxiety and has an uplifting lemony aroma.

Ylang Ylang: is calming and relaxing. It brings a feeling of self-love, confidence, joy, and peace.

Osmanthus: is one of the 10 famous traditional flowers of China. The blossoms are highly aromatic and are used in the world's rarest and most expensive perfumes. Its heady, uplifting fragrance (a very rich, sweet floral fruit bouquet) has been known to make everyone smile.

Hawaiian Sandalwood: is calming and sedative. It helps balance and harmonize the emotions and may help ease nervous tension.

⊕ **Body System(s) Affected:** The oils in this blend may help it be effective for dealing with various problems related to Emotional Balance.

Aromatic Influence: The fragrance of this blend of oils is uplifting, refreshing, and helps promote feelings of self-worth. It can help dispel feelings of depression, sorrow, and anxiety.

Safety Data: Avoid exposure to direct sunlight for up to 12 hours after use.

Forgive® *(Renewing Blend)*

Quick Facts

This blend contains tree and herb oils that are known to help soothe feelings of anger or guilt and help promote feelings of love and forgiveness.

Common Primary Uses*: ⚫⬤Acceptance, ⚫⬤Anger, ⚫⬤Blocks (Emotional), ⚫⬤Confidence, ⚫⬤Emotional Trauma, ⚫⬤Grief, ⚫⬤Guilt, ⚫⬤Loss, ⚫⬤Pity, ⚫⬤Release (Emotional), ⚫⬤Uplifting

Application:

⚫: Diffuse or inhale the aroma directly.

⬤: Apply on wrists, back of neck, over the heart area, or on the bottoms of the feet.

Single Oils in This Blend:

Spruce (Hemlock Spruce): is uplifting to the emotions, as it opens and elevates while grounding at the same time. It is often used to help enhance meditation.

Bergamot: is often used to help soothe feelings of agitation, anger, depression, and mental and emotional stress. It may help soothe anxious or depressed feelings and is uplifting and refreshing.

Juniper Berry: was used traditionally to help purify the body and spirit and helps promote feelings of health, love, and peace.

Myrrh: helps promote awareness and has an uplifting influence.

Arborvitae: has calming properties and may help enhance mental and spiritual awareness.

Nootka: is a tree indigenous to the northwest coast of North America. It was used traditionally to carve boats and important decorative items. Its aroma is believed to open the heart and spirit to emotional clearing and allow change to take place.

Thyme: is energizing in times of weakness and stress. It may also help to uplift and relieve depressed feelings.

Citronella: is stimulating and energizing and helps uplift the mind and spirit.

⊕ **Body System(s) Affected:** Hormonal System, Emotional Balance.

Safety Data: Repeated use can result in contact sensitization. Consult your doctor before using if you are pregnant, epileptic, or have a medical condition.

Companion Blends: Console, Motivate, Passion, Peace, Cheer.

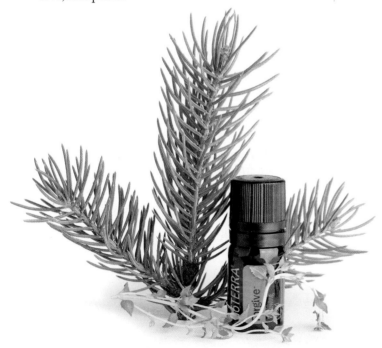

---

*See Personal Usage Guide chapter for more details on these primary uses.   ⬤=Neat, ⬤=Dilute for Children/Sensitive Skin, ⬤=Dilute

HD Clear® *(Topical Blend)*

Quick Facts

This new formulation of HD Clear contains oils that have been selected for their unique abilities to help protect the skin from bacterial and fungal proliferation and from other skin problems such as eczema and acne. This blend can be applied topically to infected areas.

Common Primary Uses*: Acne, Callouses, Dermatitis, Impetigo, Oily Skin

Application:

: Apply on location daily as needed.

Single Oils in This Blend:

Ho Wood: is known for its antiseptic properties and is often used to help clear infections and to support the revitalization of skin tissue.

Melaleuca: is one of the most studied antibacterial and antifungal oils. Melaleuca also has anti-inflammatory properties and can help support the skin in the recovery process after injuries.

Litsea Berry: has antiseptic and astringent properties and has been used for oily skin and acne.

Eucalyptus globulus: is often used for inflammation and skin infections and sores. It is used medicinally in France to treat candida and other fungal infections and has also demonstrated strong antibacterial properties.

Geranium: has antibacterial and anti-inflammatory properties and is often used to help alleviate the effects of acne and eczema. It may also help balance sebum levels in the skin.

Other Oils:

Black Cumin Seed Oil: has been used since ancient times for a myriad of health concerns. In addition to its antioxidant and anti-inflammatory properties, black cumin seed oil also has a high content of linoleic acid, an essential fatty acid used by the body to help maintain healthy skin and hair. Linoleic acid has been studied for its ability to reduce acne microcomedones (Letawe et al., 1998) and to enhance cellular migration during wound healing (Ruthig et al., 1999).

Body System(s) Affected: The oils in this blend may help it be effective for dealing with various problems related to the Skin and the Immune System.

Safety Data: Repeated use may possibly result in contact sensitization. Use with caution during pregnancy.

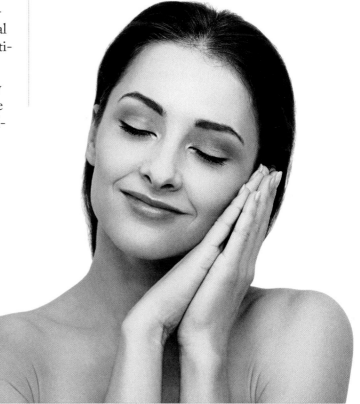

Immortelle *(Anti-Aging Blend)*

Quick Facts

This soothing blend may be useful for maintaining skin health and vitality. The oils in this blend have been studied for their abilities to help reduce inflammation, protect the skin from UV radiation, and promote healthy cellular function and proper hydration of the skin.

Common Primary Uses*: ⬢Aging, ⬢Chapped/Cracked Skin, ⬢Dry Skin, ⬢Revitalizing, ⬢Wrinkles

Application:

⬢: Apply directly on areas of concern. Use along with other natural skin care products.

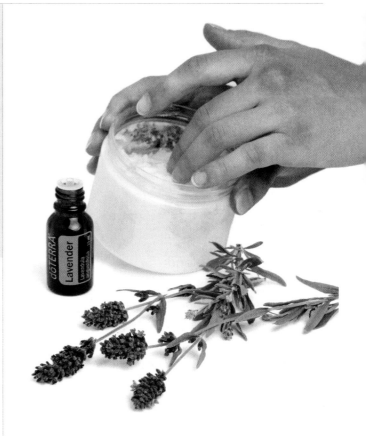

Single Oils in This Blend:

Frankincense: has been studied for its anti-inflammatory properties. Its anti-infectious property also helps protect the skin from harmful microbes. Frankincense is also soothing to the skin and nerves.

Hawaiian Sandalwood: has been found in several animal studies to protect the skin from the harmful effects of ultraviolet (UV-b) radiation. It may also be useful in skin regeneration and in stopping skin infections.

Lavender: has been studied for its ability to reduce inflammation and allergic reactions in the skin. It has also been used to help the skin recover from burns, blisters, infections, and other injuries, as well as to help reduce conditions related to dry skin.

Myrrh: is known to be soothing to the skin and is often used to relieve chapped or cracked skin. It has been studied for its anti-inflammatory properties and is also used to fight many bacterial, fungal, and viral infections of the skin.

Helichrysum: is used to help relieve skin conditions such as eczema and psoriasis. It has antioxidant properties, and is often used for tissue regeneration, pain relief, and healing. It has also been used as a natural sunscreen.

Rose: is often used to help stop the breakdown of collagen in the skin that can lead to a loss of elasticity and wrinkles. It has also been used to help prevent scarring and to help the body overcome various skin diseases and infections.

⬢ **Body System(s) Affected:** The oils in this blend may help it be effective for dealing with various problems related to the Skin.

Safety Data: Use with caution during pregnancy.

See Personal Usage Guide chapter for more details on these primary uses.   ●=Neat, ●=Dilute for Children/Sensitive Skin, ●=Dilute

150

InTune® *(Focus Blend)*

Quick Facts

This blend contains oils that have been studied and used traditionally for their abilities to promote calmness, focus, and a balanced state of mind. Many of the oils in this blend contain high levels of sesquiterpenes, which have demonstrated an ability to pass the blood-brain barrier to reach the cells of the brain.

Common Primary Uses*: ⊜⊘ADD/ADHD, ⊜⊘Anxiety, ⊜⊘Calming, ⊜Clarity, ⊜⊘Concentration, ⊜⊘Focus, ⊜⊘Hyperactivity, ⊜⊘Stress

Application:

⊜: Apply on back of neck and on bottoms of the feet.

⊘: Diffuse or inhale the aroma directly.

Single Oils in This Blend:

Amyris (West Indian Sandalwood): contains a high level of sesquiterpenes and may help promote calmness and relief from stress and tension.

Patchouli: has a sedating, calming, and relaxing influence and may be useful in relieving anxiety and depression. It also has a high level of sesquiterpenes.

Frankincense: has antidepressant and sedating properties. It is often used to help enhance memory, reduce mental fatigue, focus energy, and aid concentration.

Lime: has a refreshing aroma that is often used to help overcome exhaustion, depression, and listlessness. It may also be beneficial for anxiety.

Ylang Ylang: has demonstrated sedative properties and is often used to help aid with anxiety and depression.

Hawaiian Sandalwood: is often used as an aid in focus and meditation. It also has calming and sedative properties.

Roman Chamomile: has a calming and relaxing influence. It is often used to help safely and effectively reduce irritability and nervousness in children, especially hyperactive children.

✛ **Body System(s) Affected:** The oils in this blend may help it be effective for dealing with various problems related to Emotional Balance, the Hormonal System, and the Nervous System.

Safety Data: Repeated use may result in contact sensitization.

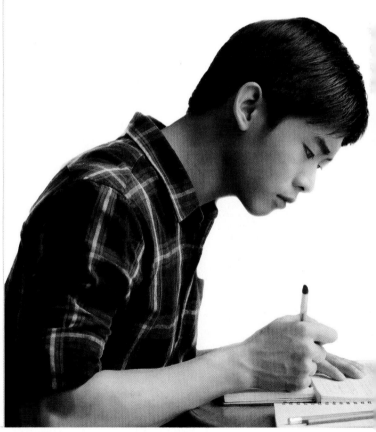

Kids: Brave™ *(Courage Blend)*

Quick Facts

Brave contains oils that are known for the ability to hesoothe anxious feelings. This blend can help promote feelings of self-worth and confidence in new and unknown situations. It is diluted in a base of fractionated coconut oil, so it is just right for young skin.

Common Primary Uses*: ⬤⬤Anxiety, ⬤⬤Courage, ⬤⬤Uplifting

Application:

⬤: Roll onto bottoms of feet, back of neck, or pulse points on wrists as needed.

⬤: Inhale the aroma directly. Roll onto a diffusing bracelet or necklace to wear throughout the day.

Single Oils in This Blend:

Orange: is uplifting to the mind and body. Its aroma has demonstrated the ability to help reduce feelings of anxiety in stressful situations.

Amyris (West Indian Sandalwood): contains a high level of sesquiterpenes and may promote calmness and relief from stress and tension.

Osmanthus: is one of the 10 famous traditional flowers of China. The highly aromatic blossoms are used in the world's rarest and most expensive perfumes. This warm, floral aroma aids concentration and focus during meditation, helping to relieve stress and declutter the mind.

Cinnamon Bark: is energizing and warming. It is often used to help combat physical and mental fatigue.

Carrier Oil in This Blend: Fractionated Coconut Oil.

⬤ **Body System(s) Affected:** The oils in this blend may help it be effective for various problems related to the Nervous System and Emotional Balance.

Aromatic Influence: Brave is warm, cheery, and uplifting. It may promote feelings of self-worth and can help dispel feelings of depression, sorrow, and anxiety.

Safety Data: Keep out of reach of younger children. Consult with a physician before use if being treated for a medical condition.

Companion Blends: Calmer, Steady, Elevation.

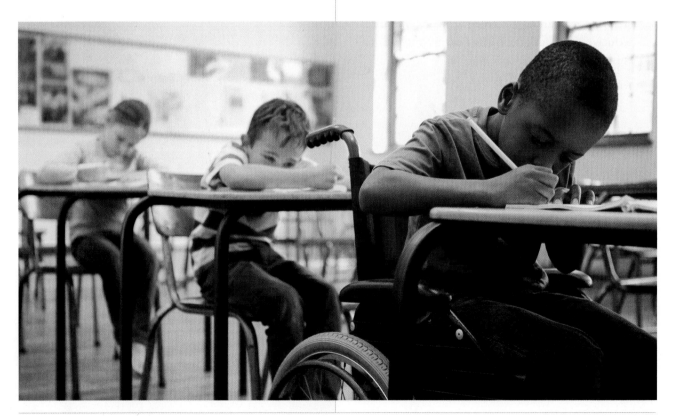

*See Personal Usage Guide chapter for more details on these primary uses.   ⬤=Neat, ⬤=Dilute for Children/Sensitive Skin, ⬤=Dilute

Kids: Calmer™ *(Restful Blend)*

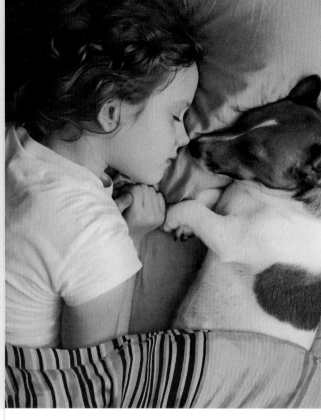

Quick Facts

Calmer is designed to help soothe and promote relaxation after a busy, stressful day. It contains oils known for their calming and sedative properties. This blend can help steady and balance the mind and emotions in preparation for a good night's sleep. It is diluted in a base of fractionated coconut oil, so it is just right for young skin.

Common Primary Uses*: Anger, Anxiety, Calming, Hyperactivity, Insomnia, Mental Fatigue, Mood Swings, Sedative, Sleep, Stress, Teeth Grinding, Tension

Application:

: Roll onto bottoms of feet, back of neck, chest, or pulse points on wrists as needed. Apply a small amount in palms, and then gently rub front and back of hands for a relaxing massage.

: Inhale the aroma directly. Roll onto a diffusing bracelet or necklace to wear throughout the day.

(Right margin tab) Essential Oil Blends

Single Oils in This Blend:

Lavender: has calming and sedative properties. It may help lift feelings of depression and anxiety.

Cananga: has calming and sedative properties. It brings a feeling of self-love, confidence, joy, and peace.

Buddha Wood: has a woody, sweet aroma that is often used for relaxing and as an aid for meditation.

Roman Chamomile: is calming and relaxing. It may help relieve muscle tension, as well as calm nerves and soothe emotions.

Carrier Oil in This Blend: Fractionated Coconut Oil.

Body System(s) Affected: The oils in this blend may help it be effective for various problems related to the Nervous System and Emotional Balance.

Aromatic Influence: Calmer is well suited for soothing nerves or emotions at the end of the day or during stressful times.

Safety Data: Keep out of reach of younger children. Consult with a physician before use if being treated for a medical condition.

Companion Blends: Brave, Steady, Serenity.

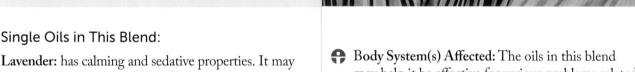

=Topical, =Aromatic, =Internal

Kids: Rescuer™ *(Soothing Blend)*

Quick Facts

Rescuer is ideal for soothing and comforting tired, achy muscles and joints at the end of a strenuous day. Oils in this blend are known for the ability to help relieve minor aches and pains. The blend is diluted in a base of fractionated coconut oil, so it is just right for young skin.

Common Primary Uses*: ⬤Back Pain, ⬤Bone Pain, ⬤Bruises, ⬤⬤Inflammation, ⬤Joint Pain, ⬤Migraines, ⬤Muscle Aches/Pain, ⬤⬤Muscle Tension, ⬤⬤Pain, ⬤⬤Stress, ⬤⬤Tension Headache, ⬤Whiplash

Application:

⬤: Roll onto tired or sore muscles at the end of the day or after strenuous activities. Roll onto legs to help soothe growing pains. Apply a small amount on the back, shoulders, and neck, gently massaging into tissues.

⬤: Inhale the aroma directly. Roll onto a diffusing bracelet or necklace to wear throughout the day.

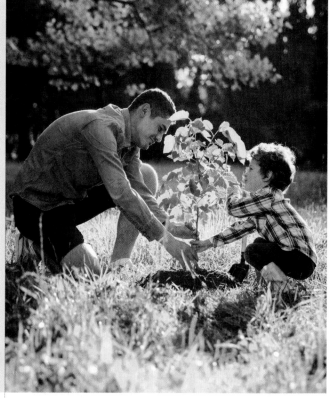

Single Oils in This Blend:

Copaiba: has anti-inflammatory and pain-relieving properties. It is often used to help soothe muscle aches and pains. Copaiba oil has also demonstrated the ability to help reduce anxious feelings.

Lavender: is well known for its ability to soothe pain from minor skin irritations and wounds. It is often used to help with headaches and muscle pain too.

Spearmint: is often used to help relieve mental strain and fatigue and to help lift one's spirit.

Zanthoxylum: is extremely high in linolool, which has demonstrated the ability to soothe pain when used both topically and aromatically.

Carrier Oil in This Blend: Fractionated Coconut Oil.

🜛 **Body System(s) Affected:** The oils in this blend may help it be effective for various problems related to the Nervous System and to Muscles and Bones.

Aromatic Influence: Rescuer has a soothing, calming influence that helps ease worried and stressful feelings.

Safety Data: Keep out of reach of younger children. Consult with a physician before use if being treated for a medical condition.

Companion Blends: Stronger, Deep Blue

---

*See Personal Usage Guide chapter for more details on these primary uses.   ⬤=Neat, ⬤=Dilute for Children/Sensitive Skin, ⬤=Dilute

Kids: Steady™ *(Grounding Blend)*

Quick Facts

Steady is comprised of oils known for their ability to help bring about a feeling of balance, peace, and relaxation. This blend can help focus the mind during times of distraction. It is diluted in a base of fractionated coconut oil, so it is just right for young skin.

Common Primary Uses*: ⊘ADD/ADHD, ⊘⊙Anxiety, ⊘⊙Balance, ⊘⊙Brain, ⊘⊙Confusion, ⊘⊙Depression, ⊘⊙Energy, ⊘⊙Fear, ⊘⊙Grief/Sorrow, ⊘⊙Jet Lag, ⊘⊙Metabolism (Balance), ⊘⊙Mood Swings

Application:

⊜: Roll onto bottoms of feet, back of neck, or pulse points on wrists as needed.

⊘: Inhale the aroma directly. Roll onto a diffusing bracelet or necklace to wear throughout the day.

Single Oils in This Blend:

Amyris (West Indian Sandalwood): is similar in nature to the more commonly known East Indian Sandalwood, including its calming and harmonizing aroma. It is often used for its sedative properties and to help relieve tension and stress.

Balsam Fir: is grounding, anchoring, and empowering. It is stimulating to the mind while relaxing to the body. It helps balancing the emotions.

Coriander: has sedative properties. Its aroma helps one relax when feeling stressed, irritable, and nervous. It may also provide a calming influence to one suffering from shock or fear.

Magnolia: has sedative properties and is often used to help with anxiety and stress. It has a soothing, steadying influence that can help relax both the body and mind.

Carrier Oil in This Blend: Fractionated Coconut Oil.

⊕ Body System(s) Affected: The oils in this blend may help it be effective for various problems related to the Nervous System and Emotional Balance.

Aromatic Influence: Steady is uplifting and empowering, while still keeping one focused and grounded.

Safety Data: Keep out of reach of younger children. Consult with a physician before use if being treated for a medical condition.

Companion Blends: Thinker, Brave, Balance

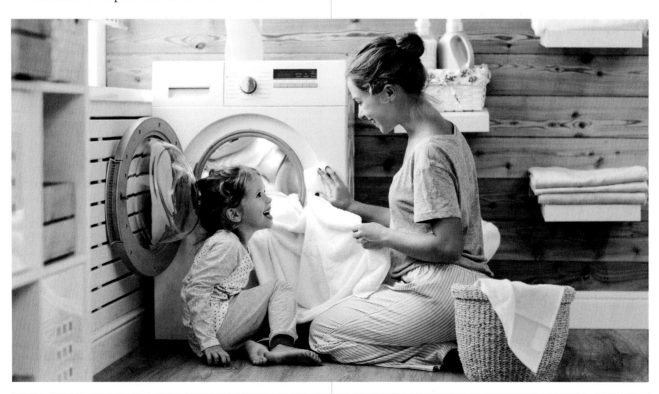

⊜=Topical, ⊘=Aromatic, ◯=Internal

Kids: Stronger™ *(Protective Blend)*

Quick Facts

Stronger is comprised of oils known to help soothe and protect the skin and body from environmental threats. This blend is diluted in a base of fractionated coconut oil, so it is just right for young skin.

Common Primary Uses*: ⬤Acne, ⬤Antibacterial, ⬤Antiseptic, ⬤⬤Candida, ⬤⬤Cleansing, ⬤Cuts/Scrapes, ⬤⬤Coughs, ⬤Insect Bites/Stings,

Application:

⬤: Roll onto distressed or irritated skin. Apply to bottoms of feet, back of neck, or pulse points on wrists as needed.

⬤: Inhale the aroma directly. Roll onto a diffusing bracelet or necklace to wear throughout the day.

Single Oils in This Blend:

Cedarwood: is calming and soothing to nervous tension It has antifungal and antiseptic properties.

Litsea: is often used in cleaning for its strong antibacterial and antiseptic properties. It may also help reduce skin blemishes.

Frankincense: has anti-inflammatory and immune-stimulating properties. An anti-infectious ability helps protect the skin from harmful microbes. It is generally soothing to the skin and nerves.

Rose: is often used to help stop the breakdown of collagen in skin that can lead to a loss of elasticity. It has also been used to help prevent scarring and to help overcome various skin diseases and infections.

Carrier Oil in This Blend: Fractionated Coconut Oil.

⬤ **Body System(s) Affected:** The oils in this blend may help it be effective for various problems related to the Immune System and Skin.

Aromatic Influence: Stronger has a bright, uplifting aroma that can help one face life's challenges head-on with feelings of resiliency.

Safety Data: Keep out of reach of younger children. Consult with a physician before using if being treated for a medical condition.

Companion Blends: Rescuer, On Guard

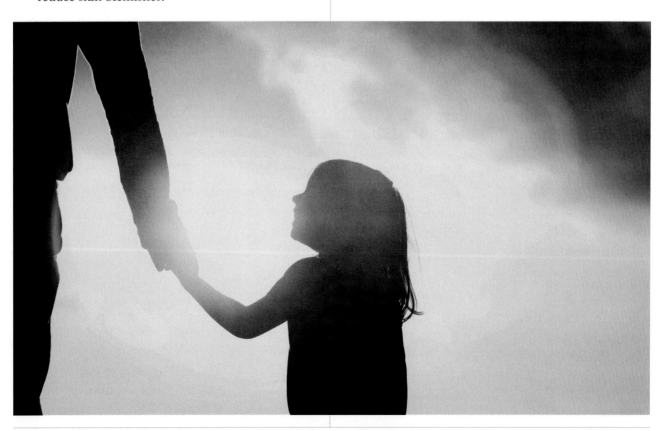

*See Personal Usage Guide chapter for more details on these primary uses.   ⬤=Neat, ⬤=Dilute for Children/Sensitive Skin, ⬤=Dilute

Kids: Thinker™ *(Focus Blend)*

Quick Facts

Thinker contains oils known for their ability to aid focus, memory, and concentration. This blend can help create a positive, nurturing atmosphere to support learning. It is diluted in a base of fractionated coconut oil, so it is just right for young skin.

Common Primary Uses*: ⬭⬯ADD/ADHD, ⬭⬯Alertness, ⬭⬯Anxiety, ⬭⬯Calming, ⬭⬯Clarity, ⬭⬯Concentration, ⬭⬯Focus, ⬭⬯Memory, ⬭⬯Stress

Application:

⬭: Roll onto temples, back of neck, or pulse points on wrists as needed to help maintain focus and concentration.

⬯: Inhale the aroma directly. Roll onto a diffusing bracelet or necklace to wear throughout the day.

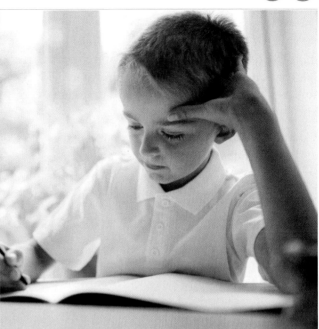

Single Oils in This Blend:

Vetiver: has calming, balancing properties and is often used to help sedate the nerves. It may also help with anxious, stressful, and worried feelings.

Clementine: is soothing and sedating and may help ease tension.

Peppermint: is well known for its energizing and invigorating properties. Stimulating to the mind, it aids memory and focus. It also helps relieve headaches and has a cooling effect on the skin.

Rosemary: is often used to help relieve feelings of nervousness, mental fatigue, or depression. It has been studied for the ability to help improve memory and concentration.

Carrier Oil in This Blend: Fractionated Coconut Oil.

Body System(s) Affected: The oils in this blend may be effective for various problems related to the Nervous System and Emotional Balance.

Aromatic Influence: Thinker blend has an energizing, motivating aroma. It can help bring clarity, focus, and alertness to the mind.

Safety Data: Keep out of reach of younger children. Consult with a physician before use if being treated for a medical condition.

Companion Blends: Steady, Calm, InTune

⬭=Topical, ⬯=Aromatic, ◯=Internal

Motivate® *(Encouraging Blend)*

Quick Facts

This blend contains a combination of mint and citrus oils that can help motivate and inspire an individual to have the courage to move forward with confidence and strength.

Common Primary Uses*: ⊘⊜Anxious Feelings, ⊘⊜Confidence, ⊘⊜Creativity, ⊘⊜Defeat, ⊘⊜Depression, ⊘⊜Expression (Self-expression), ⊘⊜Fear, ⊘⊜Happiness, ⊘⊜Positiveness, ⊘⊜Rejection

Application:

⊘: Diffuse or inhale the aroma directly.

⊜: Apply on wrists, back of neck, over the heart area, or on the bottoms of the feet.

Single Oils in This Blend:

Peppermint: is well known for its energizing and invigorating properties. It is also used to help aid with memory and focus.

Clementine: is soothing and sedating and may help ease tension.

Coriander: is often used as a gentle stimulant for those with low physical energy. It also helps one relax during times of stress and nervousness. It may also provide a calming influence.

Basil: is often used to aid with concentration and alertness and may help reduce mental fatigue. It may also help maintain an open mind and clarity of thought.

Yuzu: has been used traditionally in Japan since the eighteenth century in a bath taken at winter solstice to help warm the body and improve circulation. Yuzu oil has a calming and warming influence and is often used to help improve focus and concentration.

Melissa: has calming and sedative properties and may help balance and uplift the emotions.

Rosemary: is often used to help relieve feelings of nervous or mental fatigue or depression and has been studied for its ability to help improve memory and concentration.

Vanilla: is calming and balancing and may help ease tension.

Body System(s) Affected: Hormonal System, Emotional Balance.

Safety Data: Repeated use can result in contact sensitization. Consult your doctor before using if you are pregnant, epileptic, or have a medical condition.

Companion Blends: Console, Passion, Peace, Forgive, Cheer.

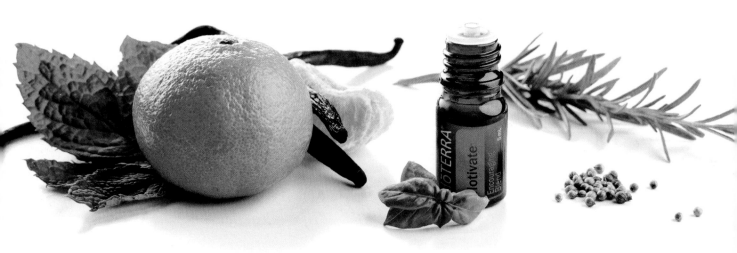

---

*See Personal Usage Guide chapter for more details on these primary uses.   ●=Neat, ●=Dilute for Children/Sensitive Skin, ●=Dilute

On Guard® *(Protective Blend)*

Quick Facts

The oils in this blend have been studied for their strong abilities to kill harmful bacteria, mold, and viruses. This blend can be diffused into the air or be used to clean and purify household surfaces.

Common Primary Uses*: ⭕Abscess (Oral), ✴Air Pollution, ⭕✴⭕Antibacterial, ⭕✴Antifungal, ⭕✴Antiviral, O⭕Bladder Infection, ⭕Candida, ⭕✴Chronic Fatigue, ⭕✴Cleansing, ⭕Cold Sores, ✴⭕Colds, ✴⭕Coughs, ⭕✴Flu, ⭕Gum Disease, ⭕Halitosis, ⭕OHypoglycemia, ⭕✴OInfection, ⭕Lupus, ✴⭕Mold, ✴⭕Mono, ⭕MRSA, ✴⭕Plague, ✴⭕Pneumonia, ⭕Scabies, O⭕✴Sore Throat, O⭕Staph Infection, ⭕Warts

Application:

⭕: Massage throat, stomach, intestines, and bottoms of feet. Dilute one drop in 15 drops of fractionated coconut oil: massage the thymus to stimulate the immune system, and massage under the arms to stimulate the lymphatic system. It is best applied to the bottoms of the feet, as it may be caustic to the skin. Dilute with fractionated coconut oil when used on sensitive/young skin.

✴: Diffuse or inhale the aroma directly.

Single Oils in This Blend:

Orange: is antibacterial, antifungal, antidepressant, and antiseptic. It is a powerful disinfectant and very effective against colds and flu.

Clove Bud: is antibacterial, antifungal, anti-infectious, antiparasitic, a strong antiseptic, antiviral, and an immune stimulant. It may influence healing and help create a feeling of protection and courage.

Cinnamon Bark: has very specific purposes: (1) it is a powerful purifier, (2) it is a powerful oxygenator, and (3) it enhances the action and the activity of other oils. It may have a stimulating and toning effect on the whole body and particularly on the circulatory system. It is antibacterial, antifungal, anti-infectious, anti-inflammatory, antimicrobial, antiparasitic, antiseptic, antispasmodic, antiviral, astringent, immune stimulant, sexual stimulant, and warming.

Eucalyptus: may have a profound antiviral effect upon the respiratory system. It also has strong antibacterial, anticatarrhal, and antiseptic properties.

Rosemary: may help balance heart function, energize the solar plexus, and reduce mental fatigue. It may improve circulation and help stimulate the nerves. It is antiseptic and anti-infectious.

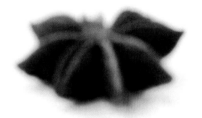 **Body System(s) Affected:** The oils in this blend may help it be effective for dealing with various problems related to the Immune System.

Aromatic Influence: Diffuse this blend of oils periodically for 20–25 minutes at a time to help protect the body against the onset of flu, colds, and viruses.

Safety Data: Repeated use can result in extreme contact sensitization. Can cause extreme skin irritation. Use with caution during pregnancy.

Essential Oil Blends

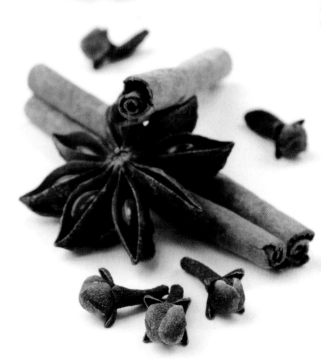

⭕=Topical, ✴=Aromatic, O=Internal

Passion® *(Inspiring Blend)*

Quick Facts

This blend contains spice and herb oils that are known to help enhance passion and excitement for life.

Common Primary Uses*: Confidence, Defeat, Expression, Fear, Joy, Rejection, Uplifting, Passion

Application:

: Diffuse or inhale the aroma directly.

: Apply on wrists, back of neck, over the heart area, or on the bottoms of the feet.

Single Oils in This Blend:

Cardamom: is uplifting, refreshing, and invigorating and may help with feelings of confusion.

Cinnamon: has warming, stimulating properties and is often used to help with low libido.

Ginger: is often used for its stimulating, warming influence. The aroma may help influence physical energy and love.

Clove: helps create a feeling of protection and courage and is often used to help with hormonal balance.

Sandalwood: helps calm, harmonize, and balance the emotions and can help relieve nervous tension.

Jasmine: has a beautiful, uplifting fragrance that symbolizes hope, happiness, and love. It is often used to help uplift and open the emotions and to help promote powerful, inspirational relationships.

Vanilla: is calming and balancing and may help ease tension.

Damiana: was used traditionally by the ancient Mayan and Aztec people to promote stronger feelings of affection. It is often used to help reduce feelings of anxiety and promote relaxation.

Carrier Oil in This Blend: Fractionated coconut oil.

Body System(s) Affected: Hormonal System, Emotional Balance.

Safety Data: Repeated use can result in contact sensitization. Consult your doctor before using if you are pregnant, epileptic, or have a medical condition.

Companion Blends: Console, Motivate, Peace, Forgive, Cheer.

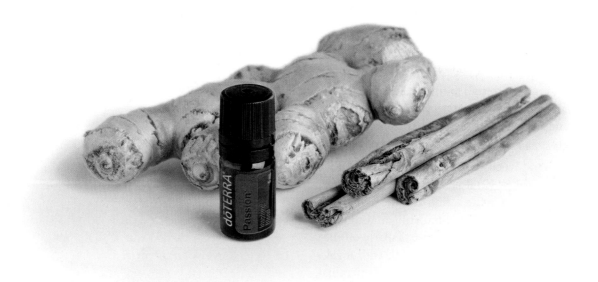

See Personal Usage Guide chapter for more details on these primary uses.   ●=Neat, ●=Dilute for Children/Sensitive Skin, ●=Dilute

160

PastTense® *(Tension Blend)*

Quick Facts

The oils in this blend are known to help relieve the pain and tension associated with headaches.

Common Primary Uses*: ⬡⟳Headaches, ⬡⟳Migraines, ⬡Muscle Tension, ⬡⟳Tension Headaches

Application:

⬡: Use a roll-on applicator to apply this blend to the temples, the forehead, the back of the neck, and to the reflex areas on the hands and feet.

⟳: Inhale the aroma directly.

Single Oils in This Blend

Wintergreen: has pain-relieving, anti-inflammatory, and antispasmodic properties. It may help with muscle and bone pain.

Lavender: may help relieve pain and inflammation. It is an antispasmodic and may help with migraine headaches and tension.

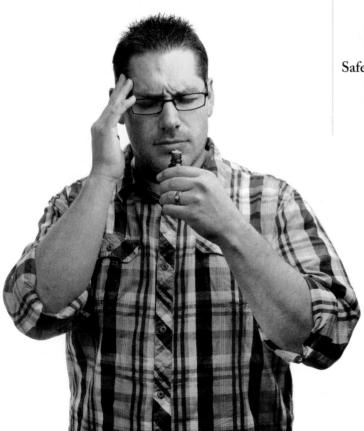

Peppermint: has pain relieving, anti-inflammatory, and antispasmodic properties. It is often used to help relieve headaches and has a cooling effect on the skin.

Frankincense: has sedative properties and may help reduce inflammation, headaches, and high blood pressure.

Cilantro: has anti-inflammatory and analgesic properties. It is a circulatory stimulant and helps alleviate aches, pains, and stiffness.

Roman Chamomile: has calming properties and is anti-inflammatory and antispasmodic. It also helps soothe the nerves.

Marjoram: is often used to soothe muscle aches and pains. It also has sedative properties and may help increase blood flow.

Basil: is often used to relieve muscle aches and pains and deep muscle spasms.

Rosemary: is often used to help relieve headaches. It may also help relieve sinus congestion and infections that can contribute to sinus headaches.

✦ **Body System(s) Affected:** The oils in this blend may help it be effective for dealing with various problems related to the Nervous System and to the Muscles and Bones.

Safety Data: Repeated use can result in extreme contact sensitization. Can cause extreme skin irritation. Use with caution during pregnancy.

Essential Oil Blends

⬡=Topical, ⟳=Aromatic, ⬡=Internal

Peace® *(Reassuring Blend)*

Quick Facts

This blend contains floral and mint oils that are known to help alleviate fearful, worried, and anxious feelings and replace them with peaceful contentment.

Common Primary Uses*: ⚫☝Anxious Feelings, ⚫☝Clearing (Emotional), ⚫☝Defeat, ⚫☝Depression, ⚫☝Fear, ⚫☝Guilt, ⚫☝Overburdened, ⚫☝Peace, ⚫☝Stress, ⚫☝Worried Feelings

Application:

⚫: Diffuse or inhale the aroma directly.

☝: Apply on wrists, back of neck, over the heart area, or on the bottoms of the feet.

Safety Data: Consult your doctor before using if you are pregnant, epileptic, or have a medical condition.

Companion Blends: Console, Motivate, Passion, Forgive, Cheer.

Single Oils in This Blend:

Vetiver: has calming, balancing properties and is often used to help sedate the nerves. It may also help with anxious, stressful, worried feelings and promote restful sleep.

Lavender: is well known for its calming, soothing properties. It helps promote consciousness, health, love, peace, and a general sense of well-being.

Ylang Ylang: has antidepressant and sedative properties. It is often used to help calm and relax.

Frankincense: is often used to help promote feelings of balance, to help with focus and meditation, and to help ease impatience and restlessness.

Clary Sage: has sedative and soothing properties and is often used to help with hormonal balance.

Marjoram: is often used to help relieve physical stress and helps promote feelings of peace and restfulness.

Labdanum: or cistus, was one of the first aromatic substances used anciently. It is stimulating to the senses and is often used to help elevate the emotions and soothe the nerves.

Spearmint: is often used to help open and release emotional blocks and to bring about a feeling of balance. It is also known to help with feelings of depression by relieving mental strain and fatigue and lifting one's spirit.

✛ **Body System(s) Affected:** Hormonal System, Emotional Balance.

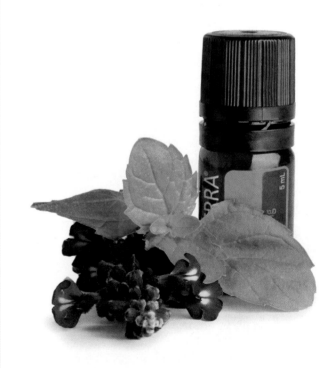

---

*See Personal Usage Guide chapter for more details on these primary uses.   ⬤=Neat, ⬤=Dilute for Children/Sensitive Skin, ⬤=Dilute

Purify *(Cleansing Blend)*

Quick Facts

Several of the oils contained in this blend are well-known and are often used to help remove odors from the air. Others have been studied for their powerful abilities to disinfect and to remove harmful microorganisms.

Common Primary Uses*: ⬡Abscess (Tooth), ⬡⬡Addictions, ⬡Airborne Bacteria, ⬡Air Pollution, ⬡Allergies, ⬡⬡Antibacterial, ⬡Boils, ⬡Bug Bites, ⬡⬡Cleansing, ⬡⬡Deodorant, ⬡⬡Deodorizing, ⬡⬡Disinfectant, ⬡Ear Infection, ⬡Infected Burns, ⬡Laundry, ⬡⬡Mice (Repel), ⬡Mildew, ⬡Skin Ulcer, ⬡Stings, ⬡Urinary Infection

Application:

⬡: Apply to reflex points on the body, ears, feet, and temples. Apply topically for infections and cleansing.

⬡: Put on cotton balls and place in air vents for an insect repellent at home or at work. Can also be added to paint to help reduce fumes. Diffuse or inhale the aroma directly.

Single Oils in This Blend:

Lemon: is antiseptic and antiviral. It may help as an air disinfectant and as a water purifier. Its uplifting aroma promotes healing and purification.

Lime: has antibacterial, antiviral, and antiseptic properties.

Siberian Fir: is highly valued for its fine fragrance, air purifying action, and ability to protect against environmental threats.

Citronella: has antiseptic, antibacterial, antispasmodic, anti-inflammatory, deodorizing, insecticidal, purifying, and sanitizing properties.

Melaleuca: may help balance heart function and act as a cleanser and detoxifier of the blood. It has antibacterial, antifungal, anti-infectious, antiseptic, antiviral, and immune-stimulant properties.

Cilantro: is relaxing, uplifting, refreshing, and may help memory. It may help with burns, bites, and stings. Cilantro and coriander are distilled from the same plant—cilantro oil, however, is distilled from the leaves of the plant, while coriander oil is distilled from the seeds of the plant.

Body System(s) Affected: The oils in this blend may help it be effective for dealing with various problems related to the Digestive System, to Emotional Balance, and to the Skin.

Aromatic Influence: This blend is great for air purification when diffused. When illness is in the home, diffuse for 1 hour and then wait for 2 hours. Repeat this pattern as desired. Diffuse in the office, barn, or garbage areas; or put it on a cotton ball, and place it in an air vent to freshen the car.

Application: Apply to reflex points on the body, ears, feet, and temples. Apply topically for infections and cleansing. Put on cotton balls and place in air vents for an insect repellent at home or at work. Can also be added to paint to help reduce fumes.

Safety Data: Repeated use can possibly result in contact sensitization. Can be irritating to sensitive skin.

Companion Blends: Citrus Bliss, On Guard.

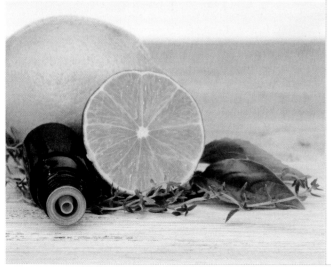

Serenity® *(Restful Blend)*

Quick Facts

This relaxing blend contains essential oils that are often used to help calm and soothe feelings of stress, excitement, and anxiety in order to help the body have a restful sleep.

Common Primary Uses*: ⊘⊘ADD/ADHD, ⊘⊘Addictions, ⊘⊘Anger, ⊘⊘Anxiety, ⊘⊘Calming, ⊘⊘Hyperactivity, ⊘⊘Insomnia, ⊘Itching, ⊘⊘Mental Fatigue, ⊘Mood Swings, ⊘⊘Sedative, ⊘⊘Sleep, ⊘⊘Stress, ⊘⊘Teeth Grinding, ⊘⊘Tension

Application:

⊘: Apply under nose and to back, feet, and back of neck. Put in bathwater. Apply to navel, feet, or back of neck for insomnia.

⊘: Wear as perfume or cologne. Diffuse or inhale the aroma directly.

Single Oils in This Blend:

Lavender: has calming and sedative properties. It may help lift feelings of depression and anxiety.

Ho Wood: is soothing to the skin, appeasing to the mind, relaxing to the body, and creates a feeling of peace and gentleness.

Cedarwood: is calming and soothes nervous tension.

Ylang Ylang: has calming and sedative properties. It brings a feeling of self-love, confidence, joy, and peace.

Sweet Marjoram: may help relax and calm the body and mind and also help promote peace.

Roman Chamomile: is calming and relaxing. It may help relieve muscle tension as well as calm nerves and soothe emotions.

Vanilla Bean Absolute: is calming and may help ease tension.

Vetiver: has calming, balancing properties and is often used to help sedate the nerves. It may also help with anxious, stressful, worried feelings and promote restful sleep.

Hawaiian Sandalwood: is calming and sedative. It helps balance and harmonize the emotions and may help ease nervous tension.

Body System(s) Affected: The oils in this blend may help it be effective for dealing with various problems related to the Nervous System and to Emotional Balance.

Aromatic Influence: This blend of oils is perfect for calming the nerves or emotions at the end of a long day or in times of stress. As the body is able to relax, more blood is able to circulate to the brain.

Companion Oils: Lavender.

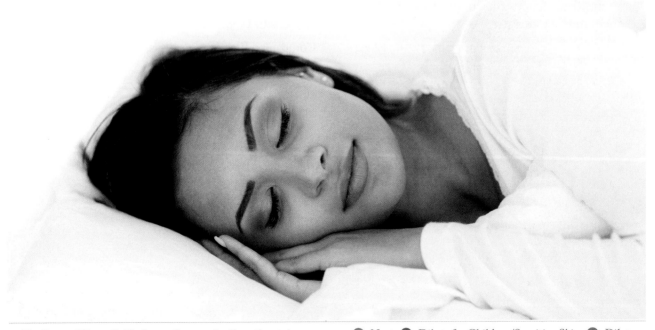

See Personal Usage Guide chapter for more details on these primary uses.   ⬤=Neat, ⬤=Dilute for Children/Sensitive Skin, ⬤=Dilute

164

Slim & Sassy® *(Metabolic Blend)*

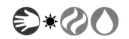

Quick Facts

This blend is designed to help control hunger and to help limit excessive calorie intake. The oils in this blend are calming to the stomach and work to improve emotional well-being. This blend is most effective when combined with exercise and healthy eating.

Common Primary Uses*: ⃝⬳Appetite Suppressant, ⃝⬳Cellulite, ⃝⬳Obesity, ⃝⬳Overeating, ⃝⬳Weight Loss

Application:

⬳: Apply on wrists, bottoms of the feet, or on area of concern.

⬳: Apply to palms of hands: cup hands over nose and mouth, and breathe deeply. Diffuse into the air.

◯: Add 8 drops of Slim & Sassy to 2 cups (500 ml) of water, and drink throughout the day between meals.

Single Oils in This Blend:

Grapefruit: is balancing and uplifting to the mind. It has been used medicinally by the French to help with cellulite and digestion.

Lemon: is invigorating, enhancing, and warming. It promotes health, healing, and energy.

Peppermint: is purifying and stimulating to the human mind. It may also help soothe digestive difficulties.

Ginger: may help increase physical energy and promote healthy digestion.

Cinnamon: enhances the action of other oils. It may improve circulation, digestion, and energy levels.

⊕ **Body System(s) Affected:** Emotional Balance, Digestive System.

Aromatic Influence: This blend of oils is calming to the stomach and uplifting to the mind.

Safety Data: Because this blend contains citrus oils, it may increase skin photosensitivity. It is best to avoid sunlight or UV rays for 12 hours after topical application. Do not apply directly in eyes, ears, or nose. Consult your doctor before using if you are pregnant or have a medical condition.

Companion Oils: Grapefruit, orange, lemongrass, thyme, lavender, Elevation, rosemary, fennel.

Essential Oil Blends

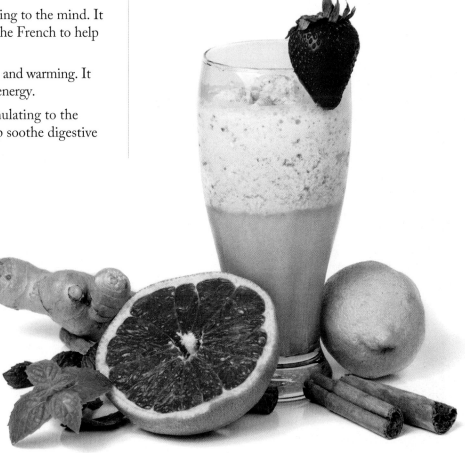

TerraShield® *(Outdoor Blend)*

Quick Facts

This blend combines essential oils that have been proven to effectively repel biting insects.

Common Primary Uses*: Bug/Insect Repellent

Application:

: Apply a small amount of this oil on the skin.

: Diffuse into the air, or place a few drops on ribbons and strings, and place near air vents, windows, or openings where bugs might come in.

Single Oils in This Blend:

Ylang Ylang: has been studied for its ability to repel mosquitoes.

Tamanu Seed: is a cold-pressed oil that has been studied for its ability to block UV rays as a natural sunscreen.

Nootka Wood: has been studied for its ability to repel fire ants and other insects.

Cedarwood: is insecticidal against adult mosquitoes and other household insects.

Catnip: repels flies and other insects.

Lemon Eucalyptus: is insecticidal. It may also help repel cockroaches, silverfish, and other insects.

Litsea: has been studied for its ability to repel mosquitoes

Vanilla Bean Absolute: has a soft, sweet aroma.

Arborvitae: has insect repellent properties, and can help protect the skin from UV radiation.

Carrier Oil in This Blend: Fractionated coconut oil.

Aromatic Influence: It is highly repellent to many flying and crawling insects and bugs.

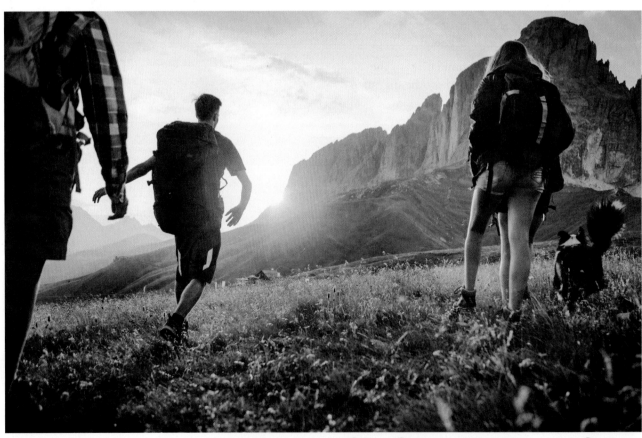

*See Personal Usage Guide chapter for more details on these primary uses. ●=Neat, ●=Dilute for Children/Sensitive Skin, ●=Dilute

Whisper® *(Blend for Women)*

Quick Facts

This exquisite blend of oils works harmoniously with an individual's unique chemistry to create an appealing aroma—without the harmful chemicals found in many of today's perfumes.

Common Primary Uses*: 🖐🍃Aphrodisiac, 🍃🖐Frigidity, 🖐🍃Hormonal Balance

Application:

🖐: Add 5–6 drops to 1 Tbs. (15 ml) of fractionated coconut oil for use in massage.

🍃: Diffuse or wear as a perfume.

Single Oils in This Blend:

Patchouli: may help calm and relax, relieving feelings of anxiety.

Bergamot: may help relieve feelings of anxiety, stress, and tension. Its aroma is uplifting and refreshing.

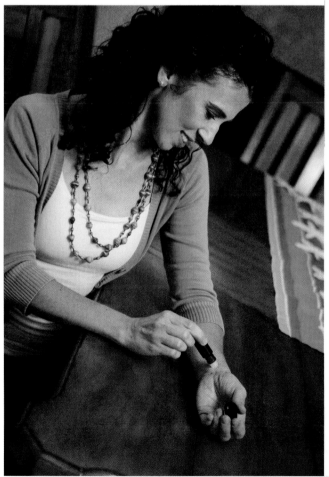

Hawaiian Sandalwood: helps to alleviate feelings of depression. It helps one accept others with an open heart, while diminishing one's own egocentricity.

Rose: is stimulating and elevating to the mind. Its beautiful fragrance is felt to be aphrodisiac-like in nature.

Jasmine: is very uplifting to the emotions. It produces feelings of confidence, energy, and optimism.

Cinnamon Bark: has antidepressant and stimulating properties.

Vetiver: is antispasmodic and locally warming. Vetiver has been valuable for relieving stress and helping people recover from emotional traumas and shock.

Ylang Ylang: has calming and sedative properties. It brings a feeling of self-love, confidence, joy, and peace.

Labdanum: is valued for its unique scent and relaxing aroma.

Cocoa Bean Extract: has a pleasurable, soothing aroma.

Vanilla Bean Extract: is calming and may help ease tension.

Carrier Oil in This Blend: Fractionated coconut oil.

➕ **Body System(s) Affected:** Emotional Balance, Skin.

Aromatic Influence: The subtle aroma of this blend enhances the aura of beauty, femininity, and allure.

Companion Blends: Elevation, ClaryCalm, Zendocrine.

Essential Oil Blends

Zendocrine® *(Detoxification Blend)*

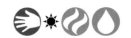

Quick Facts

This blend contains oils that have been studied for their abilities to help support organ cleansing and healthy tissue function.

Common Primary Uses*: ○◉Endocrine Support, ○◉Hormonal Balance

Application:

🖐: Massage on bottoms of feet.

🌀: Diffuse or inhale the aroma directly.

💧: Take 3–5 drops of Zendocrine in capsules either alone or with a Zendocrine Complex supplement capsule up to once a day.

Single Oils in This Blend:

Rosemary: has demonstrated strong antioxidant effects and has been used to help mitigate the effects of endocrine disorders such as diabetes and stress-related chronic fatigue.

Cilantro: has been studied for its ability to help support the liver against toxins.

Juniper Berry: is often used for its cleansing and antioxidant properties.

Tangerine: is often used for its antioxidant properties and its ability to support the digestive system.

Geranium: may help with hormonal balance, liver and kidney function, pancreas support, and the discharge of toxins from the liver.

✛ **Body System(s) Affected:** Hormonal System, Emotional Balance, Skin and Hair.

Safety Data: Because this blend contains citrus oils, it may increase skin photosensitivity. It is best to avoid sunlight or UV rays for 12 hours after topical application. Repeated use can result in contact sensitization. Consult your doctor before using if you are pregnant, epileptic, or have a medical condition.

Companion Blends: Whisper.

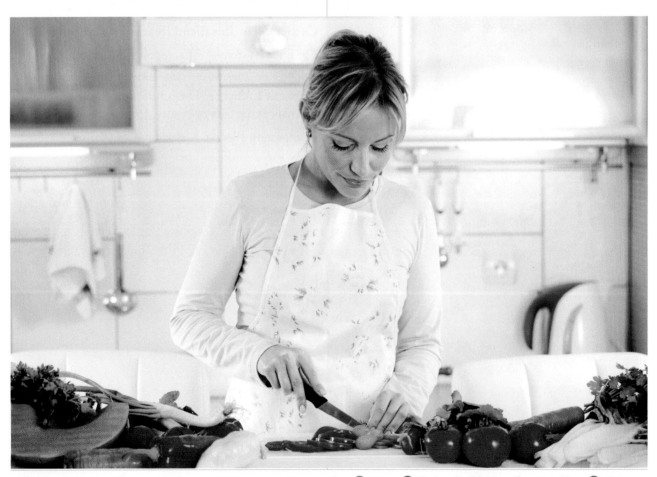

*See Personal Usage Guide chapter for more details on these primary uses.   ●=Neat, ●=Dilute for Children/Sensitive Skin, ●=Dilute

Yarrow Pom™ *(Active Botanical Nutritive)*

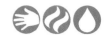

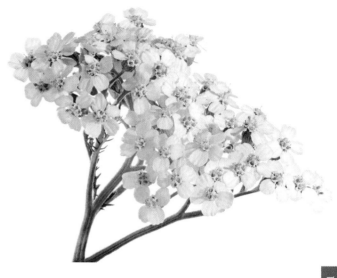

Quick Facts

This unique formulation combines the skin benefits of yarrow essential oil with the powerful antioxidant and cellular health properties of pomegranate seed oil.

Common Primary Uses*: ○Aging, ○Antioxidant, ○◉Cancer, ○Cellular Health, ○Diabetes, ○Obesity, ◉○Skin (Healing).

Application:

◉: Apply on area of concern.

◑: Inhale the aroma directly. Or apply to a diffusing bracelet or necklace to wear throughout the day.

○: Take 1–2 drops daily in a capsule or in 1 cup (250 ml) of beverage.

Single Oils in This Blend:

Yarrow: has powerful antioxidant properties. It is also anti-inflammatory and cleansing. When applied topically, it has antimicrobial properties, and it can help skin heal from sunburn, sores, and wounds.

Carrier Oils in This Blend:

Pomegranate Seed Oil: contains a high amount of punicic acid, a poly-unsaturated fatty acid. Punicic acid has been studied for its ability to help lessen insulin resistence in pre-diabetic models (Anusree et al., 2015; Vroegrijk et al., 2011). It has also shown an ability in animal tests to reduce obesity caused by high-fat diets (Keisuke et al., 2004; Vroegrijk et al., 2011). Additionally, punicic acid has been studied for its ability to inhibit human prostate (Gasmi et al., 2010) and breast cancer cells growth (Grossmann et al., 2010). It has also demonstrated anti-inflammatory and antioxidant properties (Bassaganya-Riera et al., Saha et al., 2012).

⊕ **Body System(s) Affected:** The oils in this blend may be effective for various problems related to the Cardiovascular System, Immune System, Nervous System, Emotional Balance, and Skin.

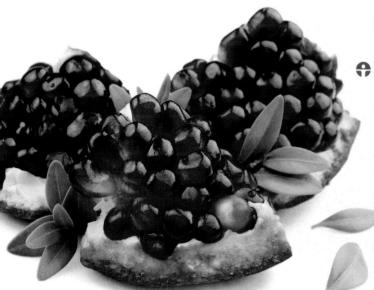

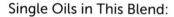

◉=Topical, ◑=Aromatic, ○=Internal

Yoga: Align *(Centering Blend)*

Quick Facts

This blend is designed to help bring order to the chaos that surrounds our daily lives, bringing alignment, focus, trust, purpose, and understanding to what matters most.

Common Primary Uses*: 🌿Focus, 🌿Yoga

Application:

🖐: Apply to the wrists, heart area, and back of neck. Apply on reflex points on the hands and feet.

🌀: Diffuse, or inhale from the hands.

Single Oils in This Blend:

Bergamot: helps relieve feelings of stress and agitation, relieves tension, and helps balance emotions.

Coriander: has sedative properties and is often used to help relax and calm during times of stress or fear.

Marjoram: is often used to help regulate blood pressure and to promote feelings of peace.

Peppermint: is uplifting and invigorating. Its aroma is purifying and stimulating to the conscious mind.

Geranium: may help with hormonal balance; has a calming influence.

Basil: is energizing and renewing and helps one maintain an open mind and clarity of thought.

Rose: is stimulating and elevating to the mind, creating a sense of well-being.

Jasmine: may help produce a feeling of confidence, energy, euphoria, and optimism. It is uplifting to the emotions and may help clarity of thought.

➕ **Body System(s) Affected:** Hormonal System, Emotional Balance.

Aromatic Influence: Helps to uplift and motivate the mind and emotions, while still keeping one centered and focused.

Safety Data: Consult your doctor before using if you are pregnant or have a medical condition.

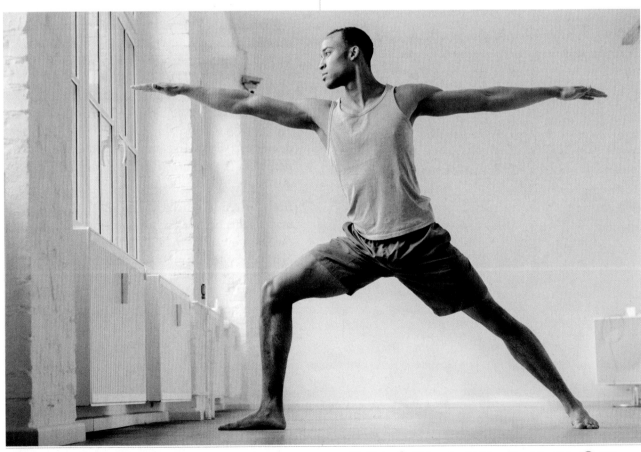

*See Personal Usage Guide chapter for more details on these primary uses.   ⬤=Neat, ⬤=Dilute for Children/Sensitive Skin, ⬤=Dilute

Yoga: Anchor *(Steadying Blend)*

Quick Facts

This blend is designed to help ground and anchor the mind and emotions to help promote a sense of courage, calmness, and assurance, allowing one a firm base from which to move onward with life.

Common Primary Uses*: ⬡Calming, ⬡Centering, ⬡Yoga

Application:

⬡: Apply on the heart, ankles, bottoms of the feet, and the base of the spine.

⬡: Diffuse, or inhale from the hands.

Single Oils in This Blend:

Lavender: is calming and soothing to the mind and emotions. It promotes consciousness, health, love, peace, and a general sense of well-being while nurturing creativity.

Cedarwood: is calming and balancing and is often used to help center and focus meditation and yoga.

Frankincense: helps soothe mental fatigue and supports the brain. It also helps to focus energy, minimize distractions, and improve concentration. It can also enhance spiritual awareness and meditation.

Cinnamon: is warming and soothing to the mind and soul.

Sandalwood: is calming and sedative and is often used to help enhance meditation. It can also help calm, harmonize, and balance the emotions.

Black Pepper: is comforting and stimulating and helps the mind overcome physical limitations.

Patchouli: is sedating, calming, and relaxing and has an effect on physical energy.

⬡ **Body System(s) Affected:** Hormonal System, Emotional Balance.

Aromatic Influence: Helps to ground the mind and emotions to a solid foundation, giving a quiet confidence to help balance the challenges of life.

Safety Data: Consult your doctor before using if you are pregnant or have a medical condition.

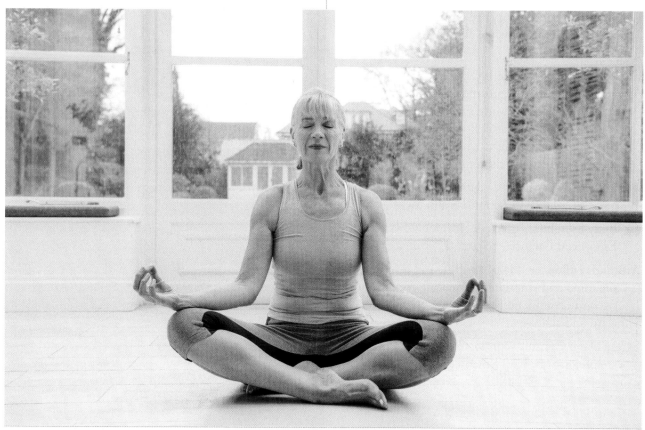

⬡=Topical, ⬡=Aromatic, ⬡=Internal

Essential Oil Blends

Yoga: Arise *(Enlightening Blend)*

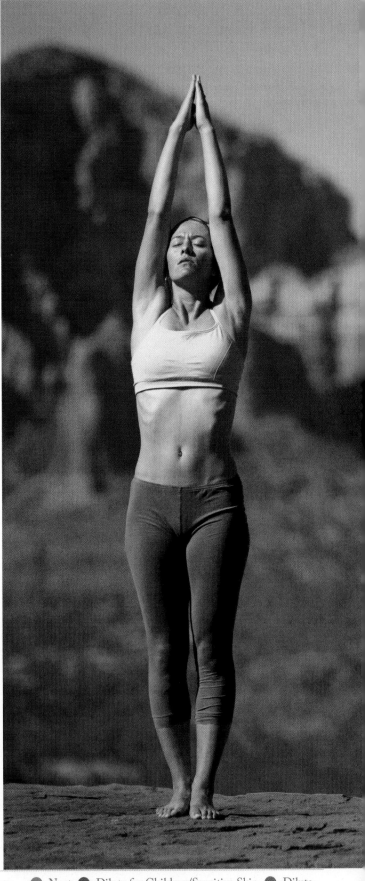

Quick Facts

This blend helps promote feelings of inspiration and joy, helping one to arise and move beyond opposition and challenges in life.

Common Primary Uses*: Inspiration, Joy, Yoga

Application:

: Apply to the wrists, heart area, and back of neck. Apply on reflex points on the hands and feet.

: Diffuse, or inhale from the hands. Wear as perfume or on aromatherapy jewelry.

Single Oils in This Blend:

Lemon: is uplifting and soothing to the mind and emotions. It helps promote physical energy and purification. Its aroma is invigorating, enhancing, and warming.

Grapefruit: helps to free the mind and spirit from physical restraints. It is balancing and uplifting to the mind and may help to relieve anxiety.

Siberian Fir: is energizing while creating a feeling of grounding, anchoring, and empowerment. It can stimulate the mind while allowing the body to relax.

Osmanthus: is one of the 10 famous traditional flowers of China. The blossoms are highly aromatic and are used in the world's rarest and most expensive perfumes. Its warm, floral aroma helps with concentration and focus while meditating, helping to relieve stress and clutter in the mind.

Melissa: has calming and sedative properties, and helps to balance the emotions and mind.

Body System(s) Affected: Hormonal System, Emotional Balance.

Aromatic Influence: Helps to uplift and inspire the mind and emotions, promoting feelings of strength, confidence, and courage to move forward and achieve.

Safety Data: Consult your doctor before using if you are pregnant or have a medical condition.

---

*See Personal Usage Guide chapter for more details on these primary uses.   ●=Neat, ●=Dilute for Children/Sensitive Skin, ●=Dilute

172

=Topical, =Aromatic, =Internal

Essential Supplements

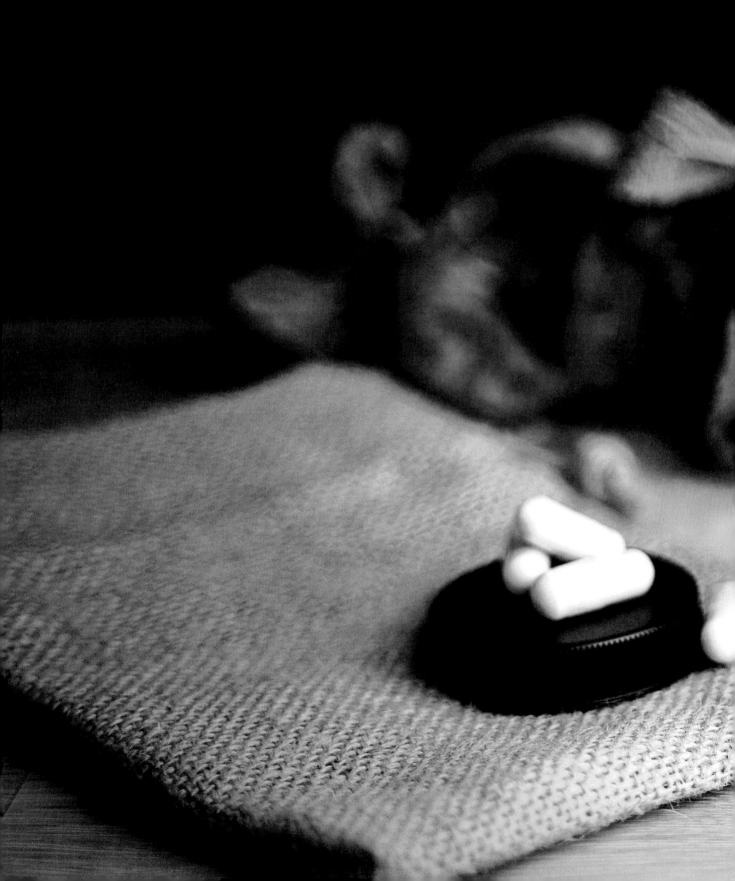

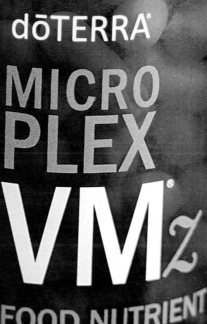

Essential Oil–Inspired Wellness Supplements

This section contains various essential oil–inspired supplements that are available commercially and the essential ingredients that each supplement contains.

For further information and research on many of the essential oils contained in these supplements, see the Essential Oils section of this book.

a2z Chewable™

Chewable Multivitamin

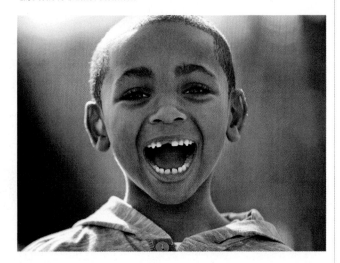

This supplement is a complete daily nutrient supplement for children and for those who have a hard time swallowing pills.

Key Ingredients:

–Vitamin and Mineral Complex:

Vitamin A (natural alpha and beta carotene): plays a role in vision, skin health, and DNA transcription.

Vitamin C (from acerola cherry fruit extract): provides stability to collagen (the main protein in connective tissue) and helps synthesize neurotransmitters and carnitine (which helps create energy through the breakdown of fatty acids).

Vitamin D_3 (as cholecalciferol): plays an important role in bone health and strength and helps modulate hormone secretion and immune function.

Vitamin E (as d-alpha tocopheryl acetate and mixed tocopherols): is a potent antioxidant and may play a role in cellular communication.

Thiamin/Vitamin B1 (as thiamine HCl): plays a critical role in generating energy from carbohydrates within the cell and is critical to healthy heart and nerve cell function.

Riboflavin/Vitamin B2: plays an important role in the creation of energy from lipids and carbohydrates in the cell as well as in the synthesis of several other important cellular chemicals.

Niacin/Vitamin B3 (as niacinamide): plays a role in cellular metabolism. Deficiency of niacin can result in dermatitis, diarrhea, confusion, and dementia.

Vitamin B6 (as pyridoxine HCl): is a necessary coenzyme to several enzymes involved in metabolism as well as to the creation of neurotransmitters such as serotonin and epinephrine.

Folic Acid: is necessary for cells to create nucleotides (the building blocks of DNA and RNA).

Vitamin B12 (as methylcobalamin): plays a key role in the synthesis of DNA by regenerating folate and is also critical to maintaining a healthy myelin sheath that preserves the normal functioning of the nervous system.

Biotin: helps metabolize fatty acids and is important to the synthesis of glucose from various substances.

Pantothenic Acid/Vitamin B5 (as d-calcium pantothenate): plays an important role in the creation of energy within the cell and in the creation of cholesterol, various fatty acids, and acetylcholine (a neurotransmitter that allows cells within the nervous system to communicate with each other).

Calcium (as calcium amino acid chelate): plays a critical role in bone structure and has a role in muscle contraction and nerve cell communication as well.

Iron (iron amino acid chelate): is part of the structure of heme (a critical part of the protein hemoglobin that allows red blood cells to transport oxygen throughout the body) as well as several other proteins. It also plays a role in several other important enzymatic reactions within the body.

Iodine (from potassium iodide): is a necessary nutrient for the creation of regulating hormones in the thyroid.

Magnesium (as magnesium amino acid chelate): is required to create many different enzymes in the body, including those that create and use ATP (cellular energy) and that create DNA and RNA.

Zinc (as zinc amino acid chelate): is an important component of many enzymes and proteins found in the body and also plays a role in cellular communication.

Copper (as copper amino acid chelate): is found in several different enzymes, including superoxide dismutase.

Manganese (as manganese amino acid chelate): is an important component in several different enzymes.

Potassium (as potassium glycinate): plays a critical role in nerve cell transmission and muscle control.

Choline (as choline bitartrate): is critical for healthy cell membrane structure and certain types of nerve cell transmissions.

Inositol: is an important part of the phospholipid structure of cell membranes and cellular messengers.

–Superfood Blend:

Pineapple (Bromelain Protease Enzymes): have been studied for their anti-inflammatory (Fitzhugh et al, 2008; Brien et al, 2004) properties and for their potential to reduce joint pain and arthritis (Walker et al, 2002).

Pomegranate Extract (Ellagic Acid): is found in raspberries, pomegranates, walnuts, and other fruits and vegetables. This well-researched polyphenol has been studied for

its ability to prevent low-density lipoprotein (LDL) oxidation (a known risk factor for cardiovascular disease) (Anderson et al, 2001; Chang et al, 2008) and atherosclerotic lesions (Yu et al, 2005), which could help prevent atherosclerosis.

Lemon Bioflavonoids: have antioxidant potential.

Spirulina: is high in amino acids, vitamin B12, and essential fatty acids.

Sunflower Oil: is high in the essential fatty acids oleic and linoleic acids.

Others: Rice Bran, Beet Greens, Broccoli, Brown Rice, Carrot, Mango, Cranberry, Rose Hips, Spinach.

–Alpha CRS+® Blend:

Tomato Fruit Extract (Lycopene): Lycopene is a red-colored pigment found in many red plants. It has been studied for its potential role in reducing the risk of prostate cancer (Giovannucci et al, 2002).

Grape Seed Extract (Proanthocyanidins): Proanthocyanidins extracted from grape seeds were found in one recent study to significantly decrease oxidized LDL in people with high cholesterol (Bagchi et al, 2003).

Marigold Flower Extract (Lutein): Lutein is created in many plants as an antioxidant and a light absorber. In humans, lutein is found in high concentration in the macula, the area of the eye where central vision occurs. Lutein supplementation has been found in at least one study to improve the visual acuity and macular pigment optical density in patients with age-related macular degeneration (Richer et al., 2004).

Companion Supplements: IQ Mega, PB Assist Jr

Alpha CRS+®

Cellular Vitality Complex

Alpha CRS+® contains important ingredients that may help to increase cellular health, vitality, and energy.

Key Ingredients:

***Boswellia serrata* Extract (beta-Boswellic Acids):** Boswellic acids are a family of water-soluble triterpene molecules extracted from the resin of plants in the genus *Boswellia*, such as frankincense. Boswellic acids have been studied for years for their strong anti-inflammatory (Ammon, 2002; Banno et al., 2006; Gayathri et al., 2007) and anticancerous (Bhushan et al., 2007; Huang et al., 2000; Liu et al., 2002) properties as well as for their potential to support joint health and to help prevent arthritis (Roy et al., 2006; Goel et al., 2010). This extract contains 6 highly bioavailable beta-boswellic acids.

Scuttelaria Root Extract (Baicalin): Baicalin is a polyphenol extracted from the scuttelaria, or Chinese skullcap, root. Besides being known for its antioxidant properties (Jung et al., 2008), baicalin has also been studied for its anticancer benefits (Zhou et al, 2008; Franek et al, 2005).

Milk Thistle Extract (Silymarin): Silymarin is a complex of polyphenols extracted from the milk thistle plant. Animal and cellular studies have suggested a toxin-protective effect on the liver from these polyphenols, especially the polyphenol silibinin (Al-Anati et al., 2009; Abenavoli et al., 2010).

Pineapple Extract (Bromelain Protease Enzymes): Bromelain protease enzymes extracted from the pineapple plant have been studied for their anti-inflammatory (Fitzhugh et al., 2008; Brien et al., 2004) properties and for their potential to reduce joint pain and arthritis (Walker et al., 2002).

Polygonum cuspidatum **Extract (Resveratrol):** Resveratrol is a polyphenol created by plants in a defensive response to bacteria or fungi. In addition to its antioxidant properties (Chakraborty et al, 2008), resveratrol has also been studied for its ability to inhibit skin (Jang et al., 1997) and leukemia (Lee et al, 2005) cancer cell growth and to improve mitochondrial function in cells (Lagouge et al, 2006).

Green Tea Leaf Extract: Green tea extract has been found to protect bone marrow cells from chromosome aberrations (Ito et al., 1989). Green tea may also decrease the risk of cardiovascular disease and some forms of cancer (Cabrera et al., 2006).

Pomegranate Fruit Extract (Ellagic Acid): Ellagic acid is found in raspberries, pomegranates, walnuts, and other fruits and vegetables. This well-researched polyphenol has been studied for its ability to prevent low-density lipoprotein (LDL) oxidation (a known risk factor for cardiovascular disease) (Anderson et al, 2001; Chang et al, 2008) and atherosclerotic lesions (Yu et al, 2005), which could help prevent atherosclerosis.

Turmeric Root Extract (Curcumin): Curcumin is a polyphenol found in turmeric root (a spice commonly used in curry). In recent studies, curcumin was found to prevent and bind amyloid-beta plaques (Yang et al., 2005) and to reduce oxidative stress and DNA damage caused by ameloid-beta in neuronal cells (Park et al., 2008). Ameloid-beta, and its accumulation in the brain in plaque form, has been hypothesized as a possible cause of Alzheimer's disease.

Grape Seed Extract (Proanthocyanidins): Proanthocyanidins extracted from grape seeds were found in one recent study to significantly decrease oxidized LDL in people with high cholesterol (Bagchi et al., 2003).

Sesame Seed Extract: Sesame seeds have been shown to possess antioxidant activity (Ben Othman et al., 2015).

Pine Bark Extract: Pine bark extract is a powerful antioxidant. A recent study found that pine bark extract may prevent alveolar bone resorption and therefore be a possible preventative agent for bone diseases (Sugimoto et al., 2015). Furthermore, pine bark extract enhances antioxidant defense capacity of low-density lipoproteins (complex particles that transport fats around the body) (Nakayama et al., 2015).

Acetyl-L-Carnitine: is a substance created by the body that transports fatty acids to the mitochondria to help break down fats into energy. Supplementation with L-carnitine (the bioactive form of carnitine) was found in several studies to reduce fatigue as well as to increase muscle mass and to decrease fat mass in certain populations (Ciacci et al., 2007; Malaguarnera et al., 2007; Pistone et al., 2003; Brass et al., 2001).

Alpha Lipoic Acid: plays an important role in the aerobic metabolism of cells. It has a strong antioxidant ability (Zembron-Lacne et al.,

2007) and has been studied for its effects on Alzheimer's disease patients (Hager et al., 2007) and as a treatment for neuropathy in diabetic patients (Ziegler et al., 2006; Tang et al., 2007). Lipoic acid and acetyl-l-carnitine have also been studied together for their ability to reduce the oxidative mitochondrial decay in the brain associated with aging (Long et al., 2009; Hagen et al., 2002).

Coenzyme Q(10): is a substance that plays a critical role in the electron transport chain that helps create cellular energy. Besides having antioxidant properties, coenzyme Q(10) has also been studied for its neuroprotective effect in Parkinson's disease (Hargreaves et al., 2008; Kooncumchoo et al., 2006; Winkler-Stuck et al., 2004) and for its ability to help alleviate symptoms of chronic heart failure (Belardinelli et al, 2005; Keogh et al., 2003) and other cardiovascular problems (Kuettner et al., 2005; Tiano et al., 2007).

Quercetin: is a polyphenol commonly found in apples, citrus fruits, green vegetables, and many berries. It has been studied for its ability to selectively kill prostate cancer cells without harming surrounding healthy cells (Paliwal et al., 2005; Aalinkeel et al., 2008).

Ginkgo Biloba Leaf Extract: Ginkgo biloba leaf extract's antioxidant activity has been shown to protect the liver against damage (Parimoo et al., 2014).

Tummy Taming Blend: An herbal blend that combines peppermint leaf, ginger root extract, and caraway seed to help keep the stomach calm.

Companion Supplements: xEO Mega, Microplex VMz

Bone Nutrient Lifetime Complex

This supplement combines bioavailable vitamins and minerals that have demonstrated a role in promoting bone health and in preventing age- and nutritional-related calcium loss and bone demineralization.

Key Ingredients:

Vitamin C (as magnesium ascorbate): provides stability to collagen (the main protein in connective tissue) and helps synthesize neurotransmit-

ters and carnitine (which helps create energy through the breakdown of fatty acids).

Vitamin D-2 (as ergocalciferol) and Vitamin D-3 (as cholacalciferol): play an important role in bone health and strength and helps modulate hormone secretion and immune function.

Biotin (as d-biotin): helps metabolize fatty acids and is important to the synthesis of glucose from various substances.

Calcium (as coral calcium): plays a critical role in bone structure, density, and strength. It has a role in muscle contraction and nerve cell communication as well.

Magnesium (as magnesium chelate): is required to create many different enzymes in the body, including those that create and use ATP (cellular energy) and that create DNA and RNA.

Zinc (as yeast): is an important component of many enzymes and proteins found in the body and also plays a role in cellular communication.

Copper (as yeast): is found in several different enzymes, including superoxide dismutase.

Manganese (as yeast): is an important component in several different enzymes.

Boron (as yeast): has been studied for its role in decreasing calcium loss and bone demineralization in women, and may play a role in hormone balance (Nielsen et al., 1987) and Vitamin D activation (Samman et al., 1998).

Companion Supplements: Phytoestrogen Lifetime Complex, ClaryCalm.

Breathe® Respiratory Drops

Respiratory Lozenge Drops

These drops combine many essential oils that are often used and studied for their abilities to help support the respiratory system.

Key Ingredients:

Lemon Essential Oil: has antiseptic properties and may help alleviate symptoms related to asthma and colds. A lemon-based spray has also been studied for its abilities to help alleviate immunological reactions related to rhinitis (Ferrara et al., 2012).

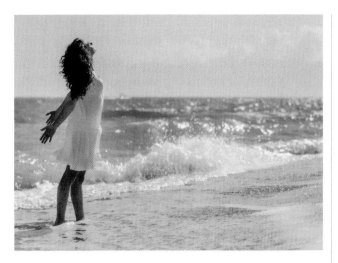

Peppermint Essential Oil: is often used for its anti-inflammatory and decongestant properties. It may help alleviate rhinitis, asthma, and other respiratory conditions.

Eucalyptus radiata **Essential Oil:** may have a profound antiviral effect upon the respiratory system. It may also help reduce inflammation of the nasal mucous membrane.

Thyme Essential Oil: has strong antibacterial and antifungal properties and is often used for asthma, bronchitis, croup, and other respiratory issues.

Melissa Essential Oil: has strong antiviral properties and is often used to help with asthma, chronic coughs, and colds.

Cardamom Essential Oil: has antiseptic and anti-inflammatory properties. It may also help with congestion and other respiratory problems.

Companion Blend: Breathe.

Copaiba Softgels

These unique softgels contain copaiba essential oil in a base of olive oil. Copaiba oil contains high levels of beta-caryophyllene, which has been studied for its ability to affect one of the two cannibinoid receptors in the body. Cannabinoid receptors—found throughout the body—are involved in a variety of physiological processes, including appetite, pain sensation, mood, and memory. The two known cannabinoid receptors are CB1 and CB2. When activated, both CB1 and CB2 help with inflammation, pain, and mood. The difference is that activation of the CB1 receptor (which is activated by marijuana) also creates a psychoactive high in the body, while activation

of the CB2 receptor does not cause any psychoactive effects. Beta-caryophyllene activates only the CB2 receptor, allowing it to powerfully affect inflammation, pain, and mood, without any psychoactive side-effects (Klauke et al., 2013; Fine et al., 2013; Cheng et al., 2014; Alberti et al., 2017).

Key Ingredients:

Copaiba Essential Oil: contains a high level of beta-caryophyllene. It is often used to help with anxiety, inflammation, aches, and pain. It also has high antioxidant properties, and it can help stimulate the circulatory and pulmonary systems.

Companion Oil: Copaiba, Deep Blue.

DDR Prime® Softgels

Essential Oil Cellular Complex

The oils in this essential oil blend have been chosen for their abilities to provide antioxidant support for the cells and to promote a healthy cellular life cycle.

Key Ingredients:

Frankincense: has anti-inflammatory and immune-stimulant properties. It is often used to help support the body's response to cancer and other cellular diseases.

Orange: contains high levels of d-Limonene, which has demonstrated potential in inhibiting cancer tumor growth (Kato et al., 1992) and has also been shown to reduce cholesterol levels in animal studies (Sorentino et al., 2005).

Litsea: has antibacterial properties, and is energizing and uplifting. It is used traditionally to help with pain and digestive issues.

Lemongrass: has anti-inflammatory and antiseptic properties. Constituents found in this oil have demonstrated an ability to inhibit cancer cell growth (Carnesecchi et al., 2001) and to induce apoptosis (cellular death) in human leukemia cells (Kumar et al., 2008).

Thyme: has strong antioxidant and antiseptic properties. It is often used to help support the brain as it ages.

Summer Savory (*Satureja hortensis*): has demonstrated antifungal (Sabzghabaee et al., 2012) and anti-inflammatory (Hajhashemi et al., 2012) properties. Studies have also demonstrated the ability of summer savory oil to decrease lipid peroxidation associated with aging in mice (Misharina et al., 2011) and to reduce DNA damage caused by oxidative stress in rat lymphocytes (Mosaffa et al., 2006). Additionally, a methanol extract of *Satureja hortensis* was found to reduce blood platelet adhesion (a risk factor in cardiovascular disease) in vitro (Yazdanparast et al., 2008).

Clove: has high antioxidant properties and is anti-infectious and helps support healthy liver and thyroid function.

Niaouli (*Melaleuca quinquenervia*): has powerful antifungal properties and is anti-inflammatory. It is often used to help protect against radiation and also to help regenerate damaged tissue.

Deep Blue Polyphenol Complex®

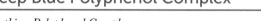

Soothing Polyphenol Complex

Like Deep Blue, this polyphenol nutritional supplement provides natural support for aching muscles, sore joints, and other occasional discomforts. The polyphenols, found in green tea, resveratrol, grape juice, and pomegranate juice, provide antioxidant power.

Key Ingredients:

Frankincense (*Boswellia serrata*) Gum Resin Extract: has long been used for its soothing properties. Frankincense is often used to help support the body's response to cancer and other cellular diseases. Boswellic acids, found in frankincense, have been studied for years for their strong anti-inflammatory properties (Ammon, 2002., Banno et al., 2006., and Gayathri et al., 2007) as well as for their potential

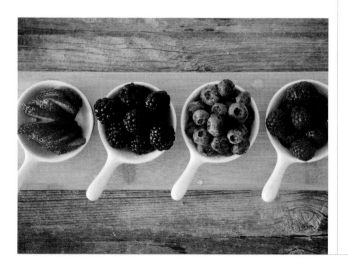

to support joint health and to help prevent arthritis (Roy et al., 2006; Goel et al., 2010).

Turmeric Root Extract (Curcumin): Curcumin is a polyphenol found in turmeric root (a spice commonly used in curry). In recent studies, curcumin was found to prevent and bind amyloid-beta plaques (Yang et al., 2005) and to reduce oxidative stress and DNA damage caused by amyloid-beta in neuronal cells (Park et al., 2008). Amyloid-beta, and its accumulation in the brain in plaque form, has been hypothesized as a possible cause of Alzheimer's disease.

Green Tea Leaf Extract: has been found to protect bone marrow cells from chromosome aberrations (Ito et al., 1989). Green tea may also decrease the risk of cardiovascular disease and some forms of cancer (Cabrera et al., 2006).

Pomegranate (*Punica granatum*) Fruit Extract: Ellagic acid is found in raspberries, pomegranates, walnuts, and other fruits and vegetables. This well-researched polyphenol has been studied for its ability to prevent low-density lipoprotein (LDL) oxidation (a known risk factor for cardiovascular disease) (Anderson et al, 2001; Chang et al, 2008) and atherosclerotic lesions (Yu et al, 2005), which could help prevent atherosclerosis.

Grape (*Vitis vinifera*) Seed Extract: Proanthocyanidins extracted from grape seeds were found in one recent study to significantly decrease oxidized LDL in people with high cholesterol (Bagchi et al, 2003).

Resveratrol (from *Polygonum cuspidatum* Extract): is a polyphenol created by plants in a defensive response to bacteria or fungi. In addition to its antioxidant properties (Chakraborty et al, 2008), resveratrol has also been studied for its ability to inhibit skin (Jang et al, 1997) and leukemia (Lee et al, 2005) cancer cell growth and to improve mitochondrial function in cells (Lagouge et al, 2006).

Tummy Taming Blend: An herbal blend with peppermint leaf, ginger root extract, and caraway seed to help keep the stomach calm.

Companion Blend: Deep Blue.

DigestTab®

Digestive Calcium Tablets

DigestTab combines the acid-neutralizing benefits of calcium carbonate with an infusion of essential oils that have been studied for their abilities to soothe digestive symptoms and support the digestive system.

Key Ingredients:

Calcium Carbonate: is alkaline in nature, is often used to help buffer occasional gastric acidity, and can help alleviate symptoms of heartburn and flatulence. It also provides a good source of dietary calcium.

Ginger Essential Oil: is warming, uplifting, and empowering. Emotionally, it may help influence physical energy, love, and courage. Because of its calming influence on the digestive system, it may help reduce feelings of nausea and motion sickness.

Peppermint Essential Oil: is an anti-inflammatory to the prostate and nerves. It is soothing, cooling, and dilating to the system. It may also be beneficial for counteracting food poisoning, vomiting, diarrhea, constipation, flatulence, halitosis, colic, nausea, and motion sickness.

Tarragon Essential Oil: may help to reduce anorexia, dyspepsia, flatulence, intestinal spasms, nervous and sluggish digestion, and genital urinary tract infection.

Fennel Essential Oil: may help improve digestive function by supporting the liver. It may also help balance the hormones.

Caraway Essential Oil: is antiparasitic and antispasmodic. It may also help with indigestion, gas, and colic.

Coriander Essential Oil: is antispasmodic and has anti-inflammatory properties. It may also help with indigestion, flatulence, diarrhea, and other spasms of the digestive tract.

Anise Essential Oil: may help calm and strengthen the digestive system.

Companion Supplements: DigestZen, DigestZen Terrazyme, DigestZen Softgels.

DigestZen® Softgels

Digestive Softgels

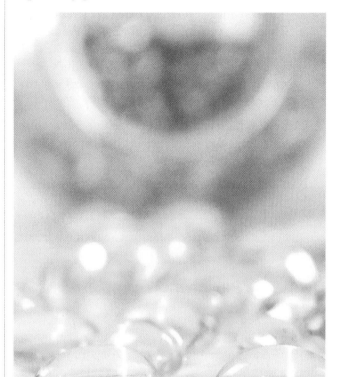

DigestZen Softgels are a convenient way to DigestZen, which contains oils that have been studied for their abilities to soothe digestive symptoms and support the digestion system.

Key Ingredients:

Ginger: is warming, uplifting, and empowering. Emotionally, it may help influence physical energy, love, and courage. Because of its calming influence on the digestive system, it may help reduce feelings of nausea and motion sickness.

Peppermint: is an anti-inflammatory to the prostate and nerves. It is soothing, cooling, and dilating to the system. It may also be beneficial for counteracting food poisoning, vomiting, diarrhea, constipation, flatulence, halitosis, colic, nausea, and motion sickness.

Tarragon: may help to reduce anorexia, dyspepsia, flatulence, intestinal spasms, nervous and sluggish digestion, and genital urinary tract infection.

Fennel: may help improve digestive function by supporting the liver. It may also help balance the hormones.

Caraway: is antiparasitic and antispasmodic. It may also help with indigestion, gas, and colic.

Coriander: is antispasmodic and has anti-inflammatory properties. It may also help with indigestion, flatulence, diarrhea, and other spasms of the digestive tract.

Anise: may help calm and strengthen the digestive system.

Companion Supplements: DigestZen, DigestTab, DigestZen Terrazyme.

DigestZen Terrazyme®

Digestive Enzyme Complex

This supplement blends food-derived enzymes and mineral cofactors that can aid in the digestion and absorption of critical nutrients that are lacking in many of today's diets.

Key Ingredients:

Protease (Aspergillus): aids in breaking proteins down into smaller amino acid units for use by the body to create necessary protein structures.

Papain (Papaya): is used to aid digestion and treat parasitic worms. Papain assists the body in breaking down proteins (meat) during digestion.

Amylase (Aspergillus): begins the process of breaking down complex carbohydrates such as starches into simpler sugars such as maltose.

Lactase (Aspergillus): is the enzyme responsible for breaking down lactose (a sugar in milk). Ingesting lactase assists in the digestion of milk and dairy products.

Lipase (Rhizopus): aids in breaking down large lipids and fats to help release energy and to create smaller units that can be used to build critical lipid-based structures such as hormones and the cell membrane.

Alpha Galactosidase (Aspergillus): aids in breaking down glycolipids and glycoproteins.

Cellulase (Trichoderma): breaks down cellulose into simpler sugars such as glucose for use as energy.

Sucrase (Saccharomyces): converts the disaccharide sucrose into fructose and glucose for use by the body for energy.

Betaine HCL: delivers hydrochloric acid to the stomach.

Glucoamylase (Aspergillus): is a digestive enzyme that breaks down starch and frees up glucose molecules for use by the body for energy.

Anti-gluten Enzyme Blend (Aspergillus): aids in breaking down gluten.

Tummy Taming Blend: An herbal blend that combines peppermint leaf, ginger root extract, and caraway seed to help keep the stomach calm.

Companion Supplements: DigestZen, DigestZen Softgels, Zendocrine Detoxification Complex.

GX Assist®

GI Cleansing Formula

GX Assist blends essential oils with caprylic acid to help support the gastrointestinal tract in eliminating pathogens.

Key Ingredients

Oregano Essential Oil: has antibacterial, antifungal, antiparasitic, and antiviral properties.

Melaleuca Essential Oil: has demonstrated strong antifungal properties as well as antibacterial, antiparasitic, and antiviral abilities. It may also help reduce inflammation.

Lemon Essential Oil: is often used for its antiseptic and antiviral properties.

Lemongrass Essential Oil: has demonstrated antiseptic and anti-inflammatory properties.

Peppermint Essential Oil: has demonstrated antibacterial and antiviral properties.

Thyme Essential Oil: is highly antibacterial, as well as antifungal.

Caprylic Acid: is a fatty acid naturally found in coconut milk, breast milk, and other sources. It has demonstrated antimicrobial properties against pathogens such as *E. Coli* (Marounek et al., 2003), *Salmonella* (Skrivanova et al., 2004; Johny et al., 2009), and *Strep* (Nair et al., 2009), among others.

IQ Mega®

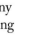

Omega-3 Fish Oil

IQ Mega provides all of the essential fatty acid benefits from fish oil without the fishy taste. It should be molecularly filtered to remove the fish aroma and

Essential Supplements

naturally flavored with orange essential oil for a great taste even kids will love.

Key Ingredients:

Fish Oil Concentrate (EPA, DHA): Eicosapentaenoic acid (or EPA) is an omega-3 fatty acid. It is largely known for its anti-inflammatory benefits but has also been found in several studies to help individuals suffering from depression (Su et al., 2008; Osher et al., 2005; Lucas et al., 2009; Frangou et al., 2006). Docosahexaenoic acid (or DHA) is another omega-3 fatty acid that is found in high concentrations in the brain and in the retina of the eye, where it is part of several important phospholipids. DHA has also been studied for its ability to help inhibit colon (Kato et al., 2002) and prostate (Shaikh et al., 2008) cancer cells. Taken together in fish oil, there is strong evidence that EPA and DHA can help with high blood pressure (Erkkila et al., 2008; Mori et al., 1999; Morris et al., 1993) and cardiovascular disease (Erkkila et al., 2004; Bucher et al., 2002), especially in high-risk individuals. When taken together by pregnant women, EPA and DHA have also been found to have beneficial effects on these women's children, such as reduced allergies (Furuhjelm et al., 2009; Dunstan et al., 2003) and improved neurological development (Helland et al., 2003).

Vitamin D: plays an important role in bone health and strength and helps modulate hormone secretion and immune function.

Vitamin E (as natural mixed tocopherols): is a potent antioxidant and may play a role in cellular communication.

Vitamin C (as ascorbyl palmitate): provides stability to collagen (the main protein in connective tissue) and helps synthesize neurotransmitters and carnitine (which helps create energy through the breakdown of fatty acids).

Orange Essential Oil: aids the digestive system and may help with indigestion and diarrhea. Contains high levels of d-Limonene, which has demonstrated a role in promoting healthy cellular function.

Rosemary Essential Oil: is often used to help support memory and mental clarity and focus.

Companion Supplement: a2z Chewable, PB Assist Jr.

Microplex VMz®

Food Nutrient Complex

This multivitamin combines natural vitamins and minerals with a complex of whole-food nutrients and minerals that are bound to a glycoprotein matrix to help enhance their bioavailability. These nutrients help support healthy cell, tissue, and system function. Additionally, this supplement contains a whole-food blend and a patented enzyme assimilation system to help further enhance nutrient bioavailability.

Key Ingredients:

Vitamin A (as retinyl palmitate and alpha and beta carotene): plays a role in vision, skin health, and DNA transcription.

Vitamin C (as calcium ascorbate and magnesium ascorbate): provides stability to collagen (the main protein in connective tissue) and helps synthesize neurotransmitters and carnitine (which helps create energy through the breakdown of fatty acids).

Vitamin D_3 (as natural cholecalciferol): plays an important role in bone health and strength and helps modulate hormone secretion and immune function.

Vitamin E (as natural mixed tocopherols and tocotrienols): is a potent antioxidant and may play a role in cellular communication.

Vitamin K (as glycoprotein matrix): is required by the liver to create the proteins involved in blood clotting and in bone structure.

Thiamin (as glycoprotein matrix): plays a critical role in generating energy from carbohydrates within the cell and is critical to healthy heart and nerve cell function.

Riboflavin (as glycoprotein matrix): plays an important role in the creation of energy from lipids and carbohydrates in the cell as well as in the synthesis of several other important cellular chemicals.

Niacin (as glycoprotein matrix): plays a role in cellular metabolism. Deficiency of niacin can result in dermatitis, diarrhea, confusion, and dementia.

Vitamin B_6 (as glycoprotein matrix): is a necessary coenzyme to several enzymes involved in metabolism as well as to the creation of neurotransmitters such as serotonin and epinephrine.

Folic Acid (as natural extract): is necessary for cells to create nucleotides (the building blocks of DNA and RNA).

Vitamin B$_{12}$ (as glycoprotein matrix): plays a key role in the synthesis of DNA by regenerating folate and is also critical to maintaining a healthy myelin sheath that preserves the normal functioning of the nervous system.

Biotin (as glycoprotein matrix): helps metabolize fatty acids and is important to the synthesis of glucose from various substances.

Pantothenic Acid (as glycoprotein matrix): plays an important role in the creation of energy within the cell and in the creation of cholesterol, various fatty acids, and acetylcholine (a neurotransmitter that allows cells within the nervous system to communicate with each other).

Calcium (as dicalcium malate and ascorbate): plays a critical role in bone structure and has a role in muscle contraction and nerve cell communication as well.

Iron (as bis-glycinate chelate): is part of the structure of heme (a critical part of the protein hemoglobin that allows red blood cells to transport oxygen throughout the body) as well as several other proteins. It also plays a role in several other important enzymatic reactions within the body.

Iodine (from kelp): is used by the thyroid gland to synthesize hormones. Deficiency in iodine can cause intellectual disability in children and other health problems.

Magnesium (as dimagnesium malate and ascorbate): is required to create many different enzymes in the body, including those that create and use ATP (cellular energy) and that create DNA and RNA.

Zinc (as bis-glycinate chelate): is an important component of many enzymes and proteins found in the body and also plays a role in cellular communication.

Selenium (as glycinate and selenomethionine): plays a role as a cofactor for several enzymes within the body, including several in the thyroid.

Copper (as bis-glycinate chelate): is found in several different enzymes, including superoxide dismutase.

Manganese (as bis-glycinate chelate): is an important component in several different enzymes.

Chromium (as nicotinate glycinate chelate): is believed to play a role in sugar and lipid metabolism within the body.

Whole-Food Blend: A blend of kale leaf extract, dandelion leaf powder, parsley leaf powder, spinach leaf powder, brocolli aerial parts powder, cabbage leaf extract, and brussels sprout immature inflorescences powder.

Active Enzyme Blend: A blend of enzymes to help transform sugars, proteins, and lipids into simpler molecules that can more easily be used by cells for structure and energy.

Tummy Taming Blend: An herbal blend with peppermint leaf, ginger root extract, and caraway seed to help keep the stomach calm.

Companion Supplements: Alpha CRS+®, xEO Mega.

Mito2Max®

Energy & Stamina Complex

This multi-nutrient supplement would be a natural alternative to unhealthy energy drinks to support stamina and increase cellular health, vitality, and energy.

Key Ingredients:

Acetyl-L-Carnitine HCL: is a substance created by the body that transports fatty acids to the mitochondria to help break down fats into energy. Supplementation with L-carnitine (the bioactive form of carnitine) was found in several studies to reduce fatigue as well as to increase muscle mass and to decrease fat mass in certain populations (Ciacci et al., 2007; Malaguarnera et al., 2007; Pistone et al., 2003; Brass et al., 2001).

Alpha Lipoic Acid: plays an important role in the aerobic metabolism of cells. It has a strong antioxidant ability (Zembron-Lacne et al., 2007) and has been studied for its effects on Alzheimer's disease patients (Hager et al., 2007) and as a treatment for neuropathy in diabetic patients (Ziegler et al., 2006; Tang et

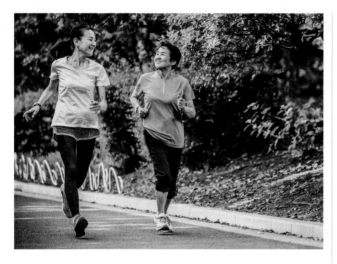

al., 2007). Lipoic acid and acetyl-l-carnitine have also been studied together for their ability to reduce the oxidative mitochondrial decay in the brain associated with aging (Long et al., 2009; Hagen et al., 2002).

Coenzyme Q(10): is a substance that plays a critical role in the electron transport chain that helps create cellular energy. Besides having antioxidant properties, coenzyme Q(10) has also been studied for its neuroprotective effect in Parkinson's disease (Hargreaves et al., 2008; Kooncumchoo et al., 2006; Winkler-Stuck et al., 2004) and for its ability to help alleviate symptoms of chronic heart failure (Belardinelli et al, 2005; Keogh et al., 2003) and other cardiovascular problems (Kuettner et al., 2005; Tiano et al., 2007).

Lychee (*Litchi chinensis*) Fruit Extract: protects against free radicals and oxidation.

Green Tea (*Camellia sinensis*) Leaf Polyphenol Extract: Green tea extract has been found to protect bone marrow cells from chromosome aberrations (Ito et al., 1989). Green tea may also decrease the risk of cardiovascular disease and some forms of cancer (Cabrera et al., 2006).

Quercetin (from *Sophorae japonica* Bud): is a polyphenol commonly found in apples, citrus fruits, green vegetables, and many berries. It has been studied for its ability to selectively kill prostate cancer cells without harming surrounding healthy cells (Paliwal et al., 2005; Aalinkeel et al., 2008).

Cordyceps (*Cordyceps sinensis*) Mycelium: have been shown in several animal studies to enhance endurance (Jung et al., 2004) by promoting enhanced ATP (cellular energy) production (Siu et al., 2004). Cordyceps have also demonstrated a high antioxidant activity (Liet al., 2001) and the ability to help restore libido in both men and women (Zhu et al., 1998).

Ginseng (*Panax quinquefolius*) Root Extract: Various components from ginseng have been studied for their abilities to help modulate the immune system, regulate blood glucose levels, and reduce tumors (Benzie et al., 2011). Ginseng is also the topic of considerable research for its potential ability to help improve memory (Qiu et al., 1995) and protect against neurodegenerative diseases, such as dementia and Alzheimer's disease (Yang et al., 2009; Shieh et al., 2008).

Ashwagandha (*Withania somnifera*) Root Extract: has demonstrated a potential to help reduce stress (Archana et al., 1999; Bhattacharya et al., 1987) and to help lower blood serum cortisol levels (Abedon, 2008). Cortisol—a hormone created by the adrenal glands—is released into the blood as the result of stress or anxiety, and it also plays a role in the body's sleep/wake cycle. When an individual is exposed to constant or chronic stress, levels of cortisol remain elevated in the body, disrupting the body's ability to relax and its ability to sleep naturally, sapping it of needed energy. Animal tests with ashwagandha root extract have also demonstrated an ability to increase energy and stamina, nearly doubling the endurance time of rats in forced swimming tests (Singh et al., 2011). Ashwagandha has also shown promising potential in helping to mitigate the damage to nerve cells found in conditions such as Huntington's disease, Parkinson's disease (Nagashyana et al., 2000), and Alzheimer's disease (Bhattacharya et al., 1995) and may help improve cognition (Singh et al., 1993). It is also a powerful antioxidant.

Companion Supplements: Alpha CRS+®, xEO Mega, Microplex VMz.

On Guard® Protecting Throat Drops

Protective Throat Drops

These drops offer the relief of a throat drop, soothing dry and scratchy throats, combined with the immune-protectant power of the essential oils that make up On Guard.

Key Ingredients:

Orange Essential Oil: is calming, uplifting, and antiseptic.

Clove Bud Essential Oil: is antibacterial, antiseptic, and may influence healing.

Cinnamon Bark Essential Oil: is antibacterial and antimicrobial. It also enhances the action and activity of other oils.

Eucalyptus radiata **Essential Oil:** is analgesic, antibacterial, and anti-infectious.

Rosemary Essential Oil: is anti-infectious, analgesic, antibacterial, anti-inflammatory, anticatarrhal, and supportive of the respiratory system.

Cassia Essential Oil: is strongly antibacterial and antimicrobial.

Myrrh Essential Oil: is anti-infectious, anti-inflammatory, antiseptic, and combats coughs and sore throats.

Companion Personal Care and Blend: On Guard Foaming Hand Wash, On Guard Natural Whitening Toothpaste, On Guard.

On Guard®+ Softgels

Protective Softgels

Combines the power of On Guard with black pepper, oregano, and melissa essential oils to help support the immune system.

Key Ingredients:

Orange Essential Oil: is calming, uplifting, and antiseptic.

Clove Bud Essential Oil: is antibacterial, antiseptic, and may influence healing.

Black Pepper Essential Oil: has antiseptic, anticatarrhal, and expectorant properties. It may help with respiratory ailments and with promoting blood flow and circulation.

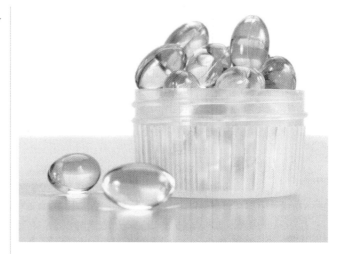

Cinnamon Bark Essential Oil: is antibacterial and antimicrobial. It also enhances the action and activity of other oils.

Eucalyptus radiata **Essential Oil:** is analgesic, antibacterial, and anti-infectious.

Oregano Essential Oil: has strong antibacterial, antifungal, and antiviral properties and is often used to help support the immune system against respiratory ailments.

Rosemary Essential Oil: is anti-infectious, analgesic, antibacterial, anti-inflammatory, anticatarrhal, and supportive of the respiratory system.

Melissa Essential Oil: is known for its antiviral properties and is often used to support the body against respiratory ailments.

Companion Supplement, Blend, and Personal Care: On Guard Foaming Hand Wash, On Guard Protecting Throat Drops, On Guard.

PB Assist®+

Probiotic Defense Formula

This supplement blends six strains of probiotic intestinal flora that can help support healthy colonies of friendly microflora in the digestive tract. These probiotics are recommended to be taken using a special double-coated capsule that protects the flora as they pass through the stomach.

Key Ingredients:

Lactobacillus acidophilus: is a bacteria that converts sugars (such as lactose in dairy products) into lactic acid. It may also help to control the

Essential Supplements

growth of *Candida albicans*, helping to prevent oral and vaginal yeast infections. It is commonly used to create yogurt.

Bifidobacterium lactis: is found in the intestines and can help support healthy digestion and immune function. It can be found in yogurt.

Lactobacillus salivarious: is a bacteria commonly found in the intestines. *L. salivarious* has been studied for its ability to help reduce inflammation and prevent the adhesion and growth of harmful bacteria in the digestive system.

Lactobacillus casei: produces lactic acid that can help promote growth of friendly microflora. It is commonly used to make cheddar cheese and other foods.

Bifidobacterium bifidum: is an intestinal bacteria that helps promote healthy digestive function.

Bifidobacterium longum: is found in the intestines and can help support healthy digestion and immune function.

Fructo-Oligosaccharide (FOS): promotes friendly bacteria growth and adhesion while inhibiting growth of pathogenic bacteria.

Companion Supplement: GX Assist.

PB Assist® Jr

Probiotic Powder

This supplement blends 6 strains of probiotic intestinal flora that can help support healthy colonies of friendly microflora in the digestive tract. These strains have been studied for their abilities to help support healthy digestion and to help protect against harmful infections that are common in childhood. These probiotics are recommended to be taken using a special micro-encapsulation that protects the flora as they pass through the stomach.

Key Ingredients:

Lactobacillus rhamnosus: has been studied for its ability to protect the gastrointestinal tract of children and adults from infections that cause diarrhea and other problems (Vanderhoof et al., 1999). It has also demonstrated an ability to help protect from respiratory tract infections (Hojsak et al., 2009) and may help reduce the severity of food allergies (Scott, 2015).

Lactobacillus salivarius: is a bacteria commonly found in the intestines. *L. salivarius* has been studied for its ability to help reduce inflammation and prevent the adhesion and growth of harmful bacteria in the digestive system.

Lactobacillus plantarum LP01 and LP02: are two strains of *Lactobacillus* normally found in the gut. *Lactobacillus plantarum* has been studied for its ability to replace gas-emitting bacteria, helping to reduce flatulence and cramping (Bixquert, 2009).

Bifidobacterium breve: has been studied for its ability to help protect the colon in individuals suffering from ulcerative colitis (Ishikawa et al., 2011).

Bifidobacterium lactis: is found in the intestines and can help support healthy digestion and immune function. It can be found in yogurt.

Fructo-Oligosaccharide (FOS): promotes friendly bacteria growth and adhesion while inhibiting growth of pathogenic bacteria.

Companion Supplements: a2z Chewable, IQ Mega.

Phytoestrogen Lifetime Complex

Phytoestrogen Complex

This complex may help women maintain a healthy estrogen balance with a potent blend of phytoestrogens (plant-derived estrogen-mimicking compounds) from soy, pomegranate, and flax seeds.

Key Ingredients:

Soy Extract (64% isoflavones with a minimum 50% genistein): Isoflavones such as genistein act as phytoestrogens in the body that bind with the estrogen receptor beta (ER-β) within cells. Unlike estrogen receptor alpha (ER-α), which is found in high concentrations in all parts of the female reproductive tract and mammary tissues, beta receptors are found in much smaller concentrations in uterine and mammary tissues (Couse et al., 1997). This seems to indicate that soy phytoestrogens do not directly act on cells in uterus and breast tissue. This can be important as over-estrogenation of cells in the mammary tissues has been linked to an increased risk for breast cancer. Isoflavones from soy have also been found to reduce levels of potentially carcinogenic estrogen metabolites in postmenopausal women (Xu et al., 2000 and Xu et al., 1998) and also to enhance levels of protective estrogen metabolites (Lu et al., 2000).

Flax Seed Extract (40% lignan): Flax seed contains several potent lignans which are metabolized by gastrointestinal bacteria into the active phytoestrogenic lignans, enterodiol and enterolactone. Both of these lignans have been studied for their antiproliferative effect on breast cancer cells (Truan et al., 2012; Mabrok et al., 2012) and evidence had been found that they may help lower blood triglyceride levels while raising levels of the good high density lipoproteins (HDL) in the blood (Zhang et al., 2008; Penalvo et al., 2012).

Pomegranate Extract (40% ellagic acid): contains strong antioxidants in addition to several phytoestrogens that are being studied for their roles in regulating hormone balance and their potential roles in reducing breast cancer growth (Strati et al., 2009).

Safety Data: If pregnant, lactating, or experiencing any health conditions, consult a physician before using.

Companion Nutrients: Bone Nutrient Lifetime Complex, ClaryCalm.

Serenity™ Restful Complex Softgels

Restful Complex

This unique supplement combines the powerful sedative and anti-anxiety effects of lavender essential oil and l-theanine with melissa, passionflower, and German chamomile extracts to help calm, soothe, and prepare the body and mind to enter a relaxed state of sleep.

Key Ingredients:

Lavender Essential Oil: is well knows for its soothing and calming influence. Clinical studies have shown that taking lavender essential oil internally has helped reduce general anxiety and feelings of stress that disrupt the body's ability to fall asleep naturally (Kasper, 2013, Woelk et al., 2010).

L-Theanine (Green Tea Extract): has been widely studied in recent years for its ability to affect the sympathetic nervous system and to help moder-

ate the body's natural stress-induced functions (Kimura et al., 2007, Tian et al., 2013).

Lemon Balm (Melissa) Extract: has been studied for its sedative and anxiety-reducing properties. (Keddedy et al., 2003 & 2006, Ballard et al., 2002).

Passionflower (*Passiflora incarnata*) Extract: has been studied for both its sedative properties (Ngan et al., 2011), and it ability to help reduce symptoms of general anxiety (Akhondzadeh et al., 2001).

German Chamomile Extract: has been studied for its ability to improve sleep quality (Adib-Hajbaghery et al., 2017, Chang et al., 2016).

Companion Blend: Serenity.

Slim & Sassy® Contrōl™ Bars

Appetite Suppressant Bars

Slim & Sassy Contrōl Bars are filled with natural ingredients to help manage weight, hunger, and well-being. One of the key ingredients found in these bars is a spinach leaf extract that has been shown to significantly reduce appetite for up to 6 hours. Slim & Sassy Contrōl Bars can be used for weight management when combined with a healthy lifestyle, exercise, and a balanced nutrition.

Key Ingredients:

Organic Brown Rice Syrup and Honey: are used as sweeteners, as an alternative to high-fructose corn syrup.

Yogurt: contains probiotics that have possible health benefits (Jacques et al., 2014). Studies have shown that yogurt may have the ability to assist in weight management (Jacques et al., 2014). Yogurt is a part of a healthy diet because of the many nutrients, including calcium, it contains.

Spinach (*Spinacia oleracea*) Leaf Extract: is packed full of a nutrient called thylakoids. Thylakoids have been shown to slow down digestion and the absorption of fats. Specifically, researchers discovered that ingesting thylakoids (in conjunction with food) suppresses food intake, raises hormones that cause a feeling of being full, and lowers blood lipid levels in rats (Albertsson et al., 2007). Thylakoids work best when consumed with dietary fat because thylakoids decrease the feeling of hunger by slowing down the digestion of fat and allowing the fat to stay longer in the intestine (Albertsson et al., 2007). This lengthened digestion time allows for the body to feel full longer. These Slim & Sassy® Contrōl™ Bars contain a small percentage of fat to work with the thylakoids and decrease hunger.

High Oleic Sunflower Oil: is very high in oleic (monounsaturated) acid. Eating foods that are high in monounsaturated fats have been found to improve blood cholesterol levels, insulin levels, and blood sugar control (Jenkins et al., 2010; Allman-Farinelli et al., 2005).

Whey Protein Crisp: provides protein, the most satiating macronutrient (Chungchunlam et al., 2014). A recent study showed that consuming whey protein produces a longer lasting feeling of being full than carbohydrates (Chungchunlam et al., 2014).

Gluten-Free Rolled Oats: contain valuable nutrients, including protein, vitamins, and minerals. In a study comparing the appetite sensations of subjects consuming either rolled oats or pinhead oats, subjects reported feeling fuller following the consumption of rolled oats compared with pinhead oats (Gonzalez et al., 2012).

Almonds: are a healthy snack option. A recent study found that woman who consumed a mid-morning almond snack consumed less food at lunch and dinner and experienced enhanced satiety following the almond snack (Hull et al., 2014).

Sunflower Seeds: provide vitamin C, iron, and calcium.

Raisins: are high in fiber and regular consumption of raisins may reduce glycemia and cardiovascular risk factors (Anderson et al., 2014). A study that evaluated after-school snack consumption in young children found that eating raisins led to lower cumulative food intake, compared to other less healthy snacks (Patel et al., 2013).

Organic Flax Meal: is nutritionally beneficial and research has found that consuming flaxseed can help prevent cardiovascular diseases, cancer, diabetes and can enhance spatial memory (Akhtar et al., 2013; Singh et al., 2011). Flax-

seed is also an antioxidant agent (Akhtar et al., 2013).

Sesame Seeds: have been shown to possess antioxidant activity (Ben Othman et al., 2015).

Chia Seeds: are packed with fiber, protein, omega-3 fatty acids, calcium, magnesium, phosphorus, and other vitamins.

Tocopherols: are potent antioxidants and may play a role in cellular communication.

Companion Products: Slim & Sassy Contrōl Instant Drink Mix and Slim & Sassy.

Slim & Sassy® Contrōl™

Appetite Suppressant Drink Mix

This powdered drink mix combines the action of Slim & Sassy with natural ingredients to help manage weight, hunger, and well-being. One of the key ingredients found in this drink mix is a spinach leaf extract that has been shown to significantly reduce appetite for up to 6 hours. This drink mix can be used for weight management when combined with a healthy lifestyle, exercise, and balanced nutrition. The drink mix can be mixed in water, a trim shake, or a favorite beverage.

Key Ingredients:

Spinach (*Spinacia oleracea*) Leaf Extract: is packed full of a nutrient called thylakoids. Thylakoids have been shown to slow down digestion and the absorption of fats. Specifically, research-

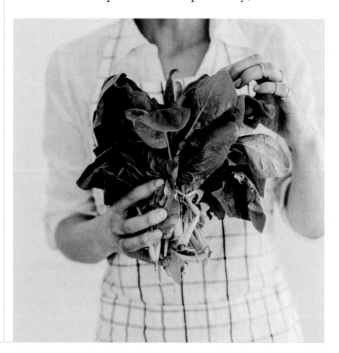

ers discovered that ingesting thylakoids (in conjunction with food) suppresses food intake, raises hormones that cause a feeling of being full, and lowers blood lipid levels in rats (Albertsson et al., 2007). Thylakoids work best when consumed with dietary fat because thylakoids decrease the feeling of hunger by slowing down the digestion of fat and allowing the fat to stay longer in the intestine (Albertsson et al., 2007). This lengthened digestion time allows for the body to feel full longer. Ideally, Slim & Sassy® Contrōl™ Instant Drink Mix, in order to work most effectively, should be consumed during a meal that contains fat.

Ground Flax (*Linum usitatissimum*) Seed Powder: is nutritionally beneficial, and research has found that consuming flaxseed can help prevent cardiovascular diseases, cancer, and diabetes and can enhance spatial memory (Akhtar et al., 2013; Singh et al., 2011). Flaxseed is also an antioxidant agent (Akhtar et al., 2013).

Grapefruit Essential Oil: is balancing and uplifting to the mind. It has been used medicinally by the French to help with cellulite and digestion. Limonene, a component of grapefruit oil, was found to reduce appetite and body weight in rats exposed to the oil for 15 minutes 3 times per week (Shen et al., 2005).

Lemon Essential Oil: is invigorating, enhancing, and warming. It promotes health, healing, and energy. Lemon oil also displays antioxidant activity (Grassmann et al., 2001).

Peppermint Essential Oil: is purifying and stimulating to the human mind. It may also help soothe digestive difficulties (Kim et al., 2005).

Ginger Essential Oil: may help increase physical energy and promote healthy digestion.

Cinnamon Essential Oil: enhances the action of other oils. It may improve circulation, digestion, and energy levels.

Potato (*Solanum tuberosum*) Tuber Extract: contains a high level of natural proteins, including the protease inhibitor PI-2. PI-2 has been shown to inhibit the digestive enzyme trypsin (Pouvreau et al., 2001). Trypsin inhibitors such as PI-2 have been studied for their ability to induce feelings of fullness by prolonging the secretion of the hormone cholycystokinin,

which acts to promote feelings of satiation (Marinangeli et al., 2012).

Companion Products: Slim & Sassy Contrōl Bars and Slim & Sassy.

Slim & Sassy® TrimShake

Trim Shake

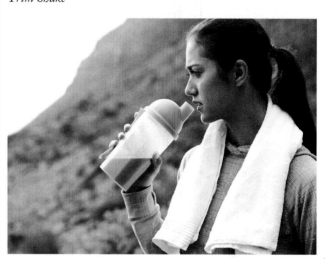

Choose a high-fiber, high-protein meal alternative drink powder with a low glycemic index and low calories. These shakes should contain extracts from the ashwagandha plant (*Withania somnifera*) that have shown potential to decrease blood serum levels of cortisol (Abedon, 2008) and to reduce stress (Archana et al., 1999; Bhattacharya et al., 1987). Cortisol—a hormone created by the adrenal glands—is released into the blood as the result of stress or anxiety, and it also plays a role in the body's sleep/wake cycle. When an individual is exposed to constant or chronic stress, levels of cortisol remain elevated in the body, disrupting the body's ability to relax and its ability to sleep naturally. Chronic stress and abnormally elevated cortisol levels have also been associated with increased cravings and with increased levels of obesity and abdominal weight (De Vriendt et al., 2009; Wallerius et al., 2003).

Key Ingredients:

Protein Blend: A blend of whey, pea, and rice proteins that helps support the body's protein needs—which is critical during exercise and dieting to help maintain and build lean body tissues such as muscle (Walker et al., 2010).

Potato Protein Extract: contains a high level of natural proteins, including the protease inhibitor PI-2. PI-2 has been shown to inhibit the digestive enzyme trypsin (Pouvreau et al., 2001). Trypsin inhibitors, such as PI-2, have been studied for their ability to induce feelings of fullness by prolonging the secretion of the hormone cholycystokinin, which acts to promote feelings of satiation (Marinangeli et al., 2012).

Fiber Blend: contains a mixture of insoluble fiber and prebiotic soluble fiber that can help promote beneficial GI tract bacteria function and elimination. These dietary fibers include maltodextrin, guar gum, and oligofructose.

Ashwagandha (*Withania somnifera*) Root and Leaf Extracts: have demonstrated a potential to help reduce stress (Archana et al., 1999; Bhattacharya et al., 1987) and to help lower blood serum cortisol levels (Abedon, 2008). Cortisol—a hormone created by the adrenal glands—is released into the blood as the result of stress or anxiety, and it also plays a role in the body's sleep/wake cycle. When an individual is exposed to constant or chronic stress, levels of cortisol remain elevated in the body, disrupting the body's ability to relax and its ability to sleep naturally. Chronic stress and abnormally elevated cortisol levels have also been associated with increased cravings and with increased levels of obesity and abdominal weight (De Vriendt et al., 2009; Wallerius et al., 2003).

Vitamins and Minerals: include nutrients that have been shown to support cellular energy levels and muscle and bone health. Key vitamins and minerals are listed below:

    Calcium (dicalcium phosphate): helps support bone density and muscle contraction.

    Magnesium (magnesium oxide): supports ATP production and use for energy.

    Vitamin C (ascorbic acid): is antioxidant and supports blood vessel and cartilage health.

    Vitamin E (vitamin E acetate): is antioxidant.

    Vitamin B7 (biotin): helps support metabolism of fats and aerobic energy generation.

    Vitamin B3 (niacinamide): helps support cellular energy creation.

    Iodine (potassium iodide): plays a role in two important thyroid hormones.

    Zinc (zinc oxide): is an important component in many critical cellular enzymes and proteins.

    Vitamin A (vitamin A acetate): plays a role in vision, skin health, and DNA transcription.

    Copper (copper gluconate): is found in several enzymes, including superoxide dismutase.

    Vitamin B5 (D-calcium pantothenate): plays a role in the metabolism of fatty acids.

    Vitamin D3: plays an important role in bone health and strength.

    Vitamin B6 (pyridoxine hydrochloride): is important in the creation of enzymes that aid in the creation of energy.

    Vitamin B2 (riboflavin): plays an important role in the creation of energy from lipids (fat) and carbohydrates in the cell.

    Vitamin B1 (thiamine mononitrate): plays a critical role in generating energy from carbohydrates within the cell.

    Vitamin B12: plays a key role in the synthesis of DNA and in nerve cell protection.

    Folic acid: is a critical nutrient for the creation of DNA and RNA in cells.

Stevia: is a natural herb with a very sweet taste (said to be many times sweeter than sugar). This naturally sweet herb has been found in at least one study to increase glucose tolerance while decreasing plasma glucose levels in normal volunteers (Curi et al., 1986).

Companion Products: Lifelong Vitality Pack, DigestZen Terrazyme, Zendocrine Detoxification Complex, Zendocrine.

Slim & Sassy® V Shake

Vegan Trim Shake

Slim & Sassy V Shake has the same high fiber and high protein content, the ashwagandha root and leaf extracts, and the potato protein extracts found in the Slim & Sassy TrimShake—but with natural, vegan-friendly options.

Key Ingredients:

Protein Blend: a blend of pea, quinoa, and amaranth proteins that helps support the body's protein needs. This support is critical during exercise and dieting to help maintain and build lean body tissues such as muscle (Walker et al., 2010).

Potato Protein Extract: contains a high level of natural proteins, including the protease inhibitor PI-2. PI-2 has been shown to inhibit the digestive enzyme trypsin (Pouvreau et al., 2001). Trypsin inhibitors such as PI-2, have been studied for their ability to induce feelings of fullness by prolonging the secretion of the hormone cholecystokinin, which acts to promote feelings of satiation (Marinangeli et al., 2012).

Fiber Blend: contains a mixture of insoluble fiber and prebiotic soluble fiber that can help promote beneficial GI tract bacteria function and elimination. These dietary fibers include soluble corn fiber, xanthan gum, citrus fiber, and tara gum.

Ashwagandha (*Withania somnifera*) Root and Leaf Extracts: have demonstrated a potential to help reduce stress (Archana et al., 1999; Bhattacharya et al., 1987) and to help lower blood serum cortisol levels (Abedon, 2008). Cortisol—a hormone created by the adrenal glands—is released into the blood as the result of stress or anxiety, and it also plays a role in the body's sleep/wake cycle. When an individual is exposed to constant or chronic stress, levels of cortisol remain elevated in the body, disrupting the body's ability to relax and its ability to sleep naturally. Chronic stress and abnormally elevated cortisol levels have also been associated with increased cravings and with increased levels of obesity and abdominal weight (De Vriendt et al., 2009; Wallerius et al., 2003).

Stevia: is a natural herb with a very sweet taste (said to be many times sweeter than sugar). This naturally sweet herb has been found in at least one study to increase glucose toler-ance while decreasing plasma glucose levels in normal volunteers (Curi et al., 1986).

Companion Supplements: Slim & Sassy TrimShake, Daily Vitality Pack, DigestZen Terrazyme, Zendocrine Detoxification Complex, Zendocrine.

TerraGreens®

Fruit & Veggie Drink Mix

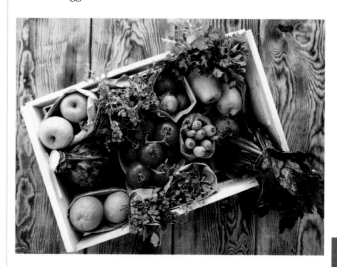

TerraGreens consist of a wide assortment of fruits and vegetables known to contain high levels of vitamins, minerals, and other important nutrients that are often missing from the diet of the average person. This drink mix can help boost overall nutrient levels in the average diet, helping to support the body in maintaining optimal health.

Key Ingredients:

Kale: is a green leafy vegetable that has a high content of vitamin C, β-carotene, nutritive fiber, phenolic compounds, and high antioxidant activity (Sikora et al., 2012).

Collard Greens: is a leafy vegetable that has a high vitamin content and has been studied for its ability to help protect against elevations of atherogenic fatty acids (Johnson et al., 2013).

Dandelion Greens: are high in vitamins A, C, and K, as well as several minerals. Dandelion greens have been studied for their ability to help manage weight (Gonzalez-Castejon et al., 2014; Zhant et al., 2008) and as an antioxidant (Choi et al., 2010).

Wheat Grass: is high in vitamins C & E (Shukla et al., 2009) and has been studied for its anti-oxidant abilities (Shyam et al., 2007).

Barley Grass: is high in flavonoids that have potent antioxidant activity (Kamiyama et al., 2012).

Guava: is high in fiber, vitamin C, and polyphenols. Guava fruit has been studied for its potential to aid with obesity (Norazmir et al., 2010) and diabetes (Huang et al., 2011).

Acerola Cherry: are small berries from South and Central America. This fruit is extremely high in vitamin C and contains other A and B vitamins as well. It has been studied for its strong antioxidant properties (Schreckinger et al., 2010; Leffa et al., 2013) and its potential to help reduce weight gain (Dias et al., 2014).

Goji Berry: contains high levels of various vitamins and minerals, as well as amino acids, polyphenols, and other nutrients. It has been studied for its antioxidant properties (Zhang et al., 2011; Bucheli et al., 2011; Reeve et al., 2010).

Lemon Essential Oil: has a great citrus flavor and has been studied for its antioxidant properties (Grassman et al., 2001) and its ability to help support the digestive system (Kime et al., 2005; Rozza et al., 2011).

Ginger Essential Oil: is well known for its ability to help soothe the digestive system and has also been studied for its abilities to help support the liver (Liu et al., 2013).

Companion Supplement: Slim & Sassy TrimShake.

TriEase® Softgels

Seasonal Blend Softgels

These softgels combine three powerful essential oils that have been studied for their abilities to help the body respond appropriately to symptoms related to seasonal allergies.

Key Ingredients:

Lemon Essential Oil: has antiseptic properties and may help alleviate symptoms related to asthma and colds. A lemon-based spray has also been studied for its abilities to help alleviate immunological reactions related to rhinitis (Ferrara et al., 2012).

Lavender Essential Oil: is anti-inflammatory and analgesic. It has been studied for its abilities to help alleviate allergic reactions (Kim et al., 1999; Ueno-Lio et al., 2014).

Peppermint Essential Oil: is often used for its anti-inflammatory and decongestant properties. It may help alleviate rhinitis, asthma, and other respiratory conditions.

Companion Blend: Breathe.

vEO Mega®

Vegan Essential Oil Omega Complex

This supplement is a vegan-friendly blend of essential fatty acids that is particularly high in beneficial omega-3 fatty acids. It also includes the potent antioxidant astaxanthin and a unique essential oil blend that helps enhance the benefits of the essential fatty acids.

Key Ingredients:

Algae Oil (DHA): Docosahexaenoic acid (or DHA) is an omega-3 fatty acid that is found in high concentrations in the brain and in the retina of the eye, where it is part of several important phospholipids. DHA has also been studied for its ability to help inhibit colon (Kato et al., 2002) and prostate (Shaikh et al., 2008) cancer cells.

Flaxseed Oil (ALA): Alpha-linolenic acid, or ALA, is an omega-3 fatty acid that is readily able to be synthesized into DHA or EPA by the human body. Eicosapentaenoic acid (or EPA) is another omega-3 fatty acid. It is largely known for its anti-inflammatory benefits but has also been found in several studies to help individuals suffering from depression (Su et al., 2008; Osher et al., 2005; Lucas et al., 2009; Frangou et al., 2006). There is strong evidence that EPA and DHA together can help with high blood pressure (Erkkila et al., 2008; Mori et al., 1999; Morris et al., 1993) and cardiovascular disease (Erkkila et al., 2004; Bucher et al., 2002), especially in high-risk individuals. When taken together by pregnant women, EPA and DHA have also been found to have beneficial effects on these women's children, such as reduced allergies (Furuhjelm et al., 2009; Dunstan et al., 2003) and improved neurological development (Helland et al., 2003).

Inca Inchi Seed Oil (ALA): Inca inchi (or sacha inchi) seeds come from a star-shaped fruit native to the Amazonian forests of Peru. The seeds have a naturally high content of the omega-3 fatty acid ALA.

Astaxanthin: Astaxanthin is a natural carotenoid that can be found in many marine plants (and in the animals that eat these plants), but it is found in the most abundance in marine algae. This dark, red-colored carotenoid pigment has been well studied for its potent antioxidant abilities (Palozza et al., 1992; Naguib et al., 2000) and has demonstrated a unique potential to cross the blood-brain barrier in mammals, making it a prime candidate for treating diseases of the central nervous system caused by oxidative damage (Tso et al., 1994).

Lutein: Lutein is created in many plants as an antioxidant and a light absorber. In humans, lutein is found in high concentration in the macula, the area of the eye where central vision occurs. Lutein supplementation has been found in at least one study to improve the visual acuity and macular pigment optical density in patients with age-related macular degeneration (Richer et al., 2004).

Lycopene: is a red-colored pigment found in many red plants. It has been studied for its potential role in reducing the risk of prostate cancer (Giovannucci et al, 2002).

Zeaxanthin: is a carotenoid pigment found in many plants such as corn and wolfberries. It has been studied for its antioxidant abilities.

Alpha & Beta Carotene: Vitamin A (alpha and beta carotene) plays a role in vision, skin health, and DNA transcription.

Borage Seed Oil (GLA): Borage seed oil has one of the highest contents of the omega-6 fatty acid gamma-linolenic acid. GLA has been studied for its ability to aid with dermatitis (Senapati et al., 2008; Kanehara et al., 2007) and other skin conditions (De Spirt et al., 2009; Chen et al., 2006).

Cranberry Seed Oil (ALA): In addition to being high in alpha-linolenic acid, cranberry seed oil is also high in vitamin E, a potent antioxidant.

Pomegranate Seed Oil (CLNA): 9cis, 11trans, 13cis-conjugated linolenic acid (or punicic acid) is a conjugated linolenic acid (CLNA) that is found in pomegranate seed oil. This isomer of linolenic acid has been studied for its antioxidant (Saha et al., 2009) and anti-inflammatory (Boussetta et al., 2009) properties.

Pumpkin Seed Oil: Pumpkin seed oil is rich in several essential fatty acids and has been studied for its potential to improve HDL cholesterol levels (Gossell-Williams et al., 2011).

Grape Seed Oil: Grape seed oil contains high levels of the essential fatty acid linoleic acid.

Vitamin D (cholecalciferol): plays an important role in bone health and strength and helps modulate hormone secretion and immune function.

Vitamin E (d-alpha & mixed tocopherols): is a potent antioxidant and may play a role in cellular communication.

Clove Bud Essential Oil: is highly antioxidant as well as anti-inflammatory. It may also help relieve pain and skin problems.

Frankincense Essential Oil: is an immune stimulant and is anti-inflammatory. It may also help with blood pressure and depression.

Thyme Essential Oil: Thymol in thyme is highly antioxidant. Thyme oil may help with depression and fatigue.

Cumin Essential Oil: is a digestive aid and may help with indigestion and flatulence.

Orange Essential Oil: aids the digestive system and may help with indigestion and diarrhea.

Peppermint Essential Oil: is anti-inflammatory and antispasmodic. It may help with intestinal cramping and spasms as well as with feelings of nausea.

Ginger Essential Oil: is calming to the digestive system. It may help alleviate feelings of nausea and indigestion.

Caraway Seed Essential Oil: is antispasmodic and antiparasitic. It may also help with indigestion and diarrhea and may be calming to the intestinal muscles.

German Chamomile Essential Oil: is anti-inflammatory and aids the digestive system. It may also aid liver function and help alleviate gastritis.

Essential Supplements

Companion Supplements: Alpha CRS+®, Microplex VMz.

xEO Mega®

Essential Oil Omega Complex

This complex is a blend of essential fatty acids. It includes essential fatty acids from both marine and land sources, the potent antioxidant astaxanthin, and an essential oil blend that helps enhance the benefits of the essential fatty acids.

Key Ingredients:

Fish Oil (as Anchovy, Sardine, and Mackerel) and Calamari Oil Concentrates (EPA, DHA, and other Omega-3s): Eicosapentaenoic acid (or EPA) is an omega-3 fatty acid. It is largely known for its anti-inflammatory benefits but has also been found in several studies to help individuals suffering from depression (Su et al., 2008, Osher et al., 2005, Lucas et al., 2009; Frangou et al., 2006). Docosahexaenoic acid (or DHA) is another omega-3 fatty acid that is found in high concentrations in the brain and in the retina of the eye, where it is part of several important phospholipids. DHA has also been studied for its ability to help inhibit colon (Kato et al., 2002) and prostate (Shaikh et al., 2008) cancer cells. Taken together in fish oil, there is strong evidence that EPA and DHA can help with high blood pressure (Erkkila et al., 2008, Mori et al., 1999, and Morris et al., 1993) and cardiovascular disease (Erkkila et al., 2004; Bucher et al., 2002), especially in high-risk individuals. When taken together by pregnant women, EPA and DHA have also been found to have beneficial effects on these women's children, such as reduced allergies (Furuhjelm et al., 2009; Dunstan et al., 2003) and improved neurological development (Helland et al., 2003).

***Echium plantagineum* Seed Oil (ALA, SDA, and GLA):** Alpha linolenic acid (ALA), stearidonic acid (SDA), and gamma linolenic acid (GLA) are fatty acids. Omega-3 fatty acids are essential nutrients for health. The body partially converts ALA, an omega-3 fatty acid, to EPA and DHA, other omega-3 fatty acids. Omega-3 fatty acids have been found to help soothe joint stiffness and pain, lower levels of depression, and protect against dementia.

Pomegranate Seed Oil: 9cis, 11trans, 13cis-conjugated linolenic acid (or punicic acid) is a conjugated linolenic acid (CLNA) that is found in pomegranate seed oil. This isomer of linolenic acid has been studied for its antioxidant (Saha et al., 2009) and anti-inflammatory (Boussetta et al., 2009) properties.

Astaxanthin: Astaxanthin is a natural carotenoid that can be found in many marine plants (and in the animals that eat these plants), but it is found in the most abundance in marine algae. This dark, red-colored carotenoid pigment has been well studied for its potent antioxidant abilities (Palozza et al., 1992; Naguib et al., 2000) and has demonstrated a unique potential to cross the blood-brain barrier in mammals, making it a prime candidate for treating diseases of the central nervous system caused by oxidative damage (Tso et al., 1994).

Lutein (from Marigold Flower): is a natural carotenoid synthesized by plants and found abundantly in green leafy vegetables (Khachik et al., 1995). Lutein has been found to be an antioxidant (Khachik et al., 1995), photoprotectant (protect the eye from oxidative stress caused by UV radiation and decrease risk of age-related macular degeneration) (Abdel-Aal et al., 2013), and a promising chemopreventive agent (Khachik et al., 1995).

Zeaxanthin (from Marigold Flower): is a natural carotenoid that has been found to have an important role in eye health (Abdel-Aal et al., 2013). Both lutein and zeaxanthin have been shown to decrease the risk of age-related macular degeneration (Abdel-Aal et al., 2013).

Lycopene (from Tomato Fruit): is a red carotene found in tomatoes, carrots, and watermelons as well as other fruits and vegetables. Lycopene has strong antioxidant activity.

Vitamin A (as alpha and beta carotene): are antioxidants. A recent study found that administration of beta-carotene for 12 weeks reduced oxidative stress in male subjects (Kasperczyk et al., 2014).

Vitamin D$_3$ (as natural cholecalciferol): plays an important role in bone health and strength and helps modulate hormone secretion and immune function.

Vitamin E (d-alpha & natural mixed tocopherols): is a potent antioxidant and may play a role in cellular communication.

Clove Essential Oil: is highly antioxidant as well as anti-inflammatory. It may also help relieve pain and skin problems.

Frankincense Essential Oil: is an immune stimulant and is anti-inflammatory. It may also help with blood pressure and depression.

Thyme Essential Oil: Thymol in thyme is highly antioxidant. Thyme oil may help with depression and fatigue.

Cumin Essential Oil: is a digestive aid and may help with indigestion and flatulence.

Orange Essential Oil: aids the digestive system and may help with indigestion and diarrhea.

Peppermint Essential Oil: is anti-inflammatory and antispasmodic. It may help with intestinal cramping and spasms as well as with feelings of nausea.

Ginger Essential Oil: is calming to the digestive system. It may help alleviate feelings of nausea and indigestion.

Caraway Essential Oil: is antispasmodic and anti-parasitic. It may also help with indigestion and diarrhea and may be calming to the intestinal muscles.

German Chamomile Essential Oil: is anti-inflammatory and aids the digestive system. It may also aid liver function and help alleviate gastritis.

Companion Supplements: Alpha CRS+®, Microplex VMz.

Zendocrine® Detoxification Complex

Detoxification Complex

This supplement is a blend of whole food–based nutrients that may help promote healthy endocrine gland functions and the filtering of toxins by the body's systems.

Key Ingredients:

Psyllium Seed Husk Powder: contains a high level of soluble fiber that can help keep the digestive tract and the colon functioning properly.

Barberry Leaf: contains the alkaloid berberine, which has been studied for its ability to aid the pancreas in regulating insulin production, thus promoting healthy blood sugar levels (Zhou et al., 2009).

Turkish Rhubarb Stem: has been used in traditional Chinese medicine to promote healthy bowel movement, aiding in clearing the intestines and colon of waste.

Kelp: is naturally high in the essential element iodine, which is necessary for proper thyroid functioning.

Milk Thistle Seed (Silymarin): Silymarin is a complex of polyphenols extracted from the milk thistle plant. Animal and cellular studies have suggested a toxin-protective effect in the liver of these polyphenols, especially the polyphenol silibinin (Al-Anati et al., 2009; Abenavoli et al., 2010).

Osha Root: was used by Native Americans as a purifier and was chewed to help resolve sore throat and upper respiratory tract ailments.

Safflower Petals: are used in traditional Chinese medicine to aid the endocrine system in promoting healthy menstrual functioning in women.

Acacia Gum Bark: is known as a natural astringent that can decrease diarrhea and bloody discharges.

Burdock Root: has been used traditionally to help clear the body of toxins and has been used as a diuretic to help eliminate uric acid. It has also been studied for its ability to help protect liver cells from toxins (Lin et al., 2000).

Clove Bud: has very potent antimicrobial (Fabio et al., 2007, Smith-Palmer et al., 2004, Hitokoto et al., 1980, and Benencia et al., 2000) and antioxidant (Chaieb et al., 2007) properties that can help protect cells from toxins.

Dandelion Root (Inulin): has been studied for its ability to protect liver cells from toxin-induced damage (Domitrović et al., 2010; Mahesh et al., 2010).

Essential Supplements

Garlic Fruit: is known for its antibacterial and antiseptic properties and has been studied for its potential to help decrease problems related to diabetes (Younis et al., 2010; Drobiova et al., 2009).

Marshmallow Root: has been used traditionally to soothe coughs and irritations of the upper respiratory tract and to soothe irritations of tissues of the gastrointestinal tract, due to its ability to both coat the mucous membrane linings and to stimulate epithelial cell function within these membranes (Deters et al., 2010).

Red Clover Leaf (Isoflavones): contains high levels of isoflavones, which are structurally similar to natural estrogens in the body. These isoflavones have been studied for their abilities to help regulate healthy estrogen-mediated functions in postmenopausal women (Lipovac et al., 2010).

Enzyme Assimilation System: A patented system that contains special enzymes and mineral cofactors that may enhance digestion and nutrient absorption in the small intestine and blood stream, including amylase (breaks complex carbohydrates into sugars), protease (breaks proteins into smaller amino acids), cellulase (breaks cellulose into sugars), and lipase (breaks fats and lipids into their component parts).

Companion Supplements: DigestZen, DigestZen Softgels, DigestZen Terrazyme.

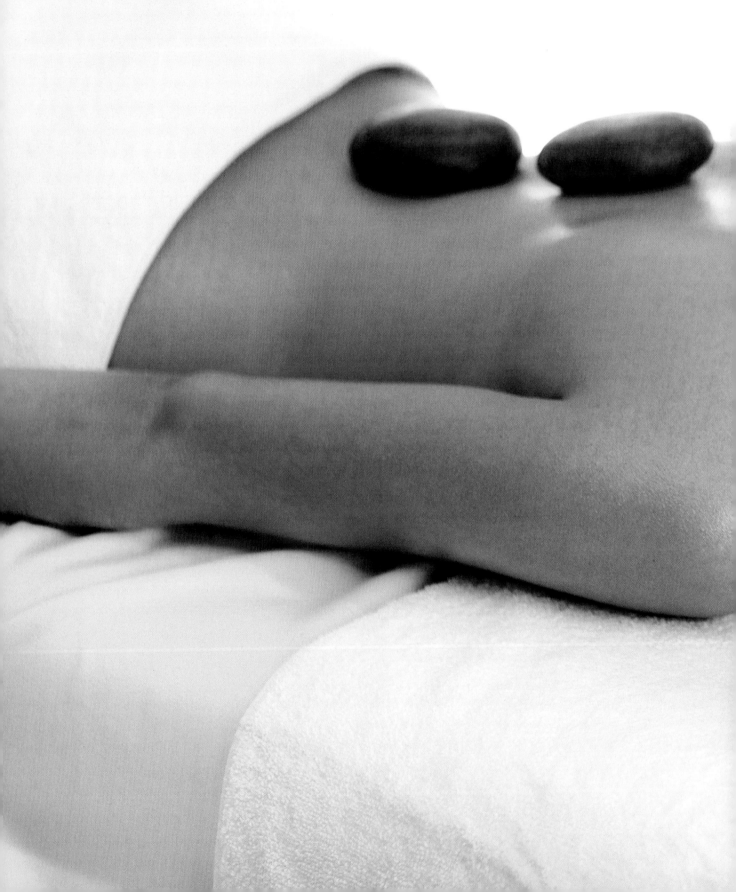

Personal Care and Spa

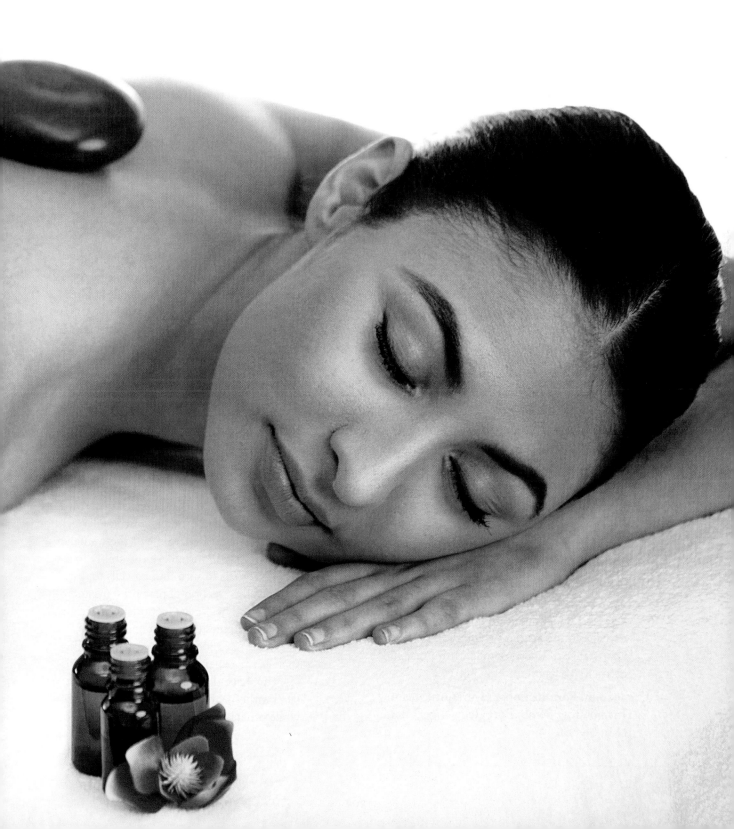

Personal Care and Spa

This section contains various essential oil–inspired personal care and spa formulations that that are available commercially. See the Essential Oils and the Essential Oil Blends sections of this book for more information on the single essential oil and blends referenced here.

Anti-Aging Eye Cream

Eye Cream

This unique cream targets fine lines and wrinkles that appear around the eyes and helps the skin in that area maintain a full, youthful appearance.

Key Ingredients:

Frankincense Essential Oil: prevents scarring, supports the immune system, and speeds the healing of wounds.

Ylang Ylang Essential Oil: is often used to help with skin problems and has a soothing, relaxing aroma.

Blue Tansy Oil: has antiseptic and soothing properties on the skin, and is often used to help with wounds.

Meadowfoam Seed Oil: has natural moisturizing properties and is easily absorbed by the skin to penetrate deeply. It also has a high content of the natural antioxidant vitamin E.

Pullulan: Is a natural biopolymer that creates a film over the skin that helps to gently tighten the skin and smooth its texture.

Red Algae Extract: contains amino acids that can help protect the skin from UVA damage, as well as polysaccharides that help to firm and smooth the skin.

Bukachiol: is a naturally occurring phenol. It has demonstrated an ability to help promote collagen production, and to help reduce photodamage in the skin, resulting in improved appearance of lines, wrinkles, firmness, and elasticity (Chaudhuri et al., 2014).

Companion Formulations: Hydrating Cream, Invigorating Scrub, Pore Reducing Toner, Skin Serum.

Anti-Aging Moisturizer

Anti-Aging Moisturizer combines several ingredients that have been studied for their abilities to combat many of the visible signs of aging by reducing wrinkles and fine lines and improving skin elasticity and tone.

Key Ingredients:

Lavender Essential Oil: is calming and balances the body wherever there is a need.

Jasmine Essential Oil: is uplifting to the emotions and helps reduce anxiety, apathy, and depression.

Geranium Essential Oil: is hydrating and helps to ease nervous tension and stress.

Frankincense Essential Oil: helps repair cells and reduce signs of aging.

Palmitoyl Oligopeptides and Tetrapeptide-7 (Matrikine Messaging): The space in between skin (and other tissue) cells is filled with water and a mixture of fibrous proteins and polysaccharides called the extracellular matrix. These proteins and polysaccharides help give skin tissue its strength and elasticity and provide a framework for new cell growth and migration. Examples of extracellular proteins commonly found in skin tissue include collagen (provides strength, volume, and rigidity) and elastin (provides flexibility and resilience).

Enzymes on the outside of the cell membranes have the ability to break down some of these extracellular proteins into smaller peptide units when activated. Some of these smaller peptide units, in turn, have the ability to send further signals to surrounding cells to start, or turn off, the creation of new proteins and other structures. These small peptide messengers are called matrikines (Maquart et al., 1999).

Studies have shown that certain matrikines, such as the tripeptide glycyl-histidyl-lysine (GHK), have the ability to activate and regulate synthesis of extracellular matrix proteins[1], while others can help stimulate the creation of an extracellular matrix framework that facilitates new cell growth and the healing of skin wounds (Siméon et al., 1999; Tran et al., 2004).

With aging, extracellular proteins and fibers begin to break down, and synthesis of new structures is limited. Because of this loss of proteins and other structures in the extracellular matrix, the skin begins to lose its rigidity, structure, resilience, and elasticity, resulting in the appearance of fine lines and wrinkles.

In vitro studies and limited clinical trials have demonstrated evidence that palmitoylated matrikines may have the ability to activate synthesis of extracellular matrix structures, such as collagen, fibronectin, and hyaluronic acid, that can lead to a fuller, tighter skin structure and can reduce the appearance of fine lines and wrinkles.

Sodium Hyaluronate (Patented Hyaluronic Acid Spherulites): Hyaluronic acid (also called hyaluronan, or hyaluronate) is not a true acid but is actually a special type of polysaccharide structure (called a glycosaminoglycan) that can form huge molecular chains that have the ability to absorb and hold water. Hyaluronic acid is found in large amounts in the extracellular matrix, where it helps provide structure and may help regulate transport of macromolecules between the cells. It is also found in the joints, where its viscous properties allow it to be used to cushion and lubricate the joint (Laurent et al., 1995).

Hyaluronic acid is also found in high concentrations in the skin tissue, where it helps provide structure, support, and turgidity in the skin. Researchers in Italy have found that hyaluronic acid content in the skin decreases with aging and is nearly absent in the skin of individuals over 60 years old (Ghersetich et al., 1994). This decline in hyaluronic acid has been hypothesized to be one of the main causes of skin issues related to aging.

Because of hyaluronic acid's unique ability to absorb water—causing it to swell to many times its original size—it has been used for years as an injectable cosmetic treatment for increasing volume in the skin in problem areas to reduce wrinkles and also for increasing volume in the lips and other areas. The unique formulation of the patented hyaluronic acid spherulites, however, actually allows

these spherulites to naturally penetrate the outer layers of the skin without the need for invasive injections. These spherulites can then absorb water, allowing them to increase the volume of the skin and also to help improve the moisture-barrier functionality of the skin so it can stay hydrated.

Grapeseed Oil: has an extremely high content of the omega-6 fatty acid, linoleic acid. Both animal studies (Darmstadt et al., 2002) and clinical trials (Darmstadt et al., 2005) have found that application of an oil high in linoleic acid can help enhance the skin-moisture barrier. Linoleic acid has also been studied for its ability to reduce acne microcomedones (Letawe et al., 1998) and to enhance cellular migration during wound healing (Ruthig et al., 1999).

Summer Snowflake Bulb Extract: Many plants and animals enter a dormant stage, where they cease many metabolic activities in order to conserve energy and resources during times of harsh environmental conditions, such as drought or freezing temperatures. This dormancy allows the plant or animal to survive these harsh conditions and continue to live longer than it would otherwise be able.

Over the past several decades, researchers have begun to discover that several substances available in the dormant parts of plants—such as within the bulb—demonstrate an ability to prevent cell growth and cell division in human tissues as well (Ceriotti et al., 1967; Jimenez et al., 1976). This can be important for skin health, as researchers have found that human cells appear to only have the ability to replicate a certain number of times, and that as they approach their limit, the cells becomes less functional (Hayflick, 1979). Because of this limitation, it has been theorized that slowing the process of cell replication can slow the process of loss of cell function associated with aging.

An extract from the bulbs of dormant Summer Snowflake flowers (Leucojum Aestivum) has shown promising potential to slow replication of skin fibroblast cells, as well as the ability to increase the activity of a potent antioxidant—mitochondrial superoxide dismutase. Both of these abilities may help promote more youthful skin cell function.

Acetyl Octapeptide-3 (Proprietary Octapeptide): Around the eyes and forehead, fine lines and wrinkles are often the result of tense, contracting muscle fibers repeatedly pulling the skin into folds and creases (often called frown lines).

Muscle fiber contraction is dependent on a complex signaling process from the motor neurons of nerve cells. Within each motor neuron are small, round structures called synaptic vesicles that each contain many copies of the signaling molecule acetylcholine. When stimulated, a protein on the synaptic vesicle wall called VAMP (vesicle-associated membrane protein) will bind with two proteins on the motor neuron cell membrane called syntaxin (or T-SNARE) and SNAP25. When these proteins bind together, the synaptic vesicle is pulled in close to the motor neuron cell membrane, and the synaptic vesicle fuses with the neuron cell membrane, opening the vesicle and releasing the acetylcholine outside of the cell. The acetylcholine then binds with a protein receptor on the cell membrane of surrounding muscle fiber cells, signaling to them to contract (Südhof, 1995, Kee et al., 1995; Pevsner et al., 1994).

The biomimetic peptide Acetyl Octapeptide-3 mimics the part of the SNAP25 protein that binds with the VAMP protein on the synaptic vesicle. Because this proprietary peptide temporarily binds with the VAMP protein, the VAMP protein is blocked from being able to bind with the proteins that allow the synaptic vesicles to release acetylcholine into the extracellular matrix. This results in the muscle fibers remaining more relaxed, preventing them from pulling the skin around the eyes and forehead into the distinctive lines and wrinkles associated with aging.

Vitamin Blend: This type of vitamin blend should include tocopherol acetate (Vitamin E—antioxidant and cellular communication) and tetrahexyldecyl ascorbate (stabilized vitamin C—provides stability to collagen).

Companion Formulations: Facial Cleanser, Invigorating Scrub, Pore Reducing Toner, Skin Serum, Immortelle, Veráge Immortelle Hydrating Serum, Veráge Moisturizer, Veráge Cleanser, Veráge Toner.

Baby: Diaper Rash Cream

This gentle cream safely and effectively creates a natural barrier to protect a baby's sensitive skin. It soothes and relieves diaper rash while moisturizing the skin.

Key Ingredients:

Lavender Essential Oil: has been studied for its ability to reduce inflammation and allergic reactions in the skin. It has also been used to help the skin recover from burns, blisters, infections, and other injuries. It aids conditions related to dry skin. Lavender is also well known for its ability to help decrease pain and inflammation (Ghelardini et al., 1999; Olapour et al., 2013).

Carrot Seed Essential Oil: is often used to help moisturize and soothe the skin.

Melaleuca Essential Oil: is antimicrobial and can be used on a wound to help fight infection. Melaleuca oil has anti-inflammatory properties, including the ability to reduce swelling, so it can help support skin in the recovery process after injuries (Brand et al., 2002; Caldefie-Chézet et al., 2006; Hart et al., 2000).

Non-Nano Zinc Oxide: gently creates a barrier on the skin, protecting it from excess moisture.

Muyao Shea Butter: is widely known as a powerful moisturizer. Shea butter has been used to heal skin conditions and reduce wrinkles. Shea butter mimics the body's natural moisturizers and is, therefore, extremely effective at treating dry skin, sunburns, wounds, skin cracks, stretch marks, and burns. This variety of shea butter has a unique fatty acid profile that helps support a baby's delicate skin.

Companion Supplements: Baby Hair and Body Wash, Baby Lotion.

Baby: Hair and Body Wash

This unique baby washcontains natural ingredients that are gentle on a baby's delicate skin. It has a soft, delicate aroma that is soothing to babies and children of all ages.

Key Ingredients:

Lavender Essential Oil: has been studied for its ability to reduce inflammation and allergic reactions in the skin. It has also been used to help the skin recover from burns, blisters, infections, and other injuries. It aids conditions related to dry skin. Lavender is also well known for its ability to help decrease pain and inflammation (Ghelardini et al., 1999; Olapour et al., 2013).

Roman Chamomile Essential Oil: is often used help soothe rashes or dry and irritated skin. It has anti-inflammatory properties and has a calming and relaxing aroma.

Vanilla Extract: has a soft, gentle aroma.

Muyao Shea Butter: is widely known as a powerful moisturizer. Shea butter has been used to heal skin conditions and reduce wrinkles. Shea butter mimics the body's natural moisturizers and is, therefore, extremely effective at treating dry skin, sunburns, wounds, skin cracks, stretch marks, and burns. This variety of shea butter has a unique fatty acid profile that helps support a baby's delicate skin.

Companion Supplements: Baby Diaper Rash Cream, Baby Lotion.

Baby: Lotion

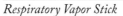

This unique lotion combines natural ingredients to help moisturize baby's skin. It contains the soft, gentle aroma of lavender and Roman chamomile essential oils blended with a hint of vanilla.

Key Ingredients:

Lavender Essential Oil: has been studied for its ability to reduce inflammation and allergic reactions in the skin. It has also been used to help the skin recover from burns, blisters, infections, and other injuries. It aids conditions related to dry skin. Lavender is also well known for its ability to help decrease pain and inflammation (Ghelardini et al., 1999; Olapour et al., 2013).

Roman Chamomile Essential Oil: is often used help soothe rashes or dry and irritated skin. It has anti-inflammatory properties and has a calming and relaxing aroma.

Vanilla Extract: has a soft, gentle aroma.

Muyao Shea Butter: is widely known as a powerful moisturizer. Shea butter has been used to heal skin conditions and reduce wrinkles.

Shea butter mimics the body's natural moisturizers and is, therefore, extremely effective at treating dry skin, sunburns, wounds, skin cracks, stretch marks, and burns. This variety of shea butter has a unique fatty acid profile that helps support a baby's delicate skin.

Coconut Oil: is often used in soaps, creams, and lotions for its moisturizing and skin-softening properties.

Apple Fruit Extract: is often used to help condition the skin and to help maintain even skin tone and texture.

Companion Supplements: Baby Diaper Rash Cream, Baby Hair and Body Wash.

Breathe® Vapor Stick

Respiratory Vapor Stick

This handy stick combines many essential oils that are often used and studied for their abilities to help support the respiratory system in an easy-to-apply solid stick.

Key Ingredients:

Lemon Essential Oil: has antiseptic properties and may help alleviate symptoms related to asthma and colds. A lemon-based spray has also been studied for its abilities to help alleviate immunological reactions related to rhinitis (Ferrara et al., 2012).

Peppermint Essential Oil: is often used for its anti-inflammatory and decongestant properties. It may help alleviate rhinitis, asthma, and other respiratory conditions.

Eucalyptus Essential Oil: may have a profound antiviral effect upon the respiratory system. It may also help reduce inflammation of the nasal mucous membrane.

Cardamom Essential Oil: has antiseptic and anti-inflammatory properties. It may also help with congestion and other respiratory problems.

Companion Supplements: Breathe, Breathe Respiratory Drops.

Brightening Gel

Skin Brightening Gel

Brightening Gel combines ingredients that have been studied for their abilities to promote even pigmenta-

Personal Care & Spa

tion and tone in the skin and to help lessen the appearance of dark spots associated with aging.

Key Ingredients:

Bergamot Essential Oil: has a bright, uplifting aroma and can help purify the skin.

Juniper Berry Essential Oil: is beneficial for relieving acne and other skin issues. Juniper berry oil is also a cleanser and purifier and helps heal wounds. This oil may also help skin retain moisture.

Melissa Essential Oil: has strong antiviral properties and is often used to help purify the skin.

Daisy Extract: Daisy has been used since ancient times for various ailments, including wounds and the common cold. Daisy flower extract is now commonly used to prevent sun spots and other undesired skin pigmentations and to help make the complexion both lighter and brighter.

Daisy flower extract contains arbutin, which can blocks pathways that lead to melanin (pigment) formation in the skin (Kim et al., 2017), resulting in a lighter, more even skin tone.

Ginger Root Extract: has antioxidant and anti-inflammatory properties that help protect the skin from damage and aging. It also may help prevent the breakdown of collagen in the skin, and helps promote an even, smooth skin tone.

Vitamin C: is a critical component to maintaining the stability of collagen in the skin. It has also been found to help protect the skin from UV radiation, prevent inflammation in the skin, and to help lighten over-pigmentation in the skin (Farris, 2005).

Companion Formulations: Anti-Aging Eye Cream, Facial Cleanser, Hydrating Cream, Invigorating Scrub, Pore Reducing Toner.

Citrus Bliss® Hand Lotion

Invigorating Blend Hand & Body Lotion

This lotion offers the same natural benefits of the regular Hand & Body Lotion, plus the added benefits of the Citrus Bliss.

Key Ingredients:

Citrus Bliss: This blend contains essential oils of orange, lemon, grapefruit, mandarin, bergamot, tangerine, and clementine, with vanilla bean extract. The oils contained in this blend have been studied for their abilities to calm and soothe tension, and also for their ability to cleanse and disinfect.

See Hand & Body Lotion for other suggested ingredients and research.

Citrus Bliss® Invigorating Bath Bar

Invigorating Bath bar

This invigorating soap combines the skin protecting abilities of sunflower, safflower, palm, coconut, and jojoba oils with naturally exfoliating oatmeal kernels and the stimulating aroma of Citrus Bliss.

Key Ingredients:

Citrus Bliss: combines the uplifting and stress-reducing benefits of many different citrus oils in a sweetly satisfying way. In addition to their elevating properties, many of the oils in this blend have been studied for their ability to cleanse and disinfect. This blend contains orange, lemon, grapefruit, mandarin, bergamot, tangerine, and clementine essential oils blended with the soothing aroma of vanilla beans.

Oatmeal (*Avena sativa*) Kernel: is widely used for its gentle exfoliating and skin soothing properties.

Sodium Cocoate (Saponified Coconut Oil): is the soap form of coconut oil (saponification is the process of transforming oils into soap). Coconut oil is often used in soaps, creams, and lotions for its moisturizing and skin-softening abilities.

Sodium Safflowerate (Saponified Safflower Oil): is the soap form of safflower oil. Safflower oil is known for its skin softening properties.

Companion Formulations: Essential Skin Care.

Correct-X®

This all natural ointment harnesses the healing power of essential oils to help soothe skin irritations and enhance the natural process of healing.

Key Ingredients:

Frankincense Essential Oil: prevents scarring, supports the immune system, and speeds the healing of wounds.

Helichrysum Essential Oil: can be used on a fresh wound to help stop bleeding. Research has shown that Helichrysum has antibacterial, antiviral, and antioxidant properties (Chinou et al., 1996; Nostro et al., 2001; Appendino et al., 2007; Nostro et al., 2003; Rosa et al., 2007).

Melaleuca Essential Oil: is antimicrobial and can be used on a wound to help fight infection. Melaleuca oil has anti-inflammatory properties, including the ability to reduce swelling and alter the secretion of chemical messengers involved in the inflammatory response (Brand et al., 2002; Caldefie-Chézet et al., 2006; Hart et al., 2000).

Cedarwood Essential Oil: is anti-inflammatory (Tumen et al., 2013). Cedarwood oil is also calming and relieves tension.

Lavender Essential Oil: is well known for its ability to help decrease pain (Ghelardini et al., 1999; Olapour et al., 2013). This oil can also be used to decrease anxiety, stress, and inflammation.

Bisabolol: is a main chemical constituent of German chamomile essential oil. Recent studies have found that bisabolol may be used to treat skin inflammation and reduce sensitivity to pain (Maurya et al., 2014; Rocha et al., 2011).

Jojoba Oil: Although called an oil, jojoba oil is actually a natural liquid wax extracted from jojoba (*Simmondsia chinensis*) plants found in the southwestern Unites States and northern Mexico. This liquid wax closely resembles the skin's natural oils (or sebum) allowing it to provide increased hydration to the skin.

Phellodendron Amurense Bark Extract: is a fundamental herb used in traditional Chinese medicine. Modern research has shown that this extract possesses anti-inflammatory properties in vitro and in vivo (Choi et al., 2014).

Deep Blue® Rub

Soothing Rub

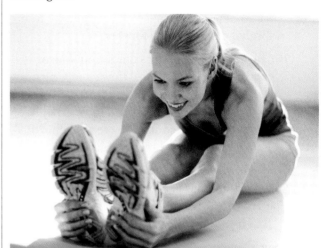

This massage and sports cream contains the Soothing essential oil blend. This blend is comprised of oils that have been studied for their abilities to help reduce muscle, joint, and bone pain and inflammation. Additionally, this moisturizing cream contains ingredients known to stimulate sensations of warmth and coolness to help soothe tissue soreness and stiffness.

Key Ingredients:

Wintergreen Essential Oil: contains 99% methyl salicylate, which gives it cortisone-like properties. It may be beneficial for arthritis, rheumatism, tendinitis, and any other discomfort that is related to the inflammation of bones, muscles, and joints.

Camphor Essential Oil: is analgesic (pain-relieving) and anti-inflammatory. It may be beneficial for arthritis, rheumatism, muscle aches and pains, sprains, and bruises.

Peppermint Essential Oil: is anti-inflammatory to the prostate and to damaged tissues. It has a soothing and cooling effect that may help with arthritis and rheumatism.

Blue Tansy Essential Oil: is analgesic and anti-inflammatory. It may also help with low blood pressure, arthritis, and rheumatism.

German Chamomile Essential Oil: is antioxidant, anti-inflammatory, and analgesic. It may also help relieve congestion and arthritis.

Helichrysum Essential Oil: may help cleanse the blood and improve circulatory functions. It is anticatarrhal in structure and nature. As a powerful anti-inflammatory, it may even help reduce inflammation in the meninges of the brain. On a spiritual level, it may help one let go of angry feelings that prevent one from forgiving and moving forward.

Osmanthus Essential Oil: comes from one of the 10 famous traditional flowers of China. The blossoms are highly aromatic and are used in the world's rarest and most expensive perfumes. It is used in Chinese medicine to "reduce phlegm and remove blood stasis."

Eucalyptus globulus **Essential Oil:** is anti-inflammatory and has pain-relieving properties. It is often used to help alleviate aches, pains, and skin infections.

Ylang Ylang: is often used to help calm and relax from exhaustion. It can help relieve anxious feelings, and soothe skin irritations.-

Menthol: is the main constituent of peppermint oil and is known for its ability to cool the body and skin.

Capsicum frutescens **Fruit Extract:** comes from a species of chili pepper. This extract causes a gentle warming sensation on the skin.

Companion Blend: Deep Blue.

Detoxifying Mud Mask

This natural earth mask combines the cleansing properties of copper, kaolin, and bentonite with skin-nourishing botanicals and natural essential oils that help purify, nourish, and soothe the skin.

Key Ingredients:

Juniper Berry Essential Oil: is beneficial for relieving acne and other skin issues. Juniper berry oil is also a cleanser and purifier and helps heal wounds. This oil may also help skin retain moisture.

Grapefruit Essential Oil: is balancing and uplifting to the mind. It is antiseptic, disinfectant, and astringent.

Myrrh Essential Oil: helps improve skin conditions, wounds, and wrinkles.

Natural Earth Clay: with kaolin and bentonite, contains essential trace minerals and helps to naturally purify and remove excess oils from the skin.

Butyrospermum parkii **(Shea) Butter:** is widely used in soaps, lotions, and creams for its natural moisturizing properties.

Lens esculenta **(Lentil) Seed Extract:** helps to minimize the appearance of pores by balancing skin sebum excretions, promoting healthy skin cells, and stimulating natural skin structure proteins (Boudier et al., 2010)

Malachite Extract: is extracted from natural malachite minerals to create a bioavailable copper complex. Copper is a natural disinfectant and helps stimulate production of the collagen and elastin fibers critical for skin structure and tone (Borkow, 2014).

Companion Formulations: Skin Care products.

Exfoliating Body Scrub

This natural body scrub combines exquisite vegetable oils that help nourish and soothe the skin with stimulating, uplifting essential oils.

Key Ingredients:

Orange Essential Oil: is often used to help aid complexion and combat the effects of dermatitis. Orange oil also contains high levels of d-limonene, which is often used for its ability to help enhance skin permeability of other key substances.

Grapefruit Essential Oil: is balancing and uplifting to the mind. It is antiseptic, disinfectant, and astringent.

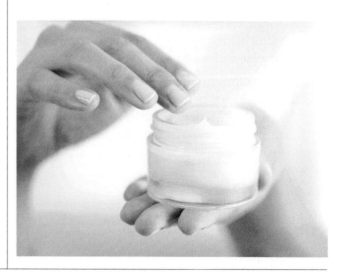

Ginger Essential Oil: has stimulating and warming properties on the skin.

Sweet Almond Oil: has natural moisturizing properties and is high in oleic and linoleic essential fatty acids, which can help soften and soothe the skin.

Sunflower Seed Oil: has natural moisturizing properties and is high in oleic and linoleic essential fatty acids, which can help soften and soothe the skin.

Macadamia Nut Oil: is high in the fatty acid palmitoleic acid. Palmitoleic acid is found naturally in breast milk and as part of the sebum of the skin. It helps moisturize the skin and may help protect the skin from bacterial infection (Wille et al., 2003). As the body ages, the percentage of palmitoleic acid in the sebum declines (Hayashi et al., 2003).

Kukui Nut Oil: is high in oleic and linoleic essential fatty acids, which can help soften and soothe the skin. Kukui nut oil was used in Hawaii for hundreds of years to help treat dry skin and other skin conditions.

Companion Formulations: Skin Care products, Refreshing Body Wash.

Facial Cleanser

This Facial Cleanser includes several ingredients that work to gently cleanse the face while leaving the skin feeling soft, smooth, and fresh.

Key Ingredients:

Melaleuca Essential Oil: promotes cleansing and purity.

Peppermint Essential Oil: is purifying and stimulating to the conscious mind.

Yucca Root Extract: Yucca root was used by Native Americans as a natural soap and cleanser. Yucca root has a high saponin content. Saponins are naturally occurring cleansers that are used as natural soaps and detergents. Yucca root also has antioxidant and anti-inflammatory properties (Cheeke et al., 2006) and was used anciently to help relieve joint pain and arthritis.

Soapbark Extract: Soapbark is a tree native to Chile that has a high content of the quillaia saponin.

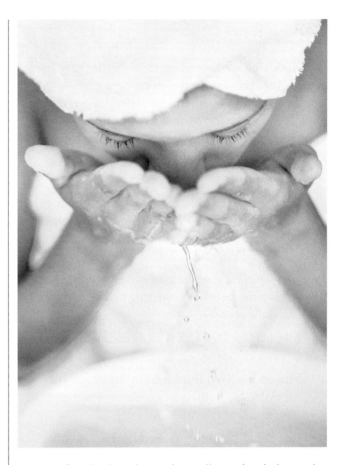

Soapbark is also traditionally used to help soothe skin sores.

Macadamia Seed Oil: has natural moisturizing properties and is high in oleic essential fatty acid, which can help soften and soothe the skin. It also contains unusually high levels of palmitoleic essential fatty acid, which is present in the skin's natural sebum and acts as a natural antibacterial agent (Wille et al., 2003).

Sodium PCA: is a sodium salt derived from a naturally occurring amino acid proline. It is a natural humectant and helps the skin retain its natural moisture levels for healthy, youthful-looking skin.

Tocopherol (Vitamin E): is a natural antioxidant and plays an important role in cellular communication in the body.

Companion Formulations: Hydrating Cream, Invigorating Scrub, Pore Reducing Toner, Skin Serum.

Personal Care & Spa

Hand & Body Lotion

This lotion blends several ingredients that have been studied for their unique moisturizing and skin-protecting abilities with natural, botanical ingredients. It should be formulated so that you can mix in your desired essential oil or blend to create your own custom lotion for many different uses.

Key Ingredients:

Sunflower Seed Oil: has natural moisturizing properties and is high in oleic and linoleic essential fatty acids, which can help soften and soothe the skin.

Coconut Oil: is often used in soaps, creams, and lotions for its moisturizing and skin-softening abilities.

Macadamia Seed Oil: is moisturizing, reparative, and cleansing.

Murumura Seed Butter: from Brazil and the Amazon basin, is an excellent moisturizer and natural emollient.

Cupuacu (Theobroma) Seed Butter: from the Amazon basin in South America, is a natural emollient and leaves a creamy feeling on the skin.

Inca Inchi Seed Oil: is high in the essential fatty acids linolenic acid and linoleic acid.

***Olea europaea* (Olive) Fruit Unsaponifiables:** contain many of the same natural compounds found in sebum—the substance secreted by the skin that helps provide protection and moisture retention for the skin's cells.

Jojoba Oil: Although called an oil, jojoba oil is actually a natural liquid wax extracted from jojoba (*Simmondsia chinensis*) plants found in the southwestern United States and northern Mexico. This liquid wax closely resembles the skin's natural oils (or sebum), allowing it to provide increased hydration to the skin.

***Bellis perennis* (Daisy) Flower Extract:** has astringent and anti-inflammatory properties.

Companion Formulations: Essential Skin Care.

HD Clear® Facial Lotion
Topical Facial Lotion

This clearing facial lotion will help to remove skin blemishes while providing lasting moisture for the skin. Using the power of essential oils, this lotion helps relieve acne and other skin blemishes.

Key Ingredients:

Melaleuca Essential Oil: has long been used to treat acne and other skin conditions because of its powerful antimicrobial properties. For example, in one study a gel with 5% melaleuca oil was found to be as effective at treating acne as a lotion with 5% benzoyl peroxide (a common chemical used to treat acne) (Bassett et al., 1990). Melaleuca oil has also been found to reduce skin swelling, oxidative stress, and speed skin recovery and healing (Brand et al., 2002; Caldefie-Chézet et al., 2006; Feinblatt et al., 1960).

Eucalyptus Essential Oil: can be used to relieve inflammation, acne, and skin infections. Eucalyptus is a powerful purifier and is known for its antibacterial, anti-infectious, and antiviral properties. It is used medicinally in France to treat candida and other fungal infections.

Geranium Essential Oil: has antibacterial and anti-inflammatory properties and is often used to help alleviate the effects of acne and eczema. It may also help balance sebum levels in the skin.

Ho Wood Essential Oil: is known for its antiseptic properties and is often used to help clear infections and to support the revitalization of skin issues.

Litsea Essential Oil: has antiseptic and astringent properties and has been used for oily skin and acne.

Vitamin B$_3$: plays a role in cellular metabolism. Deficiency in Vitamin B$_3$ can result in dermatitis, diarrhea, confusion, and dementia.

Amino Acids: are micronutrients that maintain the barrier function of the skin, nourish the skin, and support skin hydration. Topical application of micronutrients can assist the body's natural amino acids.

Black Cumin Seed Oil: has been used since ancient times for a myriad of health concerns. In addition to its antioxidant and anti-inflammatory properties, black cumin seed oil also has a high content of linoleic acid, an essential fatty acid used by the body to help maintain healthy skin and hair. Linoleic acid has been studied for its ability to reduce acne and to enhance cellular migration during wound healing.

Chaulmoogra Oil: has been used in traditional medicine to treat leprosy and other skin diseases. This oil's antibacterial properties make it beneficial for speeding wound recovery and clearing acne.

Magnolia: possesses antibacterial and anti-inflammatory effects, helping it protect against acne.

Manuka: has been found to help clear, firm, and moisturize the skin.

White Willow Bark: has been known to help prevent acne.

Companion Formulation and Blend: HD Clear Foaming Face Wash and HD Clear.

HD Clear® Foaming Face Wash

Topical Face Wash

HD Clear® Foaming Face Wash blends several ingredients that have been studied for their abilities to help clarify the skin and to create a hostile environment for detrimental skin bacteria.

Key Ingredients:

Ho Wood Essential Oil: is known for its antiseptic properties and is often used to help clear infections and to support the revitalization of skin issues.

Melaleuca Essential Oil: is one of the most studied antibacterial and antifungal oils. Melaleuca also has anti-inflammatory properties and can help support the skin in the recovery process after injuries.

Eucalyptus globulus **Essential Oil:** is often used for inflammation and skin infections and sores. It is used medicinally in France to treat candida and other fungal infections and has also demonstrated strong antibacterial properties.

Litsea Essential Oil: has antiseptic and astringent properties and has been used for oily skin and acne.

Geranium Essential Oil: has antibacterial and anti-inflammatory properties and is often used to help alleviate the effects of acne and eczema. It may also help balance sebum levels in the skin.

Lemongrass Essential Oil: is known for its antiseptic properties and is often used to help clear infections and to support the revitalization of skin tissue.

Black Cumin Seed Oil: has been used since ancient times for a myriad of health concerns. In addition to its antioxidant and anti-inflammatory properties, black cumin seed oil also has a high content of linoleic acid, an essential fatty acid used by the body to help maintain healthy skin and hair. Linoleic acid has been studied for its ability to reduce acne microcomedones (Letawe et al., 1998) and to enhance cellular migration during wound healing (Ruthig et al., 1999).

White Willow Bark Extract: has been used for centuries for its anti-inflammatory and analgesic properties. This natural extract has also been used topically as an aid for acne and acne lesions by promoting the shedding of dead skin cells from the skin's surface.

Glycyrrhiza inflata **Root Extract:** *Glycyrrhiza inflata* is a species of plant found in China that is closely related to the licorice plant. The root of this plant contains substances that have been studied for their antioxidant (Veratti et al., 2001) and anti-inflammatory (Shetty et al., 2011; Ishida et al., 2012) properties as well as for their ability to help reduce dermatitis (Saeedi et al., 2003) and to balance sebum production in the skin (Kambara et al., 2003).

Candida bombicola **Ferment:** *Candida bombicola* is a harmless yeast that has the ability to produce natural, biodegradeable biosurfactants (natural substances that act as detergents to cleanse oils and sebum from the skin) (Saerens et al., 2011).

Vitamin A: plays a critical role in the creation and growth of normal skin cells in the epidermis.

Companion Formulation and Blend: HD Clear, HD Clear Facial Lotion.

Healthy Hold Glaze

Hair Glaze

Healthy Hold Glaze combines several ingredients that have been studied for their abilities to provide a heat-activated flexible hold for hair without chemical build up, while helping to protect and strengthen the hair on the molecular level.

Key Ingredients:

Lavender Essential Oil: helps nourish the scalp and hair follicles. Medicinally, it has been used by the French to prevent hair loss.

Peppermint Essential Oil: is invigorating and helps improve the overall health of the scalp and hair.

Marjoram Essential Oil: has antiseptic properties and helps soothe the skin and muscles.

Cedarwood Essential Oil: is purifying and has properties beneficial to healthy scalp and hair growth.

Lavandin Essential Oil: has antifungal and anti-inflammatory properties and can help soothe itching and other skin discomforts.

Rosemary Essential Oil: has antioxidant properties and has shown potential for helping to alleviate dandruff and promote healthy hair growth.

Niaouli (*Melaleuca quinquenervia*) Essential Oil: has powerful antifungal and anti-inflammatory properties and may help protect against UV damage.

Eucalyptus (*E. globulus*) Essential Oil: has antiseptic and anti-inflammatory properties. It is stimulating to the tissues and helps purify.

Tangerine Essential Oil: is anti-inflammatory and has a soothing citrus aroma.

Companion Formulations: Smoothing Conditioner, Protecting Shampoo, Root to Tip Serum.

Hydrating Body Mist with Beautiful

This hydrating mist contains essential oils known to soothe and balance the skin's natural moisture levels. Additional probiotic extracts help speed the skin's replenishment process and the shedding of dead skin cells for a fuller, more youthful appearance.

Key Ingredients:

Lime Essential Oil: is often used to help revitalize skin, since it may help remove dead skin cells and tighten skin and other connective tissues. Limonene (found in lime) has been studied for its ability to promote healthy looking skin and to reduce the appearance of blemishes.

Osmanthus Essential Oil: comes from one of the 10 famous traditional flowers of China. The aromatic blossoms are used in the world's rarest and mostexpensive perfumes. The warm, floral aroma aids concentration and focus during meditation, helping to relieve stress and declutter the mind.

Bergamot Essential Oil: has a bright, uplifting aroma and can help purify the skin. It also contains limonene, which has been studied for its ability to help improve the appearance of skin.

Frankincense Essential Oil: has been studied for its anti-inflammatory and anti-infectious properties. Frankincense is also generally soothing to the skin and nerves.

Coconut Oil: is often used in soaps, creams, and lotions for its moisturizing and skin-softening properties.

Sunflower Seed Oil: has natural moisturizing properties and is high in oleic and linoleic essential fatty acids, which can help soften and soothe skin.

Passion Fruit Seed Oil: has antioxidant properties and is high in linoleic and oleic essential fatty acids.

Avocado Oil: is a unique oil high in natural proteins and vitamins A and D. It is often used in formulations to help soothe and moisturize dry or irritated skin.

Companion Formulations: Hydrating Cream, Invigorating Scrub, Facial Cleanser, Pore Reducing Toner, Skin Serum.

Hydrating Cream

Hydrating Cream combines essential oils known for their abilities to soothe and balance the skin's natural moisture levels with probiotic extracts that help speed the skin's replenishment process and the shedding of dead skin cells, giving it a more youthful, full appearance.

Key Ingredients:

Lavender Essential Oil: has been studied for its ability to reduce inflammation and allergic reactions in the skin. It has also been used to help the skin recover from burns, blisters, infections, and other injuries and to help reduce conditions related to dry skin.

Geranium Essential Oil: is soothing to the skin and may help to balance the skin's level of sebum (a fatty, waxy substance secreted by the skin that helps the skin feel moist and supple).

Frankincense Essential Oil: has been studied for its anti-inflammatory and anti-infectious properties. Frankincense is also soothing to the skin and nerves.

Jasmine Essential Oil: is often used to help soothe dry, irritated, or sensitive skin.

Lactococcus Ferment Lysate: is a solution taken from the probiotic organism *Lactococcus lactis*. This probiotic has been studied for its ability to inhibit harmful pathogens (Shuichi et al., 2015). It may also be beneficial for speeding the skin rejuvenation process and the natural shedding of dead skin cells to give the skin a more youthful appearance.

Laminaria digitata **Extract:** is rich in vitamins, amino acids, and other beneficial nutrients to help soothe and protect the skin. It is often used for its moisturizing properties.

Mugwort Extract: has been studied for its anti-inflammatory properties (Li et al., 2016), and is traditionally used to help relieve itching and irritation of the skin.

Theobroma cacao **(Cocoa) Seed Butter:** is extracted from dried cocoa beans and is widely used for its ability to help moisturize the skin.

Companion Formulations: Hydrating Body Mist with Beautiful, Invigorating Scrub, Facial Cleanser, Pore Reducing Toner, Skin Serum.

Invigorating Scrub

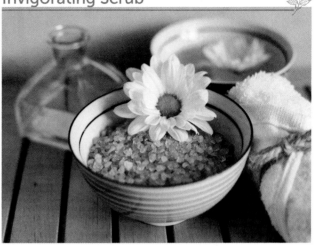

Invigorating Scrub combines fragrant and nourishing essential oils, botanical extracts, and other natural ingredients known for their ability to polish skin with naturally exfoliating jojoba wax beads.

Key Ingredients:

Grapefruit Essential Oil: is balancing and uplifting to the mind. It is antiseptic, disinfectant, and astringent.

Peppermint Essential Oil: is cooling and stimulating. It is antibacterial and invigorating.

Jojoba Beads (Hydrogenated Jojoba Oil): Although called an oil, jojoba oil is actually a natural liquid wax extracted from jojoba (*Simmondsia chinensis*) plants found in the southwestern Unites States and northern Mexico. This liquid wax closely resembles the skin's natural oils (or sebum). Hydrogenating jojoba oil (by combining this liquid wax with pressurized hydrogen) solidifies the oil, allowing the creation of a waxy bead that can be used to gently and naturally exfoliate the skin.

Mandarin Orange Extract: Mandarin orange contains a natural flavone called tangeretin. Tangeretin has been studied for its anti-inflammatory (Rodriguez et al., 2002) and antihistamine (Jang et al., 2013) properties and for its ability to reduce skin pigmentation (Yoshizaki et al., 2017).

Jasmine Flower and Leaf Extract: Jasmine is used traditionally for its anti-inflammatory and antiseptic properties. An extract from jasmine leaves has demonstrated an ability to enhance collagen synthesis in the skin, as well as an antioxidant property (Chaturvedi et al., 2013).

Greater Burdock Root Extract: Greater burdock has long been used in traditional medicine for many different conditions. It has been recently studied for its ability to promote circulation in the skin (Chan et al., 2011) and to promote quicker skin structure formation, which could help with tighter, younger-looking skin (Knott et al., 2008).

Companion Formulations: Facial Cleanser, Hydrating Cream, Pore Reducing Toner, Skin Serum.

Lip Balm

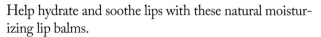

Help hydrate and soothe lips with these natural moisturizing lip balms.

Key Ingredients:

Original Blend:

> **Orange Essential Oil:** is often used to help aid complexion and combat the effects of dermatitis.
>
> **Peppermint Essential Oil:** is cooling and stimulating. It is antibacterial and invigorating to the skin.

Tropical Blend:

> **Lime Essential Oil:** has a fresh, lively fragrance that is stimulating and refreshing.
>
> **Clementine Essential Oil:** is anti-inflammatory and has a soothing citrus aroma.
>
> **Ylang Ylang Essential Oil:** is calming and relaxing to the mind and body. It brings a feeling of self-love, confidence, joy, and peace.

Herbal Blend:

> **Spearmint Essential Oil:** has an uplifting, balancing aroma, as well as antiseptic properties.
>
> **Marjoram Essential Oil:** has antiseptic properties and helps soothe the skin and muscles.
>
> **Lemon Verbena Essential Oil:** is disinfecting and uplifting. It is often used to help soften skin.

Coconut Oil: is often used in soaps, creams, and lotions for its moisturizing and skin-softening abilities.

Moringa Oil: is also known as ben oil for its high levels of behenic acid. Behenic acid is a component of the skin's natural sebum (Raghallaigh et al., 2012) and helps gives a moist, smooth feel to the lips.

Kukui Nut Oil: is high in oleic and linoleic essential fatty acids, which can help soften and soothe the skin. Kukui nut oil was used in Hawaii for hundreds of years to help treat dry skin and other skin conditions.

Companion Formulations: Essential Skin Care.

Moisturizing Bath Bar

This unique soap combines the moisturizing abilities of palm, coconut, and jojoba oils with aloe leaf juice and the stimulating aroma of bergamot and grapefruit essential oils.

Key Ingredients:

Bergamot Essential Oil: has a bright, uplifting aroma and can help purify the skin.

Grapefruit Essential Oil: is balancing and uplifting to the mind. It is antiseptic, disinfectant, and astringent.

Sodium Cocoate (Saponified Coconut Oil): is the soap form of coconut oil (saponification is the process of transforming oils into soap). Coconut oil is often used in soaps, creams, and lotions for its moisturizing and skin-softening abilities.

Vegetable Glycerin: is a natural moisturizer and humectant—helping skin and hair retain moisture by forming a protective barrier.

Jojoba Oil: Although called an oil, jojoba oil is actually a natural liquid wax extracted from jojoba (*Simmondsia chinensis*) plants found in the southwestern United States and northern Mexico. This liquid wax closely resembles the skin's natural oils (or sebum).

Aloe Leaf Juice: has been used for thousands of years for its ability to help soften, soothe, and moisturize skin.

Companion Formulations: Essential Skin Care.

Natural Deodorant

This natural deodorant combines the natural deodorizing and antibacterial properties of cypress, melaleuca, bergamot, and cedarwood essential oils in a base of beeswax, coconut oil, shea butter, and cornstarch.

Key Ingredients:

Beeswax: is a natural wax that is often used to add structure and firmness and helps provide a barrier from moisture.

Coconut Oil: is often used in soaps, creams, and lotions for its moisturizing and skin-softening abilities.

Shea Butter: is widely known as a powerful moisturizer. Shea butter has been used to heal skin conditions and reduce wrinkles. Shea butter mimics the body's natural moisturizers and is, therefore, extremely effective at treating dry skin, sunburns, wounds, skin cracks, stretch marks, and burns.

Cypress Essential Oil: has been studied for its antibacterial properties and helps revitalize the skin.

Melaleuca Essential Oil: is commonly used for its antibacterial and antifungal properties and helps soothe the skin from rashes and irritations.

Bergamot Essential Oil: has a bright, uplifting aroma and can help purify the skin.

Cedarwood Essential Oil: has strong antiseptic properties and may also help reduce inflammation and oily secretions from the skin.

On Guard® Cleaner Concentrate
Protective Cleaner

This natural cleaner combines the protective benefits of On Guard with plant-based ingredients to create a tough, yet safe and non-toxic, multi-purpose household cleaner.

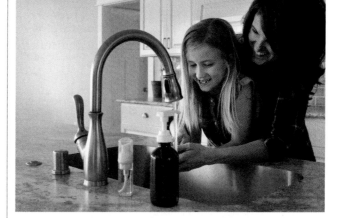

Key Ingredients:

On Guard: contains orange, clove bud, cinnamon bark, *Eucalyptus radiata*, and rosemary essential oils. These oils have all been studied for their powerful antimicrobial and antiseptic properties.

Companion Supplements, Blends, and Formulations: On Guard Foaming Hand Wash, On Guard Protecting Throat Drops, On Guard Laundry Detergent, On Guard.

On Guard® Foaming Hand Wash
Protective Hand Wash

On Guard Foaming Hand Wash combines several essential oils into a healthy, all-natural hand soap that is gentle enough for even those with sensitive skin to use. It leaves hands feeling clean, soft, and fresh while it protects against harmful microorganisms.

Key Ingredients:

Sweet Orange Essential Oil: is calming and uplifting to the mind and body.

Clove Bud Essential Oil: is antibacterial, antiviral, and disinfectant.

Cinnamon Bark Essential Oil: is antibacterial and antimicrobial. It also enhances the action and activity of other oils.

Rosemary Oil: is antibacterial, stimulates memory, and opens the conscious mind.

Companion Formulations, Blends, and Supplements: On Guard Protecting Throat Drops, On Guard Natural Whitening Toothpaste, On Guard.

On Guard® Laundry Detergent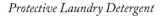

Protective Laundry Detergent

This detergent combines the natural antiseptic properties of the oils contained in On Guard with naturally based surfactants, enzymes, and stabilizers.

Key Ingredients:

On Guard: contains orange, clove bud, cinnamon bark, *Eucalyptus radiata*, and rosemary essential oils. These oils have all been studied for their powerful antimicrobial and antiseptic properties.

Naturally Sourced Enzymes: including protease (breaks down proteins), amylase (breaks down starches), cellulase (helps prevent natural fiber materials from balling), mannase (breaks down organic stains), and lipase (breaks down fat and oil stains).

Natural Surfactants

Natural Corn-Based Enzyme Stabilizer

Companion Formulations, Blends, and Supplements: On Guard Foaming Hand Wash, On Guard Protecting Throat Drops, On Guard Cleaner Concentrate, On Guard.

On Guard® Mouthwash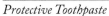

Protective Mouthwash

This natural mouthwash formulation offers the protective benefits of On Guard enhanced with peppermint, wintergreen, and myrrh essential oils.

Key Ingredients:

On Guard: contains orange, clove bud, cinnamon bark, *Eucalyptus radiata*, and rosemary essential oils. These oils have been studied for their powerful antimicrobial and antiseptic properties. Some of are also often used to help alleviate inflammation and ease gum and tooth pain.

Wintergreen Essential Oil: has analgesic (pain relieving) and disinfectant properties, and it may help with inflammation.

Myrrh Essential Oil: has antiseptic properties and is often used to help support healthy gum and mouth tissue.

Peppermint Essential Oil: contains high levels of menthol, which has been well documented in research studies for its ability to inhibit bacteria known to cause dental cavities.

Miswak Extract: Miswak (Salvadora persica) is a tree native to the Middle East and Africa. Its fibrous branches have been used for centuries as a natural toothbrush, and extracts from the wood have been found to help reduce plaque and cavities, and to improve gum health (Ezoddini-ardakani, 2010; Khalessi et al., 2004; Poureslami et al., 2007; Amoian et al., 2010).

Monk Fruit Extract: Monk fruit is a small fruit from China that contains a natural low-calorie sweetener said to be hundreds of times sweeter than sugar (sucrose).

Natural Xylitol: is a sweetener that, unlike most others, is beneficial for dental health. Xylitol has been found to help reduce cavities and remineralize tooth enamel.

Companion Formulations, Supplements, and Blends: On Guard Foaming Hand Wash, On Guard Protecting Throat Drops, On Guard Toothpaste, On Guard.

On Guard® Natural Whitening Toothpaste

Protective Toothpaste

This natural toothpaste formulation offers the protective benefits of On Guard along with peppermint, wintergreen, and myrrh essential oils.

Key Ingredients:

On Guard: contains orange, clove bud, cinnamon bark, *Eucalyptus radiata*, and rosemary essential oils. These oils have all been studied for their powerful antimicrobial and antiseptic properties. Several of these oils are also often used to help alleviate inflammation and ease gum and tooth pain.

Myrrh Essential Oil: has antiseptic properties and is often used to help support healthy gums and mouth tissues.

Peppermint Essential Oil: contains high levels of menthol, which has been well documented in research studies for its ability to inhibit bacteria known to cause dental cavities.

Calcium Hydroxyapatite: Hydroxyapatite is the main component of the hard crystal structure that makes up tooth enamel. While naturally strong, tooth enamel can be demineralized by conditions of acidity in the mouth (caused by eating sugar or acidic foods), weakening the enamel and allowing for small lesions and gaps to be created. There is some evidence that use of a polishing agent containing calcium hydroxyapatite can help restore tooth enamel from small lesions in vitro (Nishio et al., 2004).

Natural Xylitol: is a sweetener that, unlike most sweeteners, is beneficial for dental health. Xylitol has been found to reduce cavities and remineralize enamel.

Hydrated Silica: helps remove plaque.

Companion Formulations, Supplements, and Blend: On Guard Foaming Hand Wash, On Guard Protecting Throat Drops, On Guard Mouthwash, On Guard.

Pore Reducing Toner

Skin Toner

This toner includes ingredients that have been studied for their abilities to help reduce the visible size of pores while eliminating skin irritation and stress.

Key Ingredients:

Lavender Essential Oil: is calming and promotes a sense of well-being.

Ylang Ylang Essential Oil: is calming and relaxing and may help alleviate anger.

German Chamomile Essential Oil: soothes and clears the mind, creating an atmosphere of peace and patience.

Aloe Leaf Juice: has been used for thousands of years for its ability to help soften, soothe, and moisturize skin.

Watermelon Fruit Extract: is a synergistic blend of vitamins, carbohydrates, and amino acids (such as citrulline) extracted from the watermelon plant. Originating from harsh, hot climates with high amounts of sunlight, the watermelon plant developed natural protections from heat and UV radiation in order to survive.

This extract has antioxidant properties that help protect the DNA of skin cells from free radicals and the redness caused by UV radiation.

Apple Fruit Extract: is often used to help condition the skin and as a natural exfoliant that helps maintain even skin tone and texture.

Lentil Seed and Fruit Extracts: In the epidermis, the cells visible on the surface of the skin are actually converted keratinocyte cells that have lost their nucleus and have become filled with the rigid skin-barrier protein keratin. This conversion (called keratinization) is essential for creating a healthy skin barrier that helps keep moisture within the skin and that helps keep harmful microorganisms and toxins from entering the body through the skin. Occasionally, however, these keratinocyte cells do not completely convert, retaining their nuclei and not completely filling with keratin. This condition is called parakeratosis and can lead to several dermatological problems, such as psoriasis, if it happens too often (Scheinfeld et al., 2005).

Recent studies on the cosmetic concern of large, visible facial skin pores have found evidence that incomplete keratinization (or parakeratosis) is significantly more evident on individuals with larger pore sizes than on individuals with smaller pores.

The oligosaccharides found in lentil extracts are believed to help promote complete keratinization, as well as reduce excessive sebum production and promote collagen production in the skin. These 3 actions can help to reduce pore size and visibility.

Witch Hazel: has natural astringent properties that help remove excess oils and

Companion Formulations: Facial Cleanser, Hydrating Cream, Invigorating Scrub, Skin Serum.

Protecting Shampoo

Protecting Shampoo blends ingredients that have been studied for their abilities to cleanse and protect hair, especially hair that has been chemically treated or heat styled. This shampoo combines the benefits of essential oils with natural sugar beet derivatives and oat peptides

to naturally protect, repair, and condition damaged hair—and to protect hair against future damage.

Key Ingredients:

Sugar Beet Derivative (Betaine): Betaine is a natural molecule found in human skin cells, in hair, and in many other places in the plant and animal kingdom. Betaine has been found to be involved in the skin's natural protective response to UV light (Warskulat et al., 2004, 2008) and has been found to have antioxidant properties (Ganesan et al., 2010). Treatment with betaine has also demonstrated an ability to improve the tensile strength of chemically damaged hair (Woodruff, 2002).

Oat Peptides: link together to form a protective coat that can help the hair and scalp retain moisture and protect the hair from future heat and chemical damage.

Emulsion of Silica: protects hair from chemical treatments and styling damage by deeply conditioning and smoothing the cuticle.

Orange Essential Oil: is calming and uplifting to the mind and body and has a pleasant, citrusy, sweet aroma. Orange oils are well-known for their abilities to degrease and degum, making them especially effective for cleansing the hair.

Lime Essential Oil: has a fresh, lively fragrance that is stimulating and refreshing. It can be used to cleanse the hair.

Companion Formulations: Smoothing Conditioner, Healthy Hold Glaze, Root to Tip Serum.

Refreshing Body Wash

This natural body wash contains several ingredients that work to gently cleanse the skin while leaving it feeling soft, smooth, and refreshed.

Key Ingredients:

Grapefruit Essential Oil: is balancing and uplifting to the mind. It is antiseptic, disinfectant, and astringent.

Bergamot Essential Oil: has a bright, uplifting aroma and can help purify the skin.

Cedarwood Essential Oil: has strong antiseptic properties and may also help reduce inflammation and oily secretions from the skin.

Sodium Methyl Oleoyl Taurate: is a mild surfactant derived naturally from coconut oil. This mild surfactant helps break down the oils that hold dirt and grime on the skin.

Companion Formulations: Skin Care products.

Replenishing Body Butter

This body butter combines natural ingredients that help to moisturize and soothe trouble areas of the skin that take the most abuse, such as the elbows, feet, and hands.

Key Ingredients:

Orange Essential Oil: is often used to help aid complexion and combat the effects of dermatitis. Orange oil also contains high levels of d-limonene, which is often used for its ability to help enhance skin permeability of other key substances.

Douglas Fir Essential Oil: has antiseptic and sedative properties. Its beautiful aroma can help promote a sense of focus and stimulate the mind.

Frankincense Essential Oil: helps to focus energy and improve concentration and may help reduce signs of aging. It also prevents scarring, supports the immune system, and speeds the healing of wounds.

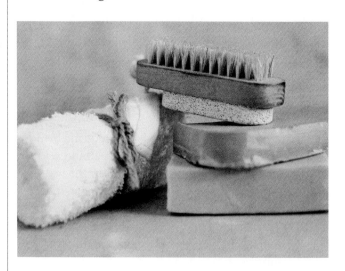

Shea Butter: is widely known as a powerful moisturizer. Shea butter has been used to heal skin conditions and reduce wrinkles. Shea butter mimics the body's natural moisturizers and is therefore extremely affective at treating dry skin, sunburns, wounds, skin cracks, stretch marks, and burns.

Avocado Oil: is a unique oil high in natural proteins and vitamins A and D. It is often used in formulations to help soothe and moisturize dry or irritated skin.

Cocoa Seed Butter: is extracted from dried cocoa beans and is widely used for its ability to help moisturize the skin.

Jojoba Oil: Although called an oil, jojoba oil is actually a natural liquid wax extracted from jojoba (*Simmondsia chinensis*) plants found in the southwestern United States and northern Mexico. This liquid wax closely resembles the skin's natural oils (or sebum).

Companion Formulations: Skin Care products.

Reveal Facial System

Two-Part Facial System

The Reveal Facial System consists of a two-part spa-grade facial care system that combines ingredients that have been studied for their abilities to help exfoliate and polish the skin and then deliver protein-building peptides to help maintain fuller, more radiant skin.

Key Ingredients:

Pumpkin Fruit Enzyme: Pumpkin fruits contain a high level of protease enzymes (enzymes that break down proteins) in order to break down the pumpkin fruit and provide nourishment for new seeds once the seeds have matured. These pumpkin-based enzymes have shown an ability in limited human studies to help break down proteins in dead skin cells without the irritation often associated with other types of enzymes or acid-based exfoliants.

Acetyl Hexapeptide-8: In vitro studies and limited clinical trials have demonstrated evidence that acetyl hexapeptide-8 has the ability to inhibit neurotransmitters involved in muscle contractions responsible for fine lines around the eyes and forehead associated with facial expressions and, therefore, may reduce the appearance of fine lines and wrinkles in these areas (Blanes-Mira et al., 2002).

Ceramide 2: Ceramides comprise a major part of the stratum corneum—a barrier found in the outer layer of the epidermis that is responsible for retaining moisture and protecting lower layers of cells within the skin. Low levels of ceramides have been associated with skin problems such as atopic dermatitis due to a breakdown or thinning of the stratum corneum (Imokawa, 2009). Topical application of ceramides such as ceramide 2 has shown potential in research studies to help increase ceramide levels in the skin and improve skin barrier function (Philippe et al., 1995).

Palmitoyl Oligopeptide and Palmitoyl Tripeptide-38 (Matrikine Messaging): The space in between skin (and other tissue) cells is filled with water and a mixture of fibrous proteins and polysaccharides called the extracellular matrix. These proteins and polysaccharides help give skin tissue its strength and elasticity and provide a framework for new cell growth and migration. Examples of extracellular proteins commonly found in skin tissue include collagen (provides strength, volume, and rigidity) and elastin (provides flexibility and resilience).

Enzymes on the outside of the cell membranes have the ability to break down some of these extracellular proteins into smaller peptide units when activated. Some of these smaller peptide units, in turn, have the ability to send further signals to surrounding cells to start, or turn off, the creation of new proteins and other structures. These small peptide messengers are called matrikines (Maquart et al., 1999).

Studies have shown that certain matrikines, such as the tripeptide glycyl-histidyl-lysine (GHK), have the ability to activate and regulate synthesis of extracellular matrix proteins (Maquart et al., 1999); others can help stimulate the creation of an extracellular matrix framework that facilitates new cell growth and the healing of skin wounds (Siméon et al., 1999; Tran et al., 2004).

With aging, extracellular proteins and fibers begin to break down, and synthesis of new structures is limited. Because of this loss of proteins and other structures in the extracellu-

Personal Care & Spa

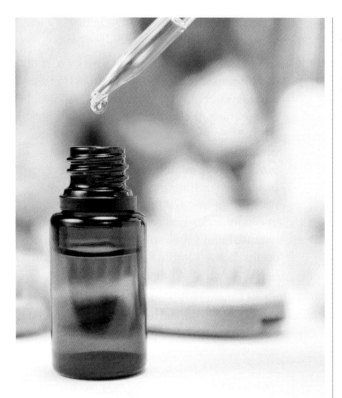

lar matrix, the skin begins to lose its rigidity, structure, resilience, and elasticity, resulting in the appearance of fine lines and wrinkles.

In vitro studies and limited clinical trials have demonstrated evidence that palmitoylated matrikines may have the ability to activate synthesis of extracellular matrix structures, such as collagen, fibronectin, and hyaluronic acid, that can lead to a fuller, tighter skin structure and can reduce the appearance of fine lines and wrinkles.

Orange Essential Oil: Orange oil is often used to help aid complexion and to help combat the effects of dermatitis. Orange oil also contains high levels of d-limonene, which is often used for its ability to help enhance skin permeability of other key substances.

Lime Essential Oil: Lime oil is often used to help revitalize skin, as it may be beneficial in helping to remove dead skin cells and helping to tighten skin and connective tissues.

Companion Formulations: Facial Cleanser, Hydrating Cream, Invigorating Scrub, Skin Serum.

Root to Tip Serum
Hair Serum

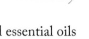

Root to Tip Serum combines beneficial essential oils with Moroccan argan oil to nourish, protect, moisturize, and revitalize the hair and scalp.

Key Ingredients:

Argan (*Argania spinosa*) Oil: is pressed from the kernels of the Moroccan argan tree. This light oil has an extremely high antioxidant capacity (Cabrera-Vique et al., 2012), with high levels of the antioxidant γ-tocopherol (vitamin E) (Charrouf et al., 2010) and the essential fatty acids linoleic acid and oleic acid (Khallouki et al., 2003). Argan oil also contains squalene (Monfalouti et al., 2010)—a substance produced naturally by the skin cells to help keep skin and hair moisturized and protected—and is rich in polyphenols and coenzyme Q_{10} (CoQ_{10}) (Venegas et al., 2011).

Lavender Essential Oil: helps nourish the scalp and hair follicles. Medicinally, it has been used by the French to prevent hair loss.

Peppermint Essential Oil: is invigorating and helps improve the overall health of the scalp and hair.

Marjoram Essential Oil: has antiseptic properties and helps soothe the skin and muscles.

Cedarwood Essential Oil: is purifying and has properties beneficial to healthy scalp and hair growth.

Lavandin Essential Oil: has antifungal and anti-inflammatory properties and can help soothe itching and other skin discomforts.

Rosemary Essential Oil: has antioxidant properties and has shown potential for helping to alleviate dandruff and promote healthy hair growth.

Niaouli (*Melaleuca quinquenervia*) Essential Oil: has powerful antifungal and anti-inflammatory properties and may help protect against UV damage.

Eucalyptus (*E. globulus*) Essential Oil: has antiseptic and anti-inflammatory properties. It is stimulating to the tissues and helps purify.

Companion Formulations: Smoothing Conditioner, Protecting Shampoo, Healthy Hold Glaze.

Rose Hand Lotion

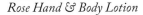

Rose Hand & Body Lotion

This lotion offers the same natural benefits of the regular Hand & Body Lotion, plus the added benefits of rose essential oil.

Key Ingredients:

Rose Essential Oil: can be used to prevent scarring; its healing properties have been used for ages. This oil can be used to help ease symptoms of aging, including wrinkles.

see Hand & Body Lotion for other suggested ingredients and research.

Serenity Bath Bar

Calming/Restful Bar

This soothing soap combines the skin protecting abilities of sunflower, safflower, palm, coconut, and jojoba oils with the moisturizing properties of shea butter and the calming aroma of Serenity.

Key Ingredients:

Serenity Essential Oil Blend: combines essential oils that are widely known—and have been studied—for their abilities to calm and soothe

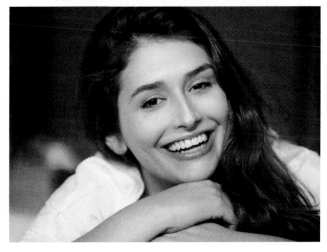

feelings of stress and anxiety in order to help the body maintain its natural state of health. This blend contains lavender, cedarwood, ho wood, ylang ylang, sweet marjoram, Roman chamomile, vanilla bean, vetiver, and sandalwood oils.

Sodium Cocoate (Saponified Coconut Oil): is the soap form of coconut oil (saponification is the process of transforming oils into soap). Coconut oil is often used in soaps, creams, and lotions for its moisturizing and skin-softening abilities.

Jojoba Oil: Although called an oil, jojoba oil is actually a natural liquid wax extracted from jojoba (*Simmondsia chinensis*) plants found in the southwestern Unites States and northern Mexico. This liquid wax closely resembles the skin's natural oils (or sebum).

Aloe Leaf Juice: has been used for thousands of years for its ability to help soften, soothe, and moisturize skin.

Companion Formulations: Skin Care products.

Smoothing Conditioner

This conditioner combines several ingredients known for their ability to help restore luminosity, shine, fullness, and overall health to hair. This formulation is designed to help smooth the outside layer of the hair strands, reducing mechanical damage caused by friction. This conditioner combines the benefits of essential oils with natural botanical extracts to naturally condition and repair damaged hair and to protect hair against future damage.

Key Ingredients:

Botanical Extracts: from Peruvian bark, yarrow, coltsfoot, barley, sandalwood, and other plants help smooth and protect the hair from heat, chemicals, and mechanical damage.

Lavender Essential Oil: helps nourish the scalp and hair follicles. Medicinally, it has been used by the French to prevent hair loss.

Peppermint Essential Oil: is invigorating and helps improve the overall health of the scalp and hair.

Marjoram Essential Oil: has antiseptic properties and helps soothe the skin and muscles.

Cedarwood Essential Oil: is purifying and has properties beneficial to healthy scalp and hair growth.

Lavandin Essential Oil: has antifungal and anti-inflammatory properties and can help soothe itching and other skin discomforts.

Rosemary Essential Oil: has antioxidant properties and has shown potential for helping alleviate dandruff and promoting healthy hair growth.

Niaouli (*Melaleuca quinquenervia*) Essential Oil: has powerful antifungal and anti-inflammatory properties and may help protect against UV damage.

Eucalyptus (*E. globulus*) Essential Oil: has antiseptic and anti-inflammatory properties. It is stimulating to the tissues and helps purify.

Companion Formulations: Protecting Shampoo, Healthy Hold Glaze, Root to Tip Serum.

Tightening Serum

Skin Tightening Serum

Tightening Serum combines ingredients that have been studied for their abilities to hydrate and tighten the skin in order to reduce the appearance of fine lines and wrinkles.

Key Ingredients:

Frankincense Essential Oil: helps to focus energy and improve concentration and may help reduce signs of aging.

Sandalwood Essential Oil: supports the cardiovascular system and may assist in skin regeneration.

Myrrh Essential Oil: helps improve skin conditions, wounds, and wrinkles.

***Acacia senegal* and Hydrolyzed Rhizobian Gums (Rhizobian & Acacia Gum Extracts):** As the skin ages, skin tissue structures such as collagen, elastin, and hyaluronic acid begin to break down or aren't synthesized by cells as quickly as before. The loss and breakage of these structural molecules in the skin tissue result in sagging, wrinkling, and less rigid skin (Ghersetich et al., 1994).

The two gum extracts consist of long polysaccharide molecules that have the ability to bind together to form a linked network of molecules. As this formulation dries, this linked network of molecules contracts, physically pulling the skin tighter to help reduce wrinkling and fine lines.

Perfluorodecalin (Proprietary Perfluorocarbon): As the skin ages, it can lose its ability to retain moisture, leading to less firm skin and increasing the visibility of fine lines and wrinkles.

Perfluorodecalin is a fluorocarbon molecule that has been studied for decades for its amazing oxygen-carrying properties and its potential to help heal wounds. When used in a cosmetic formulation during a small clinical trial, perfluorodecalin was shown to enhance the barrier function of the skin, allowing it to retain moisture and bringing about a visible reduction in fine lines and wrinkles (Stanzl et al., 1996).

***Fagus sylvatica* Bud Extract (Beech Tree Bud Extract):** As the skin ages, skin tissue structures such as collagen begin to break down or aren't synthesized by cells as quickly as before. The loss and breakage of these structural molecules in the skin tissue result in sagging, wrinkling, and less rigid skin (Ghersetich et al., 1994).

This unique beech tree bud extract contains hydroxyproline, an important component of collagen that helps it retain its unique structure and stability. This extract also contains flavonoids that help the skin retain moisture and tightness.

Betaine: Betaine is a naturally occurring substance that acts as a natural humectant to help the skin retain moisture, giving it a fuller, tighter appearance. It also can help soothe the skin, protecting it from irritation from chemicals and other irritants.

Betaine has also been studied for its abilities to help protect against heart disease and liver damage (Alfthan et al., 2004; Barak et al., 1997).

Companion Formulations: Facial Cleanser, Hydrating Cream, Invigorating Scrub, Pore Reducing Toner.

Veráge™ Cleanser

Youthful Skin Cleanser

This natural gel cleanser will reduce the appearance of skin aging by hydrating, nourishing, and smoothing the skin. To help produce a glowing youthful complexion, use this cleanser to remove makeup and dirt, deeply clean pores, and energize skin.

Key Ingredients:

Orange Essential Oil: is uplifting and invigorating and is known for its cleansing and purifying properties.

Basil Essential Oil: is cleansing and purifying. Basil oil has demonstrated strong inhibition of several multi-drug resistant bacteria (Opalchenova et al., 2003). This oil also exhibits antioxidant, anti-inflammatory, and energizing activity.

Melaleuca Essential Oil: has long been used to treat acne and other skin conditions because of its powerful antimicrobial properties. For example, in one study a gel with 5% melaleuca oil was found to be as effective at treating acne as a lotion with 5% benzoyl peroxide (a common chemical used to treat acne) (Bassett et al., 1990). Melaleuca oil has also been found to reduce skin swelling, oxidative stress, and speed skin recovery and healing (Brand et al., 2002; Caldefie-Chézet et al., 2006; Feinblatt et al., 1960).

Amino Acids and Lipids: are micronutrients that maintain the barrier function of the skin, nourish the skin, and support skin hydration. Topical application of micronutrients can assist the body's natural amino acids and lipids. Poor levels of micronutrients is associated with unhealthy looking skin.

Coconut Oil: is often used in soaps, creams, and lotions for its moisturizing and skin-softening abilities.

Olive Oil: hydrates the skin and increases skin flexibility. Olive oil also displays antioxidant properties (Budiyanto et al., 2000).

Companion Formulations and Blend: Immortelle, Veráge Immortelle Hydrating Serum, Veráge Moisturizer, Veráge Toner.

Veráge™ Immortelle Hydrating Serum

Youthful Hydrating Serum

This anti-aging hydrating serum combines the action of the Immortelle with other natural ingredients to reduce the appearance of skin aging. By emulating the natural micronutrients of the skin this serum renews the youthful properties associated with healthy skin, such as firmness, elasticity, and hydration.

Key Ingredients:

Frankincense Essential Oil: helps to focus energy and improve concentration and may help reduce signs of aging. It also prevents scarring, supports the immune system, and speeds the healing of wounds.

Hawaiian Sandalwood Essential Oil: helps to relive dry skin and hair, clear up acne, and support skin regeneration.

Lavender Essential Oil: has been studied for its ability to reduce inflammation and allergic reactions in the skin. It has also been used to help the skin recover from burns, blisters, infections, and other injuries and to help reduce conditions related to dry skin.

Myrrh Essential Oil: helps improve skin conditions, wounds, and wrinkles.

Helichrysum Essential Oil: is antibacterial, anti-inflammatory, and cleansing. It has also been used to treat dermatitis/eczema. Helichrysum can also be used to protect the skin from the sun, heal scars, and treat skin disorders.

Rose Essential Oil: can be used to prevent scarring and its healing properties have been used throughout the ages. This oil can be used to help ease symptoms of aging, including wrinkles.

Lipids: are micronutrients that maintain the barrier function of the skin, nourish the skin, and support skin hydration. Topical application of micronutrients can assist the body's natural lipids. Poor levels of micronutrients is associated with unhealthy looking skin.

Olive Oil: hydrates the skin and increases skin flexibility. Olive oil also displays antioxidant properties (Budiyanto et al., 2000).

Jojoba Oil: Although called an oil, jojoba oil is actually a natural liquid wax extracted from jojoba (*Simmondsia chinensis*) plants found in the southwestern Unites States and northern Mexico. This liquid wax closely resembles the skin's natural oils (or sebum).

Macadamia Oil: is moisturizing, reparative, and cleansing.

Companion Formulations and Blend: Immortelle, Veráge Moisturizer, Veráge Cleanser, Veráge Toner.

Veráge™ Moisturizer

Youthful Moisturizing Lotion

This moisturizing facial lotion is ideal for all skin types and provides hydration as well as skin nourishment. As the lotion hydrates deeply it helps to reduce wrinkles and smooth the skin.

Key Ingredients:

Jasmine Essential Oil: is gentle and beneficial for all types of skin. Jasmine oil can help care for dry, greasy, or irritated skin.

Geranium Essential Oil: soothes sensitive skin, hydrates dry skin, and reduces wrinkles. Geranium oil may also be beneficial for acne, balancing the sebum of skin, cleansing oily skin, and may even liven up pale skin.

Sea Buckthorn Berry Essential Oil: is beneficial for the skin, has antioxidant properties, and displays restorative properties.

Juniper Berry Essential Oil: is beneficial for relieving acne and other skin issues. Juniper berry oil is also a cleanser, purifier, and helps heal wounds. This oil may also help skin retain moisture.

Rice Bran Oil: contains antioxidants, vitamins, and nutrients. Rice bran oil is beneficial for the skin because it helps nourish, regenerate, and tone.

Shea Butter: is widely known as a powerful moisturizer. Shea butter has been used to heal skin conditions and reduce wrinkles. Shea butter mimics the body's natural moisturizers and is therefore extremely affective at treating dry skin, sunburns, wounds, skin cracks, stretch marks, and burns.

Phellodendron Amurense Bark Extract: is a fundamental herb used in traditional Chinese medicine. Modern research has shown that this extract possesses anti-inflammatory properties in vitro and in vivo (Choi et al., 2014).

Companion Formulations and Blend: Immortelle, Veráge Immortelle Hydrating Serum, Veráge Cleanser, Veráge Toner.

Veráge™ Toner

Youthful Skin Toner

This nourishing skin toner will reduce the appearance of skin aging by tightening, toning, and smoothing the skin. To help produce a youthful complexion, use this toner to increase skin glow, tone, and texture, and tighten pores.

Key Ingredients:

Ylang Ylang Essential Oil: is calming and relaxing to the mind and body. It brings a feeling of self-love, confidence, joy, and peace.

Coriander Essential Oil: is soothing and toning. Coriander oil may also regulate and help control pain. It is also rejuvenating for the skin. Coriander also helps aid muscle tone.

Cypress Essential Oil: is antibacterial, antimicrobial, relaxing, and refreshing. This oil can help regulate circulation and is revitalizing for the skin.

Palmarosa Essential Oil: is valuable for all types of skin problems because it stimulates new cell growth, regulates oil production, hydrates, moisturizes, and speeds healing.

Witch Hazel: has long been used to treat skin issues. Along with shrinking pores and removing excess oil, it can be used to cleanse, tone, and smooth skin.

Aloe: is widely known to soothe and moisturize skin.

Companion Formulations and Blend: Immortelle, Veráge Immortelle Hydrating Serum, Veráge Moisturizer, Veráge Cleanser.

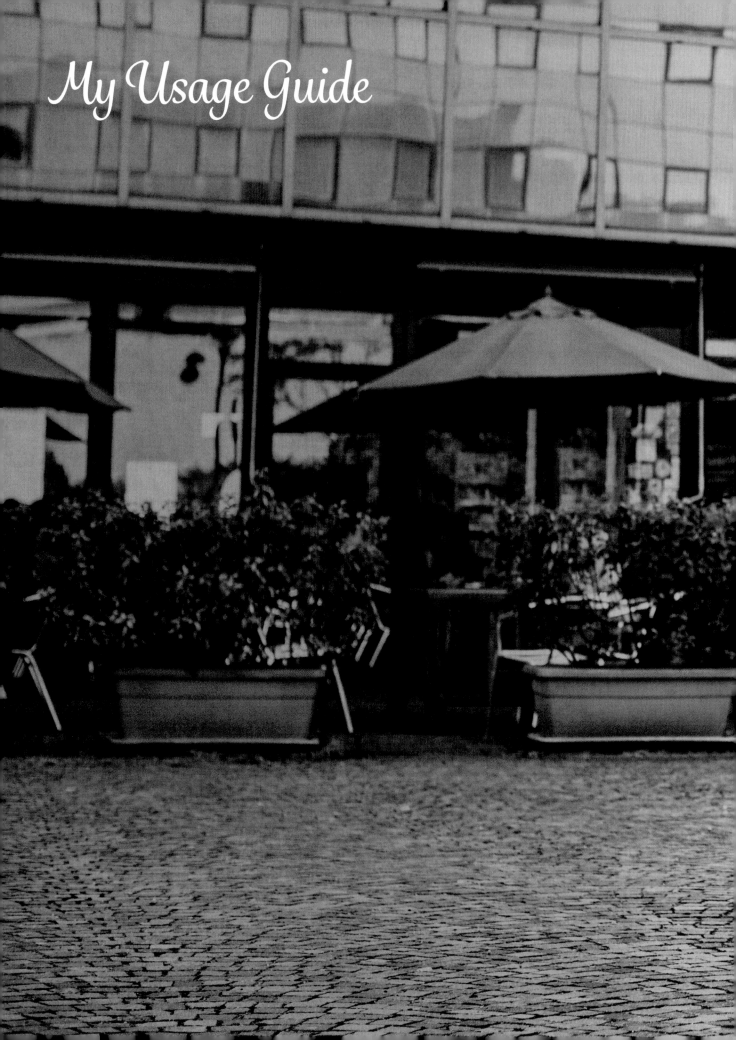

My Usage Guide

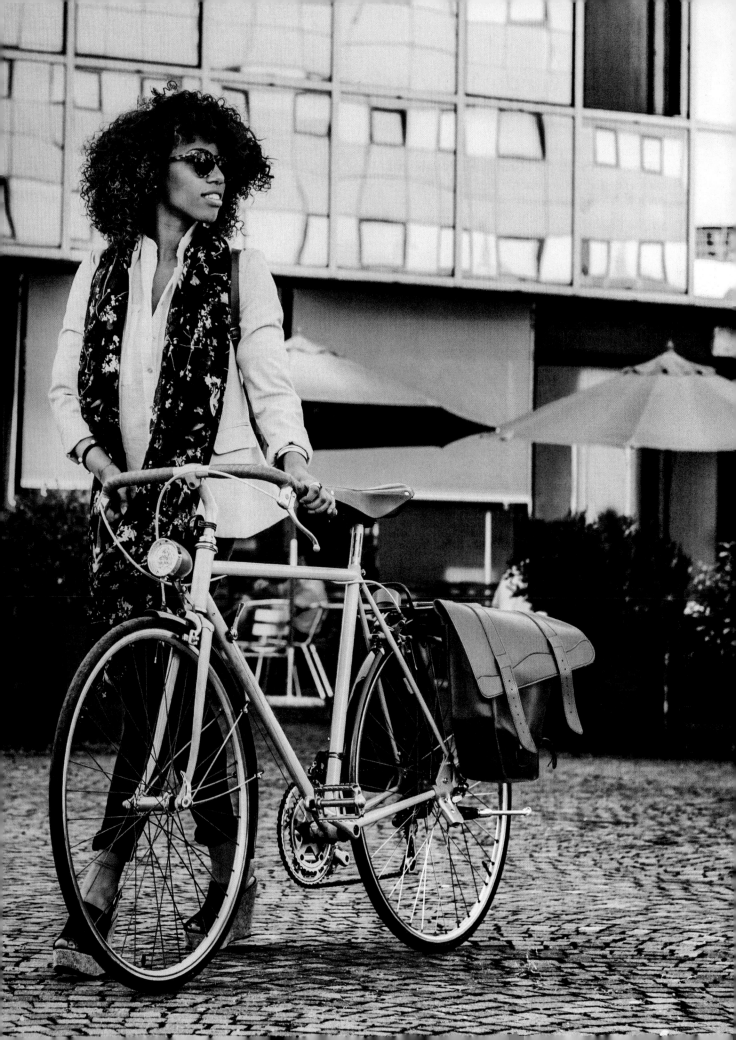

My Usage Guide: How to Use This Section

This section is a compilation of many different health conditions and the various essential oils, blends, and supplements that are commonly used and recommended for each condition.

Example Entry:

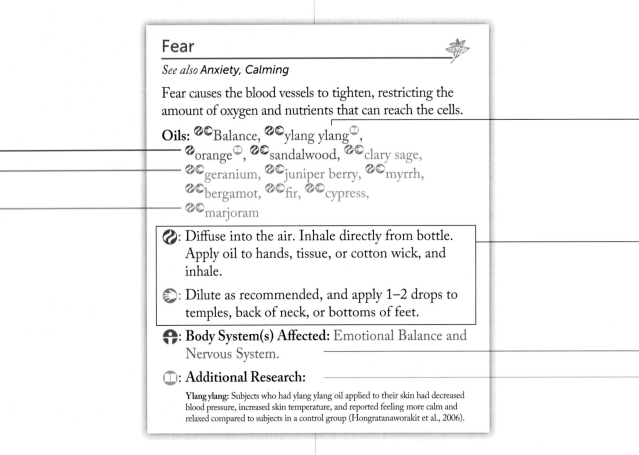

Fear

See also **Anxiety, Calming**

Fear causes the blood vessels to tighten, restricting the amount of oxygen and nutrients that can reach the cells.

Oils: Balance, ylang ylang, orange, sandalwood, clary sage, geranium, juniper berry, myrrh, bergamot, fir, cypress, marjoram

: Diffuse into the air. Inhale directly from bottle. Apply oil to hands, tissue, or cotton wick, and inhale.

: Dilute as recommended, and apply 1–2 drops to temples, back of neck, or bottoms of feet.

: **Body System(s) Affected:** Emotional Balance and Nervous System.

: **Additional Research:**

Ylang ylang: Subjects who had ylang ylang oil applied to their skin had decreased blood pressure, increased skin temperature, and reported feeling more calm and relaxed compared to subjects in a control group (Hongratanaworakit et al., 2006).

Under each **condition**, the oils, blends, and supplements have been grouped as:

• Primary Recommendations: Try these oils, blends, or supplements first.

• Secondary Recommendations: Try these oils or blends second. Supplements listed as secondary recommendations may be useful for general nutritional support of the body systems involved in prevention or healing from a specific condition.

• Other Recommendations : Oils, blends, and supplements that may also help, depending on the underlying cause.

The criteria for grouping within these categories include the recommendations of experts within the field of essential oils, supporting scientific research studies, historical uses of the oils and the herbs and plants they are derived from, and more recent French medicinal uses for the oils. However, since each individual may have different underlying causes for his or her specific condition, what may work for one individual may be different than what works for another.

Also listed under each condition are recommendations for how to use or apply these oils or supplements for that particular condition. The three main application and usage methods are aromatic, topical, and internal. The recommended methods are indicated next to each oil as a small ⊘ for Aromatic, ⊖ for Topical, and ⬤ for Internal.

⊘: Aromatic means that the oils are breathed or inhaled through the mouth and nose. This could include breathing the aroma of the oil directly from the bottle or breathing in oil that has been applied to the hands or to another material such as a tissue or cotton wick. It could also mean breathing the vapor or mist of an oil that has been diffused or sprayed into the surrounding air.

⊖: Topical means that the oils are applied directly onto the skin, hair, or other surface of the body. This can be through direct application of the oils to the skin or by using the oils in massages, baths, or within a cream, lotion, or soap. While some oils can be applied neat (without dilution), others may need to be diluted before topical application, especially for young or sensitive skin. Refer to the Single Essential Oils section of this book or the Dilution Reference Chart (following these notes) for recommended dilutions for the oils listed in this book.

⬤: Internal means that the oils or supplements are taken orally. This can be done either by adding the oil to a food or beverage that is then consumed, placing a drop of oil under the tongue, or by swallowing a capsule that has the essential oil or supplement inside.

For more information on specific ways essential oils can be applied or used, see the Science and Application of Essential Oils section in this book.

The large ⊘, ⊖, or ⬤ listed near the bottom of each entry refers to recommended application methods specific for that condition.

⬤: Listed with each entry are the main body systems primarily affected by each health condition. For more information on all of the oils and products discussed within this book and which body systems they primarily affect, see Appendix A: Body Systems Chart.

⊡: For many conditions listed in this section there is also additional supporting research.

Many entries also include **definitions** of conditions and terms (listed directly underneath the topic), **subtopics** related to that condition, and even **recipes or blends** that can be used for that condition.

Example Entry:

Below are some additional things to keep in mind as you use and apply the essential oils, blends, and supplements listed in this section.

Oils: ⊖melaleuca, ⊘⊖oregano⊡, ⊖peppermint, ⊖thyme, ⊖geranium, ⊖lavender

Blend 1: Combine 2 drops lavender, 2 drops melaleuca, and 2 drops thyme. Apply 1–2 drops on ringworm three times a day for 10 days. Then mix 30 drops melaleuca with 2 Tbs. (25 ml) fractionated coconut oil, and use daily until ringworm is gone.

—Thrush:

Thrush is another name for oral candidiasis (*see Candida above*). Thrush results in uncomfortable or painful white or yellow patches in the mouth.

Oils: ⊖melaleuca⊡, ⊖lavender, ⊖eucalyptus, ⊖marjoram, ⊖thyme

My Usage Guide: Dilution Reference Chart—Oils

Single Oil Name	Recommended Dilution Adults	Child/ Sensitive	Expectant Mother
Arborvitae	●	●:○	✕
Basil	●	●:○	✕
Bergamot	●☀	●☀☀	●☀☀
Birch	●	●:○	✕
Black Pepper	●:○○	▽	▽
Blue Tansy	●	●:○	●:○○
Cardamom	●	●	●
Cassia	●:○○○○	▽	✕
Cedarwood	●	●:○○	▽
Cilantro	●	●	●
Cinnamon	●:○○○	▽	✕
Clary Sage	●	●	▽
Clove	●:○	●:○○○○	▽
Copaiba	●	●:○	●
Coriander	●	●	●
Cypress	●	●	▽
Dill	●	●	●
Douglas Fir	●	●:○	●:○○
Eucalyptus	●	●:○	●
Fennel	●	●:○	▽
Frankincense	●	●	●
Geranium	●	●:○	●
Ginger	●☀	●:○	●
Grapefruit	●	●	●
Green Mandarin	●☀	●☀	●☀
Hawaiian Sandalwood	●	●	●
Helichrysum	●	●	●
Hinoki	●	●:○	●:○
Jasmine	●	●	●
Juniper Berry	●	●:○	●
Lavender	●	●	●
Lemon	●☀	●☀	●☀
Lemon Myrtle	●:○○○	●:○○○○	●:○○○○
Lemongrass	●	●:○	●:○
Lime	●☀	●:○☀	●☀
Litsea	●	●:○	●:○
Magnolia	●	●:○	●:○
Manuka	●	●	●:○
Marjoram	●	●:○	▽
Melaleuca	●	●	●

Single Oil Name	Recommended Dilution Adults	Child/ Sensitive	Expectant Mother
Melissa	●	●	▽
Myrrh	●	●	▽
Neroli	●	●	●:○○
Orange	●☀	●☀	●☀
Oregano	●:○○○	▽	▽
Patchouli	●	●:○	●:○
Patchouli	●	●	●
Peppermint	●	●:○	▽
Pink Pepper	●	●:○	●:○
Petitgrain	●	●:○	●
Roman Chamomile	●	●:○	●
Rose	●	●	●
Rosemary	●	●:○	✕
Sandalwood	●	●	●
Siberian Fir	●	●:○	●:○
Spearmint	●	●:○	▽
Spikenard	●	●	●
Star Anise	●	●:○	▽
Thyme	●:○○○○	▽	✕
Turmeric	●	●:○	▽
Vetiver	●	●	▽
White Fir	●	●:○	●:○
Wintergreen	●	●:○	✕
Yarrow	●	●:○	●:○
Ylang Ylang	●	●	●
Yuzu	●☀	●:○☀	●☀

My Usage Guide: Dilution Reference Chart—Blends

Oil Blend Name	Recommended Dilution		
	Adults	Child/Sensitive	Expectant Mother
AromaTouch	●	●	●
Balance	●	●	●
Brave	●	●	●
Breathe	●	●:◊	●
Calmer	●	●	●
Cheer	●	●:◊	●:◊
Citrus Bliss	●☀	●☀	●☀
ClaryCalm	●	●:◊	▽
Console	●	●	●
DDR Prime	●	●:◊	▽
Deep Blue	●	●:◊	●
DigestZen	●	●	▽
Elevation	●☀	●☀	●☀
Forgive	●	●:◊	●:◊
HD Clear	●	●	▽
Immortelle	●	●	▽
InTune	●	●:◊	●:◊
Motivate	●	●:◊	●:◊
On Guard	●	●:◊	▽
Passion	●	●:◊	●:◊
PastTense	●	●:◊	▽
Peace	●	●	●
Purify	●	●	●
Rescuer	●	●	●
Serenity	●	●	●
Slim & Sassy	●☀	●:◊☀	▽
Steady	●	●	●
Stronger	●	●	●
TerraShield	●	●	●
Thinker	●	●	●
Whisper	●	●	●
Yarrow Pom	●	●:◊	●:◊
Yoga Blends	●	●:◊	●:◊
Zendocrine	●:◊	●:◊◊◊◊	▽

 Can be used neat (without dilution)

 For ratios like this, the first drop represents the proportion of essential oil to use, and the second drop represents the proportion of carrier oil (such as fractionated coconut oil) to use. For this ratio, you would blend 1 part essential oil with 1 part carrier oil before applying.

 Use with extreme caution and dilute heavily

 Avoid

 Avoid sunlight for up to 12 hours after use

 Avoid sunlight for up to 72 hours after use

Body Systems

✛ Body Systems: Primary Single Oils

Cardiovascular System
orange, cypress

Digestive System
peppermint, ginger, lemongrass, fennel

Emotions
cypress, geranium, lavender, rose, orange, peppermint

Endocrine/Reproductive System
rosemary, peppermint, clary sage, ylang ylang, melaleuca, oregano, basil, cassia

Immune/Lymphatic System
oregano, melaleuca, rosemary, clove, frankincense, cypress, sandalwood

Muscles
marjoram, peppermint

Nervous System
peppermint, basil, lavender, lemon, grapefruit, frankincense

Respiratory System
eucalyptus, peppermint, Douglas fir, cinnamon, cardamom

Skeletal System
wintergreen, fir, cypress, juniper berry

Skin
peppermint, melaleuca, sandalwood, frankincense, lavender

✛ Body Systems: Primary Blends

Cardiovascular System
DDR Prime

Digestive System
DigestZen

Emotions
Console, Motivate, Passion, Peace, Forgive, Cheer, Balance, Citrus Bliss, Elevation, Serenity

Endocrine/Reproductive System
Zendocrine, ClaryCalm, Whisper

Immune/Lymphatic System
On Guard

Muscles
Deep Blue, AromaTouch

Nervous System
InTune

Respiratory System
Breathe, On Guard

Skeletal System
Deep Blue

Skin
HD Clear, Immortelle

Body Systems

To best support the different systems of the body, it is important to understand that essential oils produce the greatest therapeutic benefits when proper amounts (just a few drops) are used regularly. Many beginner essential oil users have the tendency to apply an overabundance of essential oils during episodes of decreased wellness. However, the human body performs best at steady levels. Many of the body systems regulate different aspects of homeostasis (derived from the Greek words for "same" and "stable") to achieve optimal wellness and health. For example, one of the key functions of the cardiovascular system is thermoregulation (the process of maintaining optimal body temperature).

To most effectively support the homeostatic function of the body systems, essential oils should be applied at steady levels. Topically applying a few drops of oil every day or continuously diffusing essential oils in the home are two powerful methods that can help support overall physical, mental, and emotional health during periods of wellness.

Essential oils are extremely beneficial and powerful. For this reason, only a few drops of essential oil are needed both during times of wellness and times of disease. To achieve the best benefit over time, apply the proper amount (only a few drops) regularly via the most focused and correct method. See the topics in this Personal Usage Guide section to better understand the correct method for applying essential oils for various conditions.

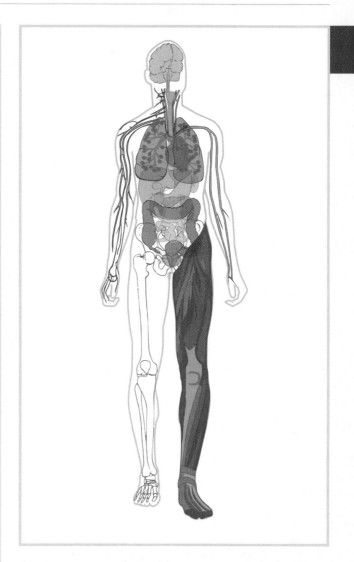

Look throughout this section for the purple tabs in the upper right-hand corner of the page to find more detailed information pages on the different body systems.

Additional Notes on Using Essential Oils

— If essential oils get into your eyes by accident or if they burn the skin a little, do not try to remove the oils with water. This will only drive the oils deeper into the tissue. It is best to dilute the essential oils on location with a pure vegetable oil (such as fractionated coconut oil).

— The FDA has approved some essential oils generically for internal use and given them the following designations: GRAS (Generally Recognized As Safe for human consumption), FA (Food Additive), or FL (Flavoring agent). *These designations are listed under Oral Use As Dietary Supplement for each single oil in the Single Essential Oils section of this book.*

— Using some oils such as lemon, orange, grapefruit, bergamot, etc., before or during exposure to direct sunlight or UV rays (tanning beds, for example) may cause a rash, pigmentation, or even severe burns. Please see the safety information under each oil in the Essential Oils chapter of this book for further information; then either dilute these oils and test a small area, or avoid their use altogether.

— Caution should be used with oils such as clary sage and fennel during pregnancy. These oils contain active constituents with hormone-like activity and could possibly stimulate adverse reactions in the mother, although there are no recorded cases in humans.

— Particular care should be taken when using cassia, cinnamon, lemongrass, oregano, and thyme, as they are some of the strongest and most caustic oils. It is best to dilute them with a pure vegetable oil.

— When a blend or recipe is listed in this section, rather than mix the oils together, it may be more beneficial to layer the oils: that is, apply a drop or two of one oil, rub it in, and then apply another oil. If dilution is necessary, a pure vegetable oil can be applied on top.
Effectiveness is in the layering.

— Less is often better: use 1–3 drops of oil and no more than 6 drops at a time. Stir, and rub on in a clockwise direction.

— When applying oils to infants and small children, dilute 1–2 drops pure essential oil with 1–3 tsp. (5–15 ml) of a pure vegetable oil (such as fractionated coconut oil). If the oils are used in the bath, always use a bath gel base as a dispersing agent for the oils. See *Children and Infants* in this section for more information about the recommended list of oils for babies and children.

— The body absorbs oils the fastest through inhalation (breathing) and second fastest through application to the feet or ears. Layering oils can increase the rate of absorption.

— The life expectancy of a cell is 120 days (4 months). When cells divide, they make duplicate cells. If the cell is diseased, new diseased cells will be made. When we stop the mutation of the diseased cells (create healthy cells), we stop the disease. Essential oils have the ability to penetrate and carry nutrients through the cell membrane to the nucleus and improve the health of the cell.

— *Use extreme caution when diffusing cassia or cinnamon,* as they may burn the nostrils if you put your nose directly next to the nebulizer of the diffuser where the mist is coming out.

— When traveling by air, you should always have your oils hand-checked. X-ray machines may interfere with the frequency of the oils.

— Keep oils away from the light and heat—although they seem to do fine in temperatures up to 90° F (30° C). If stored properly in a cool, dark environment, they can maintain their maximum potency for many years.

Symbols and Colors Used in This Section

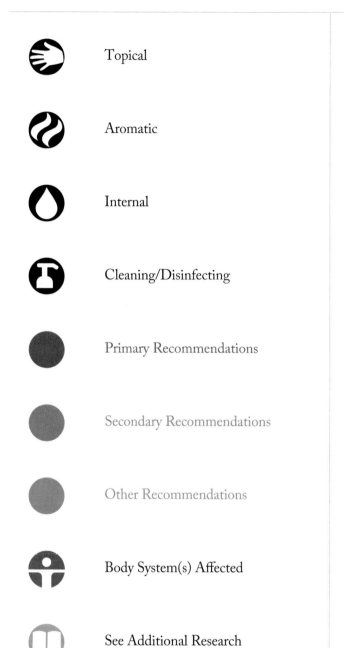

Topical

Aromatic

Internal

Cleaning/Disinfecting

Primary Recommendations

Secondary Recommendations

Other Recommendations

Body System(s) Affected

See Additional Research

My Usage Guide

ADD/ADHD

Attention deficit disorder or attention deficit/hyper-activity disorder is a psychological condition characterized by inattentiveness, restlessness, and difficulty concentrating. Although most individuals exhibit all of these symptoms at some point, ADD is characterized by a frequency and duration of these symptoms that are inappropriate to an individual's age.

> *Simple Solutions—ADD/ADHD:* Combine 3 drops lavender and 3 drops basil on a natural stone or unglazed clay pendant, and wear throughout the day.

Oils: ⊙⊘InTune, ⊙⊘Steady, ⊙⊘Thinker, ⊙⊘Serenity, ⊙vetiver, ⊙⊘lavender

Blend 1: Combine equal parts lavender and basil. Diffuse, or apply 1–3 drops on the crown of the head.

⊘: Diffuse into the air. Inhale oil directly from the bottle, or applied to a tissue or cotton wick.

⊜: Dilute as recommended, and apply 1–3 drops on the bottoms of the feet and/or on the spine.

⊕: **Body System(s) Affected:** Nervous System and Emotional Balance.

AIDS/HIV

*See also **Antiviral***

Acquired immune deficiency syndrome (AIDS) is a disease of the human immune system. AIDS progressively inhibits the effectiveness of the immune system, leaving the human body susceptible to both infections and tumors. AIDS is caused by the human immuno-deficiency virus (HIV), which is acquired by direct contact of the bloodstream or mucous membrane with a bodily fluid (such as blood, breast milk, vaginal fluid, semen, and preseminal fluid) containing HIV.

Oils: ⊙⊘helichrysum⊕, ⊙On Guard, ⊙⊘lemon, ⊙⊘bergamot⊕, ⊙Balance

⊘: Diffuse into the air. Inhale oil applied to a tissue or cotton wick.

⊜: Dilute as recommended, and apply 1–3 drops on the bottoms of the feet and/or on the spine.

⊕: **Body System(s) Affected:** Immune System.

⊡: **Additional Research:**

Helichrysum: Arzanol, extracted from helichrysum, inhibited HIV-1 replication in T cells and also inhibited the release of pro-inflammatory cytokines (chemical messengers) in monocytes (Appendino et al., 2007).

Bergamot: Bergamot extract was found to have potent antiretroviral activity towards HTLV-1 (a human retrovirus that causes T-cell leukemia and lymphoma) and HIV-1 expression in infected cells (Balestrieri et al., 2011).

Abscess

*See **Oral Conditions: Abscess***

Abuse

Abuse is the harmful treatment or use of something or someone. Abuse has many different forms: physical, sexual, verbal, spiritual, psychological, etc. Abuse in all of its forms often has long-lasting negative effects on the person or thing abused.

Oils: ⊙Elevation, ⊙lavender, ⊙melissa, ⊙sandalwood

⊜: Apply oil topically over the heart, rub on each ear, and then cup hands and inhale deeply to help release negative emotions associated with abuse.

⊕: **Body System(s) Affected:** Emotional Balance.

Acne

Acne is a skin condition, generally of the face, commonly found in adolescents and young adults. Acne is characterized by red, irritating blemishes (pimples) on the skin. Most commonly, acne is found on the oil-producing parts of the body such as the face, chest, back, upper arms, and back of neck. Acne is a blockage of a skin pore by dead skin cells, tiny hairs, and oil secreted by the sebaceous glands located near the hair follicles in the face, neck, and back. This blockage occurs deep within the skin. Acne is not currently believed to be caused by dirt on the face or by eating certain foods, and research has indicated that over-scrubbing the face may actually make acne worse.

> *Simple Solutions—Acne:* Add 2 drops melaleuca to 1 cup (250 ml) warm water, and use water to gently wash face once a day.

Oils: ⊙HD Clear, ⊙melaleuca⊕, ⊙juniper berry, ⊙copaiba, ⊙⊘manuka, ⊙Stronger, ⊙lavender,

See the *Quick Usage Chart* inside the back cover for recommended dilutions.

236

cedarwood, petitgrain, geranium, sandal-wood, thyme, vetiver, lemon, lemongrass, marjoram, patchouli

Other Products: HD Clear Foaming Face Wash and HD Clear Facial Lotion

—**Infectious:**

Oils: HD Clear, melaleuca⊕, clove

Other Products: HD Clear Foaming Face Wash and HD Clear Facial Lotion

: Dilute as recommended, and apply one of the above oils on location. Place about 10 drops of an oil in a 1–2 oz. spray bottle filled with water, and mist your face several times per day.

: **Body System(s) Affected:** Skin.

: **Additional Research:**

Melaleuca: Tea tree oil and several of its main components were found to be active against Propionibacterium acnes, a bacteria involved in the formation of acne. This oil was also found to be active against two types of staphylococcus bacteria (Raman et al., 1995).

Melaleuca: A topical gel containing 5% tea tree oil was found to be more effective than a placebo at preventing acne lesions and severity in patients suffering from acne vulgaris (Enshaieh et al., 2007).

Melaleuca: A gel with 5% tea tree oil was found to be as effective as a 5% benzoyl peroxide (a common chemical used to treat acne) lotion, with fewer side effects (Bassett et al., 1990).

Addictions

Addiction is an obsession, compulsion, or extreme psychological dependence that interferes with an individual's ability or desire to function normally. Common addictions include drugs, alcohol, coffee, tobacco, sugar, video games, work, gambling, money, explicit images, compulsive overeating, etc.

> *Simple Solutions—Addictions:* Diffuse grapefruit oil using an aromatherapy diffuser to help calm and soothe withdrawal symptoms.

—**Alcohol:**

Oils: rosemary, Purify, Serenity, juniper berry, helichrysum, lavender, orange

—**Drugs:**

Oils: Purify, Serenity, grapefruit (withdrawal)⊕, lavender, basil, eucalyptus, marjoram, orange, sandalwood, Roman chamomile, wintergreen

—**Opioid Addiction:**

Opioid addiction has become an increasingly significant problem throughout the world due to the increasing availability of natural and synthetic opioids. As of 2016, opioid overdose was among the top causes of death in individuals under the age of 50 in the United States.

Oils: Serenity, rose (withdrawal)⊕, grapefruit (withdrawal), lavender, basil, orange, sandalwood, Roman chamomile

—**Smoking:**

Oils: black pepper, clove, or On Guard on tongue

—**Sugar:**

Oils: Purify, Serenity

Technology:

When someone has a technology addiction, he or she increasingly practices a frequent and obsessive technology-related behavior despite negative consequences. Technology addictions can include online gaming, shopping, researching, and social media use, among other things.

Oils: Serenity, lavender, grapefruit

—**Withdrawal:**

Oils: lavender, grapefruit, orange, sandalwood, marjoram

—**Work:**

Oils: lavender, basil, marjoram, geranium

: Diffuse into the air. Inhale the aroma of the oil directly.

: Dilute as recommended, and apply to temples or to reflex points.

: **Body System(s) Affected:** Emotional Balance.

: **Additional Research:**

Rose: Rose oil demonstrated an ability to reduce morphine (an opioid) withdrawal symptoms in mice. (Abbasi et al., 2013).

Grapefruit and orange: Injection of limonene, a common terpene found in many citrus essential oils, inhibited behavioral manifestations of drug use on rats administered methamphetamine (METH). Examination of the nucleus accumbens of the rats revealed that limonene may produce its effects by regulating dopamine levels and serotonin receptor function (Yun, 2014).

Black pepper: Inhaled vapor of black pepper oil was found to reduce cravings for cigarettes and symptoms of anxiety in smokers deprived from smoking, compared to a control (Rose et al., 1994).

Addison's Disease

See *Adrenal Glands: Addison's Disease*

Adenitis

Adenitis is an acute or chronic inflammation of the lymph glands or lymph nodes.

> *Simple Solutions—Adenitis:* Dilute 2 drops rosemary in 1 tsp. (5 ml) fractionated coconut oil, and apply over lymph nodes daily.

Oils: �׹rosemary

☺: Dilute as recommended, and apply on location.

✺: **Body System(s) Affected:** Immune System.

Adrenal Glands

The adrenal glands are two small glands located on top of the kidneys. The inner part of the adrenal gland, called the medulla, is responsible for producing adrenalin, a hormone that helps control blood pressure, heart rate, and sweating. The outer part of the adrenal gland, called the cortex, is responsible for producing corticosteroids, hormones that help control metabolism and help regulate inflammation, water levels, and levels of electrolytes such as sodium and potassium. An imbalance in adrenal function can lead to problems such as Addison's disease (a lack of adrenal hormones in the body due to suppressed adrenal functioning) or Cushing's syndrome (an over-abundance of corticosteroids, typically due to overactive adrenal functioning).

Oils: ☺basil, ☺rosemary, ☺clove, ☺Elevation

Other Products: ○Alpha CRS+, ○Microplex VMz, ○a2z Chewable, ○xEO Mega or vEO Mega, ○IQ Mega

—Addison's Disease:

Addison's disease is a condition where the function of the adrenal glands is either severely limited or completely shut down in their ability to produce hormones. This is most often caused by an autoimmune disorder where the body's own immune system attacks the cells in the adrenal glands, but it can also be caused by cancer, tuberculosis, or other diseases. The loss of hormones from the adrenal cortex can cause extreme dehydration due to fluid loss and low levels of

sodium. Early symptoms can include tiredness, dizziness when standing up, thirst, weight loss, and dark patches of pigmentation appearing on the skin. If untreated, this disease can eventually lead to kidney failure, shock, and death.

Oils: ☺Elevation

Other Products: ○Microplex VMz, ○Alpha CRS+ (for cellular support), ○a2z Chewable, ○xEO Mega or vEO Mega, ○IQ Mega

—Cushing's Syndrome:

Cushing's syndrome is a condition where there is an over-abundance of corticosteroids (such as cortisol) in the body, typically caused by an over-production of these steroids by the adrenal glands. This over-production in the adrenal glands can be caused by a growth in the adrenal glands or by a tumor in the pituitary gland leading to the production of too much corticotropin (the hormone that stimulates production of corticosteroids in the adrenal gland). This syndrome can also be caused by taking artificial cortisone or cortisone-like substances. Symptoms of excessive corticosteroids include weight gain, muscle loss, and weakness, bruising, and osteoporosis.

Oils: ☺Elevation, ☺lemon, ☺basil, ☺On Guard

Other Products: ○Microplex VMz, ○Alpha CRS+ (for cellular support), ○a2z Chewable, ○xEO Mega or vEO Mega, ○IQ Mega

—Schmidt's Syndrome *(Polyglandular Deficiency Syndrome (or Autoimmune Polyendocrine Syndrome) Type 2)*:

This syndrome refers specifically to an autoimmune disorder that causes Addison's disease as well as decreased thyroid function. See *Addison's Disease* (above) and *Thyroid: Hypothyroidism* for oils and products to help support the adrenal glands and thyroid.

Stimulate glands: ☺basil, ☺rosemary, ☺clove, ☺geranium

Strengthen glands: ☺peppermint

☺: Apply as a warm compress over kidney area. Dilute as recommended, and apply on location or on reflex points on the feet.

◐: Take capsules as directed on package.

✺: **Body System(s) Affected:** Endocrine System.

See the *Quick Usage Chart* inside the back cover for recommended dilutions.

Aging

See also **Alzheimer's Disease, Antioxidant, Cells, Female-Specific Conditions: Menopause, Hair: Loss,** *and* **Skin: Wrinkles** *for other age-related issues.*

> *Simple Solutions—Aging:* Diffuse lemon oil for 15 minutes daily to help promote memory.

Oils: ⁰DDR Prime, ⁰Immortelle, ⁰Yarrow Pom, ⁰lemon⊕, ⁰frankincense, ⁰sandalwood

Other Products: ⁰Anti-Aging Moisturizer, ⁰Veráge Cleanser, ⁰Veráge Toner, ⁰Veráge Immortelle Hydrating Serum, ⁰Veráge Moisturizer, ⁰Facial Cleanser, ⁰Invigorating Scrub, ⁰Pore Reducing Toner, ⁰Skin Serum. ⁰Mito2Max, ⁰Alpha CRS+, ⁰xEO Mega or vEO Mega, ⁰IQ Mega, ⁰Microplex VMz, ⁰PB Assist+

◐: Take oil with food, or take capsules as directed on package.

◑: Dilute as recommended, and apply to skin. Combine with carrier oil, and massage into skin.

◒: Diffuse, or inhale from a tissue or cotton wick.

✛: **Body System(s) Affected:** Skin and Nervous System.

◉: **Additional Research:**

Lemon: Based on lemon essential oil's acetylcholinesterase inhibitory activity, butyrylcholinesterase inhibitory activity, and antioxidant power, this essential oil could be used in the management and/or prevention of neurodegenerative conditions like Alzheimer's disease (Oboh et al., 2014).

Lemon: A study using mice demonstrated that pretreatment with lemon essential oil causes an increase in antioxidant enzymatic activities and decreased lipid degradation in the hippocampus (Campelo et al., 2011). Antioxidant and bioprotective activities, like that of lemon essential oil, can reduce damage to neurons produced by neurodegenerative disease (Campelo et al., 2011).

Agitation

See **Calming**

Airborne Bacteria

See **Antibacterial**

Air Pollution

Air Pollution is the presence in the atmosphere of chemicals, biological material, or other matter that can potentially harm humans, the environment, or other living organisms.

> *Simple Solutions—Air Cleansing:* Diffuse Purify in an aromatherapy diffuser.

Oils: ◒Purify, ◒On Guard, ◒lemon, ◒lemongrass, ◒peppermint, ◒rosemary, ◒eucalyptus, ◒cypress, ◒grapefruit

—**Disinfectants**:

Oils: ◒Purify, ◒lemon, ◒eucalyptus, ◒clove, ◒grapefruit, ◒peppermint, ◒wintergreen

Blend 1: Combine lemongrass and geranium oil, and diffuse into the air⊕.

◒: Diffuse into the air.

✛: **Body System(s) Affected:** Respiratory System.

◉: **Additional Research:**

Blend 1: A formulation of lemongrass and geranium oil was found to reduce airborne bacteria by 89% in an office environment after diffusion for 15 hours (Doran et al., 2009).

Alcoholism

See **Addictions: Alcohol**

Alertness

Alertness is the state of being watchful or paying close attention. It includes being prepared to react quickly to danger, emergencies, or any other situation.

> *Simple Solutions—Alertness:* Drop 3–4 drops of peppermint oil on the shower floor when showering in the morning to help invigorate.
> Inhale the aroma of peppermint while driving to help stay alert.

Oils: ◒◑peppermint⊕, ◒◑Thinker, ◒ylang ylang⊕, ◒◑lemon, ◒◑pink pepper, ◒◑basil, ◒◑rosemary

◒: Diffuse into the air. Inhale oil applied to a tissue or cotton wick.

◑: Dilute as recommended, and apply to the temples and bottoms of the feet.

✛: **Body System(s) Affected:** Nervous System.

◉: **Additional Research:**

Peppermint: In human trials, the aroma of peppermint was found to enhance memory and increase alertness (Moss et al., 2008).

Ylang ylang: Inhaled ylang ylang oil was found to decrease blood pressure and pulse rate and to enhance attentiveness and alertness in volunteers compared to an odorless control (Hongratanaworakit et al., 2004).

My Usage Guide

A B C D E F G H I J K L M N O P Q R S T U V W X Y Z

Allergies

An allergy is a damaging immune system response to a substance that does not bother most other people. Common allergies are to food, insect bites, pollen, dust, medicine, pets, and mold. Allergy symptoms vary greatly, but common allergic responses include itching, swelling, runny nose, asthma, and sneezing. Both host factors (gender, race, heredity) and environmental factors can cause allergies.

> *Simple Solutions—Allergies:* Blend 2 drops each of lavender, lemon, and peppermint oil in 1 tsp. (5 ml) fractionated coconut oil, and apply a small amount on the temples, under the nose, and on the bottoms of the feet morning and evening when dealing with seasonal allergies.

Oils: melaleuca, lavender, lemon, peppermint, Roman chamomile, melissa, patchouli, blue tansy, eucalyptus, spikenard (skin)

Other Products: TriEase Softgels, Breathe Respiratory Drops, Breathe Vapor Stick, Microplex VMz, Alpha CRS+, a2z Chewable

—Coughing:

    Oils: Purify

—Hay Fever

    Oils: lavender, eucalyptus, rose, peppermint

Recipe 1: Apply 1 drop of peppermint on the base of the neck 2 times a day. Tap the thymus (located just below the notch in the neck) with pointer fingers. Diffuse peppermint.

Recipe 2: For allergy rashes and skin sensitivity, apply 3 drops lavender, 6 drops Roman chamomile, 2 drops myrrh, and 1 drop peppermint on location.

⬇: Dilute as recommended, and apply to sinuses and to bottoms of feet.

🌀: Diffuse into the air. Inhale oil applied to a tissue or cotton wick.

➕: **Body System(s) Affected: Respiratory System and Immune System.**

⬜: **Additional Research:**

    Melaleuca: Tea tree oil was found to reduce swelling during a contact hypersensitivity response in the skin of mice sensitized to the chemical hapten (Brand et al., 2002).

Melaleuca: Tea tree oil applied to histamine-induced edema (swelling) in mice ears was found to significantly reduce swelling (Brand et al., 2002).

Melaleuca: Tea tree oil applied to histamine-induced weal and flare in human volunteers was found to decrease the mean weal volume when compared to a control (Koh et al., 2002).

Lavender: Lavender oil was found to inhibit immediate-type allergic reactions in mice and rats by inhibiting mast cell degranulation (Kim et al., 1999).

Lemon: A study including 100 patients (ages 3–79) suffering from vasomotor allergic rhinopathy, showed that topical application of a citrus lemon-based spray resulted in a total reduction of eosinophils granulocytes and mast cells. These results suggest that the lemon-based nasal spray is a good alternative to conventional medicine for the treatment of perennial and seasonal allergic and vasomotor rhinopathy (Ferrara et al., 2012).

Peppermint: L-menthol (from peppermint) was found to inhibit production of inflammation mediators in human monocytes (a type of white blood cell involved in the immune response) (Juergens et al., 1998).

Alzheimer's Disease

See also **Brain, Memory**

Alzheimer's is a progressive and fatal disease that attacks and kills brain cells, causing a loss of memory and other intellectual capacities. Alzheimer's is most commonly diagnosed in individuals over the age of 65. As the disease progresses, sufferers often experience mood swings, long-term memory loss, confusion, irritability, aggression, and a decreased ability to communicate.

> *Simple Solutions—Alzheimer's:* Diffuse a blend of 1 part coriander and 2 parts lemon using an aromatherapy diffuser for 15 minutes daily.

Oils: coriander, lemon, cinnamon, spikenard

Supplements: Mito2Max, Alpha CRS+

—Blood-Brain Barrier:

    Studies have shown that sesquiterpenes can pass the blood-brain barrier. Oils high in sesquiterpenes include sandalwood, ginger, myrrh, vetiver, ylang ylang, and frankincense.

Oils: frankincense, sandalwood

⬤: Take oils in capsules. Take supplements as directed on package.

🌀: Diffuse oils into the air.

⬇: Dilute as recommended, and apply over brain stem area on back of neck.

➕: **Body System(s) Affected: Nervous System.**

⬜: **Additional Research:**

    Coriander: Inhalation of coriander volatile oil was found to possess antianxiety, antidepressant, and antioxidant properties in Alzheimer's disease conditions in a rat model of beta-amyloid Alzheimer's disease (Cioanca et al., 2014).

See the *Quick Usage Chart* inside the back cover for recommended dilutions.

Coriander: Repeated inhalation of coriander oil was found to prevent memory impairment and oxidative damage in a rat model of beta-amyloid Alzheimer's disease, when compared to control (Cioanca et al., 2013).

Lemon: Based on lemon essential oil's acetylcholinesterase inhibitory activity, butyrylcholinesterase inhibitory activity, and antioxidant power, this essential oil could be used in the management and/or prevention of neurodegenerative conditions like Alzheimer's disease (Oboh et al., 2014).

Alpha CRS+: In a recent study at UCLA, the polyphenol curcumin was found to inhibit amyloid beta accumulation and to cross the blood-brain barrier of mice and bind amyloid plaques. Amyloid beta plaques are theorized to have a role in the development of Alzheimer's disease (Yang et al., 2005).

Alpha CRS+: Curcumin was found to reduce the effects of amyloid beta-caused oxidative stress and DNA damage in neuronal cells (Park et al., 2008).

Sandalwood: A blend of ethanol extracts from 8 herbs, including sandalwood, orally administered to a mice model of Alzheimer's disease was shown to improve amyloid β protein-induced memory impairment, suppress amyloid β protein levels, and diminish plaque deposition in the brain as much as that of donepezil treatment. This study suggests that the 8-herb blend may develop as a therapeutic drug for treatment of Alzheimer's disease patients (Jeon et al., 2011).

Cinnamon: An aqueous cinnamon extract was found to inhibit beta-amyloid oligomer and fibril formation and alleviate Alzheimer's disease symptoms in the Drosophila and mouse models of Alzheimer's disease (Frydman-Marom et al., 2011).

Amnesia

See **Memory**

Analgesic

See **Pain**

Aneurysm

See also **Blood**

An aneurysm is a swelling or dilation of a blood vessel in the area of a weakened blood vessel wall.

> *Simple Solutions   Aneurysm:* Diffuse a blend of 5 drops frankincense, 1 drop helichrysum, and 1 drop cypress in an aromatherapy diffuser.

Oils: cypress, melaleuca, clary sage, helichrysum, frankincense

Herbs: Cayenne pepper, garlic, hawthorn berry

: Dilute as recommended, and apply to temples, heart, and reflex points for heart on the feet.

: Diffuse into the air. Inhale oil applied to a tissue or cotton wick.

: **Body System(s) Affected: Cardiovascular System.**

Anger

See **Calming**

Angina

See **Cardiovascular System: Angina**

Animals

Only 1–2 drops of oil are necessary on most animals, as they respond more quickly to the oils than do humans. Fractionated coconut oil can be added to extend the oil over larger areas and to heavily dilute the essential oil for use on smaller animals, especially cats.

—Bleeding:

   Oils: helichrysum, geranium

—Bones (Pain):

   Oils: wintergreen, Deep Blue, lemongrass

—Calm:

   Oils: Serenity, lavender, Citrus Bliss

—Cancer, Skin

   Oils: sandalwood, frankincense

—Cats:

   Valerie Worwood says that you can treat a cat like you would a child (*see* **Children/Infants**). Dilute oils heavily with carrier oil. *Avoid melaleuca, and use oils with extreme caution.*

—Colds and Coughs:

   Oils: eucalyptus, melaleuca (not for cats). Apply on fur or stomach.

—Cows:

   Oils: For scours, use 5 drops DigestZen on stomach (dilute with fractionated coconut oil to cover a larger area). Repeat 2 hours later.

—Dogs:

   –Anxiety/Nervousness

      Oils: Serenity, lavender, Balance. Rub 1–2 drops between hands, and apply to muzzle, between toes, on tops of feet for the dog to smell, and on edges of ears.

   –Arthritis:

      Oils: frankincense

      Blend 1: Blend equal parts rosemary, lavender, and ginger. Dilute with fractionated coconut oil, and apply topically on affected joints.

–Bone Injury:

> Oils: ⬡wintergreen

–Dermatitis:

> Oils: ⬡melaleuca⬡. Note: Some adverse effects have been reported with the use of larger amounts of melaleuca oil on some species of dogs. Contact a veterinarian before using melaleuca on a dog. For smaller dogs, use only a small amount of oil, heavily diluted.

–Heart Problems:

> Oils: ⬡peppermint (on paws), ⬡On Guard (apply on back with warm compress)

–Sleep:

> Oils: ⬡lavender (on paws), ⬡Serenity (on stomach)

–Stroke:

> Oils: ⬡frankincense (on brain stem/back of neck), ⬡Balance (on each paw)

–Ticks and Bug Bites:

> Oils: ⬡Purify (drop directly on tick, or dilute and apply to wound)

–Travel Sickness:

> Oils: ⬡peppermint (dilute, and rub on stomach)

—Earache:

> Blend 2: Combine 1 drop melaleuca, 1 drop lavender, and 1 drop Roman chamomile in 1 tsp. (5 ml) fractionated coconut oil. Apply 1–2 drops to inside and outside of ear.

—Ear Infections:

> Oils: ⬡Purify. Dip cotton swab in oil, and apply to inside and front of ear.

—Fleas:

> Oils: ⬡lemongrass, ⬡eucalyptus. Add 1–2 drops of oil to shampoo.

—Horses:

> –Anxiety/Nervousness

> > Oils: ⬡Serenity. Rub 1–2 drops between hands, and apply to nose, knees, tongue, and front of chest.

–Hoof Rot:

> Blend 3: Combine 1 drop Roman chamomile, 1 drop thyme, and 1 drop melissa in 1 tsp. (5 ml) fractionated coconut oil, and apply on location.

–Infection:

> Oils: ⬡On Guard

–Leg Fractures:

> Oils: ⬡ginger. Dilute oil, and apply oil to leg with a hot compress wrapped around the leg. Massage leg after the fracture is healed with a blend of ⬡rosemary and ⬡thyme diluted with fractionated coconut oil. This may strengthen the ligaments and prevent calcification.

–Muscle Tissue

> Oils: Apply equal parts ⬡lemongrass and ⬡lavender on location, and wrap to help regenerate torn muscle tissue.

–Wounds:

> Oils: ⬡helichrysum

—Parasites:

> Oils: ⬡lavender, ⬡DigestZen, ⬡cedarwood. Rub on paws to help release parasites.

⬡: Apply as directed above. Dilute as recommended, and apply on location.

⬡: Diffuse into the air.

⬡: **Additional Research:**

Sandalwood: Sandalwood oil was found to decrease skin papilloma (tumors) in mice (Dwivedi et al., 1997).

Sandalwood: Alpha-santalol, derived from sandalwood EO, was found to delay and decrease the incidence and multiplicity of skin tumor (papilloma) development in mice (Dwivedi et al., 2003).

Sandalwood: Various concentrations of alpha-santalol (from sandalwood) were tested against skin cancer in mice. All concentrations were found to inhibit skin cancer development (Dwivedi et al., 2005).

Sandalwood: A solution of 5% alpha-santalol (from sandalwood) was found to prevent skin-tumor formation caused by ultraviolet-b (UVB) radiation in mice (Dwivedi et al., 2006).

Sandalwood: Oral sandalwood oil use enhanced GST activity (a protein in cell membranes that can help eliminate toxins) and acid-soluble SH levels. This suggests a possible chemopreventive action on carcinogenesis (Banerjee et al., 1993).

Sandalwood: Pre-treatment with alpha-santalol before UVB (ultraviolet-b) radiation significantly reduced skin tumor development and multiplicity and induced proapoptotic and tumor-suppressing proteins (Arasada et al., 2008).

Frankincense: An acetone extract of frankincense was found to decrease arthritic sores, reduce paw edema (swelling), and suppress pro-inflammatory cytokines (cellular messengers) (Fan et al., 2008).

Melaleuca: A cream with 10% tea tree oil was found to be more effective at treating dermatitis in dogs than a commercially available skin cream (Reichling et al., 2004).

See the Quick Usage Chart inside the back cover for recommended dilutions.

Lime, Lavender, Marjoram, Oregano, Peppermint, Helichrysum: Malacalm, a commercially available mixture containing lime, lavender, marjoram, oregano, peppermint, and helichrysum essential oils, was clinically successful at treating *Malassezia pachydermatis* (a fungal skin infection) in dogs (Nardoni et al., 2014).

Oregano: Four out of seven cats with the fungus mycoses (*Microsporum canis*) recovered both clinically and culturally with topical application of diluted oregano oil for a month (Mugnaini et al., 2012).

Anorexia

See Eating Disorders: Anorexia

Antibacterial

See also Disinfectant

The term antibacterial refers to anything that kills bacteria or that limits its ability to grow or reproduce.

> *Simple Solutions—Antibacterial:* Add 5 drops of On Guard to a damp rag, and use to wipe down surfaces.

Oils: On Guard, melaleuca, thyme, cinnamon, Stronger, peppermint, Purify, litsea, pink pepper, lemon myrtle, lime, lemongrass, helichrysum, geranium, rosemary, clove, oregano, turmeric, Breathe, cypress, arborvitae, cedarwood, basil, cassia, lemon, eucalyptus, grapefruit, marjoram, clary sage, lavender, frankincense, juniper berry

Blend 1: For an antibiotic blend, place 12 drops of On Guard, 6 drops oregano, and 2 drops frankincense in a size "00" capsule, and ingest every 4–8 hours.

Other Products: On Guard+ Softgels, On Guard Foaming Hand Wash & Correct-X to help eliminate bacteria on the skin, On Guard Cleaner Concentrate to help eliminate bacteria from household surfaces, PB Assist+, PB Assist Jr, GX Assist to help support the intestinal tract against harmful bacteria.

—Airborne Bacteria:

Oils: cinnamon, lemongrass, geranium, On Guard, Purify, Stronger, oregano

—Cleansing:

Oils: Purify

Common Bacterial Infections

- Bacterial Meningitis
- Eye Infections
- Otitis Media (Middle Ear Infection)
- Strep Throat
- Upper Respiratory Tract Infection
- Tuberculosis
- Pneumonia
- Gastritis
- Food Poisoning
- Urinary Tract Infections
- Lyme Disease
- Sexually Transmitted Diseases
- Skin Infections

—MRSA (Methicillin Resistant *Staphylococcus aureus*):

Oils: melaleuca, oregano, geranium, On Guard, frankincense, peppermint, lemon myrtle, lemon, thyme, cinnamon, clove, eucalyptus, lemongrass, orange, grapefruit, lavender

Recipe 1: Place 2–5 drops each of oregano, On Guard, and frankincense (followed by lemon and peppermint) on bottoms of feet every 2 hours.

—Staph (*Staphylococcus aureus*) Infection:

Oils: On Guard, melaleuca, oregano, helichrysum, thyme, geranium, Purify, lavender Note: peppermint may make a staph infection more painful.

Other Products: On Guard+ Softgels

⊖: Dilute as recommended, and apply on location. Dilute and apply to liver area and bottoms of the feet. Use hand wash as directed on packaging.

◐: Place 1–2 drops of oil under the tongue, or place oils in empty capsules and swallow. Take supplements as directed.

⊘: Diffuse into the air. Combine a few drops in a small spray bottle with distilled water, and spray into the air.

⊕: **Body System(s) Affected: Immune System.**

▭ **Additional Research:**

Melaleuca: Tea tree oil was found to disrupt the cellular membrane and inhibited respiration in *Candida albicans*, Gram-negative *E. coli*, and Gram-positive *Staphylococcus aureus* (Staph) (Cox et al., 2000).

Melaleuca: In a human trial, most patients receiving treatment with Melaleuca alternifolia oil placed topically on boils experienced healing or reduction of symptoms; while of those receiving no treatment (control), half required surgical intervention, and all still demonstrated signs of the infection (Feinblatt et al., 1960).

Melaleuca: Gram-positive strains of *Staphylococcus aureus* and *Enterococcus faecalis* were shown to have very low frequencies of resistance to tea tree oil (Hammer et al., 2008).

Melaleuca: Tea tree, peppermint, and sage oils were found to inhibit oral bacteria, with thymol and eugenol being the most active components of these oils (Shapiro et al., 1994).

Melaleuca: Cinnamon oil exhibited a strong antimicrobial activity against two detrimental oral bacteria. Manuka, tea tree, and the component thymol also exhibited antimicrobial potency (Filoche et al., 2005).

Melaleuca: MRSA (methicillin-resistant staph) and MSSA (methicillin-sensitive staph) in biofilms (plaque/microcolonies) were eradicated by a 5% solution of tea tree oil, as were 5 of 9 CoNS (coagulase-negative staph) (Brady et al., 2006).

Melaleuca: 66 isolates of *Staphylococcus aureus* (Staph), including 64 methicillin-resistant (MRSA) and 33 mupirocin-resistant strains, were inhibited by tea tree essential oil (Carson et al., 1995).

Melaleuca: A combination of Citricidal and geranium oil demonstrated strong antibacterial effects on MRSA. Geranium and tea tree demonstrated strong antibacterial effects on *Staphylococcus aureus* (Edwards-Jones et al., 2004).

Melaleuca: Tea tree oil and its component terpinen-4-ol demonstrated antibacterial activity against *Staphylococcus aureus* (Staph) bacteria, superior to the activities of several antibiotic drugs—even against antibiotic-resistant strains (Ferrini et al., 2006).

Melaleuca: Tea tree oil demonstrated ability to kill *Staphylococcus aureus* (Staph) bacteria both within biofilms and in the stationary growth phase at concentrations below 1% (Kwieciński et al., 2009).

Melaleuca: Turpin-4-ol, found in tea tree oil, was found to effectively inhibit MRSA and CoNS, while not exhibiting toxicity to human fibroblast cells (Loughlin et al., 2008).

Thyme: Tea tree, peppermint, and sage oils were found to inhibit oral bacteria, with thymol and eugenol being the most active components of these oils (Shapiro et al., 1994).

Thyme: Cinnamon oil exhibited a strong antimicrobial activity against two detrimental oral bacteria. Manuka, tea tree, and the component thymol also exhibited antimicrobial potency (Filoche et al., 2005).

Thyme: Cinnamon bark, lemongrass, and thyme oils were found to have the highest level of activity against common respiratory pathogens among 14 essential oils tested (Inouye et al., 2001).

Thyme: Thyme oil demonstrated a strong antibacterial effect against Staph and *E. coli* bacteria (Mohsenzadeh et al., 2007).

Thyme: Oils with aldehydes or phenols as major components demonstrated a high level of antibacterial activity (Inouye et al., 2001).

Cinnamon: Cinnamon oil exhibited a strong antimicrobial activity against two detrimental oral bacteria. Manuka, tea tree, and the component thymol also exhibited antimicrobial potency (Filoche et al., 2005).

Cinnamon: Cinnamon bark, lemongrass, and thyme oils were found to have the highest level of activity against common respiratory pathogens among 14 essential oils tested (Inouye et al., 2001).

Peppermint: Tea tree, peppermint, and sage oils were found to inhibit oral bacteria, with thymol and eugenol being the most active components of these oils (Shapiro et al., 1994).

Peppermint: Peppermint and spearmint oil inhibited resistant strains of Staphylococcus, *E. coli*, Salmonella, and *Helicobacter pylori* (Imai et al., 2001).

Peppermint: Peppermint and rosemary oils were each found to be more effective at preventing dental biofilm (plaque) formation than chlorhexidine (an antiseptic) (Rasooli et al., 2008).

Litsea: Essential oil from the fruit of *Litsea cubeba* demonstrated an excellent antibacterial property (Su et al., 2016).

Pink pepper: Schinus molle essential oil was found to demonstrate antibacterial properties against several strains of gram-positive and gram-negative bacteria (Martins et al., 2014; Guerra-Boone et al., 2013; Gundidza, 1993).

Lemongrass: Cinnamon bark, lemongrass, and thyme oils were found to have the highest level of activity against common respiratory pathogens among 14 essential oils tested (Inouye et al., 2001).

Lemongrass: A formulation of lemongrass and geranium oil was found to reduce airborne bacteria by 89% in an office environment after diffusion for 15 hours (Doran et al., 2009).

Lemongrass: Lemongrass and lemon verbena oil were found to be bactericidal to *Helicobacter pylori* at very low concentrations. Additionally, it was found that this bacteria did not develop a resistance to lemongrass oil after 10 passages, while this bacteria did develop resistance to clarithromycin (an antibiotic) under the same conditions (Ohno et al., 2003).

Helichrysum: Helichrysum oil was found to exhibit definite antibacterial activity against six tested Gram (+/-) bacteria (Chinou et al., 1996).

Helichrysum: Helichrysum was found to inhibit both the growth and some of the enzymes of the *Staphylococcus aureus* (staph) bacteria (Nostro et al., 2001).

Geranium: A combination of Citricidal and geranium oil demonstrated strong antibacterial effects on MRSA. Geranium and tea tree demonstrated strong antibacterial effects on *Staphylococcus aureus* (Edwards-Jones et al., 2004).

Geranium: A formulation of lemongrass and geranium oil was found to reduce airborne bacteria by 89% in an office environment after diffusion for 15 hours (Doran et al., 2009).

Rosemary: Peppermint and rosemary oils were each found to be more effective at preventing dental biofilm (plaque) formation than chlorhexidine (an antiseptic) (Rasooli et al., 2008).

Oregano: Oregano oil was found to inhibit MRSA (Nostro et al., 2004).

Cypress: Cypress essential oil was found to possess antibacterial activity against *Staphlococcus aureus*, *Klebsiella pneumoniae*, and *Salmonella indica* when tested for antimicrobial properties against 13 microorganisms (Selim et al., 2014).

Cassia: Cinnamaldehyde, the main constituent of cassia oil, showed strong growth inhibiting activity toward five human intestinal bacteria in vitro (Lee et al., 1998).

Arborvitae: Arborvitae essential oil vapor and liquid displayed bactericidal activity against seven bacteria (including three Gram-positive organisms, Bacillus subtilis, Streptococcus pyogenes, and *Enterococcus fecalis*, and four Gram-negative organisms, *Acinetobacter baumannii*, *Hemophilus influenzae*, *Salmonella enteritidis*, and *Escherichia coli*) as well as the bacterial spores of Bacillus subtilis (Hudson et al., 2011).

Lavender: Scanning electron microscopy analysis and zeta potential measurement revealed that lavender essential oil's antibacterial action against multidrug-resistant *Escherichia coli* occurs via two mechanisms: alteration of outer membrane permeability and possible inhibition of bacterial quorum sensing (Yap et al., 2014).

Anticatarrhal

See Congestion: Catarrh

See the *Quick Usage Chart* inside the back cover for recommended dilutions.

Anticoagulant

See Blood: Clots

Antidepressant

See Depression

Antifungal

Fungi are a broad range of organisms such as yeast, mold, and mushrooms. While many fungi are safe and beneficial, some create mycotoxins, which are chemicals that can be toxic to plants, animals, and humans. Examples of fungi that can be detrimental to humans include black mold, *Candida*, and ringworm.

> *Simple Solutions—Antifungal:* Diffuse On Guard in an aromatherapy diffuser.

> *Simple Solutions—Antifungal:* Mix 20 drops On Guard with ¼ cup (50 ml) water in a small spray bottle, spray on surfaces, and wipe down.

> *Simple Solutions—Nails:* Apply melaleuca oil to toenails to help keep a clean appearance.

Oils: melaleuca, oregano, thyme, cinnamon, clove, On Guard, arborvitae, lavender, peppermint, rosemary, lemon, turmeric, Stronger, spikenard, lemon myrtle, Purify, blue tansy, patchouli, lemongrass, pink pepper, juniper berry, geranium

Other Products: On Guard Foaming Hand Wash, On Guard Cleaner Concentrate, PB Assist+, PB Assist Jr, GX Assist

—Athlete's Foot:

Athlete's foot (tinea pedis) is a fungal infection that develops on the skin of the feet. This infection causes itching, redness, and scaling of the skin, and in severe cases it can cause painful blistering or cracking of the skin.

> *Simple Solutions—Athlete's Foot:* Mix 25 drops melaleuca with 2 Tbs. (15 g) cornstarch, and sprinkle a small amount in shoes each night.

Oils: melaleuca, oregano, turmeric, cypress, thyme, geranium, lavender

—Candida:

Candida refers to a genus of yeast that are normally found in the digestive tract and on the skin of humans. These yeast are typically symbiotically beneficial to humans. However, several species of *Candida*, most commonly *Candida albicans*, can cause infections such as vaginal candidiasis or thrush (oral candidiasis) that cause localized itching, soreness, and redness *(see Vaginal: Candida for further application methods)*. In immune system–compromised individuals, these infection-causing species of *Candida* can spread further, leading to serious, life-threatening complications.

Oils: melaleuca, oregano, clove, On Guard, Stronger, peppermint, thyme, dill, cilantro, lavender, lemon myrtle, eucalyptus, rosemary, spikenard, DigestZen

—Mold:

Mold are a type of microscopic multi-cellular fungi that grow together to form filaments. Mold is found throughout the world and can survive in extreme conditions. While most mold does not adversely affect humans, an over-abundance of mold spores can cause allergies or other problems within the respiratory system. Additionally, some types of mold produce toxins that can be harmful to humans or to animals.

Oils: On Guard, clove, thyme, cinnamon, oregano, rosemary, Purify

—Ringworm:

Ringworm (or tinea) is a fungal infection of the skin that can cause itching, redness, and scaling of the skin. The name comes from the ring-shaped patches that often form on the skin.

Oils: melaleuca, oregano, turmeric, peppermint, thyme, bergamot, geranium, lavender

Blend 1: Combine 2 drops lavender, 2 drops melaleuca, and 2 drops thyme. Apply 1–2 drops on ringworm three times a day for 10 days. Then mix 30 drops melaleuca with 2 Tbs. (25 ml) fractionated coconut oil, and use daily until ringworm is gone.

Primary Recommendations • Secondary Recommendations • Other Recommendations / ✷=Aromatic, ✷=Topical, ○=Internal

—Thrush:

Thrush is another name for oral candidiasis (*see Candida above*). Thrush results in uncomfortable or painful white or yellow patches in the mouth.

Oils: ⊕melaleuca⊕, ⊕lavender, ⊕eucalyptus, ⊕marjoram, ⊕thyme

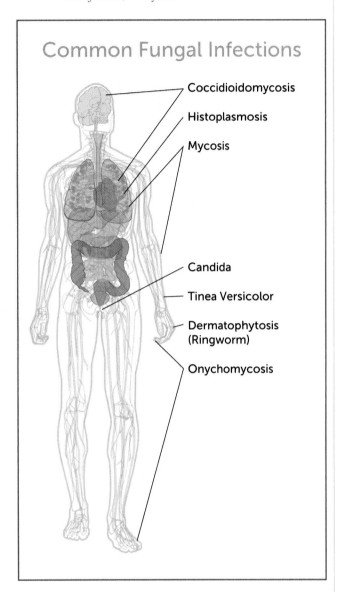

Common Fungal Infections

- Coccidioidomycosis
- Histoplasmosis
- Mycosis
- Candida
- Tinea Versicolor
- Dermatophytosis (Ringworm)
- Onychomycosis

🔄: Dilute as recommended, and apply on location. Apply as a warm compress over affected area.

🌀: Diffuse into the air.

⊙: Take capsules as directed on package.

⊕: **Body System(s) Affected:** Immune System.

📖: **Additional Research:**

Melaleuca: Tea tree oil was found to inhibit 301 different types of yeasts isolated from the mouths of cancer patients suffering from advanced cancer, including 41 strains that are known to be resistant to antifungal drugs (Bagg et al., 2006).

Melaleuca: Eleven types of Candida were found to be highly inhibited by tea tree oil (Banes-Marshall et al., 2001).

Melaleuca: Tea tree oil was found to disrupt the cellular membrane and to inhibit respiration in *Candida albicans* (Cox et al., 2000).

Melaleuca: Melaleuca oil at concentrations of .16% was found to inhibit the transformation of C. albicans from single-cell yeast to the pathogenic mycelial (multi-cellular strands) form (D'Auria et al., 2001).

Melaleuca: Tea tree oil was found to alter the membrane properties and functions of *Candida albicans* cells, leading to cell inhibition or death (Hammer et al., 2004).

Melaleuca: Terpinen-4-ol, a constituent of tea tree oil, and tea tree oil were found to be effective against several forms of vaginal Candida infections in rats, including azole-resistant forms (Mondello et al., 2006).

Melaleuca: Melaleuca oil inhibited several Candida species in vitro (Vazquez et al., 2000).

Melaleuca: Patients with tinea pedis (athlete's foot) were found to have a higher rate of cure and a higher clinical response when treated topically with 25 or 50% tea tree oil solution compared to control (Satchell et al., 2002).

Melaleuca: When applied as a coating to protect oranges after harvest, a mixture containing chitosan and melaleuca essential oil was found to reduce fungal growth by 50% (Cháfer et al., 2012).

Oregano: In a test of nine oils, clove, followed by cinnamon, oregano, and mace oil, was found to be inhibitory to two toxin-producing fungi. It was also shown that whole and ground cloves stored with grain reduced the amount of aflatoxin contamination (Juglal et al., 2002).

Oregano: The vapor of oregano oil was found to be fungicidal against the Trichophyton mentagrophytes fungi (a fungus that causes a skin infection known as Malabar itch) (Inouye et al., 2006).

Oregano: Mice infected with *Candida albicans* who were fed origanum oil or carvacrol diluted in olive oil had an 80% survival rate after 30 days, while infected mice fed olive oil alone all died after 10 days (Manohar et al., 2001).

Oregano: Cinnamon, thyme, oregano, and cumin oils inhibited the production of aflatoxin by aspergillus fungus (Tantaoui-Elaraki et al., 1994).

Thyme: Cinnamon, thyme, oregano, and cumin oils inhibited the production of aflatoxin by aspergillus fungus (Tantaoui-Elaraki et al., 1994).

Thyme: Thyme oil was found to inhibit Candida species by causing lesions in the cell membrane, as well as inhibiting germ tube (an outgrowth that develops when the fungi is preparing to replicate) formation (Pina-Vaz et al., 2004).

Thyme: Eugenol from clove and thymol from thyme were found to inhibit the growth of Aspergillus flavus and Aspergillus versicolor at concentrations of .4 mg/ml or less (Hitokoto et al., 1980).

Cinnamon: In a test of nine oils, clove, followed by cinnamon, oregano, and mace oil, was found to be inhibitory to two toxin-producing fungi. It was also shown that whole and ground cloves stored with grain reduced the amount of aflatoxin contamination (Juglal et al., 2002).

Cinnamon: Cinnamon, thyme, oregano, and cumin oils inhibited the production of aflatoxin by aspergillus fungus (Tantaoui-Elaraki et al., 1994).

Cinnamon: Vapor of cinnamon bark oil and cinnamic aldehyde was found to be effective against fungi involved in respiratory tract mycoses (fungal infections) (Singh et al., 1995).

Clove: In a test of nine oils, clove, followed by cinnamon, oregano, and mace oil, was found to be inhibitory to two toxin-producing fungi. It was also shown that whole and ground cloves stored with grain reduced the amount of aflatoxin contamination (Juglal et al., 2002).

Clove: Eugenol from clove and thymol from thyme were found to inhibit the growth of Aspergillus flavus and Aspergillus versicolor at concentrations of .4 mg/ml or less (Hitokoto et al., 1980).

Clove: Clove oil was found to have very strong radical scavenging activity (antioxidant). It was also found to display an antifungal effect against tested Candida strains (Chaieb et al., 2007).

Arborvitae: Arborvitae essential oil vapor and liquid displayed antifungal activity against two commonly encountered fungi (the medically important yeast *Candida albicans*, and the filamentous mold Aspergillus niger)(Hudson et al., 2011).

Lavender: Lavandula oil demonstrated antifungal activity against three pathogenic fungi (Behnam et al., 2006).

Lavender: Lavender oil demonstrated both fungistatic (stopped growth) and fungicidal (killed) activity against *Candida albicans* (D'Auria et al., 2005).

See the Quick Usage Chart inside the back cover for recommended dilutions.

Dill: Dill essential oil was demonstrated to induce apoptosis (cell death) in *Candida albicans* in a metacaspase-dependent manner (Chen et al., 2014).

Cilantro: Cilantro essential oil was found to have fungicidal effect against *Candida albicans* and other yeasts. The oil appeared to act by binding to membrane ergosterol, rendering the cell membrane more permeable and ultimately causing cell death (Freires Ide et al., 2014).

Peppermint: Peppermint oil was found to have a higher fungistatic and fungicidal activity against various fungi (including Candida) than the commercial fungicide bifonazole (Mimica-Dukić et al., 2003).

Bergamot: Bergamot essential oil is active in vitro against several common species of ringworm (Sanguinetti et al., 2007).

Rosemary: Rosemary oil was found to inhibit aflatoxin production by aspergillus fungi (a highly toxic and carcinogenic substance produced by these fungi) (Rasooli et al., 2008).

Lemon: Lemon oil was found to be an effective antifungal agent against two bread-mold species (Caccioni et al., 1998).

Turmeric: Ar-turmerone (a component of turmeric oil) was found to inhibit the growth of several fungi responsible for skin conditions such as ringworm and tinea (Mukda et al., 2013).

Cassia: Cassia essential oil was found to have a strong inhibitory effect against *Aspergillus* mold in vitro and in grapes (Kocevski et al., 2013).

Antihemorrhaging

See Blood: Hemorrhaging

Antihistamine

See Allergies

Anti-Infectious

See Infection, Antibacterial, Antiviral, Antifungal

Anti-Inflammatory

See Inflammation

Antimicrobial

See Antibacterial, Antifungal, Antiviral

Antioxidant

As part of its normal metabolic processes, the body uses and creates oxidative molecules, each capable of transferring electrons to itself from other molecules or substances. This type of reaction can create molecules known as free radicals (Davies, 1995). If left unchecked in the body, these free radicals can bind or react with different molecular structures, altering their abilities to function normally. Under normal, healthy conditions, the body's own systems are able to create or metabolize enough antioxidant materials to neutralize the ability of these oxidative molecules to

create free radicals. But when the body comes under stress—including physical stress, psychological stress, poor nutrition, or disease—the amount of oxidative molecules being produced can increase, and the delicate balance between oxidative molecules and antioxidants can be thrown off, potentially overwhelming the body's own antioxidant mechanisms. This "oxidative stress" (Sies, 1997) creates a condition optimal for the formation of many free radicals, which in turn can potentially cause enough damage to the cell's normal structures to cause cell death, mutation, or loss of its ability to function normally within the body (Rhee, 2006; Vertuani et al., 2004).

> *Simple Solutions—Antioxidant:* Add 2 drops clove to olive oil in an empty capsule, and swallow.

Oils: ⭕DDR Prime, 🌀clove⊕, ⭕🌀thyme⊕, 🌀rosemary⊕, ⭕Yarrow Pom, 🌀peppermint⊕, ⭕🌀yarrow⊕, 🌀melaleuca⊕, 🌀helichrysum⊕, 🌀copaiba⊕, ⭕🌀turmeric, 🌀Purify, 🌀On Guard, 🌀Breathe, 🌀Deep Blue, 🌀cinnamon, 🌀frankincense, 🌀oregano⊕, 🌀Roman chamomile, 🌀petitgrain, 🌀spikenard

Other Products: ⭕Alpha CRS+ or ⭕a2z Chewable, which contains polyphenols that act as powerful antioxidants, such as quercetin⊕, epigallocatechin gallate⊕, ellagic acid⊕, resveratrol⊕, baicalin⊕, and others⊕. ⭕Mito2Max. ⭕TerraGreens for a whole food source of essential nutrients and antioxidants.

⭕: Take capsules as directed. Use oils recommended as flavoring agents in cooking. Place 1–3 drops of oil in an empty capsule, and ingest it as a dietary supplement.

🌀: Diffuse into the air. Inhale directly from bottle. Apply oil to hands, tissue, or cotton wick, and inhale.

🌀: Dilute as recommended, and apply on the skin and reflex points on the feet. Dilute in a carrier oil, and massage into the skin. Apply as a hot compress.

➕: **Body System(s) Affected:** Immune System.

📖: **Additional Research:**

Clove: Clove oil was found to have very strong radical scavenging activity (antioxidant). It was also found to display an antifungal effect against tested Candida strains (Chaieb et al., 2007).

Clove: Various essential oils demonstrated an antioxidant effect toward skin lipid squalene oxidized by UV irradiation, with a blend of thyme and clove oil demonstrating the highest inhibitory effect (Wei et al., 2007).

Thyme: Extracts from eucalyptus and thyme were found to have high nitrous oxide scavenging abilities and inhibited nitrous oxide production in macrophage cells. This could possibly explain their role in aiding respiratory inflammatory diseases (Vigo et al., 2004).

Thyme: Older rats whose diets were supplemented with thyme oil were found to have a higher level of the antioxidant enzymes superoxide dismutase and glutathione peroxidase in the heart, liver, and kidneys than older rats without this supplementation (Youdim et al., 1999).

Thyme: Aging rats fed thyme oil or the constituent thymol were found to have higher levels of the antioxidant enzymes superoxide dismutase and glutathione peroxidase in the brain than aging rats not fed the oil or constituent (Youdim et al., 2000).

Rosemary: Extracts from rosemary were found to have high antioxidant properties. Rosmarinic acid and carnosic acid from rosemary were found to have the highest antioxidant activities of studied components of rosemary (Almela et al., 2006).

Rosemary: An ethanol extract of rosemary was found to have an antiproliferative effect on human leukemia and breast carcinoma cells, as well as an antioxidant effect (Cheung et al., 2007).

Rosemary: Extracts from rosemary were found to have high antioxidant levels. Additionally, a methanol extract with 30% carnosic acid, 16% carnosol, and 5% rosmarinic acid were found to be effective against gram-positive and negative bacteria, and yeast (Moreno et al., 2006).

Rosemary: In patients with chronic bronchitis, rosemary, basil, fir, and eucalyptus oils were found to demonstrate an antioxidant effect. Lavender was found to promote normalization of lipid levels (Siurin, 1997).

Peppermint: Peppermint oil was found to be an effective antibacterial and antioxidant agent (Mimica-Dukić et al., 2003).

Peppermint: Peppermint oil fed to mice prior to exposure to gamma radiation was found to decrease levels of damage from oxidation when compared to mice not pretreated with peppermint (Samarth et al., 2006).

Peppermint: Peppermint extract fed orally to mice demonstrated the ability to protect the testes from gamma radiation damage (Samarth et al., 2009).

Yarrow: Yarrow essential oil demonstrated antioxidant and antimicrobial activity against several pathogenic bacteria and fungi (Candan et al., 2003).

Melaleuca: Melaleuca alternifolia oil was found to reduce reactive oxygen species (ROS) production in neutrophils (a type of white blood cell), indicating an antioxidant effect and decreased Interleukin 2 (a chemical messenger that helps trigger an inflammatory response) secretion, while increasing the secretion of Interleukin 4 (a chemical messenger involved in turning off the inflammatory response) (Caldefie-Chézet et al., 2006).

Melaleuca: Melaleuca alternifolia oil was found to mediate the Reactive Oxygen Species (ROS) production of leukocytes (white blood cells), indicating a possible anti-inflammatory activity (Caldefie-Chézet et al., 2004).

Copaiba: The overproduction of oxygen radicals, specifically NO and H_2O_2, and cytokines (both involved in the etiology of MS) by mouse splenocytes was significantly inhibited by copaiba oil (Dias et al., 2014).

Helichrysum: Arzanol (extracted from helichrysum), at non-cytotoxic concentrations, showed a strong inhibition of TBH-induced oxidative stress in VERO cells (Rosa et al., 2007).

Oregano: The antioxidant activity of oregano essential oil added to extra virgin olive oil at 0.05% was found to retard the lipid oxidation process in olive oil and prolong the olive oil's shelf life (Asensio et al., 2011).

Quercetin: Quercetin was found to increase plasma antioxidant status in healthy volunteers who took it as a supplement over four weeks (Boots et al., 2008).

Epigallocatechin gallate: Epigallocatechin-3-gallate (EGCG) supplementation was found to improve the antioxidant status of heat-stressed Japanese quail (Tuzcu et al., 2008).

Epigallocatechin gallate: Epigallocatechin-3-gallate (EGCG) was found to improve body weight and increase enzymatic and non-enzymatic antioxidants in bleomycin-induced pulmonary fibrosis in rats (Sriram et al., 2008).

Ellagic acid: Ellagic acid supplementation was found to significantly decrease mitochondrial and microsomal lipid peroxidation in endrin-induced hepatic lipid peroxidation (Bagchi et al., 1993).

Resveratrol: Resveratrol was found to act as an antioxidant and to reverse the anti-apoptotic effects of repetitive oxidative stress on lung fibroblasts in vitro (Chakraborty et al., 2008).

Baicalin: Baicalin was found to be an effective antioxidant, and to counteract oxidative stress induced to retinal cells and brain membranes of rats (Jung et al., 2008).

Other Polyphenols: Extracts from bilberry and blueberry were found to have higher ORAC values than strawberry, cranberry, elderberry, or raspberry and were found to significantly inhibit both H_2O_2 and TNF alpha induced VEGF expression by human keratinocytes (Roy et al., 2002).

Other Polyphenols: Catechins and procyanidins extracted from various berries were found to provide substantial antioxidant protection (Maatta-Riihinet et al., 2005).

Other Polyphenols: Oral supplementation of bilberry extract was found to reduce the degree of oxidative stress and kidney damage by potassium bromate oxidization in mice (Bao et al., 2008).

Antiparasitic

See **Parasites**

Antirheumatic

See **Arthritis: Rheumatoid Arthritis**

Antiseptic

See **Antibacterial, Antifungal, Antiviral**

Antiviral

The term "antiviral" refers to something that is able to inhibit or stop the development, function, or replication of an infection-causing virus.

> *Simple Solutions—Cold Sores:* **Combine 4 tsp. (5 g) beeswax pellets, 1 Tbs. (10 g) cocoa butter, and 3 Tbs. (45 ml) jojoba oil, and melt in the microwave (30 seconds at a time, stirring in between) or in a double boiler. Cool slightly, and add 5 drops melissa, 5 drops peppermint, and 5 drops helichrysum essential oil. Pour in small jars or lip balm containers, and allow to cool completely. Apply a small amount of balm on cold sores as needed.**

Oils: 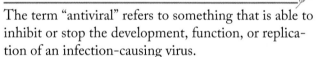helichrysum, melaleuca, clove, On Guard, melissa, Breathe, lime, cinnamon, lemon, oregano, peppermint, eucalyptus, thyme, orange, grapefruit, clary sage, juniper berry, myrrh, pink pepper, geranium, lavender, sandalwood, rosemary, cypress

Other Products: On Guard+ Softgels, On Guard Foaming Hand Wash to help protect against

See the *Quick Usage Chart* inside the back cover for recommended dilutions.

skin-borne microorganisms, 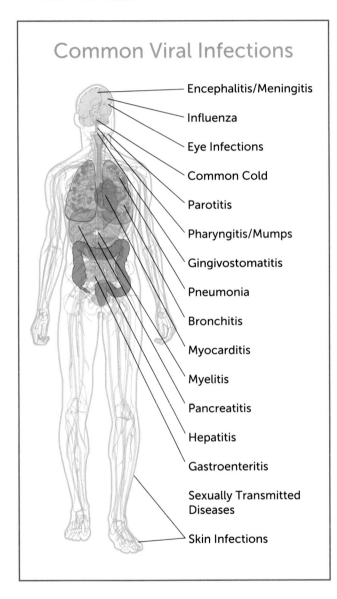On Guard Cleaner Concentrate to help eliminate microorganisms from household surfaces. **O**On Guard Protecting Throat Drops to soothe irritated and sore throats. **O**Alpha CRS+, **O**a2z Chewable, **O**xEO Mega or vEO Mega, **O**IQ Mega, **O**Microplex VMz to help support the immune system.

—**Airborne Viruses:**

Oils: On Guard

Common Viral Infections

Encephalitis/Meningitis
Influenza
Eye Infections
Common Cold
Parotitis
Pharyngitis/Mumps
Gingivostomatitis
Pneumonia
Bronchitis
Myocarditis
Myelitis
Pancreatitis
Hepatitis
Gastroenteritis
Sexually Transmitted Diseases
Skin Infections

—**Ebola Virus:**

Oils: cinnamon, oregano

—**Epstein-Barr Virus:**

Oils: On Guard

—**Herpes Simplex:**

Oils: peppermint, clove, helichrysum, melaleuca, lavender, eucalyptus, cypress, lemon

—**HIV:** *See also* AIDS

Oils: helichrysum, On Guard, lemon, Balance

—**Respiratory:**

Oils: eucalyptus, On Guard

—**Spine:**

Blend 1: 5 drops oregano and 5 drops thyme. Apply to bottoms of feet and along the spine.

: Dilute as recommended, and apply on location or to reflex points on the bottoms of the feet. Use hand wash as directed on packaging.

: Diffuse into the air. Inhale oil applied to a tissue or cotton wick.

: Take capsules as directed on package.

: **Body System(s) Affected:** Immune System.

: **Additional Research:**

Helichrysum: Arzanol, extracted from helichrysum, inhibited HIV-1 replication in T cells and also inhibited the release of pro-inflammatory cytokines (chemical messengers) in monocytes (Appendino et al., 2007).

Helichrysum: Helichrysum was found to have significant antiviral activity against the herpes virus at non-cytotoxic concentrations (Nostro et al., 2003).

Melaleuca: Tea tree and eucalyptus oil demonstrated an ability to inhibit the Herpes simplex virus (Schnitzler et al., 2001).

Clove: Eugenol (found in clove oil) was found to be virucidal to Herpes simplex and to delay the development of herpes-induced keratitis (inflammation of the cornea) in mice (Benencia et al., 2000).

Melissa: Melissa oil demonstrated inhibition of Herpes simplex type 1 and 2 viruses (Schnitzler et al., 2008).

Peppermint: Peppermint oil demonstrated a direct virucidal activity against herpes type 1 and 2 viruses (Schuhmacher et al., 2003).

Eucalyptus: Tea tree and eucalyptus oil demonstrated an ability to inhibit the Herpes simplex virus (Schnitzler et al., 2001).

Menthol, thymol, methyl salicylate, and eucalyptol: A trial including 80 subjects with *Herpes labialis* showed that rinsing with an essential oil containing mouthrinse resulted in effectively zero recoverable virions at 30 seconds post rinse and a significant reduction in saliva viral presence 30 minutes post rinse, suggesting that an essential oil mouthrinse can reduce viral contamination of saliva (Meiller et al., 2005).

Anxiety

Anxiety is the body's way of preparing itself to deal with a threat or to deal with future stressful events. While this response is normal and happens as part of the body's natural response to stress, this response can also happen at inappropriate times or too frequently, as in the case of anxiety disorders. Anxiety can include both physical and mental symptoms such as fear, nervousness, nausea, sweating, increased blood pressure and heart rate, feelings of apprehension or dread, difficulty concentrating, irritability, restlessness, panic attacks, and many others.

Simple Solutions—Anxiety: Diffuse lavender in an aromatherapy diffuser when feeling anxious.

Simple Solutions—Anxiety: Combine 5 drops orange and 10 drops lemon with 1 tsp. (5 ml) water in a small spray bottle, and spray into the air and inhale as needed.

Oils: lavender, orange, lemon, copaiba, rose, magnolia, Peace, InTune, Serenity, Calmer, Brave, Steady, Thinker, Motivate, AromaTouch, Elevation, Balance (on back of neck) and Breathe (on chest), neroli, blue tansy, ylang ylang, melissa, frankincense, sandalwood, cedarwood, juniper berry, Citrus Bliss, bergamot, geranium, lime, clary sage, basil, cypress, marjoram, Douglas fir

Other Products: Therapeutic Bath Salts. Add 1–2 drops of essential oil to ¼ cup (50 g) bath salts, and dissolve in warm bathwater for an anxiety-relieving bath.

: Diffuse into the air. Inhale directly from bottle. Apply oil to hands, tissue, or cotton wick, and inhale.

: Place 1–2 drops in 1 Tbs. (15 ml) fractionated coconut oil, and massage into the skin. Dilute as recommended, and apply to back of neck, temples, or reflex points on feet. Add 1–2 drops to ¼ cup (50 g) bath salts, and dissolve in warm bathwater.

: **Body System(s) Affected:** Nervous System and Emotional Balance.

: **Additional Research:**

Lavender: Exposure to lavender odor was found to decrease anxiety in gerbils in the elevated plus maze, with a further decrease in anxiety in females after prolonged (2 week) exposure (Bradley et al., 2007).

Lavender: Subjects receiving a lozenge containing lavender oil, hops extract, lemon balm, and oat were found to have increases in alpha 1, alpha 2, and beta 1 electrical output (Dimpfel et al., 2004).

Lavender: In patients admitted to an intensive care unit, those receiving lavender aromatherapy reported a greater improvement in mood and perceived levels of anxiety compared to those receiving massage or a period of rest (Dunn et al., 1995).

Lavender: Female patients being treated for chronic hemodialysis demonstrated less anxiety when exposed to lavender aroma compared to control (Itai et al., 2000).

Lavender: Lavender oil was found to demonstrate anticonflict effects in mice similar to the anxiolytic (antianxiety) drug diazepam (Umezu, 2000).

Lavender: Patients waiting for dental treatment were found to be less anxious and to have a better mood when exposed to the odor of lavender or orange oil as compared to control (Lehrner et al., 2005).

Lavender and Roman Chamomile: A study with 56 percutaneous coronary intervention patients in an intensive care unit found that an aromatherapy blend of lavender, Roman chamomile, and neroli decreased anxiety and improved sleep quality when compared to conventional nursing intervention (Cho et al., 2013).

Orange: Patients waiting for dental treatment were found to be less anxious and to have a better mood when exposed to the odor of lavender or orange oil as compared to control (Lehrner et al., 2005).

Orange: Bitter orange peel oil taken orally by mice was found to reduce anxiety, increase sleeping time, and increase the time before a chemically induced seizure started (Carvalho-Freitas et al., 2002).

Orange: Female patients waiting for dental treatment were found to be less anxious, more positive, and more calm when exposed to orange oil odor than patients who were not exposed to the orange oil odor (Lehrner et al., 2000).

Orange: Dental patients (aged 6–9 years) displayed reduced salivary cortisol, pulse rate, and anxiety while undergoing dental treatments when inhaling wild orange essential oil, compared to no aroma (Jafarzadeh et al., 2013).

Orange: Healthy male subjects displayed reduced anxiety after five minutes of inhalation of orange essential oil compared to the inhalation of melaleuca essential oil or distilled water when submitted to an anxiety inducing situation (Goes et al., 2012).

Orange: Rats subjected to the elevated plus-maze following exposure to the aroma of orange essential oil for five minutes displayed reduced anxiety as compared to exposure to melaleuca essential oil (Faturi et al., 2010).

Lemon: Lemon oil was found to have an antistress effect on mice involved in several behavioral tasks (Komiya et al., 2006).

Copaiba: In the elevated plus maze, copaiba oil was found to demonstrate anxiolitic effects on rats comparable to the antianxiety drug diazepam (Curio et al., 2009).

Rose: Inhalation and a warm foot bath with rose oil was found to decrease anxiety levels in women during the first stage of labor (Kheirkhah et al., 2014).

Rose: Self-massage with rose oil was found to help decrease pain and anxiety in women experiencing menstrual pain (Kim et al., 2011).

Melissa: Results of a clinical trial indicate that a combination of melissa and valerian oils may have anxiety-reducing properties at some doses (Kennedy et al., 2006).

Bergamot: Inhalation of bergamot essential oil produced similar anxiolytic results as acute injection of an antianxiety drug, diazepam, administered to mice subjected to two behavioral measurements of anxiety (the elevated plus maze test and the hole-board test) (Saiyudthong et al., 2011). Bergamot essential oil also reduced the corticosterone response to stress exposure of the mice (Saiyudthong et al., 2011).

Clary Sage: Dietary administration of clary sage oil (from conception) was found to have an anti-anxiety and submissive effect on mice, when compared to administration of sunflower oil (from conception and weaning) and clary sage (from weaning) (Gross et al., 2013).

Cassia: A single treatment of cassia extract decreased anxiety in mice by causing a change of serotonin receptors in the dorsal raphe nucleus (Jung et al., 2012).

Cypress: In rats, *Chamaecyparis obtusa* essential oil (a Japanese plant belonging to the same botanical family as cypress essential oil) decreased anxiety-related behaviors caused by the early life stress of maternal separation. This decrease in anxiety was comparable to the effects of fluoxetine, a drug commonly used to treat depression and anxiety disorders. The same study found that cytokine gene expression in the hippocampus was altered by the inhalation of *Chamaecyparis obtusa* (Park et al., 2014).

Aromatherapy Massage: Results from a randomized, controlled trial suggest that aromatherapy massage can be an effective therapeutic option for the short-term management of mild to moderate anxiety and depression in patients with cancer (Wilkinson et al., 2007).

Carvacrol in thyme and oregano: Carvacrol is a monoterpenic phenol found in thyme and oregano. Oral administration of carvacrol produced antianxiety-like effects in mice (Melo et al., 2010).

See the Quick Usage Chart inside the back cover for recommended dilutions.

Apathy

See Depression

Aphrodisiac

An aphrodisiac is a substance used to stimulate feelings of love or sexual desire. Many books of aromatherapy tout the aphrodisiac qualities of a number of oils. Perhaps an aphrodisiac to one individual may not be to another. The most important factor is to find an oil that brings balance to the mind and body. A balanced individual is more likely to extend love.

> *Simple Solutions—Aphrodisiac:* Blend 2 Tbs. (25 ml) jojoba oil with 10 drops ylang ylang, 6 drops patchouli, 5 drops clove, 6 drops orange, and 2 drops clary sage.

> *Simple Solutions—Aphrodisiac:* Dissolve 2 drops ylang ylang, 2 drops clary sage, 1 drop lemongrass, and 2 drops sandalwood in 2 tsp. (10 ml) of pure grain (or perfumer's) alcohol. Combine with water in a 1 oz. spray bottle. Mist into the air and on bed linens.

Oils: sandalwood, ylang ylang, rose, jasmine, Whisper, cinnamon, ginger, clary sage

: Diffuse into the air. Dissolve 2–3 drops in 2 tsp. (10 ml) pure grain or perfumer's alcohol, combine with distilled water in a 1–2 oz. spray bottle, and spray into the air or on clothes or bed linens.

: Dilute as recommended and wear on temples, neck, or wrists as a perfume or cologne. Combine 3–5 drops of your desired essential oil with 1 Tbs. (15 ml) fractionated coconut oil to use as a massage oil. Combine 1–2 drops with ¼ cup (50 g) Therapeutic Bath Salts, and dissolve in warm bathwater for a romantic bath.

: **Body System(s) Affected:** Emotional Balance.

Appetite

Appetite is the body's desire to eat, expressed as hunger. Appetite is important in regulating food intake to provide the body with the necessary nutrients to sustain life and maintain energy.

> *Simple Solutions—Appetite:* Diffuse grapefruit in an aromatherapy diffuser to help quell cravings.

—Loss of Appetite:

Oils: lavender, ginger, lemon, orange

—Suppressant:

Oils: Slim & Sassy, grapefruit

Other Products: Slim & Sassy TrimShakes

: Add 8 drops of Slim & Sassy to 2 cups (500 ml) of water, and drink throughout the day between meals. Drink Trim or V Shake 1–2 times a day as a meal alternative.

: Diffuse into the air. Inhale oil applied to a tissue or cotton wick.

: **Body System(s) Affected:** Digestive System, Nervous System, and Endocrine System.

: **Additional Research:**

Lavender: Lavender oil was found to inhibit sympathetic nerve activity while exciting parasympathetic nerve activity and increasing appetite and weight gain in rats. Linalool, a component of lavender, was shown to have similar effects (Shen et al., 2005).

Grapefruit: The scent of grapefruit oil and its component, limonene, was found to affect the autonomic nerves by exciting sympathetic nerve activity and inhibiting parasympathetic nerve activity. It was also found to reduce appetite and body weight in rats exposed to the oil for 15 minutes three times per week (Shen et al., 2005).

Arteries

See also Blood, Cardiovascular System

Arteries are the vessels of the circulatory system that function to carry blood away from the heart.

—Arterial Vasodilator:

A vasodilator is a substance that causes a blood vessel to dilate (increase in diameter) through the relaxation of the endothelial cells lining the vessel walls. This gives the blood more room to flow and lowers blood pressure.

Oils: eucalyptus, rosemary, marjoram

—Atherosclerosis:

Atherosclerosis is a hardening of the arteries due to a build-up of plaques along the arterial wall.

Oils: lemon, lavender, rosemary, ginger, cedarwood, thyme, juniper berry, wintergreen

: Dilute as recommended, and apply to carotid arteries in neck, over heart, and reflex points on the feet.

⟳: Diffuse into the air. Inhale directly from bottle. Apply oil to hands, tissue, or cotton wick, and inhale.

⊕: **Body System(s) Affected:** Cardiovascular System

⊡: **Additional Research:**

Eucalyptus: Treatment of rats with 1,8-cineole (or eucalyptol found in eucalyptus and rosemary) demonstrated an ability to lower mean aortic pressure (blood pressure), without decreasing heart rate, through vascular wall relaxation (Lahlou et al., 2002).

Rosemary: Treatment of rats with 1,8-cineole (or eucalyptol found in eucalyptus and rosemary) demonstrated an ability to lower mean aortic pressure (blood pressure), without decreasing heart rate, through vascular wall relaxation (Lahlou et al., 2002).

Lemon: Lemon oil and one of its components, gamma-terpinene, were found to inhibit oxidation of low-density lipoprotein (LDL). Oxidation of LDL has been found to increase the risk of atherosclerosis and cardiac disease (Grassmann et al., 2001).

Lavender: Inhalation of lavender and monarda oils was found to reduce cholesterol content and atherosclerotic plaques in the aorta (Nikolaevski et al., 1990).

Arthritis

See also **Inflammation, Joints**

Arthritis is the painful swelling, inflammation, and stiffness of the joints.

> *Simple Solutions—Arthritis:* Blend 3 drops frankincense, 4 drops peppermint, and 2 drops marjoram with 1 Tbs. (15 ml) fractionated coconut oil. Massage gently on affected joints each day. If desired, 10 drops Deep Blue may be substituted for the above oils.

Oils: frankincense, rosemary, marjoram, Deep Blue, manuka, eucalyptus, fir, peppermint, lavender, cypress, juniper berry, ginger, Roman chamomile, helichrysum, cedarwood, wintergreen, basil, clove

Blend 1: Combine equal parts wintergreen and Deep Blue. Apply on location.

Other Products: Alpha CRS+

—Arthritic Pain:

Oils: Deep Blue, wintergreen, ginger

—Osteoarthritis:

Osteoarthritis is a degenerative arthritis where the cartilage that provides lubrication between the bones in a joint begins to break down, becoming rough and uneven. This causes the bones in the joint to wear and create rough deposits that can become extremely painful.

Oils: rosemary, marjoram, Deep Blue, geranium, wintergreen, thyme, basil, lavender, eucalyptus

Other Products: Alpha CRS+

—Rheumatoid Arthritis:

Rheumatoid arthritis is arthritis caused by inflammation within the joint, causing pain and possibly causing the joint to degenerate.

Oils: marjoram, lavender, cypress, Deep Blue, geranium, bergamot, clove, ginger, manuka, lemon, rosemary, wintergreen, cinnamon, eucalyptus, oregano (chronic), peppermint, Roman chamomile, thyme

Other Products: Alpha CRS+

⟿: Dilute as recommended, and apply on location. Apply as a warm compress over affected area. Dilute 1–2 drops in 1 Tbs. (15 ml) fractionated coconut oil, and use as a massage oil. Add 1–2 drops to ¼ cup (50 g) Therapeutic Bath Salts, and dissolve in warm bathwater for a soaking bath.

⟳: Diffuse into the air.

⊕: **Body System(s) Affected:** Muscles and Skeletal System.

⊡: **Additional Research:**

Frankincense: An acetone extract of frankincense was found to decrease arthritic scores, reduce paw edema (swelling), and suppress pro-inflammatory cytokines (cellular messengers) (Fan et al., 2005).

Rosemary, Marjoram, Eucalyptus, Peppermint, Lavender: In patients suffering from arthritis, it was found that a blend of lavender, marjoram, eucalyptus, rosemary, and peppermint blended with carrier oils reduced perceived pain and depression compared to control (Kim et al., 2005).

Alpha CRS+: Epigallocatechin-3-gallate was found to ameliorate experimental rheumatoid arthritis in the short term (Morinobu et al., 2008).

Clove: Eugenol and ginger oil taken orally were found to reduce paw and joint swelling in rats with induced severe arthritis (Sharma et al., 1994).

Ginger: Eugenol and ginger oil taken orally were found to reduce paw and joint swelling in rats with induced severe arthritis (Sharma et al., 1994).

Eugenol (found in cassia, cinnamon, and clove): Eugenol was found to ameliorate experimental arthritis in mice by inhibiting mononuclear cell infiltration into the knee joints and lowering cytokine levels (Grespan et al., 2012).

Cinnamon: The polyphenol fraction from cinnamon bark was found to improve inflammation and pain in animal models of inflammation and rheumatoid arthritis (Rathi et al., 2013).

Coriander: Coriander extract produced a dose-dependent inhibition of joint swelling in two mice models of induced arthritis (Nair et al., 2012).

Asthma

Asthma is a disease that causes the lung's airways to narrow, making it difficult to breathe. Episodes (or attacks) of asthma can be triggered by any number of

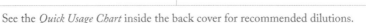

See the *Quick Usage Chart* inside the back cover for recommended dilutions.

252

things, including smoke, pollution, dust mites, and other allergens. Asthma causes reoccurring periods of tightness in the chest, coughing, shortness of breath, and wheezing.

> *Simple Solutions—Asthma:* Gently massage 2 drops lavender on chest.

Oils: eucalyptus, frankincense, peppermint, thyme, Breathe, Douglas fir, oregano, lemon, myrrh, lavender, geranium, cypress, clary sage, ylang ylang, rose, helichrysum, marjoram, rosemary

—Attack

Oils: Breathe, eucalyptus, frankincense (calming), lavender, marjoram

: Diffuse into the air. Inhale directly from bottle. Apply oil to hands, tissue, or cotton wick, and inhale.

: Dilute as recommended and apply to the chest, throat, or back. Add 2–3 drops to 1 Tbs. (15 ml) fractionated coconut oil, and massage onto chest, shoulders, and back.

: **Body System(s) Affected:** Respiratory System.

: **Additional Research:**

Eucalyptus: Extracts from eucalyptus and thyme were found to have high nitrous oxide (NO) scavenging abilities and inhibited NO production in macrophage cells. This could possibly explain their role in aiding respiratory inflammatory diseases (Vigo et al., 2004).

Eucalyptus: Therapy with 1,8 cineole (eucalyptol, found in eucalyptus) in both healthy and bronchitis-afflicted humans was shown to reduce production of LTB4 and PGE2, both metabolites of arachidonic acid (a known chemical messenger involved in inflammation), in white blood cells (Juergens et al., 1998).

Peppermint: L-menthol (found in peppermint) was found to inhibit production of inflammation mediators in human monocytes (a type of white blood cell involved in the immune response) (Juergens et al., 1998).

Lavender: Long-term inhalation of lavender oil was found to suppress allergic airway inflammation and mucous cell hyperplasia in a mouse model of acute asthma (Ueno-Iio et al., 2014).

Laurel Leaf (Bay) in Breathe: Magnolialide, extracted from laurel leaf, was found to inhibit key factors in the development and amplification of type I hypersensitivity responses (implicated in the cause of allergic asthma)(Lee, T. et al., 2013).

Athlete's Foot

See Antifungal: Athlete's Foot

Attention Deficit Disorder

See ADD/ADHD

Autism

Autism is a developmental disorder that impairs the normal development of communication, sociality, and human interaction.

—Reduce Anxiety/Fear: *See also Anxiety*

Oils: geranium, clary sage, bergamot

—Stimulate the Senses: *See also Stimulating*

Oils: peppermint, basil, lemon, rosemary

: Add 1–2 drops to 1 Tbs. (15 ml) fractionated coconut oil, and massage into skin.

: **Body System(s) Affected:** Nervous System.

Comments: Only apply these oils when the autistic child is willing and open to receive them. If the experience is forced or negative, the autistic child will associate these oils with a negative experience when used again.

Auto-Immune Diseases

See Grave's Disease, Hashimoto's Disease, Lupus

Awake

See Alertness, Jet Lag

Babies

See Children and Infants

Back

Oils: Deep Blue, Balance, Rescuer, cypress, eucalyptus, geranium, lavender, Roman chamomile, oregano, peppermint, rosemary, juniper berry, thyme

> *Simple Solutions—Backache:* Combine 3 drops peppermint with 1 drop wintergreen in 1 tsp. (5 ml) fractionated coconut oil. Gently massage on lower back to help soothe muscle aches.

—Calcified Spine

Calcification occurs when calcium builds up in tissue and causes the tissue to harden. As people age, calcification can cause the ligaments of the spine to thicken and harden, making the spinal canal narrow and creating pressure on the spinal nerve.

Oils: ⬡Deep Blue, ⬡geranium, ⬡rosemary

—Deteriorating Spine:

Deteriorating disc disease occurs as people age and their spinal discs begin to deteriorate. As deterioration progresses, movement becomes restricted, and pain in the neck and back increases. Although most commonly associated with aging, disc deterioration can be caused by back injuries as well.

Oils: ⬡Deep Blue

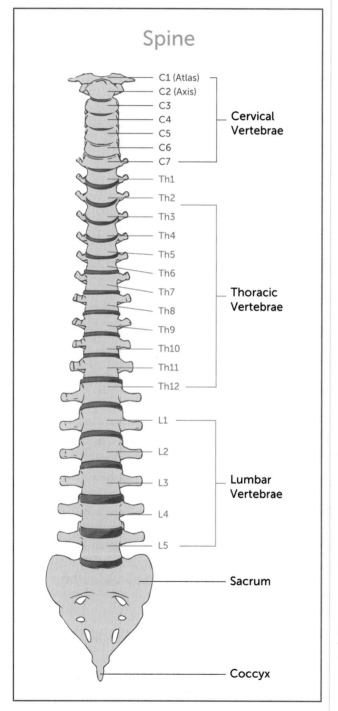

Spine

- C1 (Atlas)
- C2 (Axis)
- C3
- C4
- C5 — Cervical Vertebrae
- C6
- C7
- Th1
- Th2
- Th3
- Th4
- Th5
- Th6
- Th7 — Thoracic Vertebrae
- Th8
- Th9
- Th10
- Th11
- Th12
- L1
- L2
- L3 — Lumbar Vertebrae
- L4
- L5
- Sacrum
- Coccyx

—Herniated Discs:

In between the bones of the spine are cushioning discs that keep the spine flexible and act as shock absorbers. A herniated disc is caused when one of the discs of the spine is damaged and either bulges or breaks open. When the herniated disc presses on a nerve, it causes pain in the buttock, thigh, and calf. Herniated discs can be caused by spinal injuries or by the wear and tear that come with age as the discs begin to dry out

Oils: ⬡Deep Blue, ⬡Balance (3 drops on location), ⬡peppermint, ⬡cypress (strengthens blood capillary walls, improves circulation, anti-inflammatory)

—Lumbago/Lower Back Pain:

Oils: ⬡sandalwood, ⬡Deep Blue

—Muscular Fatigue:

Oils: ⬡clary sage, ⬡marjoram, ⬡lavender, ⬡rosemary

—Pain:

Oils: ⬡Balance, ⬡Deep Blue, ⬡Rescuer

Blend 1: Combine 5–10 drops each of lavender, eucalyptus, and ginger, and apply 2–3 drops on location or as a warm compress.

Blend 2: Combine 5–10 drops each of peppermint, rosemary, and basil, and apply 2–3 drops on location or as a warm compress.

—Stiffness:

Oils: ⬡marjoram, ⬡Balance

—Viruses Along Spine:

Oils: ⬡oregano, ⬡eucalyptus

⬡: Dilute as recommended, and apply along the spine, on affected muscles, or on reflex points on the feet. Dilute 1–3 drops in 1 Tbs. (15 ml) fractionated coconut oil, and massage into muscles on the back or along the spine. Apply as a warm compress over affected area.

⬡: **Body System(s) Affected:** Muscles and Skeletal System.

Bacteria

See Antibacterial

See the *Quick Usage Chart* inside the back cover for recommended dilutions.

254

Balance

Oils: Balance, Steady, frankincense, vetiver, ylang ylang, cedarwood

—Electrical Energies:

Oils: Balance, frankincense

Application Methods:

: Dilute as recommended, and apply on location. Apply 3–6 drops of Balance to the bottom of each foot, and, if desired, apply some to the neck and shoulders. Hold the palm of each hand to the bottom of each corresponding foot (left to left and right to right) for 5–15 minutes to help balance electrical energies.

: Diffuse into the air.

: **Body System(s) Affected:** Emotional Balance.

Baldness

See Hair: Loss

Bath

Using essential oils in the bath can be a wonderful way to receive and possibly enhance the benefits of the oils.

Oils: lavender, geranium, Roman chamomile, ylang ylang

Some common ways to use essential oils in the bath include the following:

Direct: Add 1–3 drops of oil directly to bathwater while the bath is filling. Oils will be drawn to your skin quickly from the top of the water, so use non-irritating oils such as lavender, ylang ylang, etc., or dilute the oil with fractionated coconut oil to safe topical application dilutions.

Bath Gel: To disperse the oil throughout the bathwater, add 5–10 drops of your favorite essential oil to 1 Tbs. (15 ml) unscented bath and shower gel.

Bath Salts: For a relaxing mineral bath, add 1–5 drops of your desired essential oil to ¼–½ cup (50–125 g) of Therapeutic Bath Salts or Epsom salt; mix well. Dissolve salts in warm bathwater while the tub is filling.

: **Body System(s) Affected:** Skin.

Bed Wetting

See Bladder: Bed Wetting

Bell's Palsy

See Nervous System: Bell's Palsy

Birthing

See Pregnancy/Motherhood

Bites/Stings

See also Insects/Bugs: Repellent

> *Simple Solutions—Bee Sting:* Combine 2 drops Roman chamomile with ¼ tsp. (2 g) baking soda and a few drops of water to make a paste. Scrape stinger from skin if still there, and apply paste on location. Cover with a cool, damp cloth; hold on location for 5–10 minutes.

Oils: thyme, basil, lemon, cinnamon, lavender

—Allergic:

Oils: Purify

—Bees and Hornets

Oils: Roman chamomile, basil, Purify, lavender, lemongrass, lemon, peppermint, thyme

Recipe 1: Remove the stinger, and apply a cold compress of Roman chamomile to the area for several hours or for as long as possible.

—Gnats and Midges:

Oils: lavender

Recipe 2: Mix 3 drops thyme in 1 tsp. (5 ml) cider vinegar or lemon juice. Apply to bites to stop irritation.

—Mosquitoes:

Oils: lavender, helichrysum

—Snakes:

Oils: basil

—Spiders:

Oils: basil, Purify (with melaleuca), lavender, lemongrass, lemon, peppermint, thyme

Recipe 3: Mix 3 drops lavender and 2 drops Roman chamomile with 1 tsp. (5 ml) alcohol. Apply to area 3 times per day.

—**Ticks:**

Oils: After getting the tick out, apply 1 drop lavender every 5 minutes for 30 minutes.

Removing Ticks:

Do not apply mineral oil, Vaseline, or anything else to remove the tick, as this may cause it to inject the spirochetes into the wound.

Be sure to remove the entire tick. Get as close to the mouth as possible, and firmly tug on the tick until it releases its grip. Don't twist. If available, use a magnifying glass to make sure that you have removed the entire tick.

Save the tick in a jar, and label it with the date, where you were bitten on your body, and the location or address where you were bitten for proper identification by your doctor, especially if you develop any symptoms.

Do not handle the tick.

Wash hands immediately.

Check the site of the bite occasionally to see if any rash develops. If it does, seek medical advice promptly.

—**Wasps:**

Recipe 4: Combine 1 drop basil, 2 drops Roman chamomile, 2 drops lavender, and 1 tsp. (5 ml) apple cider vinegar. Apply to area 3 times a day.

🌀: Dilute as recommended, and apply on location.

🧍: **Body System(s) Affected:** Skin.

Bladder

See also **Urinary Tract**

The urinary bladder is a hollow organ that collects urine before it is disposed by urination. The bladder sits on the pelvic floor.

> *Simple Solutions—Bed Wetting:* Combine 5 drops cypress and 3 drops ylang ylang with 2 Tbs. (25 ml) water in a small spray bottle. Mist on pillow and sheets just before bedtime.

—**Bed Wetting and Incontinence:**

Oils: 🌀cypress (rub on abdomen at bedtime), 🌀ylang ylang⊕.

—**Cystitis/Infection:**

Oils: 🌀lemongrass, 🅾🌀On Guard, 🌀sandalwood, 🌀juniper berry, 🌀thyme, 🌀cedarwood, 🌀basil, 🌀cinnamon, 🌀clove, 🌀eucalyptus, 🌀frankincense, 🌀lavender, 🌀bergamot, 🌀fennel, 🌀marjoram, 🌀oregano

Other Products: 🅾On Guard+ Softgels

🌀: Dilute as recommended, and apply on abdomen and on reflex points on the feet. Add 1–2 drops to warm bathwater; bathe for 10–15 minutes.

⬤: Add 1 drop to 1 cup (250 ml) juice or water; drink 3 times a day.

🧍: **Body System(s) Affected:** Digestive System.

⊕: **Additional Research:**

Ylang ylang: Ylang ylang oil induced relaxation in rat (in vitro) and rabbit (in vivo) bladder smooth muscle, suggesting that ylang ylang may be effective at alleviating an overactive bladder (Kim et al., 2003).

Bleeding

See **Blood: Bleeding**

Blister

> *Simple Solutions—Blisters:* Apply 1 drop lavender oil on blister once or twice a day as needed.

Oils: 🌀lavender

🌀: Apply oil to blister as often as needed.

Bloating

See **Digestive System: Bloating**

Blood

Blood is the fluid inside the body that transports oxygen and nutrients to the cells and carries waste away from the cells. It also transports cells involved in the immune and inflammatory response, hormones and other chemical messengers that regulate the body's functions, and platelets that help facilitate the blood clotting necessary to repair damaged blood vessels. Blood is primarily composed of plasma (water with dissolved nutrients,

See the *Quick Usage Chart* inside the back cover for recommended dilutions.

256

minerals, and carbon dioxide) that carries red blood cells (the most numerous type of cells in blood, responsible for transporting oxygen), white blood cells (cells involved in the immune system and immune response), and platelet cells. Blood is circulated in the body by the pumping action of the heart propelling blood through various blood vessels. Proper and healthy circulation and function of blood throughout the body is critical for health and even for the sustaining of life.

> *Simple Solutions—Bleeding:* Add 3 drops helichrysum to ½ cup (125 ml) cool water in a bowl. Dampen a small rag in the mixture. Apply on bleeding area and apply pressure to help stop.

—**Blood Pressure**

Oils: ^Olemon (will regulate pressure—either raise or lower as necessary), lime

–**High (hypertension)**

Oils: ylang ylang, marjoram, eucalyptus, lavender, clove, clary sage, lemon, wintergreen **Note:** Avoid rosemary, thyme, and possibly peppermint.

Bath 1: Place 3 drops ylang ylang and 3 drops marjoram in bathwater, and bathe in the evening twice a week.

Blend 1: Combine 10 drops ylang ylang, 5 drops marjoram, and 5 drops cypress in 2 Tbs. (25 ml) fractionated coconut oil. Rub over heart and reflex points on left foot and hand.

Blend 2: Combine 5 drops geranium, 8 drops lemongrass, and 3 drops lavender in 2 Tbs. (25 ml) fractionated coconut oil. Rub over heart and reflex points on left foot and hand.

–**Low**

Oils: rosemary, blue tansy

: Diffuse into the air. Inhale the aroma directly.

: Place 1–2 drops of oil under the tongue or place 1–3 drops of oil in an empty capsule; ingest up to 3 times per day.

: Dilute as recommended, and apply on location, on reflex points on feet and hands, and over heart.

—**Bleeding (stops):**

Oils: helichrysum, geranium, yarrow, rose

: Dilute as recommended, and apply on location.

—**Broken Blood Vessels**

Oils: helichrysum, grapefruit

: Dilute as recommended, and apply on location, on reflex points on feet and hands, and over heart.

—**Cholesterol:**

Cholesterol is a soft, waxy substance found in the bloodstream and in all of the body's cells. The body requires some cholesterol to function properly, but high levels of cholesterol narrow and block the arteries and increase the risk of heart disease.

Oils: helichrysum

: Dilute as recommended, and apply on reflex points on feet and hands, and over heart.

—**Circulation:** *See Cardiovascular System*

—**Cleansing**

Oils: helichrysum, geranium, Roman chamomile

: Dilute as recommended, and apply on reflex points on feet and hands, and over heart.

—**Clots:**

Blood clots occur as a natural bodily defense to repair damaged blood vessels and to keep the body from losing excessive amounts of blood. However, clotting can become dangerous if an internal blood clot breaks loose in the circulatory system and blocks the flow of blood to vital organs.

Oils: clove, fennel, thyme, grapefruit

: Place 1–2 drops of oil under the tongue or place 1–3 drops of oil in an empty capsule; ingest up to 3 times per day.

: Dilute as recommended, and apply on location, on reflex points on feet and hands, and over heart.

: Diffuse into the air. Inhale the aroma directly.

—**Hemorrhaging:**

Hemorrhaging is excessive or uncontrollable blood loss.

Oils: helichrysum, ylang ylang, rose

: Dilute as recommended, and apply on location.

—**High Blood Sugar:** *See Diabetes*

—Low Blood Sugar:

The term "blood sugar" refers to the amount of glucose in the bloodstream. When the blood glucose drops below its normal level, this is called "low blood sugar" or "hypoglycemia." Since glucose is such an important source of energy for the body, low blood sugar can result in light-headedness, hunger, shakiness, weakness, confusion, nervousness, difficulty speaking, and anxiety.

Oils: ⊘On Guard, ⊘cinnamon, ⊘clove, ⊘thyme

Other Products: ⭘On Guard+ Softgels

⊜: Dilute as recommended, and apply on location, on reflex points on feet and hands, and over heart.

—Stimulates Blood Cell Production

Oils: ⭘⊘peppermint⊡, ⭘⊘lemon

⭘: Place 1–2 drops of oil under the tongue or place 1–3 drops of oil in an empty capsule; ingest up to 3 times per day. Take supplement as directed.

⊜: Dilute as recommended, and apply on location, on reflex points on feet and hands, and over heart.

—Vessels: *See Arteries, Capillaries, Veins*

⊕: **Body System(s) Affected:** Cardiovascular System.

⊡: **Additional Research:**

Ylang ylang: Subjects who had ylang ylang oil applied to their skin had decreased blood pressure, increased skin temperature, and reported feeling more calm and relaxed than did subjects in a control group (Hongratanaworakit et al., 2006).

Ylang ylang: Inhaled ylang ylang oil was found to decrease blood pressure and pulse rate and to enhance attentiveness and alertness in volunteers compared to an odorless control (Hongratanaworakit et al., 2004).

Ylang ylang, lavender, marjoram: Eighty-three hypertensive or prehypertensive subjects were divided into the following three groups: a study group (exposed to an essential oil blend containing lavender, ylang ylang, marjoram, and neroli), a placebo group (exposed to artificial fragrance), and a control group (no interventions). The study group was found to have an immediate and long-term decrease in home blood pressure (Kim et al., 2012).

Marjoram: Treatment of rats with 1,8-cineole (or eucalyptol, found in eucalyptus, rosemary, and marjoram) demonstrated an ability to lower mean aortic pressure (blood pressure), without decreasing heart rate, through vascular wall relaxation (Lahlou et al., 2002).

Eucalyptus: Treatment of rats with 1,8-cineole (or eucalyptol, found in eucalyptus, rosemary, and marjoram) demonstrated an ability to lower mean aortic pressure (blood pressure), without decreasing heart rate, through vascular wall relaxation (Lahlou et al., 2002).

Rosemary: Oral treatment with rosemary essential oil on primary hypotensive subjects was found to increase blood pressure values when compared to the subjects' placebo treatments before and after rosemary treatment (Fernández et al., 2014).

Clove: Clove oil demonstrated an ability to prevent the aggregation of platelets that can lead to blood clots and thrombosis both in vivo and in vitro (Saeed et al., 1994).

Fennel: Both fennel oil and its constituent, anethole, were found to significantly reduce thrombosis (blood clots) in mice. They were also found to be free from the prohemorrhagic (increased bleeding) side effect that aspirin (acetylsalicylic acid) has (Tognolini et al., 2007).

Peppermint: In mice exposed to whole-body gamma irradiation, only 17% of mice who had been fed peppermint oil died, while 100% of mice who did not receive peppermint oil died. It was also found that the mice pre-fed peppermint oil were able to return blood cell levels to normal after 30 days, while the control mice were not able to (and consequently died), suggesting a protective or stimulating effect of the oil on blood stem cells (Samarth et al., 2004).

Body Systems

*See **Cardiovascular System, Digestive System, Endocrine System, Lymphatic System, Muscles, Skeletal System, Nervous System, Respiratory System, Skin***

Boils

*See also **Antibacterial***

A boil is a skin infection that forms in a hair follicle or oil gland. The boil starts as a red, tender lump that after a few days forms a white or yellow point in the center as it fills with pus. Boils commonly occur on the face, neck, armpits, buttock, and shoulders and can be very painful.

> *Simple Solutions—Boils:* Add 5 drops melaleuca oil and 2 drops lavender to 2 cups (500 ml) clean hot water in a bowl. Soak a clean washcloth with the solution, and use to wash infected area twice a day.

Oils: ⊘melaleuca⊡, ⊘lavender, ⊘Purify, ⊘lemongrass, ⊘lemon, ⊘frankincense, ⊘clary sage

⊜: Dilute as recommended, and apply on location.

⊕: **Body System(s) Affected:** Skin and Immune System.

⊡: **Additional Research:**

Melaleuca: In a human trial, most patients receiving treatment with *Melaleuca alternifolia* oil placed topically on boils experienced healing or reduction of symptoms; while of those receiving no treatment (control), half required surgical intervention, and all still demonstrated signs of the infection (Feinblatt, 1960).

Bones

*See **Skeletal System***

Bowel

*See **Digestive System***

Brain

The brain is the central part of the nervous system. It is responsible for processing sensory stimuli and for directing appropriate behavioral responses to each stimulus, or set of stimuli. The brain also stores memories and is the center of thought.

See the *Quick Usage Chart* inside the back cover for recommended dilutions.

258

Oils: ⊘☉lavender⊕, ○☉lemon⊕, ⊘☉lemongrass, ⊘☉clary sage, ⊘☉cypress, ⊘☉geranium

Other Products: ○xEO Mega or vEO Mega or ○IQ Mega for omega-3 fatty acids essential for proper brain function, ○Microplex VMz for vitamins and minerals critical for brain health.

⊘: Diffuse into the air. Inhale directly from bottle. Apply oil to hands, tissue, or cotton wick, and inhale.

☉: Dilute as recommended, and rub onto the brain stem area, back of neck, temples, behind ears down to jaw, or on reflex points on the feet. Apply as a cold compress.

○: Take capsules as directed on package. Place 1–2 drops of oil under the tongue; or place 1–2 drops of oil in an empty capsule and swallow the capsule.

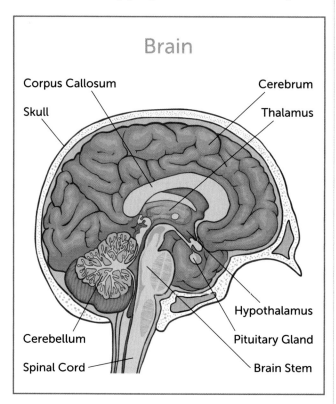

Brain

Corpus Callosum
Skull
Cerebrum
Thalamus
Cerebellum
Spinal Cord
Hypothalamus
Pituitary Gland
Brain Stem

—Activates Right Brain

Oils: ⊘☉geranium, ⊘☉grapefruit, ⊘☉helichrysum, ⊘☉wintergreen, ⊘☉Roman chamomile

⊘: Diffuse into the air. Inhale directly from bottle. Apply oil to hands, tissue, or cotton wick, and inhale.

☉: Dilute as recommended, and rub onto the brain stem area, or on reflex points on the feet.

—Aging:

Oils: ○☉thyme⊕, ⊘☉frankincense, myrrh⊕, rose⊕

○: Place 1–2 drops of oil under the tongue or place 1–2 drops of oil in an empty capsule; swallow capsule.

☉: Dilute as recommended, and rub onto the brain stem area, back of neck, temples, behind ears down to jaw, or on reflex points on the feet.

—Broken Blood Vessels: *See Blood: Broken Blood Vessels*

—Concentration: *See Concentration*

—Concussion:

A concussion is a type of brain injury that causes temporary or permanent impairment in the brain's functioning. Concussions most commonly occur as a result of a blow to the head. Concussion symptoms include headaches, dizziness, blurred vision, vomiting, disorientation, difficulty focusing attention, ringing in the ears, selective memory loss, etc.

Oils: ⊘☉frankincense⊕, ☉cypress

⊘: Diffuse into the air. Inhale directly from bottle. Apply oil to hands, tissue, or cotton wick, and inhale.

☉: Dilute as recommended, and rub onto the brain stem area, back of neck, temples, behind ears down to jaw, or on reflex points on the feet. Apply as a cold compress.

—Injury

Oils: ⊘☉frankincense⊕, ⊘☉bergamot⊕, ⊘☉peppermint⊕, ⊘☉lemon⊕, ⊘☉Balance, ⊘☉lemongrass

⊘: Diffuse into the air. Inhale the aroma of the oil directly.

☉: Dilute as recommended, and rub onto the brain stem area, back of neck, temples, behind ears down to jaw, or on reflex points on the feet.

—Integration

Oils: ⊘☉Balance, ⊘☉Steady, ⊘☉helichrysum, ⊘☉geranium, ⊘☉clary sage, ⊘☉cypress, ⊘☉lemongrass

⊘: Diffuse into the air. Inhale the aroma of the oil directly.

A B C D E F G H I J K L M N O P Q R S T U V W X Y Z

⬱: Dilute as recommended, and rub onto the brain stem area, back of neck, temples, behind ears down to jaw, or on reflex points on the feet.

—**Learning and Memory:** *See Memory*

—**Mental Fatigue:**

Oils: ⬡⬢frankincense

—**Myelin Sheath:**

The myelin sheath is an insulating layer of protein and fatty substances that forms around nerves (including those in the brain), increasing the speed of nerve impulses. Damage to the myelin sheath interrupts these nerve impulses and can cause diseases such as multiple sclerosis, peripheral neuropathy, central pontine myelinolysis, and other neurological diseases.

Oils: ⬡⬢peppermint, ⬡⬢frankincense, ⬡⬢lemongrass, ⬡⬢juniper berry, ⬡⬢Balance, ⬡⬢geranium

Other Products: ᴼxEO Mega or vEO Mega or ᴼIQ Mega, which contains the omega-3 fatty acid DHA that helps support the myelin sheath

⬭: Diffuse into the air. Inhale directly from bottle. Apply oil to hands, tissue, or cotton wick, and inhale.

⬱: Apply as a cool compress over the brain stem area, back of neck, temples, behind ears down to jaw, or on reflex points on the feet.

—**Oxygenate:**

Oils: ⬡eucalyptus⊕, ⬡rosemary⊕, ⬡⬢helichrysum, ⬡⬢sandalwood, ⬡marjoram⊕

Recipe 1: Place 3 drops each of helichrysum and sandalwood on the back of the neck, on the temples, and behind the ears down to the jaw once or twice a day.

⬭: Diffuse into the air. Inhale the aroma directly.

⬱: Dilute as recommended, and rub onto the brain stem area, back of neck, temples, behind ears down to jaw, or on reflex points on the feet.

⬤: **Body System(s) Affected:** Nervous System.

—**Stroke:** *See Stroke*

—**Tumor:** *See Cancer: Brain*

⬚: **Additional Research:**

Lavender: Subjects who smelled a cleansing gel with lavender aroma were more relaxed and able to complete math computations faster (Fielt et al., 2005).

Lavender: Subjects exposed to 3 minutes of lavender aroma were more relaxed and were able to perform math computations faster and more accurately. Subjects exposed to rosemary aroma were more alert and completed math computations faster (but not more accurately) (Diego et al., 1998).

Lemon: Several constituents of lemon oil and their metabolites (chemicals made from these constituents by the body) were found to increase the release of monoamines (various chemicals responsible for neurotransmission and neuromodulation) in rat brain tissue, indicating a possible effect on brain nerve cell behavior (Fukumoto et al., 2006).

Lemon: Pretreatment of human and rat astrocyte cells (cells found in the nerve and brain that support the blood-brain barrier and help repair the brain and spinal cord following injuries) with lemon oil was found to inhibit heat-shock—induced apoptosis (Koo et al., 2002).

Thyme: Aging rats fed thyme oil or the constituent thymol were found to have higher levels of the antioxidant enzymes superoxide dismutase and glutathione peroxidase in the brain than did aging rats not fed the oil or constituent (Youdim et al., 2000).

Rose: The chloroform extract of *Rosa damascena* was found to cause neurite outgrowth activity in rat cortical neurons subjected to neurotic atrophy conditions. These findings suggest that *Rosa damascena* possesses neuronal protective properties that may benefit persons with dementia (Awale et al., 2011).

Myrrh: Three new cadinane sesquiterpenes isolated from myrrh resin were found to have neuroprotective activities against 1-methyl-4-phenylpyridinium induced neuronal cell death in a human derived cell line cells (Xu et al., 2011).

Frankincense: Incensole acetate, isolated from frankincense resin, was found to demonstrate an anti-inflammatory and neuroprotective effect in mice with a closed head injury (Moussaieff et al., 2008).

Bergamot: Bergamot essential oil was found to exert neuroprotective effects against brain injury in rats with induced cerebral ischemia (Amantea et al., 2009).

Bergamot: Bergamot essential oil was found to reduce excitotoxic neuronal damage caused by exposure of human neuroblastoma cells to NMDA in vitro, displaying the neuroprotection capabilities of bergamot oil (Corasaniti et al., 2007).

Peppermint: Pretreatment of human and rat astrocyte cells (cells found in the nerve and brain that support the blood-brain barrier and help repair the brain and spinal cord following injuries) with peppermint oil was found to inhibit heat shock—induced apoptosis of these cells (Koo et al., 2001).

Eucalyptus: Imaging of the brain demonstrated that inhalation of 1,8-cineol (eucalyptol, a constituent of many essential oils, especially eucalyptus, rosemary, and marjoram) increased global cerebral blood flow after an inhalation time of 20 minutes (Nasel et al., 1994).

Rosemary: Imaging of the brain demonstrated that inhalation of 1,8-cineol (eucalyptol, a constituent of many essential oils, especially eucalyptus, rosemary, and marjoram) increased global cerebral blood flow after an inhalation time of 20 minutes (Nasel et al., 1994).

Marjoram: Imaging of the brain demonstrated that inhalation of 1,8-cineol (eucalyptol, a constituent of many essential oils, especially eucalyptus, rosemary, and marjoram) increased global cerebral blood flow after an inhalation time of 20 minutes (Nasel et al., 1994).

(-)-Linalool (found in basil, bergamot, cinnamon, clary sage, coriander, cypress, eucalyptus, fennel (sweet), geranium, ginger, helichrysum, jasmine, lavender, lemon, lemongrass, lime, marjoram, oregano, peppermint, rosemary, tangerine, thyme, wild orange, and ylang ylang essential oils): In two mice models of chronic pain, inflammatory pain and neuropathic pain, (-)-linalool was able to promote marked and long-lasting reduction in sensitivity to pain when compared to the control (Batista et al., 2010).

Bergamot: Using a mouse model of neuropathic pain, researchers discovered that injections of bergamot or linalool (a main chemical constituent of bergamot) provided reduction of pain symptoms by inhibiting phosphorylation of the spinal ERK pathway (Kuwahata et al., 2013).

Breast

See also Cancer: Breast. For issues related to lactation and motherhood, see Pregnancy/Motherhood

Oils: ⬢clary sage, ⬢geranium, ⬢lemongrass, ⬢fennel, ⬢cypress, ⬢vetiver

---

See the *Quick Usage Chart* inside the back cover for recommended dilutions.

—Enlarge and Firm:

Oils: ⊘clary sage

⊜: Dilute as recommended, and apply on location or on reflex points on feet.

⊕: **Body System(s) Affected:** Endocrine System.

Breathing

See Respiratory System: Breathing

Bronchitis

See also Antibacterial, Antifungal, Antiviral, Congestion, Inflammation, Respiratory System

Bronchitis is the inflammation of the bronchi (the tubes that lead from the trachea to the lungs). Symptoms include coughing, breathlessness, and thick phlegm.

> *Simple Solutions—Bronchitis:* Apply 2 drops of eucalyptus on the chest.

Oils: ⊘⊘eucalyptus⊕, ⊘⊘thyme⊕, ⊘⊘fir, ⊘⊘basil, ⊘⊘Breathe, ⊘⊘Douglas fir, ⊘⊘manuka, ⊘⊘On Guard, ⊘⊘clary sage, ⊘⊘cypress, ⊘⊘cedarwood, ⊘⊘melaleuca, ⊘⊘marjoram, ⊘⊘peppermint, ⊘⊘rosemary, ⊘⊘wintergreen, ⊘⊘myrrh, ⊘⊘clove, ⊘⊘frankincense, ⊘⊘ginger, ⊘⊘lavender, ⊘⊘lemon, ⊘⊘sandalwood, ⊘⊘bergamot

—Chronic

Oils: ⊘⊘eucalyptus, ⊘⊘oregano, ⊘⊘sandalwood

—Children

Oils: ⊘⊘eucalyptus, ⊘⊘melaleuca, ⊘⊘lavender, ⊘⊘Roman chamomile, ⊘⊘rosemary

—Clear Mucus:

Oils: ⊘⊘sandalwood, ⊘⊘thyme, ⊘⊘bergamot, ⊘⊘On Guard

⊘: Diffuse into the air. Inhale directly from bottle. Apply oil to hands, tissue, or cotton wick, and inhale.

⊜: Dilute as recommended, and apply to chest, sinuses, neck, or reflex points on the feet. Add 2–3 drops to water; gargle.

⊕: **Body System(s) Affected:** Respiratory System.

⊡: **Additional Research:**

Eucalyptus: Extracts from eucalyptus and thyme were found to have high nitrous oxide scavenging abilities and inhibited nitrous oxide production in macrophage cells. This could possibly explain their role in aiding respiratory inflammatory diseases (Vigo et al., 2004).

Eucalyptus: Eucalyptus oil was found to have an anti-inflammatory and mucin-inhibitory effect in rats with lipopolysaccharide-induced bronchitis (Lu et al., 2004).

Eucalyptus: Therapy with 1,8 cineole (eucalyptol) in both healthy and bronchitis-afflicted humans was shown to reduce production of LTB4 and PGE2 (both metabolites of arachidonic acid, a known chemical messenger involved in inflammation) in white blood cells (Juergens et al., 1998).

Thyme: Extracts from eucalyptus and thyme were found to have high nitrous oxide scavenging abilities and inhibited nitrous oxide production in macrophage cells. This could possibly explain their role in aiding respiratory inflammatory diseases (Vigo et al., 2004).

Bruises

See also Capillaries

A bruise is an injury to tissue that results in blood capillaries breaking and spilling blood into the tissue. This can cause swelling, soreness, and a visible discoloration when the bruise is near the skin.

> *Simple Solutions—Bruises:* Add 5 drops helichrysum to 1 tsp. (5 ml) fractionated coconut oil in a small roll-on bottle, and apply over the bruised area.

Oils: ⊘helichrysum, ⊘geranium, ⊘fennel, ⊘Deep Blue (for pain), ⊘Rescuer, ⊘On Guard, ⊘lavender

⊜: Dilute as recommended, and apply 1–2 drops on location.

⊕: **Body System(s) Affected:** Skin and Cardiovascular System.

Bugs

See Insects/Bugs

Bulimia

See Eating Disorders: Bulimia

Bunions

See Bursitis: Bunion

Burns

A burn is an injury to tissue caused by heat, chemicals, or radiation. The tissue most often affected by burns is the skin. Minor burns can cause redness and pain over a small area and do not break the skin. For minor heat burns, immediately immerse the affected skin in cool water to stop the heat from causing more damage to the tissue. More serious burns that involve areas of the body larger than the palm of the hand or that involve blistering, swelling, intense pain that lasts for more than a day, or visible skin damage should be attended to by a medical professional. Skin damaged by burns is more prone to developing infection as it cannot act as a barrier against invading microorganisms.

> *Simple Solutions—Burns:* For minor burns, gently apply 1–2 drops of lavender oil, and cover with a cloth soaked in cool water. If the burn covers large areas of the body, is blistering, or has visible skin damage, seek immediate medical attention.

Oils: ⬡lavender, ⬡geranium, ⬡melaleuca, ⬡peppermint, ⬡helichrysum, ⬡Roman chamomile

Other Products: ⊙Microplex VMz to help replace minerals depleted from the skin and tissues surrounding a burn.

—Infected:

  Oils: ⬡Purify

—Pain:

  Oils: ⬡lavender

—Healing:

  Oils: ⬡lavender

  Blend 1: Blend together 1 drop geranium and 1 drop helichrysum; apply on location.

—Peeling:

  Oils: ⬡lavender

—Sunburn:

> *Simple Solutions—Sunburn:* Mix 10 drops lavender oil with ¼ cup (50 ml) cool water in a small spray bottle. Shake well, and spray on location to help soothe.

  Oils: ⬡lavender, ⬡melaleuca, ⬡Roman chamomile, ⬡manuka

  Recipe 1: Place 10 drops lavender in a 4 oz. misting spray bottle filled with distilled water. Shake well, and spray on location to aid with pain and healing.

—Sun Screen:

  Oils: ⬡helichrysum

⬭: Dilute as recommended, and apply on location. Add 2–3 drops oil to 2 Tbs. (25 ml) water in a spray bottle; shake well, and mist on location.

⬤: **Body System(s) Affected:** Skin.

Bursitis

Bursitis is the inflammation of the fluid-filled sack located close to joints that provides lubrication for tendons, skin, and ligaments rubbing against the bone. Bursitis is caused by infection, injury, or diseases such as arthritis and gout. Bursitis causes tenderness and pain which can limit movement.

> *Simple Solutions—Bursitis:* Apply 1 drop cypress oil on location. Alternate holding a hot and cold damp rag over the area every 5 minutes for 20 minutes total.

Oils: ⬡Balance, ⬡fir, ⬡basil, ⬡cypress, ⬡Deep Blue, ⬡ginger, ⬡Roman chamomile, ⬡marjoram, ⬡juniper berry, ⬡wintergreen

Recipe 1: Apply 1–3 drops each of Balance, fir, and basil on location. Alternate cold and hot packs (10 min. cold and then 15 min. hot) until pain subsides.

Recipe 2: Apply 6 drops marjoram on shoulders and arms, and wait 6 minutes. Then apply 3 drops of wintergreen, and wait 6 minutes. Then apply 3 drops cypress.

—Bunion:

  A bunion is bursitis of the big toe. It is often caused by constrictive shoes that force the big toe to point inward and the base of the big toe to jut outward. This misplacement can irritate the bursa at the base of the toe and cause it to become inflamed, causing further irritation.

  Oils: ⬡cypress, ⬡juniper berry

⬭: Dilute as recommended, and apply 1–2 drops on location.

⬤: **Body System(s) Affected:** Immune System, Muscles, and Skeletal System.

Callouses

See Skin: Callouses

Calming

See also Anxiety

> *Simple Solutions—Calming:* Diffuse Serenity in an aromatherapy diffuser.

See the *Quick Usage Chart* inside the back cover for recommended dilutions.

262

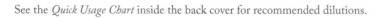

> *Simple Solutions—Calming:* Combine 5 drops ylang ylang, 6 drops lavender, and 2 drops Roman chamomile with ¼ cup (50 ml) water in a small spray bottle. Mist into the air to help calm children.

Oils: ⊘⊜lavender⚬, ⊘⊜InTune, ⊘⊜ylang ylang⚬, ⊘⊜melissa⚬, ⊘⊜Serenity, ⊘⊜Calmer, ⊘⊜Thinker, ⊘⊜cedarwood, ⊘⊜yuzu⚬, ⊘⊜blue tansy, ⊘⊜hinoki⚬, ⊘⊜magnolia, ⊘⊜Anchor, ⊘⊜green mandarin, ⊘yarrow, ⊘Citrus Bliss, ⊘⊜myrrh, ⊘⊜juniper berry

—Agitation:

Oils: ⊘⊜lavender⚬, ylang ylang⚬, ⊘⊜geranium⚬, ⊘⊜bergamot, ⊘⊜Serenity, ⊘⊜sandalwood, ⊘⊜cedarwood, ⊘⊜Balance, ⊘⊜marjoram, ⊘⊜myrrh, ⊘⊜clary sage, ⊘⊜rose, ⊘⊜frankincense, ⊘⊜Elevation

—Anger:

Oils: ⊘⊜Serenity, ⊘⊜lavender, ⊘⊜ylang ylang, ⊘⊜Balance, ⊘⊜Elevation, ⊘⊜bergamot, ⊘⊜geranium, ⊘⊜cedarwood, ⊘⊜frankincense, ⊘⊜sandalwood, ⊘⊜cypress, ⊘⊜lemon, ⊘⊜myrrh, ⊘⊜marjoram, ⊘⊜helichrysum, ⊘⊜rose, ⊘⊜orange

—Hyperactivity:

Oils: ⊘⊜InTune, ⊘⊜lavender⚬, ⊘⊜Calmer, ⊘⊜Serenity, ⊘⊜Balance, ⊘⊜Thinker, ⊘⊜Roman chamomile, ⊘Citrus Bliss

—Sedative:

Oils: ⊘⊜lavender⚬, ⊘⊜Serenity, ⊘⊜Calmer, ⊘Citrus Bliss, ⊘⊜bergamot⚬, ⊘⊜ylang ylang⚬, ⊘⊜cedarwood, ⊘⊜geranium, ⊘⊜vetiver, ⊘⊜juniper berry, ⊘⊜frankincense, ⊘⊜sandalwood, ⊘⊜orange, ⊘⊜rose, ⊘⊜lemongrass, ⊘⊜clary sage, ⊘⊜marjoram

⊘: Diffuse into the air. Inhale directly from bottle. Apply oil to hands, tissue, or cotton wick, and inhale.

⊜: Dilute as recommended, and apply 1–2 drops to back of neck, temples, chest, shoulders, back, or reflex points on the feet. Place 1–2 drops in 1 Tbs. (15 ml) fractionated coconut oil, and massage into the back, shoulders, neck, or arms.

⊕: **Body System(s) Affected:** Emotional Balance.

⊙: **Additional Research:**

Lavender: *Lavandula angustifolia* essential oil demonstrated ability to inhibit GABA-A receptor channels of rat brain cells (Huang et al., 2008).

Lavender: Inhaling lavender oil was found to be effective at alleviating agitated behaviors in older Chinese patients suffering from dementia (Lin et al., 2007).

Lavender: Female patients waiting for dental treatment were found to be less anxious, more positive, and more calm when exposed to orange oil odor than were patients who were not exposed to the orange oil odor (Lehrner et al., 2000).

Lavender: Exposure to inhaled lavender oil and to its constituents, linalool and linalyl acetate, was found to decrease normal movement in mice as well as to return mice to normal movement rates after caffeine-induced hyperactivity (Buchbauer et al., 1991).

Lavender: Swiss mice fed lavender oil diluted in olive oil were found to be more sedate in several common behavioral tests (Guillemain et al., 1989).

Lavender: Linalool, found in several essential oils, was found to inhibit induced convulsions in rats by directly interacting with the NMDA receptor complex (Brum et al., 2001).

Ylang ylang: In human trials, the aroma of peppermint was found to enhance memory and to increase alertness, while ylang ylang aroma was found to increase calmness (Moss et al., 2008).

Ylang ylang: Subjects who had ylang ylang oil applied to their skin had decreased blood pressure, increased skin temperature, and reported feeling more calm and relaxed, as compared to subjects in a control group (Hongratanaworakit et al., 2006).

Yuzu: In a limited trial, the aroma of yuzu essential oil was found to affect parasympathetic nervous system activity and to have a mood-balancing effect on women experiencing premenstrual emotional symptoms (Matsumoto et al., 2016; Matsumoto et al., 2017).

Hinoki: Inhaling hinoki oil was found to decrease heart rate and blood pressure and to affect the autonomic nervous system and stimulate a positive mood state in a limited human trial (Chen et al., 2015).

Melissa: Melissa (lemon balm) oil applied topically in a lotion was found to reduce agitation and to improve quality of life factors in patients suffering severe dementia, as compared to those receiving a placebo lotion (Ballard et al., 2002).

Geranium: Geraniol and eugenol, two components of rose oil (among others), were found to demonstrate antianxiety effects on mice in several tests (Umezo et al., 2008).

Ylang ylang: In healthy control subjects, inhalation of ylang ylang aroma significantly reduced the P300 (an event-related potential interpreted to reflect attentional allocation and working memory) amplitude when compared to inhalation without aroma. These results suggest that ylang ylang produces a relaxing effect on cognition (Watanabe et al., 2013).

Bergamot: A study using 114 subjects found that listening to soft music and/or inhaling *Citrus bergamia* essential oil were effective methods of relaxation, as indicated by a shift of the autonomic balance toward parasympathetic (Peng et al., 2009).

Cancer

Cancer can be any of many different conditions where the body's cells duplicate and grow uncontrollably, invade healthy tissues, and possibly spread throughout the body. It is estimated that 95% of cancers result from damage to DNA during a person's lifetime rather than from a pre-existing genetic condition (American Cancer Society, 2008). The most important factor leading to this DNA damage is DNA mutation. DNA mutation can be caused by radiation, environmental chemicals we take into our bodies, free radical damage, or DNA copying or division errors. If the body is working properly, it can correct these mutations either by repairing the DNA or by causing the mutated cell to die. When the DNA mutation is severe enough that it allows the cell to bypass these controls, however, the mutated DNA can be copied to new cells that continue to replicate and create more and more new cells uncontrollably, leading to a cancerous growth within an individual.

Oils: frankincense, sandalwood, lavender, DDR Prime, arborvitae, Yarrow Pom, rosemary, lemongrass, clove, basil, geranium, clary sage, citrus oils, rose

Other Products: Alpha CRS+ contains multiple nutrients that have been studied for their abilities to combat different types of cancer, including polyphenols (such as resveratrol, baicalin, EGCG, quercetin, ellagic acid, and catechin) and coenzyme Q10. xEO Mega or vEO Mega or IQ Mega and Microplex VMz to help support cellular and immune function.

Note: Healthcare professionals are emphatic about avoiding heavy massage when working with cancer patients. Light massage may be used—but never over the trauma area.

—Bone:

    Oils: frankincense

—Brain:

    Oils: frankincense, myrrh, clove

    Recipe 1: Combine 15 drops frankincense, 6 drops clove, and 1 Tbs. (15 ml) fractionated coconut oil. Massage lightly on spine every day. Diffuse 15 drops frankincense and 6 drops clove for 30 minutes, three times a day.

    Recipe 2: Diffuse frankincense, and massage the brain stem area lightly with frankincense neat.

—Breast:

    Oils: rosemary, lavender, frankincense, arborvitae, Yarrow Pom, clary sage, clove, basil, sandalwood, oregano, lemongrass, marjoram

—Cervical:

    Oils: frankincense, geranium, fir, cypress, clove, lavender, lemon

—Colon:

    Oils: lavender, geranium, frankincense, arborvitae, lemongrass

—Leukemia:

    Oils: frankincense, lemongrass, rosemary, clary sage, clove

—Liver:

    Oils: frankincense, lemongrass, lavender, rosemary

—Lung:

    Oils: frankincense (apply to chest, or mix 15 drops with 1 tsp. (5 ml) fractionated coconut oil for nightly rectal retention enema), lavender

—Prostate

    Oils: frankincense (blend 15 drops with 1 tsp. (5 ml) fractionated coconut oil for nightly rectal retention enema), arborvitae, Yarrow Pom

—Skin/Melanoma:

    Oils: Hawaiian sandalwood, arborvitae, frankincense, citrus oils

—Throat:

    Oils: frankincense, lavender

—Uterine:

    Oils: geranium, frankincense

: Dilute as recommended, and apply 1–5 drops on location and on reflex points on the feet and hands. Apply as a warm compress over affected area.

: Diffuse into the air. Inhale oil directly or applied to hands, tissue, or a cotton wick.

: Take capsules as recommended on package. Place 1–2 drops of oil under the tongue or add 1–3 drops of oil in an empty capsule; swallow capsule. Repeat up to twice daily as needed.

: **Body System(s) Affected:** Immune System.

: **Additional Research:**

Frankincense: An extract from *Boswellia carterii* was found to induce apoptosis (cell death) in 2 leukemia cell lines (Hunan et al., 1999).

Frankincense: An extract from frankincense was found to produce apoptosis in human leukemia cells (Bhushan et al., 2007).

Frankincense: β-elemene—a sesquiterpene found in curcumin and *Boswellia frereana* and black pepper essential oils—is currently being studied for its promising potential to induce apoptosis and inhibit cancer cell proliferation in ovarian (Zou et al, 2013), liver (Dai et al, 2013), breast (Zhang et al., 2013; Ding et al., 2013), bladder (Li et al, 2013), lung (Li et al., 2013; Chen et al., 2012), and brain (Li et al., 2013) cancer cell lines, both on its own and in combination with cisplatin chemotherapy.

Frankincense: Ethanol extract of *Boswellia serrata* demonstrated antiproliferative effects on 5 leukemia and two brain tumor cell lines. It was more potent than one type of boswellic acid (AKBA) on three leukemia cell lines (Hostanska et al., 2002).

See the *Quick Usage Chart* inside the back cover for recommended dilutions.

264

Frankincense: β-elemene was found to induce apoptosis in brain tumor cells (Li et al., 2013).

Frankincense: Derivatives of β-elemene were found to induce apoptosis in human leukemia cells (Yu et al., 2011).

Frankincense: Proliferation of human hepatoma cells was found to be inhibited by β-elemene in vitro (Dai et al., 2013).

Frankincense: β-elemene, found in *Boswellia frereana* and black pepper essential oils, was found to have anti-lung cancer properties (Chen et al., 2012).

Frankincense: β-elemene was found to decrease MCF-7 human breast cancer cell migration and invasion (Zhang et al., 2013).

Sandalwood: Oral sandalwood oil use enhanced GST activity (a protein in cell membranes that can help eliminate toxins) and acid-soluble SH levels. This suggests a possible chemopreventive action on carcinogenesis (Banerjee et al., 1993).

Sandalwood: Alpha-santalol was found to induce apoptosis in human skin cancer cells (Kaur et al., 2005).

Sandalwood: A solution of 5% alpha-santalol (from sandalwood) was found to prevent skin-tumor formation caused by ultraviolet-b (UVB) radiation in mice (Dwivedi et al., 2006).

Sandalwood: Various concentrations of alpha-santalol (from sandalwood) were tested against skin cancer in mice. All concentrations were found to inhibit skin cancer development (Dwivedi et al., 2005).

Sandalwood: Alpha-santalol, derived from sandalwood EO, was found to delay and decrease the incidence and multiplicity of skin tumor (papilloma) development in mice (Dwivedi et al., 2003).

Sandalwood: Sandalwood oil was found to decrease skin papilloma (tumors) in mice (Dwivedi et al., 1997).

Sandalwood: Pretreatment with alpha-santalol (found in sandalwood) before UVB (ultraviolet-b) radiation significantly reduced skin tumor development and multiplicity and induced proapoptotic and tumor-suppressing proteins (Arasada et al., 2008).

Sandalwood: Sandalwood oil was found to induce apoptosis and cell arrest in several types of cancer cell lines and in animal models of skin cancer (Santha et al., 2015).

Lavender: In tests for mutagenicity, both tea tree and lavender oils were found to not be mutagenic. In fact, lavender oil was found to have strong antimutagenic activity, reducing mutations of cells exposed to a known mutagen (Evandri et al., 2005).

Lavender: Perillyl alcohol (found in caraway, lavender, and mint), EGCG (polyphenol from green tea), squalene (a triterpene derived from sharks and other vegetable material), and EPA (an essential fatty acid from fish or microalgae) were found to inhibit hyperproliferation of mammary epithelial cells prior to tumorigenisis (Katdare et al., 1997).

Lavender: Rats fed diets containing perillyl alcohol (derived from lavender plants) were found to have less incidence of colon tumors and less multiplicity of tumors in the colon compared to control. Colon tumors of animals fed perillyl alcohol were found to exhibit increased apoptosis of cells compared to control (Reddy et al., 1997).

Lavender: Mice treated with perillyl alcohol (found in lavender and mint plants) had a 22% reduction in tumor incidence and a 58% reduction in tumor multiplicity during a mouse lung tumor bioassay (Lantry et al., 1997).

Lavender: Rats with liver tumors that were treated with perillyl alcohol had smaller tumor sizes than untreated rats due to apoptosis in cancer cells in treated rats (Mills et al., 1995).

Arborvitae: Hinokitiol was found to induce autophagic signaling in murine breast and colorectal tumor cells in vitro (Wang et al., 2014).

Arborvitae: Mice implanted with human colon cancer tumor cells saw a decrease in tumor size and weight when treated with β-thujaplicin (hinokitiol) (Lee et al., 2013).

Arborvitae: Hinokitiol demonstrated inhibition of cell growth and DNA synthesis in human melanoma cells in vitro (Liu et al., 2009).

Rosemary: Rosemary extract injected in rats was found to decrease mammary adenocarcinomas in rats (Singletary et al., 1996).

Rosemary: An ethanol extract of rosemary was found to have an antiproliferative effect on human leukemia and breast carcinoma cells, as well as an antioxidant effect (Cheung et al., 2007).

Rosemary: Carnosic acid (derived from rosemary) was found to inhibit the proliferation of human leukemia cells in vitro (Steiner et al., 2001).

Rosemary: Rosemary extracts induced CYP (cytochrome 450) activity in liver cells, suggesting a possibility of increased ability to remove toxins (Debersac et al., 2001).

Lemongrass: Citral (found in lemongrass, melissa, and verbena oils) was found to induce apoptosis in several cancer cell lines (hematopoietic cells=stem cells that create blood cells) (Dudai et al., 2005).

Lemongrass: Lemongrass oil was found to inhibit multiple cancer cell lines, both in vitro and in vivo, in mice (Sharma et al., 2009).

Lemongrass: Geraniol (found in geranium and lemongrass oil, among others) was found to inhibit colon cancer cell growth while inhibiting DNA synthesis in these cells (Carnesecchi et al., 2001).

Lemongrass: Lemongrass oil and its constituent, isointermedeol, were found to induce apoptosis in human leukemia cells (Kumar et al., 2008).

Lemongrass: An extract from lemongrass was found to inhibit hepatocarcinogenesis (liver cancer genesis) in rats (Puatanachokchai et al., 2002).

Clove: Beta-caryophyllene (found in clove) was found to increase the anticancer activities of paclitaxel (a chemotherapy drug derived from the yew tree) (Legault et al., 2007).

Clary Sage: Sclareol, a chemical constituent found in clary sage essential oil, was found to reduce regulatory T cells frequency and also tumor size in a mouse model of breast cancer, suggesting that sclareol can enhance the effect of cancer therapy as an immunostiumlant (Noori et al., 2013).

Basil: Basil extract was found to inhibit the growth of MCF-7 breast cancer cells, possess antioxidant activity, and protect against DNA damage (Al-Ali et al., 2013).

Basil: Basil and its component, linalool, were found to reduce spontaneous mutagenesis in bacteria cells (Berić et al., 2008).

Geranium: Geraniol (found in geranium and lemongrass oil, among others) was found to inhibit colon cancer cell growth while inhibiting DNA synthesis in these cells (Carnesecchi et al., 2001).

Clary Sage: Sclareol, from clary sage oil, was found to have a cytostatic effect in human leukemia cell lines (Dimas et al., 1999).

Clove: Eugenol, a major chemical constituent of clove essential oil, was found to induce apoptosis in human leukemia cells via reactive oxygen species generation (Yoo et al., 2005).

Citrus oils: In a study of older individuals, it was found that there was a dose-dependent relationship between citrus peel (which are high in d-limonene) consumption and a lower degree of squamous cell carcinoma (SCC) of the skin (Hakim et al., 2000).

Resveratrol: Resveratrol was found to act as an antioxidant and antimutagen in addition to inhibiting several types of cancer cells (Jang et al., 1997).

Resveratrol: Human leukemia cells were found to be irreversibly inhibited by resveratrol, while the effects of resveratrol on nonmalignant human lymphoblastoid cells was largely reversible, suggesting a selective growth inhibition of leukemia cells (Lee et al., 2008).

Resveratrol: A combination of resveratrol, quercetin, and catechin administered orally was found to reduce primary tumor growth of breast cancer tumors in nude mice (Schlachterman et al., 2008).

Baicalin: Baicalin was found to inhibit cyclobutane pyrimidine dimers (a precursor to skin cancer) in fibroblast cells exposed to UVB radiation (Zhou et al., 2008).

Baicalin: Baicalin was found to inhibit several different breast cancer cell lines (Franek et al., 2005).

Baicalin: Baicalin was found to inhibit two prostate cancer cell lines in vitro (Miocinovic et al., 2005).

EGCG: The polyphenol EGCG from green tea was found to inhibit the ability of bronchial tumor cells to migrate in vitro (Hazgui et al., 2008).

EGCG: EGCG was found to inhibit pancreatic cancer growth, invasion, metastasis and angiogenesis (ability to create blood vessels) in mice (Shankar et al., 2008).

Quercetin: A combination of resveratrol, quercetin, and catechin administered orally was found to reduce primary tumor growth of breast cancer tumors in nude mice (Schlachterman et al., 2008).

Quercetin: A combination of low-frequency ultrasound followed by treatment with quercetin was found to selectively kill cancerous skin and prostate cancer cells, while having no effect on nonmalignant skin cells (Paliwal et al., 2005).

Quercetin: Quercetin was found to inhibit and induce apoptosis in cancerous prostate cells, but not in normal prostate epithelial cells in vitro (Aalinkeel et al., 2008).

Quercetin: In a large human study, it was found that increased flavonoid intake in male smokers was found to decrease the risk of developing pancreatic cancer (Bobe et al., 2008).

Quercetin: Flavonol intake was found to reduce the risk of developing pancreatic cancer among smokers (Nothlings et al., 2007).

Quercetin: Flavonol intake (including flavonols such as epicatechin, catechin, quercetin, and kaempferol) was found to be inversely associated with lung cancer among tobacco smokers (Cui et al., 2008).

Ellagic acid: Oral supplementation with ellagic acid was found to decrease the number of induced esophageal tumors in rats, compared to a control (Mandal et al., 1990).

Catechin: A combination of resveratrol, quercetin, and catechin administered orally was found to reduce primary tumor growth of breast cancer tumors in nude mice (Schlachterman et al., 2008).

Catechin: In a large human study, it was found that increased flavonoid intake in male smokers was found to decrease the risk of developing pancreatic cancer (Bobe et al., 2008).

Catechin: Flavonol intake was found to reduce the risk of developing pancreatic cancer among smokers (Nothlings et al., 2007).

Catechin: Flavonol intake (including flavonols such as epicatechin, catechin, quercetin, and kaempferol) was found to be inversely associated with lung cancer among tobacco smokers (Cui et al., 2008).

Myrrh: Treatment with elemene (found in myrrh oil) was found to increase survival time and to reduce tumor size in patients with malignant brain tumor, as compared to treatment with chemotherapy (Tan et al., 2000).

Geranium: Geraniol (found in geranium and lemongrass oil, among others) was found to inhibit colon cancer cell growth while inhibiting DNA synthesis in these cells (Carnesecchi et al., 2001).

Hawaiian Sandalwood: Alpha-santalol was found to induce apoptosis in human skin cancer cells (Kaur et al., 2005).

Hawaiian Sandalwood: A solution of 5% alpha-santalol (from sandalwood) was found to prevent skin-tumor formation caused by ultraviolet-b (UVB) radiation in mice (Dwivedi et al., 2006).

Hawaiian Sandalwood: Various concentrations of alpha-santalol (from sandalwood) were tested against skin cancer in mice. All concentrations were found to inhibit skin cancer development (Dwivedi et al., 2005).

Hawaiian Sandalwood: Alpha-santalol, derived from sandalwood EO, was found to delay and decrease the incidence and multiplicity of skin tumor (papilloma) development in mice (Dwivedi et al., 2003).

Hawaiian Sandalwood: Sandalwood oil was found to decrease skin papilloma (tumors) in mice (Dwivedi et al., 1997).

Hawaiian Sandalwood: Pretreatment with alpha-santalol (found in sandalwood) before UVB (ultraviolet-b) radiation significantly reduced skin tumor development and multiplicity and induced proapoptotic and tumor-suppressing proteins (Arasada et al., 2008).

Candida

See Antifungal: Candida

Canker Sores

Canker sores are small, round sores that develop in the mouth, typically inside the lips and cheeks or on the tongue.

> *Simple Solutions—Canker Sores:* Combine 1 drop melaleuca with ½ tsp. (2.5 ml) olive oil 1 tsp. (5 g) baking soda. Apply a small amount on location.

Oils: ⬡melaleuca, ⬡oregano, ⬡On Guard, ⬡Roman chamomile, ⬡myrrh

🜄: Dilute as recommended, and apply 1 drop on location.

⊕: **Body System(s) Affected:** Skin.

Capillaries

Capillaries are the small, thin blood vessels that allow the exchange of oxygen and other nutrients from the blood to cells throughout the body and allow the exchange of carbon dioxide and other waste materials from these tissues back to the blood. The capillaries connect the arteries (that carry blood away from the heart) and veins (that carry blood back to the heart).

—**Broken Capillaries:**

Oils: ⬡geranium, ⬡cypress, ⬡oregano, ⬡thyme, ⬡Roman chamomile

Blend 1: Apply 1 drop lavender and 1 drop Roman chamomile on location.

🜄: Dilute as recommended, and apply 1–2 drops on location.

⊕: **Body System(s) Affected:** Cardiovascular System.

Carbuncles

See Boils

Cardiovascular System

The cardiovascular—or circulatory—system is the system responsible for transporting blood to the various tissues throughout the body. It is comprised of the heart and blood vessels such as arteries, veins, and capillaries.

Oils: ⬡⬢orange, ⬡⬢cypress, ⬡⬢cinnamon, ⬡⬢copaiba, ⬡⬢sandalwood, ⬡⬢thyme ⊕, ⬢⬡neroli

Other Products: ⬤Alpha CRS+ and ⬤a2z Chewable contain several polyphenols (including proanthocyanidin polyphenols from grape seed⊕, the polyphenols EGCG⊕, and ellagic acid⊕) and coenzyme Q10⊕, which have been found to have beneficial cardiovascular effects.

🜄: Dilute oils as recommended, and apply oils to carotid arteries, heart, feet, under left ring finger, above elbow, behind ring toe on left foot, and to reflex points on the feet. Add 1–2 drops to

See the *Quick Usage Chart* inside the back cover for recommended dilutions.

bathwater for a bath. Add 1–2 drops to 1 Tbs. (15 ml) fractionated coconut oil for massage oil, and massage on location or on chest, neck, or feet.

🕭: Diffuse into the air. Inhale oil applied to hands, tissue, or cotton wick.

—Angina:

Angina is pain in the chest due to a lack of blood flow to the heart. Angina is felt as a squeezing, tightening, aching, or pressure in the chest. The pain can also extend to the arms, back, jaw, neck, and teeth.

Oils: ⚬⚬ginger, ⚬⚬orange (for false angina)

🖐: Massage gently onto chest and feet, and apply on carotid artery.

🕭: Diffuse into the air.

—Arrhythmia:

Arrhythmia is any abnormal heart rhythm. *See also Palpitations and Tachycardia below.*

Oils: ⚬⚬ylang ylang⊕, ⚬⚬lavender, ⚬⚬Deep Blue, ⚬⚬neroli

🕭: Diffuse into the air. Inhale the aroma.

🖐: Dilute oils as recommended, and apply oils to carotid arteries, heart, feet, under left ring finger, above elbow, behind ring toe on left foot, and to reflex points on the feet.

—Atherosclerosis:

Atherosclerosis is a hardening of the arteries due to a buildup of plaques (called atheromas) along the arterial wall.

Oils: ○⚬⚬lemon⊕, ⚬lavender⊕, ○⚬melissa⊕, ○⚬dill⊕, ○DDR Prime, ⚬rosemary, ⚬ginger, ⚬thyme, ⚬wintergreen

🕭: Diffuse into the air.

◐: Take 1–2 drops under the tongue or in a capsule or with water.

🖐: Massage gently onto chest and feet, and apply on carotid artery.

—Blood Pressure: *See Blood: Blood Pressure*

—Cardiotonic:

Oils: ⚬⚬lavender, ⚬⚬thyme

🖐: Dilute oils as recommended, and apply oils to carotid arteries, heart, feet, under left ring finger, above elbow, behind ring toe on left foot, and to reflex points on the feet.

🕭: Diffuse into the air. Inhale the aroma.

—Circulation:

Oils: ⚬⚬cypress, ⚬⚬copaiba, ⚬⚬thyme, ⚬⚬peppermint, ⚬⚬clary sage, ⚬⚬wintergreen, ⚬⚬Citrus Bliss, ⚬⚬rosemary, ⚬⚬geranium, ⚬⚬cinnamon, ⚬⚬helichrysum, ⚬⚬neroli, ⚬⚬Serenity, ⚬⚬basil

🖐: Add 1–2 drops to 1 Tbs. (15 ml) fractionated coconut oil for massage oil, and massage on location or on chest, neck, or feet.

🕭: Diffuse into the air. Inhale the aroma.

—Heart:

Oils: ⚬⚬ylang ylang, ⚬⚬marjoram ⚬⚬geranium, ⚬⚬cypress, ⚬Balance, ⚬⚬ginger, ⚬⚬lavender, ⚬⚬rosemary, ⚬Deep Blue

🖐: Dilute oils as recommended, and apply oils to carotid arteries, heart, feet, under left ring finger, above elbow, behind ring toe on left foot, and to reflex points on the feet.

🕭: Diffuse into the air. Inhale the aroma.

—Heart Tissue

Oils: ⚬⚬marjoram, ⚬⚬lavender, ⚬⚬peppermint, ⚬⚬rosemary, ⚬cinnamon, ⚬rose

🖐: Dilute oils as recommended, and apply oils to carotid arteries, heart, feet, under left ring finger, above elbow, behind ring toe on left foot, and to reflex points on the feet.

🕭: Diffuse into the air. Inhale the aroma.

—High Cholesterol: *See Cholesterol*

—Hypertension: *See Blood: Blood Pressure*

—Palpitations:

Palpitations are rapid and forceful contractions of the heart.

Oils: ⚬⚬ylang ylang, ⚬⚬orange, ⚬⚬lavender, ⚬⚬melissa, ⚬⚬peppermint

🖐: Dilute oils as recommended, and apply oils to carotid arteries, heart, feet, under left ring finger, above elbow, behind ring toe on left foot, and to reflex points on the feet.

🕭: Diffuse into the air. Inhale the aroma.

—Phlebitis:

Phlebitis is the inflammation of a superficial vein, typically in the legs or groin area. Wearing

Cardiovascular System

The cardiovascular—or circulatory—system is the system responsible for transporting blood to the various tissues throughout the body. It is comprised of the heart and blood vessels such as arteries, veins, and capillaries.

The cardiovascular system distributes necessary oxygen and nutrients to body tissues while simultaneously transporting carbon dioxide and waste materials to the lungs and excretory organs to be excreted. The cardiovascular system also supports the immune system, allowing immune cells to travel in the blood stream to cells throughout the body. Thermoregulation—the body's ability to keep a constant temperature—and fluid balance are two other important functions supported by the cardiovascular system.

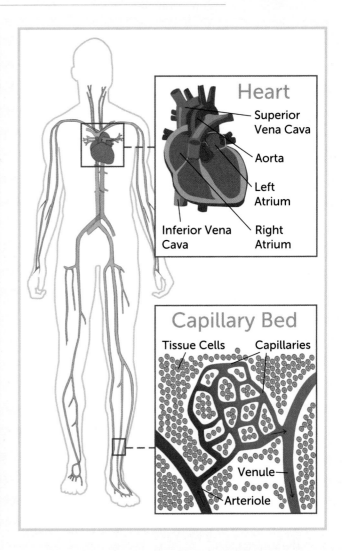

Heart
- Superior Vena Cava
- Aorta
- Left Atrium
- Inferior Vena Cava
- Right Atrium

Capillary Bed
- Tissue Cells
- Capillaries
- Venule
- Arteriole

Oils for Cardiovascular Support

Oils: orange, cypress, cinnamon, sandalwood, thyme

Common Cardiovascular Issues

Cardiovascular: Angina, Aneurysms, Arrhythmia, Atherosclerosis, Bleeding, Cholesterol, Clots, Coronary Artery Disease, Hemorrhaging, High Blood Pressure (Hypertension), Low Blood Pressure, Palpitations, Phlebitis, Shock, Tachycardia

support hose or a compression bandage over the affected area can help aid in healing.

Oils: helichrysum, lavender, cypress, geranium, grapefruit, Balance

: Add 1–2 drops to 1 Tbs. (15 ml) fractionated coconut oil for massage oil, and gently massage on location or on feet.

: Diffuse into the air. Inhale the aroma.

—Prolapsed Mitral Valve:

Oils: marjoram

: Dilute oils as recommended, and apply oils to carotid arteries, heart, feet, under left ring finger, above elbow, behind ring toe on left foot, and to reflex points on the feet.

: Diffuse into the air. Inhale the aroma.

—Tachycardia:

Tachycardia is an abnormally rapid resting heart rate, indicating a possible over-working of the heart.

Oils: lavender, ylang ylang, orange, spikenard, neroli

: Dilute oils as recommended, and apply oils to carotid arteries, heart, feet, under left ring finger, above elbow, behind ring toe on left foot, and to reflex points on the feet.

: Diffuse into the air. Inhale the aroma.

: **Body System(s) Affected:** Cardiovascular System.

: **Additional Research:**

Thyme: Older rats whose diets were supplemented with thyme oil were found to have a higher level of the antioxidant enzymes superoxide dismutase and glutathione peroxidase in the heart, liver, and kidneys, as compared to older rats without this supplementation (Youdim et al., 1999).

Grape seed: An extract of proanthocyanidin polyphenols from grape seed taken as a supplement was found to significantly reduced oxidize LDL (a risk factor for cardiovascular disease) in people with high cholesterol (Bagchi et al., 2003).

EGCG: People who habitually consumed beverages containing EGCG were found to have significantly lower incidences of cardiovascular events (Basu et al., 2007).

EGCG: Supplementation with EGCG was found to lower blood pressure in humans (Brown et al., 2008).

EGCG: EGCG was found to reduce heart weight and cardiac marker enzyme activities in induced heart attacks in rats (Devika et al., 2008).

Ellagic acid: Ellagic acid was found to reduce induced LDL oxidization in vitro (Anderson et al., 2001).

Ellagic acid: Ellagic acid was found to significantly inhibit oxidized LDL proliferation of rat aortic smooth muscle cells (Chang et al., 2008).

Ellagic acid: Supplementation with ellagic acid was found to significantly reduce the amount of atherosclerotic lesions in rabbits fed a high-cholesterol diet (Yu et al., 2005).

Coenzyme Q10: In patients with coronary artery disease, supplementation with CoQ10 was found to improve extracellular superoxide dismutase activity, endothelium-dependent vasodilation, and peak oxygen volume capacity at a level significantly higher as compared to control (Tiano et al., 2007).

Coenzyme Q10: Oral supplementation with CoQ10 was found to improve endothelial function (cells that line the blood vessels) and aerobic capacity of the cardiovascular system in patients with chronic heart failure (Belardinelli et al., 2006).

Coenzyme Q10: Supplementation with CoQ10 was found to improve endothelial dysfunction of the brachial artery in 25 male patients with manifest endothelial dysfunction (Kuettner et al., 2005).

Coenzyme Q10: Chronic heart failure patients receiving CoQ10 supplementation were found to have an improvement in left-ventricle contractility without any side effects (Belardinelli et al., 2005).

Ylang ylang: Inhaled ylang ylang oil was found to decrease blood pressure and pulse rate and to enhance attentiveness and alertness in volunteers compared to an odorless control (Hongratanaworakit et al., 2004).

Lemon: Lemon oil and one of its components, gamma-terpinene, were found to inhibit oxidation of low-density lipoprotein (LDL). Oxidation of LDL has been found to increase the risk of atherosclerosis and cardiac disease (Grassmann et al., 2001).

Lavender: Inhalation of lavender and monarda oils was found to reduce cholesterol content and atherosclerotic plaques in the aorta (Nikolaevski et al., 1990).

Melissa: Melissa essential oil was found to have hypolipidemic effects in transgenic mice. Mice orally administered Melissa essential oil for two weeks had lower plasma triglyceride concentrations and altered metabolic pathways. These results indicate that melissa oil could be beneficial in preventing hypertriglyceridemia, one of the main contributors to the development of cardiovascular disease (Jun et al., 2012).

Dill: Different fractions of *Anethum graveolens* extract improved hypercholesterolemia in rats fed a high fat diet. Hypercholesterolemia has been found to be a risk factor for the development of atherosclerosis (Bahramikia et al., 2009).

Basil: Short-term oral administration of the hydroalcoholic extract of basil leaves to rats was found to protect the muscular tissue of the heart against a chemically induced heart attack (Fathiazad et al., 2012).

Carpal Tunnel Syndrome

Carpal tunnel syndrome is a painful condition of the hand, wrist, and fingers. This condition is caused by inflamed carpal ligaments in the wrist causing pressure on the median nerve. The carpal ligaments can become inflamed due to one of many possible factors: wrist trauma or injury, fluid retention, work stress, or certain strenuous wrist activities. Symptoms include tingling or numbness of the fingers and hand, pain starting in the wrist and extending to the arm or shoulder or to the palms or fingers, a general sense of weakness, and difficulty grasping small objects.

Simple Solutions—CTS: Blend 3 drops basil, 3 drops marjoram, 2 drops lemongrass, and 2 drops cypress with 1 Tbs. (15 ml) fractionated coconut oil. Massage a small amount gently into the arm from the shoulder to the fingertips.

Oils: frankincense, basil, marjoram, lemongrass, oregano, cypress, eucalyptus, lavender

Recipe 1: Apply 1 drop basil and 1 drop marjoram on the shoulder, and massage oils into the skin. Then apply 1 drop lemongrass on the wrist and 1 drop oregano on the rotator cuff in the shoulder, and massage into the skin. Next apply 1 drop marjoram and 1 drop cypress on the wrists and 1 drop cypress on the neck down to the shoulder, and massage into the skin. Lastly, apply peppermint from the shoulder down the arm to the wrist and then out to the tips of each finger, and massage into the skin.

⊜: Dilute oils as recommended, and apply oils on area of concern. Add 1–2 drops to 1 Tbs. (15 ml) fractionated coconut oil for massage oil, and massage on location.

⊕: **Body System(s) Affected:** Immune System and Skeletal System.

Cartilage

See Skeletal System: Cartilage, Muscles: Cartilage Injury

Cataracts

See Eyes: Cataracts

Catarrh

See Congestion: Catarrh

Cavities

See Oral Conditions: Cavities

Cells

Oils: ⵔDDR Prime, ⵔⵔYarrow Pom

Other Products: ⵔAlpha CRS+, ⵔMicroplex VMz and ⵔa2z Chewable for antioxidant support to help protect cells and DNA and for necessary nutrients, ⵔMito2Max for cellular energy support, and ⵔxEO Mega or vEO Mega or ⵔIQ Mega for omega-3 fatty acids necessary for cellular health.

—DNA & Mutation:

DNA is the genetic material of the cell. DNA contains all of the codes that enable the cell to build the materials needed for proper structure and function. Mutation of DNA can lead to cell death or to cancer.

—Antimutagenic Oils:

Oils: ⵔⵔpeppermint⊕, ⵔⵔlavender⊕, ⵔⵔrosemary⊕, ⵔⵔbasil⊕, ⵔⵔfennel⊕

○: Take 3–5 drops in an empty capsule, or with food and beverage. Take up to twice per day as needed.

⊜: Dilute oils as recommended, and apply oils on area of concern. Add 1–2 drops to 1 Tbs. (15 ml) fractionated coconut oil for massage oil, and massage on location.

⊘: Diffuse into the air. Inhale oil applied to hands, tissue, or cotton wick.

◑: **Additional Research:**

Peppermint: Infusions from peppermint and valerian were shown to have antimutagenic properties on fruit flies exposed to the mutagen hydrogen peroxide (Romero-Jiménez et al., 2005).

Lavender: In tests for mutagenicity, both tea tree and lavender oils were found to not be mutagenic. In fact, lavender oil was found to have strong antimutagenic activity, reducing mutations of cells exposed to a known mutagen (Evandri et al., 2005).

Rosemary: An ethanol extract of rosemary demonstrated a protective effect against the oxidative damage to DNA in cells exposed to H_2O_2 and light-excited methylene blue (Slamenova et al., 2002).

Basil: Basil and its component linalool were found to reduce spontaneous mutagenesis in bacteria cells (Berić et al., 2008).

Fennel: Oral pretreatment with fennel essential oil was found to inhibit in vivo genotoxicity of cyclophosphamide (an important chemotherapy medication with adverse effects) in mouse bone marrow and sperm. These findings suggest that fennel could be used as an adjuvant in chemotherapeutic applications to help diminish adverse effects (Tripathi et al., 2013).

Cellulite

See also Weight

Cellulite refers to deposits of fat under the skin of the thighs, abdomen, and buttocks that cause the skin to appear dimpled.

> *Simple Solutions—Cellulite:* Combine 5 drops grapefruit with 1 tsp. (5 ml) jojoba oil in a small roll-on container, and apply on location.

Oils: ⵔⵔSlim & Sassy, ⵔgrapefruit, ⵔrosemary, ⵔbasil, ⵔorange, ⵔlemon, ⵔlime, ⵔcypress, ⵔjuniper berry, ⵔlavender, ⵔoregano, ⵔfennel, ⵔgeranium

Recipe 1: Add 5 drops grapefruit and 5 drops lemon to 1 gallon (4 L) drinking water. Adjust to taste, and drink throughout the day.

○: Add 8 drops of Slim & Sassy to 2 cups (500 ml) of water, and drink throughout the day between meals.

⊜: Dilute as recommended, and apply 1–2 drops on location. Add 1–2 drops to 1 Tbs. (15 ml) fractionated coconut oil, and massage on location.

⊕: **Body System(s) Affected:** Skin and Digestive System.

See the *Quick Usage Chart* inside the back cover for recommended dilutions.

270

Charley Horse

See **Muscles: Cramps/Charley Horses**

Chemicals

See **Detoxification**

Chilblains

See also **Inflammation, Lupus**

Chilblains are inflammatory swelling, itching, redness, or blisters that appear on hands and feet from exposure to cold. They usually appear seasonally with cold weather and clear up in 1–3 weeks, especially if the weather gets warmer. Chilblains may also be associated with other conditions, such as lupus.

> *Simple Solutions—Chilblains:* Combine 3 drops frankincense and 2 drops cypress with 1/2 cup (250 g) Epsom salt, and dissolve in warm (not hot) bathwater. Soak the affected area for 20–30 minutes.

Oils: frankincense, myrrh, Deep Blue, lavender, eucalyptus, cypress, rosemary, copaiba

: Dilute as recommended, and apply 1–2 drops on location. Add 1–2 drops to 1 tsp. (5 ml) fractionated coconut oil in a roll-on vial, and apply on location.

: **Body System(s) Affected:** Skin, Muscles and Bones.

Childbirth

See **Pregnancy/Motherhood**

Childhood Diseases

See also **Antiviral, Antibacterial**

—Chicken Pox: *See also* Shingles

Chicken pox is a common childhood illness caused by the virus varicella zoster. Symptoms of chicken pox include mild fever, weakness, and a rash. The rash appears as red spots that form into blisters that eventually burst and then crust over. Chicken pox can occur between 10 and 21 days after contact with the virus and is contagious up to 5 days before and 5 days after the rash appears. Chicken pox is highly contagious and can be contracted by anyone, but it is most common in children under the age of 15.

> *Simple Solutions—Chicken Pox:* Combine 10 drops lavender and 10 drops Roman chamomile with ½ cup (125 ml) calamine lotion. Mix and apply a small amount twice a day over affected areas.

Oils: lavender, melaleuca, Roman chamomile, eucalyptus, lemon, bergamot

Recipe 1: Add 2 drops lavender to 1 cup (200 g) baking soda. Dissolve in warm bathwater, and bathe to help relieve itching.

—Measles:

Measles is a viral infection of the respiratory system that causes coughing, runny nose, red eyes, fever, and a rash on the skin.

> *Simple Solutions—Measles:* Diffuse eucalyptus radiata in an aromatherapy diffuser.

Oils: eucalyptus, melaleuca, lavender

—Mumps:

Mumps is a viral infection that causes fever, chills, headache, and painful swelling of the saliva glands.

> *Simple Solutions—Mumps:* Apply 1 drop melaleuca on swollen glands once a day.

Oils: melaleuca, lavender, lemon

—Rubella (German Measles):

Rubella, or German measles, is a viral infection that causes rash, fever, runny nose, and joint pain.

Oils: melaleuca, lavender

—Whooping Cough:

Whooping cough, or pertussis, is a bacterial infection that causes cold-like symptoms, followed by severe coughing fits.

> *Simple Solutions—Whooping Cough:* Mix 2 drops each of cinnamon, hyssop, and thyme, and place in a water-misting aromatherapy diffuser. Run once or twice a day for 15 minutes. Use only 1 drop of each for very young children.

A
B
C
D
E
F
G
H
I
J
K
L
M
N
O
P
Q
R
S
T
U
V
W
X
Y
Z

Oils: ⬡oregano, ⬡⬡basil, ⬡⬡thyme, ⬡clary sage, ⬡cypress, ⬡lavender, ⬡Roman chamomile, ⬡grapefruit, ⬡eucalyptus, ⬡melaleuca, ⬡peppermint, ⬡rose

⬥: Dilute as recommended, and apply on location or on chest, neck, back, or reflex points on the feet. Add 1–2 drops to 4 cups (1 L) warm water, and use water for a sponge bath.

⬥: Diffuse into the air. Diffuse other antiviral oils such as lemon as well. *See Antiviral.*

⬥: **Body System(s) Affected:** Immune System.

⬥: **Additional Research:**

> **Eucalyptus:** A plaque reduction assay showed that eucalyptus essential oil possessed a mild antiviral activity against mumps virus (Cermelli et al., 2008).

Children and Infants

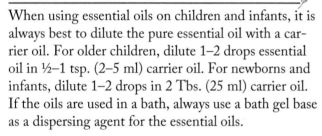

When using essential oils on children and infants, it is always best to dilute the pure essential oil with a carrier oil. For older children, dilute 1–2 drops essential oil in ½–1 tsp. (2–5 ml) carrier oil. For newborns and infants, dilute 1–2 drops in 2 Tbs. (25 ml) carrier oil. If the oils are used in a bath, always use a bath gel base as a dispersing agent for the essential oils.

Keep the oils out of children's reach. If an oil is ever ingested, give the child an oil-soluble liquid such as milk, cream, or half-and-half. Then call your local poison control center, or seek emergency medical attention. A few drops of pure essential oil shouldn't be life-threatening, but it is best to take these precautions.

Several oils that are generally considered safe for children include cypress, frankincense, geranium, ginger, lavender, lemon✴, marjoram, melaleuca, orange✴, rosemary▽, sandalwood, thyme, and ylang ylang.

✴: These oils are photosensitive; always dilute, and do not use when skin will be exposed soon to direct sunlight.

▽: This oil should never be used undiluted on infants or children.

Oils: ⬡⬡Brave, ⬡⬡Calmer, ⬡⬡Rescuer, ⬡⬡Steady, ⬡⬡Stronger, ⬡⬡Thinker

Other Products: ⬡Baby Hair and Body Wash, ⬡Baby Lotion, ⬡Diaper Rash Cream

—**Colic:**

Colic is any extended period of crying and fussiness that occurs frequently in an infant. While the exact cause is not known, it has been speculated that the cause may be from indigestion, the buildup of gas, lactose intolerance, or a lack of needed probiotic bacteria in the intestines.

> *Simple Solutions—Colic:* Blend 1 drop each of Roman chamomile, lavender, and geranium with 2 Tbs. (25 ml) almond oil. Apply a small amount on the stomach and back.

Oils: ⬡fennel⊕, ⬡⬡star anise, ⬡marjoram, ⬡bergamot, ⬡ylang ylang, ⬡ginger, ⬡Roman chamomile, ⬡rosemary, ⬡melissa

⬥: Dilute 1–2 drops of oil in 2 Tbs. (25 ml) fractionated coconut oil, and massage a small amount of this blend gently on stomach and back.

—**Common Cold:** *See Antiviral*

A cold is a viral infection that causes a stuffy or runny nose, congestion, cough, and sneezing.

> *Simple Solutions—Colds:* Diffuse thyme oil using an aromatherapy diffuser.

Oils: ⬡⬡thyme, ⬡⬡lemon, ⬡⬡cedarwood, ⬡⬡Stronger, ⬡⬡sandalwood, ⬡⬡rosemary, ⬡⬡rose

⬥: Dilute 1–2 drops of oil in 2 Tbs. (25 ml) fractionated coconut oil, and massage a little on neck and chest.

⬥: Diffuse into the air.

—**Constipation:**

Constipation is when feces becomes too hard and dry to expel easily from the body.

Oils: ⬡rosemary⊕, ⬡ginger, ⬡orange

⬥: Dilute 1–2 drops of oil in 2 Tbs. (25 ml) fractionated coconut oil, and massage on stomach and feet.

—**Cradle Cap:**

Cradle cap is a scaling of the skin on the head that commonly occurs in young infants. The scaling is yellowish in color and often disappears by the time the infant is a few months old.

See the *Quick Usage Chart* inside the back cover for recommended dilutions.

Simple Solutions—Cradle Cap: Blend 2 drops geranium with 2 Tbs. (25 ml) olive oil. Apply a small amount on the head no more than once per day as needed.

Recipe 1: Combine 2 Tbs. (25 ml) almond oil with 1 drop lemon and 1 drop geranium. Apply a small amount of this blend on the head.

—Croup:

Croup is a viral respiratory infection that causes inflammation of the area around the larynx (voice box) and a distinctive-sounding cough. Often, taking an infant or child outside to breathe cool night air can help open the restricted airways, as can humidity.

Oils: marjoram, thyme, Stronger, sandalwood

: Diffuse into the air.

: Dilute 1–2 drops in 2 Tbs. (25 ml) fractionated coconut oil, and massage on chest and neck.

—Crying:

Oils: ylang ylang, lavender, Roman chamomile, Brave, Calmer, geranium, cypress, frankincense

: Diffuse into the air.

: Dilute 1–2 drops in 2 Tbs. (25 ml) fractionated coconut oil. Massage.

—Diaper Rash:

Diaper rash is a red rash of the skin in the diaper area caused by prolonged skin exposure to the moisture and different pH of urine and feces. Often, more frequent bathing of the area and diaper changes will help alleviate the rash.

Simple Solutions—Diaper Rash: Blend 1 drop Roman chamomile, 1 drop lavender, and 1 tsp. (5 ml) fractionated coconut oil in a small roll-on bottle. Apply on location.

Oils: lavender

Other Products: Diaper Rash Cream

Blend 2: Combine 1 drop Roman chamomile and 1 drop lavender with 1 tsp. (5 ml) fractionated coconut oil, and apply on location.

: Dilute 1–2 drops in 2 Tbs. (25 ml) fractionated coconut oil, and apply a small amount of this mixture on location.

—Digestion (sluggish):

Oils: lemon, orange

: Dilute 1–2 drops in 2 Tbs. (25 ml) fractionated coconut oil, and massage a small amount on feet and stomach.

—Dry Skin:

Oils: sandalwood

Other Products: Baby Hair and Body Wash, Baby Lotion

: Dilute 1–2 drops in 2 Tbs. (25 ml) fractionated coconut oil, and apply a small amount on location.

—Earache:

Oils: melaleuca, Stronger, Roman chamomile, lavender, thyme

Blend 3: Combine 2 Tbs. (25 ml) fractionated coconut oil with 2 drops lavender, 1 drop Roman chamomile, and 1 drop melaleuca. Put a drop on a cotton ball or cotton swab, and apply in ear, behind the ear, and on reflex points on the feet.

: Dilute 1–2 drops in 2 Tbs. (25 ml) fractionated coconut oil, and apply a small amount behind the ear. Place a drop on a cotton ball, and place in the ear.

—Fever:

Oils: lavender, peppermint, Stronger

: Dilute 1–2 drops in 2 Tbs. (25 ml) fractionated coconut oil, and massage a small amount on the neck, feet, behind ears, and on back.

: Diffuse into the air.

—Flu:

Flu, or influenza, is a viral infection that affects the respiratory system. Symptoms may include coughing, sneezing, fever, runny nose, congestion, muscle aches, nausea, and vomiting.

Oils: cypress, lemon, Stronger

: Dilute 1 drop oil in an unscented bath gel, and use for a bath.

: Diffuse into the air.

—**Hyperactive:** *See Calming, ADD/ADHD*

—**Jaundice:**

Jaundice is a condition where the liver cannot clear the pigment bilirubin quickly enough from the blood, causing the blood to deposit the bilirubin into the skin and whites of the eyes, turning them a yellowish color.

Oils: geranium, lemon, rosemary

: Dilute 1–2 drops in 2 Tbs. (25 ml) fractionated coconut oil, and massage a small amount on the liver area and on the reflex points on the feet.

—**Premature:**

Since premature babies have very thin and sensitive skin, it is best to avoid the use of essential oils.

—**Rashes:**

Oils: lavender, Roman chamomile, sandalwood

Other Products: Baby Lotion

: Dilute 1–2 drops in 2 Tbs. (25 ml) fractionated coconut oil, and apply a small amount on location.

—**Teeth Grinding:**

Oils: lavender, Calmer, Serenity

: Dilute 1–2 drops in 2 Tbs. (25 ml) fractionated coconut oil, and massage a small amount on the feet.

: Diffuse into the air.

—**Tonsillitis:**

Tonsillitis is inflammation of the tonsils, two lymph-filled tissues located at the back of the mouth that help provide immune support. These may become inflamed due to a bacterial or viral infection.

Oils: melaleuca, lemon, Stronger, Roman chamomile, lavender, ginger

: Dilute 1–2 drops in 2 Tbs. (25 ml) fractionated coconut oil, and apply a small amount to tonsils and lymph nodes.

—**Thrush:** *See also Antifungal*

Thrush is an oral fungal infection caused by *Candida albicans*. It causes painful white-colored areas to appear in the mouth.

Oils: melaleuca, Stronger, lavender, thyme, lemon, geranium

: Dilute 1–2 drops in 2 Tbs. (25 ml) fractionated coconut oil, and apply a small amount on location.

: **Additional Research:**

Fennel: Fennel seed oil was found to be superior to a placebo in decreasing intensity of infantile colic in a randomized placebo-controlled trial including 121 infants. The oil was administered four times a day and consumption was limited to a maximum of 12 mg/kg/day of fennel seed oil (Alexandrovich et al., 2003).

Fennel and melissa: Colic improved in breastfed infants within 1 week of administering a phytotherapeutic agent containing *Matricariae recutita*, *Foeniculum vulgare*, and *Melissa officinalis* when compared to a placebo containing vitamins (Savino et al., 2005).

Rosemary: The use of rosemary, lemon, and peppermint oils in massage demonstrated an ability to reduce constipation and increase bowel movements in elderly subjects, compared to massage without the oils (Kim et al., 2005).

Melaleuca: Tea tree oil was found to inhibit 301 different types of yeasts isolated from the mouths of cancer patients suffering from advanced cancer, including 41 strains that are known to be resistant to antifungal drugs (Bagg et al., 2006).

Melaleuca: Eleven types of *Candida* were found to be highly inhibited by tea tree oil (Banes-Marshall et al., 2001).

Lavender: Lavender oil demonstrated both fungistatic (stopped growth) and fungicidal (killed) activity against *Candida albicans* (D'Auria et al., 2005).

Thyme: Thyme oil was found to inhibit *Candida* species by causing lesions in the cell membrane as well as inhibiting germ tube (an outgrowth that develops when the fungi is preparing to replicate) formation (Pina-Vaz et al., 2004).

Chills

See Fever, Warming Oils

Cholera

Cholera is a potentially severe bacterial infection of the intestines by the *Vibrio cholerae* bacteria. This infection can cause severe diarrhea, leading to dehydration that can cause low blood pressure, shock, or death. Rehydration with an oral rehydration solution is the most effective way to prevent dehydration. If no commercially prepared oral rehydration solution is available, a solution made from 1 tsp. (5 g) salt, 8 tsp. (35 g) sugar, and 4 cups (1 L) clean water (with some mashed fresh banana, if available, to add potassium) can work in an emergency.

Simple Solutions—Cholera: Add 1 drop rosemary to 1 tsp. (5 ml) fractionated coconut oil, and apply on the stomach twice a day.

Oils: rosemary, clove

: Dilute as recommended, and apply to stomach and on reflex points on the feet.

: **Body System(s) Affected:** Immune System and Digestive System.

See the *Quick Usage Chart* inside the back cover for recommended dilutions.

274

Cholesterol

Cholesterol is an important lipid that comprises part of the cell membrane and myelin sheath and that plays a role in nerve cell function. It is created by the body and can be found in many foods we eat. An imbalance of certain types of cholesterol in the blood has been theorized to play a role in the formation of plaques in the arteries (atherosclerosis).

Simple Solutions—Cholesterol: Add 5 drops lemongrass and 5 drops dill to 2 Tbs. (25 ml) olive oil in a small dropper bottle. Massage over stomach and bottoms of feet daily. Add a small amount of this blend to a capsule, and swallow.

Oils: ⁰lemongrass⊕, ⊘clary sage, ⊘helichrysum, ⁰⊘dill⊕, ⊘lavender⊕, ⁰⊘juniper berry⊕

◐: Dilute as recommended, and apply to liver area and reflex points on the feet.

◐: Place 1–2 drops in a capsule, and swallow.

◔: Diffuse into the air.

✛: **Body System(s) Affected:** Cardiovascular System.

▥: **Additional Research:**

> **Lemongrass:** Supplementation with lemongrass capsules was found to reduce cholesterol in some subjects (Elson et al., 1989).
>
> **Dill:** Different fractions of *Anethum graveolens* extract improved hypercholesterolemia in rats fed a high fat diet. Hypercholesterolemia has been found to be a risk factor for the development of atherosclerosis (Bahramikia et al., 2009).
>
> **Lavender:** Inhalation of lavender and monarda oils was found to reduce cholesterol content and atherosclerotic plaques in the aorta (Nikolaevski et al., 1990).
>
> **Juniper Berry:** Oral administration of juniper berry essential oil to rats fed a high cholesterol diet resulted in increased antioxidant enzyme activities in the rat heart tissue (Gumral et al., 2013).
>
> **Camphene (found in coriander, frankincense, ginger, lavender, lime, peppermint, roman chamomile, rose, rosemary, spearmint, fir):** Injection of camphene, a constituent found in many essential oils, was found to reduce plasma cholesterol and triglycerides in naïve and hyperlipidemic rats. Camphene's mechanism of action was different than that of statins (drugs used to lower cholesterol levels) (Vallianou et al., 2011).

Chronic Fatigue

Chronic fatigue syndrome refers to a set of debilitating symptoms that may include prolonged periods of fatigue that are not alleviated by rest, difficulty concentrating, muscle and joint pain, headaches, and sore throats that cannot be explained by any other known medical condition. While the exact cause of chronic fatigue syndrome is not known, some have theorized that it is caused by a virus (such as the Epstein-Barr virus) left in the body after an illness.

Simple Solutions—Chronic Fatigue: Combine 3 drops peppermint with 1 cup (250 g) Epsom salt. Dissolve ½ cup (125 g) in warm bathwater for a soothing bath.

Oils: ◔◐On Guard, ◔◐peppermint, ◔◐basil, ◔◐lemongrass, ◐◔DigestZen, ◔◐rosemary, ◔◐lavender

Other Products: ⁰Mito2Max, ⁰Alpha CRS+ or ⁰a2z Chewable to help support healthy cellular energy levels. ⁰xEO Mega or vEO Mega or ⁰IQ Mega, and ⁰Microplex VMz to help supply necessary nutrients to support cell and immune function.

◐: Dilute as recommended, and apply 1–2 drops to sore muscles or joints, to the back, or to the feet. Add 1–2 drops to warm bathwater for a bath.

◐: Take capsules as directed on package. Add 1–2 drops of oil to an empty capsule; swallow.

◔: Diffuse into the air. Inhale directly from bottle. Apply oil to hands, tissue, or cotton wick, and inhale.

✛: **Body System(s) Affected:** Immune System, Nervous System, and Emotional Balance.

Cigarettes

*See **Addictions: Smoking***

Circulatory System

*See **Cardiovascular System***

Cirrhosis

*See **Liver: Cirrhosis***

Cleansing

*See also **Housecleaning***

Oils: ◔◐Purify, ◔◐On Guard, ◔◐Stronger, ◐melaleuca

Other Products: ◐On Guard Foaming Hand Wash to cleanse hands and protect against harmful microorganisms.

—Cuts:

   Oils: ◐lavender, ◐melaleuca, ◔◐Stronger

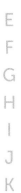

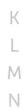
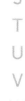
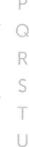

A B C D E F G H I J K L M N O P Q R S T U V W X Y Z

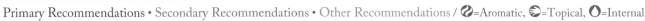

—Master Cleanse or Lemonade Diet:

Combine 2 Tbs. (25 ml) fresh lemon or lime juice (approximately ½ lemon), 2 Tbs. (25 ml) grade B maple syrup, and ¹/₁₀ tsp. (150 mg) cayenne pepper (or to taste) with 1¼ cups (300 ml) distilled water. If you have diabetes, use black strap molasses instead of the maple syrup. Drink 6–12 glasses of this mixture daily, with an herbal laxative tea taken first thing in the morning and just before retiring at night. Refer to the booklet *The Master Cleanser* for more specifics and for suggestions of how to come off of this cleanse.

🌿: Dilute as recommended, and apply on location. Dilute 1–3 drops in 1 Tbs. (15 ml) fractionated coconut oil, and use as massage oil. Use hand wash as directed on packaging.

☯: Diffuse into the air.

Colds

See also Antiviral, Coughs, Congestion

A cold is a viral infection that causes a stuffy or runny nose, congestion, cough, sore throat, or sneezing.

> *Simple Solutions—Colds:* Blend 5 drops lemon and 5 drops thyme in 1 Tbs. (15 ml) jojoba oil. Apply a small amount to the throat, forehead, chest, and back of neck 2–3 times per day.

Oils: ☯🌿thyme, ☯🌿lemon, ☯🌿On Guard, ☯🌿melaleuca, ☯🌿hinoki, ☯🌿sandalwood, 🌿eucalyptus, ☯🌿rosemary, ☯🌿lime, ☯🌿peppermint (for nasal congestion), ☯🌿Breathe (for respiratory congestion), ☯🌿Douglas fir, 🌿ginger, ☯🌿copaiba, ☯🌿basil, ☯🌿lavender, ☯🌿orange, ☯🌿oregano

Other Products: ⭘Breathe Respiratory Drops, ☯🌿Breathe Vapor Stick, ⭘On Guard+ Softgels. ⭘Microplex VMz for nutrients essential to support cellular and immune system health.

Recipe 1: When you first notice a sore throat, apply a tiny amount of melaleuca to the tip of the tongue, and then swallow. Repeat this a few times every 5–10 minutes. Then massage a couple of drops on the back of the neck.

🌿: Dilute as recommended, and apply 1–2 drops to throat, temples, forehead, back of neck, sinus area, below the nose, chest, or reflex points on the feet.

☯: Diffuse into the air. Place 1–2 drops in a bowl of hot water, and inhale the vapors. Inhale directly from bottle. Apply oil to hands, tissue, or cotton wick, and inhale.

💧: Take capsules as directed on package. Place 1–2 drops of oil under the tongue or place 1–2 drops of oil in an empty capsule, and swallow.

➊: **Body System(s) Affected:** Immune System.

Cold Sores

See also Antiviral, Herpes Simplex

Cold sores are blisters or sores in the mouth area caused by an infection of the herpes simplex virus.

> *Simple Solutions—Cold Sores:* Combine 4 tsp. (5 g) beeswax pellets, 1 Tbs. (10 g) cocoa butter, and 3 Tbs. (45 ml) jojoba oil, and melt in the microwave (30 seconds at a time, stirring in between) or in a double boiler. Cool slightly, and add 5 drops melissa, 5 drops peppermint, and 5 drops helichrysum essential oil. Pour into small jars or lip balm containers, and allow to cool completely. Apply a small amount of balm on cold sores as needed.

Oils: 🌿melaleuca☐, 🌿melissa☐, 🌿peppermint☐, 🌿lemon, 🌿On Guard, 🌿geranium, 🌿lavender, 🌿bergamot

🌿: Dilute as recommended, and apply 1–2 drops on location.

➊: **Body System(s) Affected:** Immune System and Skin.

☐: **Additional Research:**

Melaleuca: Tea tree and eucalyptus oil demonstrated an ability to inhibit the Herpes simplex virus (Schnitzler et al., 2001).

Melissa: Melissa oil demonstrated inhibition of herpes simplex type 1 and type 2 viruses (Schnitzler et al., 2008).

Peppermint: Peppermint oil demonstrated a direct virucidal activity against herpes type 1 and type 2 viruses (Schuhmacher et al., 2003).

Colic

See Children and Infants: Colic

Colitis

See Colon: Colitis

Colon

See also Cancer: Colon, Digestive System

See the Quick Usage Chart inside the back cover for recommended dilutions.

The colon, or large intestine, is the last part of the digestive system. Its function is to extract water and vitamins created by friendly bacterial flora from the material moving through the digestive system.

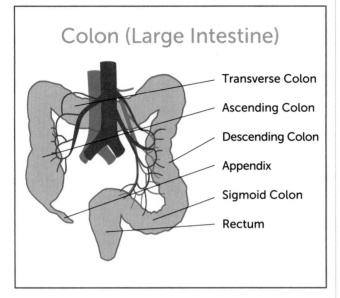

Colon (Large Intestine)

- Transverse Colon
- Ascending Colon
- Descending Colon
- Appendix
- Sigmoid Colon
- Rectum

Oils: ⊗O DigestZen, ⊗O peppermint

Other Products: O PB Assist+ or O PB Assist Jr to help restore friendly flora to the intestinal wall. O GX Assist to help the digestive system eliminate pathogens. O DigestZen Softgels to help support healthy digestion. O Zendocrine Zendocrine Detoxification Complex to help support healthy colon functioning.

—**Cancer:** *See Cancer: Colon*

—**Colitis:**

Colitis is inflammation of the large intestine or colon. The exact cause is not known but may involve an auto-immune response. Symptoms can include abdominal pain, tenderness, frequent need to expel stools, diarrhea, and possibly bloody stools and fever in the case of ulcerative colitis.

Oils: ⊗O DigestZen, ⊗⊘ helichrysum, ⊗⊘ peppermint⊕, ⊗⊘O thyme⊕, O oregano⊕, O rosemary⊕, ⊗⊘ clove

Other Products: O DigestZen Softgels to help support healthy digestion.

—**Diverticulitis:**

Diverticulitis is the inflammation of a diverticula (a small balloon-like sac that sometimes forms along the wall of the large intestine, especially in older individuals), typically due to infection. It

causes pain in the abdomen and tenderness on the lower-left-hand part of the stomach.

Oils: ⊗ cinnamon, ⊗ lavender

—**Polyps:** *See also Cancer: Colon*

Polyps are tumors that arise from the bowel surface and protrude into the inside of the colon. Most polyps eventually transform into malignant cancer tumors.

Oils: O⊗ peppermint

⊗: Dilute as recommended, and apply 1–2 drops on lower abdomen or on reflex points on the feet. Use 1–2 drops in warm bathwater for a bath.

O: Take capsule as directed on package. Place 1–2 drops in an empty capsule; swallow.

⊘: Diffuse into the air. Inhale directly from bottle. Apply oil to hands, tissue, or cotton wick, and inhale.

✛: **Body System(s) Affected:** Digestive System.

🕐: **Additional Research:**

Peppermint: L-menthol was found to inhibit production of inflammation mediators in human monocytes (a type of white blood cell involved in the immune response) (Juergens et al., 1998).

Rosemary: Rosemary essential oil was found to be effective in reducing colon tissue lesions and colitis indices when administered orally or intraperitoneally to rats induced with colitis, suggesting that rosemary has anti-colitic activity (Minaiyan et al., 2011).

Thyme and oregano: Oral administration of thyme and oregano oil at a dose of 0.2% thyme and 0.1% oregano was found to be effective in decreasing the mortality rate, accelerating body weight gain recovery, and significantly reducing the macroscopic damage of colonic tissue of mice with induced colitis (Bukovska et al., 2007).

Coma

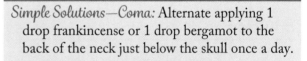

Simple Solutions—Coma: Alternate applying 1 drop frankincense or 1 drop bergamot to the back of the neck just below the skull once a day.

Oils: ⊗ frankincense, ⊗ Balance, ⊗ sandalwood, ⊗ cypress, ⊗ peppermint

⊗: Dilute as recommended, and massage 1–2 drops on the brain stem area, mastoids (behind ears), temples, and bottoms of feet.

✛: **Body System(s) Affected:** Nervous System.

Complexion

See Skin

Concentration (Poor)

> *Simple Solutions—Concentration:* Apply 5 drops InTune to a natural stone or unglazed clay pendant, and wear throughout the day.

Oils: InTune, Thinker, lavender⊕, lemon⊕, Douglas fir, petitgrain, peppermint, orange, cedarwood, cypress, juniper berry, eucalyptus, rosemary, sandalwood, ylang ylang

Other Products: xEO Mega or vEO Mega or IQ Mega, which contains omega-3 fatty acids necessary for proper brain cell function.

: Apply on back of neck and bottoms of feet.

: Diffuse into the air. Apply, and inhale from hands, tissue, or cotton wick.

: Take capsules as directed on package.

: **Body System(s) Affected:** Emotional Balance.

: **Additional Research:**

Lavender: Subjects who smelled a cleansing gel with lavender aroma were more relaxed and able to complete math computations faster (Field et al., 2005).

Lavender: Subjects exposed to 3 minutes of lavender aroma were more relaxed and able to perform math computations faster and more accurately. Subjects exposed to rosemary aroma were more alert and completed math computations faster (but not more accurately) (Diego et al., 1998).

Lemon: Daily inhalation of lemon essential oil aroma for five minutes was found to have a positive effect on learning in mice (Ogeturk et al., 2010).

Concussion

See Brain: Concussion

Confusion

> *Simple Solutions—Confusion:* Inhale the aroma of frankincense directly from the bottle.

Oils: InTune, frankincense, sandalwood, Balance, Steady, rosemary, peppermint, juniper berry, marjoram, cedarwood, basil, ylang ylang, fir, thyme, geranium, rose, ginger

: Apply on back of neck and bottoms of feet.

: Diffuse into the air. Inhale directly from bottle. Apply oil to hands, tissue, or cotton wick, and inhale.

: **Body System(s) Affected:** Emotional Balance.

Congestion

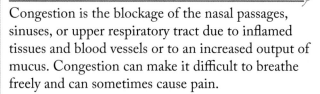

Congestion is the blockage of the nasal passages, sinuses, or upper respiratory tract due to inflamed tissues and blood vessels or to an increased output of mucus. Congestion can make it difficult to breathe freely and can sometimes cause pain.

> *Simple Solutions—Chest & Throat:* Combine 6 Tbs. (75 g) coconut oil and 1.5 Tbs. (7 g) beeswax pellets, and melt in a microwave (30 seconds at a time, stirring in between) or double boiler. Let cool slightly, and add 20 drops eucalyptus, 15 drops lemon, and 20 drops peppermint. Pour into small jars or salve containers, and allow to cool completely. Apply a small amount of salve on the chest and throat as needed.

> *Simple Solutions—Congestion:* Diffuse Breathe in an aromatherapy diffuser.

> *Simple Solutions—Congestion:* Drop 2 drops eucalyptus and 1 drop peppermint on the floor of the shower while showering, and inhale the vapors.

Oils: eucalyptus⊕, peppermint, Breathe, Douglas fir, cinnamon, juniper berry, cypress, melaleuca, cedarwood, cardamom, ginger, rosemary, fennel, citrus oils, patchouli

—Catarrh:

Catarrh refers to the secretion of mucus and white blood cells from the mucous membranes in the sinuses and nasal passages in response to an infection.

Oils: cypress, helichrysum, Breathe, On Guard, eucalyptus, Douglas fir, frankincense, myrrh, rosemary, ginger

—Expectorant:

An expectorant is an agent that helps dissolve thick mucus in the trachea, bronchi, or lungs for easier elimination.

Oils: eucalyptus⊕, marjoram, frankincense, helichrysum, cardamom

—Mucus:

Mucus is the substance produced by epithelial cells to coat the mucous membranes in the respiratory tract, digestive tract, and reproductive system. Mucus plays an important role in

See the Quick Usage Chart inside the back cover for recommended dilutions.

helping to protect these surfaces from different substances or from microorganisms they come in contact with. When one of these surfaces becomes infected or inflamed, an excess of mucus is often produced. An excess of mucus can lead to difficulty breathing in the sinuses, nasal passages, or respiratory tract. For oils to help combat an excess of mucus, see the entries above.

Oils: ⊘◯DigestZen (with ginger—helps digest old mucus)

🜄: Dilute 1–2 drops in 1 Tbs. (15 ml) fractionated coconut oil, and massage on chest, neck, back, and feet.

🌀: Diffuse into the air. Place 1–2 drops in a bowl of hot water, and inhale the vapor. Inhale directly from bottle. Apply oil to hands, tissue, or cotton wick, and inhale.

◯: Add 1–2 drops of each oil to an empty capsule; swallow.

🧍: **Body System(s) Affected:** Respiratory System.

⬭: **Additional Research:**

Eucalyptus: Eucalyptus oil was found to have an anti-inflammatory and mucin-inhibitory effect in rats with lipopolysaccharide-induced bronchitis (Lu et al., 2004).

Conjunctivitis

See Eyes: Pink Eye

Connective Tissue

See Skeletal System: Cartilage, Muscles

Constipation

See Digestive System: Constipation

Convulsions

See Seizure: Convulsions

Cooling Oils

Typically, oils that are high in aldehydes and esters can produce a cooling effect when applied topically or diffused.

Simple Solutions—Congestion: Diffuse Breathe in an aromatherapy diffuser.

Oils: ⊘⊘peppermint, ⊘⊘eucalyptus, ⊘⊘melaleuca, ⊘⊘lavender, ⊘⊘Roman chamomile, ⊘⊘citrus oils

🜄: Dilute as recommended, and apply 1–2 drops on location. Add 1–2 drops to bathwater, and bathe. Add 1–2 drops to basin of cool water, and sponge over skin.

🌀: Diffuse into the air.

🧍: **Body System(s) Affected:** Skin.

Corns

See Foot: Corns

Coughs

A cough is a sudden explosive release of air from the lungs to help clear an excess of mucus, an irritant, or other materials from the airway. Coughing can be caused by foreign material entering the airway or by an infection, asthma, or other medical problem. Proper hydration or steam inhalation can help loosen thick secretions, making them easier to eliminate.

Simple Solutions—Cough: Mix 1 drop eucalyptus and 1 drop lemon with 1 Tbs. (15 ml) honey. Mix about ⅓ of the honey mixture with 1 cup (250 ml) warm water, and drink slowly.

Simple Solutions—Cough: Diffuse Breathe in an aromatherapy diffuser.

Simple Solutions—Cough: Combine 1 drop each eucalyptus, melaleuca, and lemon with 1 tsp. (5 ml) jojoba oil, and apply over chest and back.

Oils: ⊘⊘Breathe, ⊘⊘melaleuca, ⊘⊘eucalyptus, ⊘⊘Douglas fir, ⊘⊘frankincense, ⊘⊘On Guard, ⊘⊘cardamom, ⊘⊘Stronger, ⊘⊘peppermint, ⊘⊘fir, ⊘⊘juniper berry, ⊘⊘cedarwood, ⊘⊘sandalwood, ⊘⊘thyme, ⊘⊘myrrh, ⊘⊘ginger

Other Products: ⊘⊘Breathe Vapor Stick, ◯Breathe Respiratory Drops, ◯On Guard+ Softgels. ◯On Guard Protecting Throat Drops to soothe irritated and sore throats.

—Allergy:

Oils: ⊘Purify

—Severe:

    Oils: 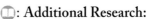frankincense

: Diffuse into the air. Use throat drops as directed on package.

: Dilute as recommended, and apply 1–2 drops on the throat and chest.

: Take supplements as directed on packaging.

: **Body System(s) Affected:** Respiratory System.

Cradle Cap

See Children and Infants: Cradle Cap

Cramps

See Digestive System: Cramps, Female-Specific Conditions: Menstruation, Muscles: Cramps/Charley Horses

Crohn's Disease

Crohn's disease is a chronic inflammation of part of the intestinal wall, thought to be caused by an over-active immune response. It can cause abdominal pain, diarrhea, nausea, and loss of appetite.

> *Simple Solutions—Crohn's Disease:* Apply 1–2 drops of DigestZen over the stomach and bottoms of the feet.

Oils: peppermint, DigestZen, basil

: Add 1–2 drops of oil to an empty capsule; swallow.

: Dilute as recommended and apply on stomach and feet.

: **Body System(s) Affected:** Digestive System.

: **Additional Research:**

Peppermint: A combination of peppermint and caraway oil was found to reduce visceral hyperalgesia (pain hypersensitivity in the gastrointestinal tract) after induced inflammation in rats (Adam et al., 2006).

Cuts

See also Wounds, Antibacterial, Blood: Bleeding

> *Simple Solutions—Cuts:* Apply 1 drop of helichrysum on cut to help stop bleeding. Add 1 drop each of lavender, melaleuca, and basil to a bowl of warm water, and use the water to wash the area around the cut.

Oils: 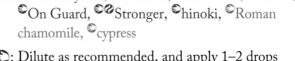helichrysum, lavender, melaleuca, basil, On Guard, Stronger, hinoki, Roman chamomile, cypress

: Dilute as recommended, and apply 1–2 drops on location.

: **Body System(s) Affected:** Skin.

: **Additional Research:**

Basil: Basil (*Ocimum gratissimum*) oil was found to facilitate the healing process of wounds in rabbits to a greater extent than two antibacterial preparations, Cicatrin and Cetavlex (Orafidiya et al., 2003).

Cystitis

See Bladder: Cystitis/Infection

Dandruff

See Hair: Dandruff

Decongestant

See Congestion

Degenerative Disease

A degenerative disease is a disease where the affected tissues or organs are damaged due to internal mechanisms rather than infection. Quite a few different diseases can be categorized as degenerative diseases, including Alzheimer's disease, cancer, Parkinson's disease, atherosclerosis, diabetes, osteoporosis, rheumatoid arthritis, and many others. To mitigate degenerative diseases, support the cells and tissues through proper nutrition, reducing stress, exercising regularly, and eliminating toxins. See specific conditions in this guide for oils and other products that can support the body for each condition.

Delivery

See Pregnancy/Motherhood: Delivery

Dental Infection

See Oral Conditions

See the *Quick Usage Chart* inside the back cover for recommended dilutions.

280

Deodorant

> *Simple Solutions—Deodorant:* Melt 1 Tbs. (5 g) beeswax pellets and 3 Tbs. (40 g) coconut oil in a microwave (30 seconds at a time, stirring in between) or in a double boiler. Stir in ¼ cup (30 g) cornstarch, ¼ cup (50 g) baking soda, and 5 drops vitamin E oil. Add 5 drops melaleuca and 5 drops lavender. Pour into empty deodorant containers, and allow to cool and harden. Apply once or twice a day as needed.

Oils: Purify, melaleuca, lavender, geranium, eucalyptus, cedarwood, cypress, Elevation, Serenity, Breathe, Whisper, spikenard

Other Products: Natural Deodorant

: Apply deodorant under the arms. Dilute oils as recommended, and apply 1–2 drops on the skin. Dilute 2–3 drops in 1 Tbs. (15 ml) fractionated coconut oil, and apply under the arms. Add 2–3 drops to ½ cup (65 g) cornstarch and ¼ cup (50 g) baking soda, and apply under the arms, on the feet, or on other areas of the body.

: **Body System(s) Affected:** Skin.

Deodorizing

Oils: Purify, peppermint, cedarwood, clary sage

: Diffuse into the air. Dissolve 8–10 drops in 1 tsp. (5 ml) perfumer's or pure grain alcohol (such as vodka), and combine with distilled water in a 1 oz. spray bottle. Spray into the air or on affected surface.

Depression

Depression is a disorder marked by excessive sadness, energy loss, feelings of worthlessness, irritableness, sudden weight loss or gain, trouble sleeping, and loss of interest in activities normally enjoyed. These symptoms can continue for weeks or months if not treated and can destroy an individual's quality of life.

> *Simple Solutions—Depression:* Inhale lemon oil directly from the bottle for a quick pick-me-up.

Oils: lemon, frankincense, Motivate, Cheer, InTune, Console, lavender, bergamot, petitgrain, Elevation, Balance, Steady, Peace, Citrus Bliss, melissa, clary sage, rosemary, ylang ylang, grapefruit, Serenity, lime, geranium, ginger, juniper berry, basil, sandalwood, patchouli

—**Postpartum Depression:** *See Pregnancy/Motherhood: Postpartum Depression*

—**Sedatives:**

Oils: lavender, ylang ylang, petitgrain, melissa, Roman chamomile, sandalwood, cedarwood, rose, clary sage, cypress, juniper berry, frankincense, bergamot, marjoram

: Diffuse into the air. Inhale directly from bottle. Apply oil to hands, tissue, or cotton wick, and inhale.

: Dilute as recommended, and apply 1–2 drops to temple or forehead. Add 5–10 drops to 1 Tbs. (15 ml) fractionated coconut oil, and use as massage oil. Add 1–3 drops to warm bathwater, and bathe.

: Add 1–2 drops to 1 cup (250 ml) distilled water or ½ cup (125 ml) rice or almond milk, and drink. Add 1–2 drops to empty capsule, and swallow.

: **Body System(s) Affected:** Nervous System.

: **Additional Research:**

Lemon: Lemon oil vapor was found to have strong antistress and antidepressant effects on mice subjected to several common stress tests (Komiya et al., 2006).

Lemon: Lemon oil and its component, citral, were found to decrease depressed behavior in a similar manner to antidepressant drugs in rats involved in several stress tests (Komori et al., 1995).

Lemon: In 12 patients suffering from depression, it was found that inhaling citrus aromas reduced the needed doses of antidepressants, normalized neuroendocrine hormone levels, and normalized immune function (Komori et al., 1995).

Frankincense: Incensole acetate was found to open TRPV receptors in mice brains, indicating a possible channel for emotional regulation (Moussaieff et al., 2008).

Lavender: In patients suffering from arthritis, it was found that a blend of lavender, marjoram, eucalyptus, rosemary, and peppermint blended with carrier oils was found to reduce perceived pain and depression compared to control (Kim et al., 2005).

Lavender: Female students suffering from insomnia were found to sleep better and to have a lower level of depression during weeks they used a lavender fragrance when compared to weeks they did not use a lavender fragrance (Lee et al., 2006).

Lavender: Swiss mice fed lavender oil diluted in olive oil were found to be more sedate in several common tests (Guillemain et al., 1989).

Lavender: Exposure to inhaled lavender oil and to its constituents, linalool and linalyl acetate, was found to decrease normal movement in mice as well as to return mice to normal movement rates after caffeine-induced hyperactivity (Buchbauer et al., 1991).

Lavender: *Lavandula angustifolia* essential oil demonstrated ability to inhibit GABA-A receptor channels of rat brain cells (Huang et al., 2008).

Lavender: Inhaling lavender oil was found to lower agitation in older adults suffering from dementia (Lin et al., 2007).

Bergamot: In 12 patients suffering from depression, it was found that inhaling citrus aromas reduced the needed doses of antidepressants, normalized neuroendocrine hormone levels, and normalized immune function (Komori et al., 1995).

Citrus Bliss: In 12 patients suffering from depression, it was found that inhaling citrus aromas reduced the needed doses of antidepressants, normalized neuroendocrine hormone levels, and normalized immune function (Komori et al., 1995).

Clary sage: Clary sage essential oil displayed antidepressant-like effects via the dopaminergic pathway in rats submitted to the forced swim test (a common stress test) (Seol et al., 2010).

Rosemary: Many fractions of *Rosmarinus officinalis*, including its essential oil, were found to have antidepressant-like effects on mice submitted to two stress tests after oral administration of the rosemary plant fractions (Machado et al., 2013).

Ylang ylang: Transdermal absorption of ylang ylang essential oil altered physiological stress responses, like blood pressure and skin temperature, and subjects reported being more calm and relaxed than the control group (Hongratanaworakit et al., 2006).

Grapefruit: In 12 patients suffering from depression, it was found that inhaling citrus aromas reduced the needed doses of antidepressants, normalized neuroendocrine hormone levels, and normalized immune function (Komori et al., 1995).

Melissa: Melissa (lemon balm) oil applied topically in a lotion was found to reduce agitation and improve quality of life factors in patients suffering severe dementia compared to those receiving a placebo lotion (Ballard et al., 2002).

Dermatitis

See Skin: Dermatitis/Eczema

Despair

See Depression

Detoxification

Detoxification is the act of clearing toxins out of the body. These toxins may be addictive drugs, alcohol, or any other harmful substance.

Oils: helichrysum, rosemary, juniper berry, coriander

: Dilute as recommended, and apply to liver area, intestines, and reflex points on the feet.

: **Additional Research:**

Rosemary: Rosemary extracts induced CYP (cytochrome 450) activity in liver cells, suggesting a possibility of increased ability to remove toxins (Debersac et al., 2001).

Coriander: Coriander extract was found to have a protective role against lead toxicity in rat brain (Velaga et al., 2014).

Diabetes

Diabetes is a disease characterized by the body's inability to properly produce or use the hormone insulin. Insulin, produced in the pancreas, helps regulate the level of sugars in the blood, as well as the conversion of starches and sugar into the energy necessary for life. Common diabetes symptoms include a frequent need to drink and urinate, blurred vision, mental fatigue, and possibly weight gain (depending on the type). Over time, diabetes can lead to additional complica-

tions, such as strokes, heart disease, kidney failure, and even the necessity of removing a limb.

Oils: cinnamon, rosemary, geranium, basil, Yarrow Pom, ylang ylang, eucalyptus, On Guard, cypress, juniper berry, dill, cassia, ginger, fennel, lavender

Blend 1: Combine 8 drops clove, 8 drops cinnamon, 15 drops rosemary, and 10 drops thyme with ¼ cup (50 ml) fractionated coconut oil. Put on feet and over pancreas.

Blend 2: Combine 5 drops cinnamon and 5 drops cypress. Rub on feet and pancreas.

Other Products: On Guard+ Softgels

—Pancreas Support:

Oils: cinnamon, geranium

—Sores (Diabetic):

Those suffering from diabetes have to be especially careful about sores of any kind, especially those on the feet and hands. Diabetes decreases blood flow, so wounds heal much slower. Many who suffer from diabetes experience decreased sensation in their hands and feet, making it more difficult to even notice an injury right away. Even a small sore left untreated can turn into an ulcer, ultimately making amputation necessary.

Oils: lavender, Balance

: Place 1–2 drops of oil under the tongue or place 1–2 drops in empty capsule and swallow. Take supplements as directed on packaging.

: Dilute as recommended, and apply on back, chest, feet, and over pancreas.

: Diffuse into the air.

: **Body System(s) Affected:** Endocrine System.

: **Additional Research:**

Cinnamon: Cinnamon bark extract supplementation for three months was found to significantly improve blood glucose control in Chinese patients with type 2 diabetes taking gliclazide (a prescribed antidiabetic medication) (Lu, T. et al., 2012).

Cinnamon: Cinnamaldehyde (the major constituent of cinnamon oil) produced protective action against alloxan-induced diabetic nephropathy in rats (Mishra et al., 2010).

Cinnamon: Cinnamaldehyde (found in cinnamon oil) was found to significantly reduce blood glucose levels in diabetic wistar rats (Subash et al., 2007).

Cinnamon: Oral administration of cinnamon oil was found to significantly reduce blood glucose levels in diabetic KK-Ay mice (Ping et al., 2010).

Cinnamon: Cinnamon polyphenols were found to restore pancreatic function and exert hypoglycemic and hypolipidemic effects in a diabetic mouse model (Li, R. et al., 2013).

See the Quick Usage Chart inside the back cover for recommended dilutions.

Rosemary: Oral rosemary extract was found to decrease blood glucose levels, while increasing insulin levels in alloxan-diabetic rabbits (Bakirel et al., 2008).

Basil: Results from a clinical trial showed that basil leaf extract decreased fasting and postprandial blood glucose in diabetes mellitus patients, suggesting that basil could be used as a dietary therapy in mild to moderate cases of type 2 diabetes mellitus (Agrawal et al., 1996) .

Melissa: Oral supplementation of melissa essential oil significantly reduced plasma glucose levels compared with the control group, and increased glucose tolerance in a type 2 diabetic mouse model (Chung et al., 2010).

Dill: Dill seed extract suppressed high-fat diet-induced hyperlipidemia through hepatic PPAR-α activation in diabetic obese mice (Takahashi et al., 2013).

Helichrysum and Grapefruit: Helichrysum and grapefruit extracts were found to improve postprandial glycemic control in a dietary model of insulin resistance in rats (da la Garza et al., 2013).

Cassia: In vitro data suggest that the constituents of cassia may be appropriate for the treatment of diabetic complications (like cataract and retinopathy) because of the constituents' ability to inhibit aldose reductase and thus prevent the conversion of glucose to corbitol (Lee, 2002).

D-Limonene (found in lime, lemon, bergamot, dill, grapefruit, lavender, lemongrass, Roman chamomile, tangerine, and wild orange essential oils): In a recent study oral intake of D-limonene ameliorated insulin resistance in mice fed a high-fat diet (Jing et al., 2013).

Diaper Rash

See Children and Infants: Diaper Rash

Diarrhea

See Digestive System: Diarrhea

Digestive System

The human digestive system is the series of organs and glands that process food. The digestive system breaks down food, absorbs nutrients for the body to use as fuel, and excretes as bowel movements the part that cannot be broken down.

Oils: peppermint, ginger, lemongrass (purifies), DigestZen, fennel, turmeric, wintergreen, marjoram (stimulates), oregano, rosemary, clary sage, copaiba, neroli, cardamom, grapefruit, basil, lemon, cinnamon, clove, juniper berry, orange, bergamot

Regimen 1: Use GX Assist for 10 days to help support the digestive system in eliminating pathogenic microorganisms, followed by PB Assist+ or PB Assist Jr for 5 days to help rebuild friendly flora to aid digestion and prevent pathogenic bacteria.

Other Products: DigestZen Softgels to help support healthy digestion. Terrazyme for healthy digestion, enzymatic function, and cellular metabolism. Alpha CRS+, xEO Mega or vEO Mega, IQ

Mega, Microplex VMz, a2z Chewable to provide essential nutrients, vitamins, and minerals for digestive system cellular support.

◯: Take capsules as directed on package. Add 1–2 drops of oil to 2 cups (500 ml) of water, and drink. Add oils as flavoring to food. Place 1–2 drops of oil in an empty capsule, and swallow.

◔: Dilute oil as recommended, and apply 1–2 drops on stomach or reflex points on feet. Dilute 1–2 drops in 1 Tbs. (15 ml) fractionated coconut oil, and massage over abdomen and lower back. Apply as a warm compress over affected area.

◉: Diffuse into the air. *See Negative Ions* for oils that produce negative ions when diffused to help stimulate the digestive system. Inhale oil directly or applied to hands, tissue, or cotton wick.

—Bloating:

Bloating is an abnormal swelling, increase in diameter, or feeling of fullness and tightness in the abdominal area as gas and liquid are trapped inside. Common causes of bloating can include overeating, menstruation, constipation, food allergies, and irritable bowel syndrome.

> *Simple Solutions—Bloating:* Combine 5 drops fennel with 1 tsp. (5 ml) fractionated coconut oil in a small roll-on bottle, and apply on stomach once or twice a day as needed.

Oils: DigestZen

Other Products: DigestTab, DigestZen Softgels

◔: Dilute as recommended, and apply to stomach and to reflex points on the feet.

◉: Diffuse into the air.

—Constipation:

Constipation is a condition characterized by infrequent or difficult bowel movements. A person is considered constipated if he or she has fewer than three bowel movements a week or if the stools are hard and difficult to expel. Common causes of constipation include a lack of fiber, dehydration, ignoring the urge to have a bowel movement, depression, medications, large dairy intake, stress, and abuse of laxatives.

Digestive System

The human digestive system is the series of organs and glands that process food. The digestive system breaks down food, absorbs nutrients for the body to use as fuel, and excretes as bowel movements the part that cannot be broken down.

The digestive system consists of the gastrointestinal tract (GI tract) and accessory organs. The GI tract, or the series of joined hollow organs through which food passes, consists of the mouth, esophagus, stomach, small intestine, and large intestine. Accessory organs associated with the digestive system also assist with the digestion of food, but food does not pass through these organs. Instead, accessory organs assist with secreting digestive enzymes, storing digestive fluids, and producing bile. For example, accessory organs include the tongue, salivary glands, liver, gallbladder, and pancreas

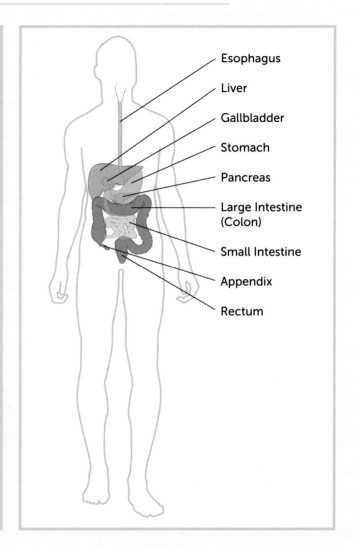

- Esophagus
- Liver
- Gallbladder
- Stomach
- Pancreas
- Large Intestine (Colon)
- Small Intestine
- Appendix
- Rectum

Oils for Digestive Support

Oils: ○◐◑peppermint◔, ○◐◑ginger◔, ◐◑lemongrass (purifies)◔, ○◐◑DigestZen, ○◐◑fennel, ○◐◑turmeric, ○◐◑wintergreen◔, ○◐◑marjoram (stimulates), ○◐◑oregano◔, ○◐◑rosemary◔, ◐◑clary sage, ◐○copaiba, ◑neroli, ○◐◑cardamom, ○◐◑grapefruit, ○◐◑basil, ○◐◑lemon◔, ◐◑cinnamon, ○◐◑clove, ◐◑juniper berry, ○◐◑orange, ○◐◑bergamot

Common Digestive Issues

Digestive: Bloating, Cirrhosis, Constipation, Cramps (Abdominal), Diarrhea, Gas/Flatulence, Gastritis, Gastroesophageal Reflux Disease (GERD), Giardia, Heartburn, Hepatitis, Indigestion, Irritable Bowel Syndrome, Jaundice, Nausea/Upset Stomach, Parasites, Ulcers

Simple Solutions—Constipation: Combine 1 drop each of rosemary, lemon, and peppermint with 1 tsp. (5 ml) fractionated coconut oil, and massage gently on stomach and back.

Oils: ⚬rosemary⚬, ⚬lemon⚬, ⚬peppermint⚬, ⚬marjoram, ⚬DigestZen, ⚬ginger, ⚬fennel, ⚬orange, ⚬copaiba, ⚬rose, ⚬juniper berry, ⚬sandalwood

Other Products: ⚬DigestZen Softgels to help support healthy digestion.

🖐: Dilute as recommended, and apply oils on abdomen. Add 1–2 drops to 1 Tbs. (15 ml) fractionated coconut oil, and massage onto abdomen.

⬤: Take capsules as directed.

—Cramps (Abdominal):

Cramps are sudden, involuntary muscle contractions that often cause severe pain. Abdominal cramps are commonly caused by stress, menstruation, mild food poisoning, and *Irritable Bowel Syndrome (below).*

Oils: ⚬⚬DigestZen, ⚬⚬basil, ⚬clary sage

Other Products: ⚬DigestZen Softgels to help support healthy digestion.

Recipe 1: Flavor water with 5 drops DigestZen, and drink for stomach pains and cramps.

⬤: Place 3 drops DigestZen and 3 drops basil in an empty capsule; swallow. Take capsules as directed.

🖐: Dilute as recommended, and massage oil onto abdomen over area of pain.

—Diarrhea:

Diarrhea is an abnormal increase in the frequency of bowel movements, marked by loose, watery stools. Diarrhea is defined as more than three bowel movements a day. Cases of diarrhea that last more than two days can become a serious problem and cause dehydration. Rehydration with an oral rehydration solution is the most effective way to prevent dehydration. If no commercially prepared oral rehydration solution is available, a solution made from 1 tsp. (5 g) salt, 8 tsp. (35 g) sugar, and 4 cups (1 L) clean water (with some mashed fresh banana, if available, to add potassium) can work in an emergency. Diarrhea is usually caused by a viral, parasitic, or bacterial infection.

Simple Solutions—Diarrhea: Blend 3 drops peppermint and 2 drops fennel with 1 tsp. (5 ml) fractionated coconut oil in a small roll-on bottle, and apply over stomach as needed.

Oils: ⚬⚬peppermint, ⚬⚬ginger, ⚬geranium, ⚬⚬DigestZen, ⚬orange, ⚬patchouli, ⚬melaleuca, ⚬sandalwood, ⚬copaiba, ⚬lavender, ⚬Roman chamomile, ⚬cypress, ⚬eucalyptusm, ⚬neroli

Other Products: ⚬DigestZen Softgels to help support healthy digestion.

—Children:

Oils: ⚬geranium, ⚬ginger, ⚬sandalwood

⬤: Place 1–2 drops in an empty capsule, and swallow. Take supplement as directed.

🖐: Dilute as recommended, and apply 1–2 drops on abdomen. Apply as a warm compress over affected area.

—Gas/Flatulence:

Simple Solutions—Gas/Flatulence: Combine 5 drops fennel with 1 tsp. (5 ml) fractionated coconut oil in a small roll-on bottle, and apply on stomach once or twice a day as needed.

Oils: ⚬⚬lavender, ⚬⚬ginger, ⚬⚬star anise, ⚬peppermint, ⚬⚬cardamom, ⚬eucalyptus, ⚬bergamot, ⚬myrrh, ⚬juniper berry, ⚬⚬petitgrain, ⚬neroli, ⚬copaiba, ⚬rosemary

Other Products: ⚬DigestTab, ⚬DigestZen Softgels to help support healthy digestion.

⬤: Place 1–2 drops in an empty capsule, and swallow. Take supplement as directed.

🖐: Dilute as recommended, and apply 1–2 drops on stomach, abdomen, or reflex points on the feet

—Gastritis: *See also Inflammation*

Gastritis is inflammation of the stomach lining.

Oils: ⚬⚬DigestZen, ⚬⚬peppermint, ⚬lemongrass⚬, ⚬⚬fennel

Other Products: ⚬DigestZen Softgels to help support healthy digestion.

⬤: Add 1 drop of oil to rice or almond milk; take as a supplement. Place 1–2 drops in an empty capsule; swallow capsule. Take supplement as directed.

🖐: Dilute as recommended, and apply 1–2 drops on stomach. Apply as a warm compress over stomach.

—GERD (Gastroesophageal Reflux Disease):

Gastroesophageal reflux disease (GERD) is a digestive disease that causes stomach acid to frequently flow back into the tube connecting the mouth and stomach (esophagus). This backwash (acid reflux) can irritate the lining of the esophagus.

Oils: ✆lemon⊕, ✆green mandarin⊕

—Giardia:

Giardia are parasites that infect the gastrointestinal tract of humans and animals. The form of *Giardia* that affects humans causes severe diarrhea. *See Diarrhea above* for information on rehydration.

Oils: ○✆lavender⊕

⚪: Place 1–2 drops in an empty capsule; swallow capsule.

🖐: Dilute as recommended, and apply 1–2 drops on abdomen or reflex points on the feet.

—Heartburn:

Heartburn is a painful burning sensation in the chest or throat. It occurs as a result of backed up stomach acid in the esophagus. Heartburn is often brought on by certain foods, medication, pregnancy, and alcohol.

> *Simple Solutions—Heartburn/Indigestion:* Add 1 drop peppermint to 1 tsp. (5 ml) honey. Dissolve in 1 cup (250 ml) warm water, and drink slowly.

Oils: ✆lemon, ✆peppermint, ✆○DigestZen

Blend 1: Blend 2 drops lemon, 2 drops peppermint, and 3 drops sandalwood in 1 Tbs. (15 ml) fractionated coconut oil. Apply to breast bone in a clockwise motion using the palm of the hand. Apply to reflex points on the feet.

Other Products: ○DigestTab, ○DigestZen Softgels to help support healthy digestion.

🖐: Dilute as recommended, and apply 1–2 drops to chest.

⚪: Add 1 drop of oil to rice or almond milk; take as a supplement. Place 1–2 drops in an empty capsule; swallow capsule. Take supplement as directed.

—Indigestion:

The term "indigestion" is used to describe abdominal discomfort felt after a meal. Symptoms of indigestion include belching, bloating, nausea, heartburn, a feeling of fullness, and general abdominal discomfort. Indigestion can be caused by overeating or eating too fast, alcoholic or carbonated drinks, particular foods, etc.

Oils: ○✆✆peppermint, ○✆✆ginger, ○✆star anise, ○✆✆turmeric, ○✆DigestZen, ✆✆lavender, ✆✆orange, ✆○✆lime, ✆✆thyme, ✆✆myrrh, ✆✆grapefruit, ✆✆petitgrain, ✆neroli

Other Products: ○DigestZen Softgels to help support healthy digestion. ○DigestTab, ○Terrazyme for healthy digestion, enzymatic function, and cellular metabolism.

⚪: Add 1–2 drops of oil to 1 cup (250 ml) of almond or rice milk; drink. Place 1–2 drops of oil in an empty capsule; swallow capsule. Take capsules as directed on package.

🖐: Dilute oil as recommended, and apply 1–2 drops on stomach or reflex points on feet. Dilute 1–2 drops in 1 Tbs. (15 ml) fractionated coconut oil, and massage over abdomen and lower back. Apply as a warm compress over stomach area.

🌀: Diffuse into the air.

—Intestines:

The intestines are the largest organs in the digestive track. The intestines include the small intestine, which begins just below the stomach and is responsible for digesting and absorbing nutrients from the food, and the large intestine, which begins at the end of the small intestine and is responsible for reabsorbing water and some vitamins before the undigested food and waste is eliminated.

Oils: ✆○basil, ✆○marjoram, ✆○ginger, ✆○rose⊕, ✆○rosemary

Other Products: ○GX Assist to help the digestive system eliminate pathogens. ○PB Assist+ or ○PB Assist Jr to provide friendly intestinal flora to aid digestion and help prevent pathogenic bacteria. ○Terrazyme for healthy digestion, enzymatic function, and cellular metabolism.

See the Quick Usage Chart inside the back cover for recommended dilutions.

**: Dilute oil as recommended, and apply 1–2 drops on stomach or reflex points on feet. Dilute 1–2 drops in 1 Tbs. (15 ml) fractionated coconut oil, and massage over abdomen and lower back. Apply as a warm compress over affected area.

**: Take capsules as directed on package. Add 1–2 drops of oil to 2 cups (500 ml) of water; drink. Add oils as flavoring to food. Place 1–2 drops of oil in a capsule, and swallow.

—Intestinal Parasites:
See Parasites: Intestinal

—Irritable Bowel Syndrome:

Irritable bowel syndrome is an intestinal disorder characterized by reoccurring diarrhea, bloating, gas, constipation, cramping, and abdominal pain. Irritable bowel syndrome is one of the most commonly diagnosed disorders by doctors.

Oils: peppermint, DigestZen

**: Add 2 drops of each oil to 1 cup (250 ml) distilled water, and drink 1–2 times per day. Place 2 drops of each oil in an empty capsule; swallow capsule.

**: Dilute 1–2 drops in 1 Tbs. (15 ml) fractionated coconut oil, and apply over the abdomen with a hot compress.

—Nausea/Upset Stomach:

Oils: DigestZen, ginger, peppermint, lavender, ClaryCalm, clove

Other Products: DigestZen Softgels to help support healthy digestion.

**: Place 1–2 drops in an empty capsule; swallow capsule. Place 1 drop in 1 cup (250 ml) rice or almond milk, and drink. Take supplement as directed.

**: Dilute as recommended, and apply behind ears, on stomach, or on reflex points on the feet.

**: Diffuse into the air. Inhale directly from bottle. Apply oil to hands, tissue, or cotton wick, and inhale.

—Parasites: *See Parasites*

—Stomach:

The stomach is the organ mainly responsible for breaking food apart using strong acids. It is located below the esophagus and before the intestines.

Oils: basil, peppermint, lemongrass, ginger, DigestZen

Other Products: DigestZen Softgels to help support healthy digestion.

**: Place 1–2 drops in an empty capsule, and swallow. Take supplement as directed.

**: Dilute as recommended, and apply 1–2 drops on stomach, abdomen, or reflex points on the feet

—Ulcers: *See Ulcers*

: Body System(s) Affected: Digestive System.

: Additional Research:

Peppermint: A combination of peppermint and caraway oil was found to reduce visceral hyperalgesia (pain hypersensitivity in the gastrointestinal tract) after induced inflammation in rats (Adam et al., 2006).

Peppermint: Peppermint oil was found to be as effective as Buscopan (an antispasmodic drug) at preventing spasms during a barium enema (a type of enema used to place barium in the colon for X-ray imaging purposes) (Asao et al., 2003).

Peppermint: The use of rosemary, lemon, and peppermint oils in massage demonstrated an ability to reduce constipation and increase bowel movements in elderly subjects, compared to massage without the oils (Kim et al., 2005).

Peppermint: Peppermint oil in enteric-coated capsules was found to relieve symptoms of irritable bowel syndrome better than a placebo in patients suffering from IBS (Rees et al., 1979).

Peppermint: Patients with IBS symptoms who took a peppermint-oil formulation in an enteric-coated capsule were found to have a significantly higher reduction of symptoms than did patients taking a placebo (Liu et al., 1997).

Peppermint: Children suffering from irritable bowel syndrome (IBS) who received peppermint oil in enteric-coated capsules (encapsulated so the capsules wouldn't open until they reached the intestines) reported a reduced severity of pain associated with IBS (Kline et al., 2001).

Peppermint: In irritable bowel syndrome patients without bacterial overgrowth, lactose intolerance, or celiac disease, peppermint oil was found over 8 weeks to reduce IBS symptoms significantly more than a placebo (Capello et al., 2007).

Peppermint: An enteric-coated capsule with peppermint and caraway oil was found to reduce pain and symptoms in patients with non-ulcer dyspepsia (indigestion), compared to a control (May et al., 1996).

Ginger: Ginger root given one hour before major gynecological surgery resulted in lower nausea and fewer incidences of vomiting compared to control (Nanthakomon et al., 2006).

Ginger: Ginger root given orally to pregnant women was found to decrease the severity of nausea and frequency of vomiting compared to control (Vutyavanich et al., 2001).

Ginger: In a trial of women receiving gynecological surgery, women receiving ginger root had less incidences of nausea than did those receiving a placebo. Ginger root has similar results to the antiemetic drug (a drug effective against vomiting and nausea) metoclopramide (Bone et al., 1990).

Lemongrass: Lemongrass and lemon verbena oil were found to be bactericidal to *Helicobacter pylori* (a pathogen responsible for gastroduodenal disease) at very low concentrations. Additionally, it was found that this bacteria did not develop a resistance to lemongrass oil after 10 passages, while this bacteria did develop resistance to clarithromycin (an antibiotic) under the same conditions (Ohno et al., 2003).

Lemon/Green Mandarin: Oral administration of d-limonene over several days was found to significantly reduce symptoms of gastroesophageal reflux compared to a placebo in a limited human trial (Sun, 2007).

Wintergreen: Methyl salicylate (found in wintergreen or birch oils) was found to inhibit leukotriene C4 (a chemical messenger involved in inflammatory response), while also demonstrating gastroprotective effects against ethanol-induced gastric injury in rats (Trautmann et al., 1991).

Oregano: Oregano oil administered orally was found to improve gastrointestinal symptoms in 7 of 11 patients who had tested positive for the parasite

Blastocystis hominis and was also found to cause disappearance of this parasite in 8 cases (Force et al., 2000).

Rosemary: The use of rosemary, lemon, and peppermint oils in massage demonstrated an ability to reduce constipation and increase bowel movements in elderly subjects, compared to massage without the oils (Kim et al., 2005).

Lemon: The use of rosemary, lemon, and peppermint oils in massage demonstrated an ability to reduce constipation and increase bowel movements in elderly subjects, compared to massage without the oils (Kim et al., 2005).

Lavender: Essential oil from *Lavandula angustifolia* demonstrated ability to eliminate protozoal pathogens *Giardia duodenalis*, *Trichomonas vaginalis*, and *Hexamita inflata* at concentrations of 1% or less (Moon et al., 2006).

Rose: Rose essential oil and its main constituents were found to inhibit rat isolated ileum (a section of the small intestine), suggesting that rose oil can be used as an antispasmodic remedy for treatment of abdominal spasm (Sadraei et al., 2013).

Disinfectant

A disinfectant is any substance that destroys microorganisms on non-living surfaces.

Oils: lemon, Purify, grapefruit, lemongrass, geranium

Other Products: On Guard Foaming Hand Wash to cleanse hands and protect against harmful microorganisms.

Blend 1: Add 10 drops lavender, 20 drops thyme, 5 drops eucalyptus, and 5 drops oregano to a large bowl of water. Use to disinfect small areas.

: Add 1–2 drops of oil to a wet cloth, and use to wipe down counters and other surfaces. Use hand wash as directed on packaging.

: Diffuse into the air.

: **Body System(s) Affected:** Immune System and Skin.

: **Additional Research:**

Lemongrass: A formulation of lemongrass and geranium oil was found to reduce airborne bacteria by 89% in an office environment after diffusion for 15 hours (Doran et al., 2009).

Geranium: A formulation of lemongrass and geranium oil was found to reduce airborne bacteria by 89% in an office environment after diffusion for 15 hours (Doran et al., 2009).

Diuretic

A diuretic is a substance that increases the rate of urination and fluid elimination from the body.

Oils: lemongrass, rosemary, cedarwood, lavender, patchouli, grapefruit, cypress, fennel, orange, lemon, oregano, juniper berry, marjoram

: Dilute as recommended, and apply oils to kidney area on back and to bottoms of feet.

: **Body System(s) Affected:** Digestive System.

Diverticulitis

See Colon: Diverticulitis

Dysentery

See also Antibacterial, Digestive System: Diarrhea

Dysentery is severe, frequent diarrhea, often with blood or mucus, that occurs due to infection by bacteria or amoeba. Dysentery can be fatal due to dehydration if left untreated. *See Digestive System: Diarrhea* for information on rehydrating the body.

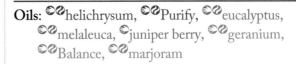

> *Simple Solutions—Dysentery:* Blend 3 drops peppermint and 2 drops myrrh with 1 tsp. (5 ml) fractionated coconut oil, and apply on stomach. Use rehydration solution (see above), and seek medical attention.

Oils: myrrh, eucalyptus, lemon, Roman chamomile, cypress, clove (amoebic), melissa

: Dilute as recommended, and apply on abdomen and on bottoms of feet.

: **Body System(s) Affected:** Digestive System.

Dyspepsia

See Digestive System: Indigestion

Ears

Oils: helichrysum, Purify, eucalyptus, melaleuca, juniper berry, geranium, Balance, marjoram

—Earache:

> *Simple Solutions—Earache:* Add 1 drop each of basil and melaleuca to a cotton ball. Hold the cotton over the ear canal (not in the ear canal) for 30 minutes.

Oils: basil, melaleuca, helichrysum

—Hearing in a Tunnel:

Oils: Purify

—Infection:

Oils: melaleuca, Purify, lavender

See the *Quick Usage Chart* inside the back cover for recommended dilutions.

288

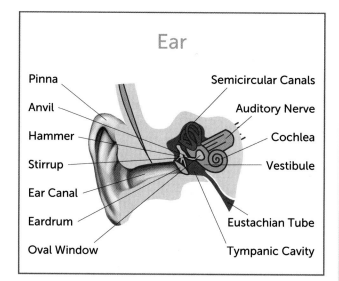

Ear

Pinna · Anvil · Hammer · Stirrup · Ear Canal · Eardrum · Oval Window

Semicircular Canals · Auditory Nerve · Cochlea · Vestibule · Eustachian Tube · Tympanic Cavity

—Inflammation:

Oils: ⬡eucalyptus

—Tinnitus:

Tinnitus is a ringing or other audible noise in the ears caused by ear infection, wax buildup, or a block in the eustachian tube.

Simple Solutions—Tinnitus: Add 1 drop helichrysum to a cotton ball. Hold the cotton over the ear canal (not in the ear canal) for 30 minutes.

Oils: ⬡helichrysum, ⬡juniper berry

⬡: Caution: Never put oils directly into the ear canal. Dilute as recommended, and apply 1–2 drops on surface of the ear and behind the ear on the mastoid bone. Apply 1 drop oil to small cotton ball, and place over opening to ear canal (do not press into the ear canal). Place 1 drop oil on cotton swab, and swab around the ear canal.

⬡: Diffuse into the air.

⬡: **Body System(s) Affected:** Skin, Immune System, Nervous System, and Respiratory System.

Eating Disorders

Simple Solutions—Eating Disorders: Diffuse grapefruit in an aromatherapy diffuser to help soothe the mind when feeling withdrawals from food or compulsive behaviors.

—Anorexia:

Anorexia is a psychological disorder where a person becomes obsessed with body size and weight, often depriving him or herself of food to avoid gaining weight.

Oils: ⬡grapefruit, ⬡Citrus Bliss

⬡: Diffuse into the air. Inhale directly from bottle. Apply oil to hands, tissue, or cotton wick, and inhale.

—Bulimia:

Bulimia is a disorder categorized by periods of overeating, or binging, followed by periods of self-induced vomiting, fasting, or abuse of laxatives and diuretics to purge the body of the food or to compensate for the overeating.

Oils: ⬡grapefruit, ⬡Citrus Bliss

⬡: Diffuse into the air. Inhale directly from bottle. Apply oil to hands, tissue, or cotton wick, and inhale.

—Overeating:

Overeating is eating too much food for the body. It can include binging (eating so much at one time that the stomach is overly filled and uncomfortable or painful) or chronic overeating (eating more than the body needs over a long period of time). Consistently overeating can lead to obesity and other health problems.

Oils: ⬡⬡Slim & Sassy, ⬡grapefruit⬡, ⬡lemon⬡, ⬡peppermint, ⬡ginger

Other Products: ⬡Slim & Sassy TrimShakes

⬡: Add 8 drops of Slim & Sassy to 2 cups (500 ml) of water, and drink throughout the day between meals. Drink Trim or V Shake 1–2 times per day as a meal alternative.

⬡: Diffuse into the air. Inhale directly from bottle. Apply oil to hands, tissue, or cotton wick, and inhale.

⬡: **Body System(s) Affected:** Nervous System, Digestive System, and Emotional Balance.

⬡: **Additional Research:**

Grapefruit: The scent of grapefruit oil and its component, limonene, was found to affect the autonomic nerves and to reduce appetite and body weight in rats exposed to the oil for 15 minutes three times per week (Shen et al., 2005).

Lemon: The scent of grapefruit oil and its component, limonene, was found to affect the autonomic nerves and to reduce appetite and body weight in rats exposed to the oil for 15 minutes three times per week (Shen et al., 2005).

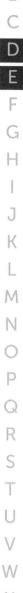

My Usage Guide

A B C D E F G H I J K L M N O P Q R S T U V W X Y Z

Eczema

See Skin: Dermatitis/Eczema

Edema

See also Allergies, Diuretic, Inflammation

Edema is swelling caused by the abnormal accumulation of fluids in a tissue or body cavity. This can be caused by an allergic reaction, inflammation, injury, or as a signal of problems with the heart, liver, or kidneys.

Oils: grapefruit, lemongrass, cypress, geranium, rosemary, cedarwood, juniper berry

: Dilute as recommended, and apply 1–2 drops on location.

: Add 1–2 drops to 1 cup (250 ml) of water, and drink every 3 hours.

: **Body System(s) Affected:** Cardiovascular System, Endocrine System, and Immune System.

Elbow

See Joints: Tennis Elbow

Emergency Oils

The following oils are recommended to have on hand in case of an emergency:

Clove: Use as an analgesic (for topical pain relief) and a drawing salve (to pull toxins/infection from the body). Good for acne, constipation, headaches, nausea, and toothaches.

Frankincense: Enhances effect of any other oil. It facilitates clarity of mind, accelerates all skin recovery issues, and reduces anxiety and mental and physical fatigue. Reduces hyperactivity, impatience, irritability, and restlessness. Helps with focus and concentration.

Lavender: Use for agitation, bruises, burns (can mix with melaleuca), leg cramps, herpes, heart irregularities, hives, insect bites, neuropathy, pain (inside and out), bee stings, sprains, sunburn (combine with frankincense), and sunstroke. Relieves insomnia, depression, and PMS and is a natural antihistamine (asthma or allergies).

Lemon: Use for arthritis, colds, constipation, coughs, cuts, sluggishness, sore throats, sunburn, and wounds. It lifts the spirits and reduces stress and fatigue. Internally it counteracts acidity, calms an upset stomach, and encourages elimination.

Lemongrass: Use for sore and cramping muscles and charley horses (with peppermint; drink lots of water). Apply to bottoms of feet in winter to warm them.

Melaleuca: Use for bug bites, colds, coughs, cuts, deodorant, eczema, fungus, infections (ear, nose, or throat), microbes (internally), psoriasis, rough hands, slivers (combine with clove to draw them out), sore throats, and wounds.

Oregano: Use as heavy-duty antibiotic (internally with olive oil or coconut oil in capsules or topically on bottoms of feet—follow up with lavender and peppermint). Also for fungal infections and for reducing pain and inflammation of arthritis, backache, bursitis, carpal tunnel syndrome, rheumatism, and sciatica. Always dilute.

Peppermint: Use as an analgesic (for topical pain relief, bumps, and bruises). Can also be used for circulation, fever, headache, indigestion, motion sickness, nausea, nerve problems, or vomiting.

AromaTouch: Use for relaxation and stress relief. It is soothing and anti-inflammatory and enhances massage.

Breathe: Use for allergies, anxiety, asthma, bronchitis, congestion, colds, coughs, flu, and respiratory distress.

Deep Blue: Use for pain relief. Works well in cases of arthritis, bruises, carpal tunnel, headaches, inflammation, joint pain, migraines, muscle pain, sprains, and rheumatism. Follow with peppermint to enhance effects.

DigestZen: Use for all digestion issues such as bloating, congestion, constipation, diarrhea, food poisoning (internal), heartburn, indigestion, motion sickness, nausea, and stomachache. Also works well on diaper rash.

On Guard: Use to disinfect all surfaces. It eliminates mold and viruses and helps to boost the immune system (bottoms of feet or internally; use daily).

Purify: Use for airborne pathogens, cuts, germs (on any surface), insect bites, itches (all types and

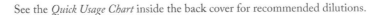

See the *Quick Usage Chart* inside the back cover for recommended dilutions.

290

varieties), and wounds. Also boosts the immune system.

TerraShield: Deters all flying insects and ticks from human bodies and pets.

Emotions

See also Anxiety, Calming, Depression, Fear, Grief/Sorrow, Stress: Emotional Stress, Uplifting

To put it simply, emotions are the way we currently feel. These feelings come in response to what we see, smell, hear, feel, taste, think, or have experienced and can affect our future thoughts and behavior. While much is still being discovered about the complex psychological and physiological processes involved in emotions, researchers have discovered that emotions involve many different systems in the body, including the brain, the sensory system, the endocrine/hormonal system, the autonomic nervous system, the immune system, and the release or inhibition of neurotransmitters (such as dopamine) in the brain. Recent research has also begun to uncover compelling evidence that various essential oils and their components have the ability to affect each one of these systems, making the use of essential oils an intriguing tool for helping to balance emotions in the human body.

Oils: Console, Motivate, Passion, Peace, Forgive, Cheer, AromaTouch, Balance, Citrus Bliss, Elevation, Serenity, ClaryCalm, Whisper, Zendocrine, cypress, geranium, lavender, rose, orange, peppermint, neroli

—**Acceptance:**

Oils: Forgive, Elevation

—**Alertness:** *See also Alertness*

Oils: peppermint, ylang ylang, black pepper, juniper berry, cinnamon

—**Anger:**

Oils: Serenity, Forgive, lavender, Console, InTune, ylang ylang, melissa, Elevation, Balance, helichrysum

—**Anxious:** *See also Anxiety*

Oils: Peace, lavender, orange, lemon, neroli, InTune, Serenity,

Motivate, AromaTouch, Elevation, Balance (on back of neck), Breathe (on chest)

—**Balance:**

Oils: Balance, AromaTouch, Citrus Bliss, geranium, juniper berry, lavender, neroli, orange, sandalwood, vetiver

—**Blocks:**

Oils: Forgive, cypress, frankincense, helichrysum, sandalwood, Balance

—**Clearing:**

Oils: Elevation, Peace, juniper berry, Balance

—**Coldness:**

Oils: Cheer, myrrh, ylang ylang

—**Concentration:** *See also Concentration*

Oils: InTune, Arise, lavender, lemon, peppermint, neroli

—**Confidence:**

Oils: Elevation, Motivate, Whisper, Passion, cedarwood, Forgive, orange

—**Creativity:**

Oils: frankincense, sandalwood, Elevation, Motivate, Cheer, cypress, lemon

—**Defeated:**

Oils: Motivate, Passion, Peace, cypress, fir, Elevation, juniper berry, Balance

—**Depression:** *See also Depression*

Oils: Motivate, Cheer, lemon, frankincense, InTune, Console, lavender, bergamot, Elevation, Balance, Peace, Citrus Bliss

—**Emotional Trauma:**

Oils: sandalwood, Forgive

—**Expression (self-expression):**

Oils: Balance, Elevation, Motivate, Passion

To put it simply, emotions are the way we currently feel. These feelings come in response to what we see, smell, hear, feel, taste, think, or have experienced and can affect our future thoughts and behavior. While much is still being discovered about the complex psychological and physiological processes involved in emotions, researchers have discovered that emotions involve many different systems in the body, including the brain, the sensory system, the endocrine/hormonal system, the autonomic nervous system, the immune system, and the release or inhibition of neurotransmitters (such as dopamine) in the brain. Recent research has also begun to uncover compelling evidence that various essential oils and their components have the ability to affect each one of these systems, making the use of essential oils an intriguing tool for helping to balance emotions in the human body.

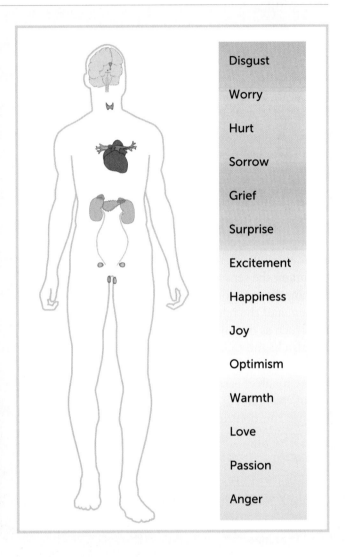

Disgust

Worry

Hurt

Sorrow

Grief

Surprise

Excitement

Happiness

Joy

Optimism

Warmth

Love

Passion

Anger

Oils for Emotional Support

Oils: Console, Motivate, Passion, Peace, Forgive, Cheer, AromaTouch, Balance, Citrus Bliss, Elevation, Serenity, ClaryCalm, Whisper, Zendocrine, cypress, geranium, lavender, rose, orange, peppermint

Common Emotional Issues

Emotional: Acceptance, Anger, Anxious Feelings, Balance (Emotional), Blocks (Emotional), Coldness, Confidence, Creativity, Defeat, Depressed Feelings, Emotional Blocks, Emotional Trauma, Expression (Self-Expression), Fear, Grief/Sorrow, Guilt, Happiness/Joy, Loss, Overwhelmed, Peace, Pity, Positiveness, Rejection, Release, Stress (Emotional), Suicidal, Uplifting, Worry

—**Fear**: *See also Fear*

Oils: Peace, Balance, ylang ylang, orange, sandalwood, Serenity, Motivate, Elevation, Passion

—**Focus**: *See Concentration*

—**Grief/Sorrow**: *See also Grief/Sorrow*

Oils: Cheer, Console, lemon, Elevation, Balance, Forgive, lavender, bergamot, orange, Citrus Bliss, grapefruit, wintergreen

—**Guilt**:

Oils: Peace, Elevation, Forgive, Deep Blue (on outer earlobes)

—**Happiness/Joy**:

Oils: Elevation, Cheer, Console, Citrus Bliss, Motivate, Passion, lemon, orange, spearmint, sandalwood, bergamot

—**Loss**:

Oils: Elevation, Forgive, tangerine, orange

—**Mind (open)**:

Oils: frankincense, sandalwood, Balance

—**Negative Emotions**:

Oils: Elevation, Citrus Bliss, orange, grapefruit, Balance, fir, wintergreen, lavender

—**Overburdened/Overwhelmed**:

Oils: Peace, Balance, Citrus Bliss, orange

—**Peace**:

Oils: Serenity, lavender, Peace, InTune, ylang ylang, melissa, neroli

—**Pity (self-pity)**:

Oils: Elevation, Forgive, Citrus Bliss, orange

—**Positive (feeling)**:

Oils: Elevation, Motivate, Cheer, basil, peppermint, frankincense, cedarwood, juniper berry

—**Rejection**:

Oils: Motivate, Passion, Balance, lavender, geranium

—**Release**:

Oils: Forgive, Roman chamomile

—**Stress**: *See also Stress: Emotional Stress*

Oils: Elevation, Peace, clary sage, bergamot, Serenity

—**Suicidal**:

Oils: Elevation, AromaTouch, Citrus Bliss, Serenity

—**Uplifting**: *See also Uplifting*

Oils: Cheer, lemon, orange, Elevation, Brave, Console, Passion, Citrus Bliss, Forgive

—**Worried**:

Oils: Peace, bergamot, neroli, Serenity, Elevation, Balance, AromaTouch

: Inhale directly from bottle. Diffuse into the air. Apply oil to hands, tissue, or cotton wick, and inhale.

: Massage oils on back, chest, and/or legs. Gently massage 1–2 drops of oil into the outer lobes of the ear (avoid the ear canal). Add 1–2 drops of oil to a bath or shower gel or to bath salts, and use during a bath or shower.

: Add 1–2 drops to 1 cup (250 ml) distilled water or to ½ cup (125 ml) rice or almond milk before drinking. Add 1–2 drops to an empty capsule, and swallow.

: **Body System(s) Affected**: Emotional Balance and Nervous System.

: **Additional Research**:

Peppermint: In human trials, the aroma of peppermint was found to enhance memory and increase alertness (Moss et al., 2008).

Ylang ylang: Inhaled ylang ylang oil was found to decrease blood pressure and pulse rate and to enhance attentiveness and alertness in volunteers compared to an odorless control (Hongratanaworakit et al., 2004).

Ylang ylang: In human trials, the aroma of peppermint was found to enhance memory and to increase alertness, while ylang ylang aroma was found to increase calmness (Moss et al., 2008).

Ylang ylang: Subjects who had ylang ylang oil applied to their skin had decreased blood pressure, increased skin temperature, and reported feeling more calm and relaxed, as compared to subjects in a control group (Hongratanaworakit et al., 2006).

Lavender: *Lavandula angustifolia* essential oil demonstrated ability to inhibit GABA-A receptor channels of rat brain cells (Huang et al., 2008).

Primary Recommendations • Secondary Recommendations • Other Recommendations / =Aromatic, =Topical, =Internal

A B C D E F G H I J K L M N O P Q R S T U V W X Y Z

Lavender: Inhaling lavender oil was found to be effective at alleviating agitated behaviors in older Chinese patients suffering from dementia (Lin et al., 2007).

Lavender: Exposure to lavender odor was found to decrease anxiety in gerbils in the elevated plus maze, with a further decrease in anxiety in females after prolonged (2 week) exposure (Bradley et al., 2007).

Lavender: Subjects receiving a lozenge containing lavender oil, hops extract, lemon balm, and oat were found to have increases in alpha 1, alpha 2, and beta 1 electrical output (Dimpfel et al., 2004).

Lavender: In patients admitted to an intensive care unit, those receiving lavender aromatherapy reported a greater improvement in mood and perceived levels of anxiety compared to those receiving massage or a period of rest (Dunn et al., 1995).

Lavender: Female patients being treated for chronic hemodialysis demonstrated less anxiety when exposed to lavender aroma compared to control (Itai et al., 2000).

Lavender: Lavender oil was found to demonstrate anti-conflict effects in mice similar to the anxiolytic (antianxiety) drug diazepam (Umezu, 2000).

Lavender: Subjects who smelled a cleansing gel with lavender aroma were more relaxed and able to complete math computations faster (Field et al., 2005).

Lavender: Subjects exposed to 3 minutes of lavender aroma were more relaxed and able to perform math computations faster and more accurately. Subjects exposed to rosemary aroma were more alert and completed math computations faster (but not more accurately) (Diego et al., 1998).

Lavender: In patients suffering from arthritis, it was found that a blend of lavender, marjoram, eucalyptus, rosemary, and peppermint blended with carrier oils was found to reduce perceived pain and depression compared to control (Kim et al., 2005).

Lavender: Female students suffering from insomnia were found to sleep better and to have a lower level of depression during weeks they used a lavender fragrance when compared to weeks they did not use a lavender fragrance (Lee et al., 2006).

Lavender: Swiss mice fed lavender oil diluted in olive oil were found to be more sedate in several common tests (Guillemain et al., 1989).

Melissa: Melissa (lemon balm) oil applied topically in a lotion was found to reduce agitation and to improve quality of life factors in patients suffering from severe dementia, as compared to those receiving a placebo lotion (Ballard et al., 2002).

Orange: Bitter orange peel oil taken orally by mice was found to reduce anxiety, increase sleeping time, and increase the time before a chemically induced seizure started (Carvalho-Freitas et al., 2002).

Orange: Female patients waiting for dental treatment were found to be less anxious, more positive, and more calm when exposed to orange oil odor than patients who were not exposed to the orange oil odor (Lehrner et al., 2000).

Lemon: Rats exposed long-term to lemon essential oil were found to demonstrate different anxiety and pain threshold levels than untreated rats. It was also found that exposure to lemon oil induced chemical changes in the neuronal circuits involved in anxiety and pain (Ceccarelli et al., 2004).

Lemon: Lemon oil was found to have an antistress effect on mice involved in several behavioral tasks (Komiya et al., 2006).

Lemon: Lemon oil vapor was found to have strong antistress and antidepressant effects on mice subjected to several common stress tests (Komiya et al., 2006).

Lemon: Lemon oil and its component, citral, were found to decrease depressed behavior in a similar manner to antidepressant drugs in rats involved in several stress tests (Komori et al., 1995).

Lemon: In 12 patients suffering from depression, it was found that inhaling citrus aromas reduced the needed doses of antidepressants, normalized neuroendocrine hormone levels, and normalized immune function (Komori et al., 1995).

Lemon: Lemon odor was found to enhance the positive mood of volunteers exposed to a stressor (Kiecolt-Glaser et al., 2008).

Frankincense: Incensole acetate was found to open TRPV receptors in mice brains, indicating a possible channel for emotional regulation (Moussaieff et al., 2008).

Emphysema

Emphysema is a chronic pulmonary disease where airflow is restricted through the lungs due to destruction (typically caused by airborne toxins such as those in cigarette smoke) of the wall of the alveoli (small air sacs in the lungs where oxygen and carbon dioxide is exchanged with the blood). This destruction of the alveolar wall causes the alveoli to collapse when air is expelled from the lungs, trapping air inside.

> *Simple Solutions—Emphysema:* Add 1 drop eucalyptus to 1 tsp. (5 ml) fractionated coconut oil, and apply on chest and back.

Oils: eucalyptus, Breathe

: Diffuse into the air.

: Dilute as recommended, and apply 1–2 drops to chest and back. Apply as a warm compress on chest.

: **Body System(s) Affected:** Respiratory System and Cardiovascular System.

Endocrine System

See also **Adrenal Glands, Ovaries, Pancreas, Pineal Gland, Pituitary Gland, Testes, Thymus, Thyroid**

See Endocrine System Chart on previous page.

The endocrine system is the series of hormone-producing glands and organs that help regulate metabolism, reproduction, blood pressure, appetite, and many other body functions. The endocrine system is mainly controlled by the hypothalamus region of the brain that either produces hormones that stimulate the other endocrine glands directly, or that stimulates the pituitary gland located just below it to release the hormones needed to stimulate the other endocrine glands. These hormones are released into the bloodstream, where they travel to other areas of the body to either stimulate other endocrine glands or to stimulate tissues and organs of the body directly. Some essential oils may act as hormones or stimulate the endocrine system to produce hormones that have a regulating effect on the body.

Oils: Zendocrine, rosemary, cinnamon

Other Products: Zendocrine Zendocrine Detoxification Complex to help support healthy endocrine cleansing and filtering.

—Hormonal Balance:

Oils: clary sage, clove, ylang ylang

Other Products: Phytoestrogen Lifetime Complex

See the *Quick Usage Chart* inside the back cover for recommended dilutions.

–**Female**:

  Oils: ⊘⊘ClaryCalm, ⊘⊘Whisper

–**Sexual Energy**:

  Oils: ⊘⊘ylang ylang

○: Take capsules as directed on package. Place 1–2 drops of oil under the tongue, or add 3–5 drops of essential oil to an empty capsule; swallow capsule.

⊘: Diffuse into the air. Inhale directly from bottle. Apply oil to hands, tissue, or cotton wick, and inhale.

⊜: Dilute as recommended, and apply 1–2 drops to the reflex points on the feet, lower back, thyroid, liver, kidneys, gland areas, the center of the body, or both sides of the spine and clavicle area. Add 1–2 drops to 1 Tbs. (15 ml) fractionated coconut oil, and use as massage oil.

⊕: **Body System(s) Affected:** Endocrine System.

Endometriosis

Endometriosis is a chronic disorder in women where endometrium cells (cells from the lining of the uterus) grow outside of the uterus—typically around the ovaries, the ligaments that support the uterus, or the peritoneal (abdominal) cavity. These cells are often still responsive to the monthly hormone cycle that effects the changes in the uterus and can cause abnormal abdominal pain and irregularities in the menstrual cycle.

Oils: ⊜geranium, ⊜cypress, ⊜clary sage, ⊜On Guard, ⊜eucalyptus, ⊜Whisper

⊜: Dilute as recommended, and apply 1–2 drops on lower abdomen or on feet. Apply as a warm compress. Place 1–2 drops in warm bathwater, and bathe.

⊕: **Body System(s) Affected:** Reproductive System.

Endurance

Simple Solutions—Endurance: Add 1 drop peppermint to a small bottle of water, and drink 15 minutes before exercising.

Oils: ⊘○peppermint▭

Other Products: ○Mito2Max, ○Alpha CRS+, ○a2z Chewable, ○xEO Mega or vEO Mega, ○IQ Mega, ○Microplex VMz to provide nutrients and antioxidants that help support healthy cellular function and energy levels.

⊘: Diffuse into the air. Inhale directly from bottle. Apply oil to hands, tissue, or cotton wick, and inhale.

○: Take capsules as directed on package.

▭: **Additional Research:**

Peppermint: A quasi experiment comparing exercise performance before and after consumption of mineral water containing peppermint essential oil for 10 days found that exercise performance improved after consumption of peppermint oil (including increases in respiratory efficiency, energy expenditure, time to exhaustion, and distance during exercise and decreases in resting and exercise heart rates) (Meamarbashi et al., 2013).

Energy

Simple Solutions—Energy: Inhale peppermint directly from the bottle for a quick energy boost.

Oils: ⊘○⊜peppermint▭, ⊘⊜fir, ⊘⊜Elevation, ⊘⊜Balance, ⊘⊜Steady, ⊘⊜lemon, ⊘⊜litsea, ⊘⊜basil, ⊘⊜thyme, ⊘⊜rosemary, ⊘⊜orange, ⊘⊜lemongrass, ⊘⊜eucalyptus

Other Products: ○Mito2Max, ○Alpha CRS+, ○a2z Chewable, ○xEO Mega or vEO Mega, ○IQ Mega, ○Microplex VMz to provide nutrients and antioxidants that help support healthy cellular function and energy levels.

–**Exhaustion**:

  Oils: First, work with one or more of the following nervous system oils to help calm and relax: ⊜lavender, ⊜ylang ylang, ⊜Roman chamomile, ⊜frankincense, ⊜clary sage. Secondly, use an energizing oil such as ⊜lemon, ⊜sandalwood, ⊜rosemary, ⊘⊜lime, ⊜basil, ⊜grapefruit.

–**Fatigue**:

  Oils: ⊘⊜rosemary (nervous fatigue), ⊘⊜thyme (general fatigue)

  –**Mental Fatigue**:

    Oils: ⊘⊜Serenity, ⊘⊜Calmer, ⊘⊜lemongrass, ⊘⊜basil, ⊜petitgrain

    Blend 1: Blend equal parts basil and lemongrass together. Apply to temples, back of neck, and feet. Diffuse into the air.

  –**Physical Fatigue**:

    Oils: ⊘⊜Serenity

–**Physical**:

  Oils: ⊘lemon, ⊘cinnamon, ⊘bergamot

A B C D E F G H I J K L M N O P Q R S T U V W X Y Z

The endocrine system is the series of hormone-producing glands and organs that help regulate metabolism, reproduction, blood pressure, appetite, and many other body functions. The endocrine system is mainly controlled by the hypothalamus region of the brain that either produces hormones that stimulate the other endocrine glands directly or that stimulates the pituitary gland located just below it to release the hormones needed to stimulate the other endocrine glands. These hormones are released into the bloodstream, where they travel to other areas of the body to either stimulate other endocrine glands or to stimulate tissues and organs of the body directly. Some essential oils may act as hormones or stimulate the endocrine system to produce hormones that have a regulating effect on the body.

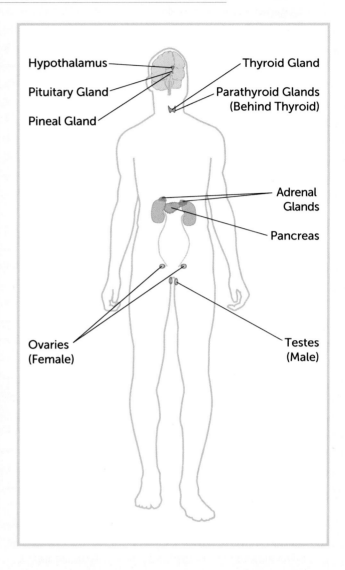

Oils for Endocrine/Reproductive Support

Endocrine Oils: Zendocrine, rosemary, cinnamon

Female-Specific Oils: ClaryCalm, Whisper, Balance, peppermint, clary sage, ylang ylang, Roman chamomile, bergamot, fennel, lavender, rose

Male Specific Oils: melaleuca, oregano, basil, clary sage, cassia, eucalyptus, lavender, cypress

Common Endocrine/Reproductive Issues

Endocrine: Addison's Disease, Cushing's Syndrome, Diabetes, Goiter, Grave's Disease, Hashimoto's Disease, Hormone Imbalance, Hyperthyroidism, Hypothyroidism, Pancreatitis, Schmidt's Syndrome

Female-Specific: Hot Flashes, Ovarian Cyst, Menopause, Menstrual Disorders, PMS, Postpartum Depression, Pregnancy

Male Specific: Impotence, Prostate Enlargement

—Sexual:

Oils: ᵉylang ylang

🔄: Diffuse into the air. Inhale directly from bottle. Apply oil to hands, tissue, or cotton wick, and inhale.

🖐: Dilute 1–2 drops in 1 Tbs. (15 ml) fractionated coconut oil, and massage into muscles. Place 1–2 drops in warm bathwater, and bathe. Dilute as recommended, and apply 1–2 drops on temples, back of neck, liver area, or feet.

🌑: Take capsules as directed on package.

✛: **Body System(s) Affected:** Nervous System and Emotional Balance.

🔔: **Additional Research:**

Peppermint: A quasi experiment comparing exercise performance before and after consumption of mineral water containing peppermint essential oil for 10 days found that exercise performance improved after consumption of peppermint oil (including increases in respiratory efficiency, energy expenditure, time to exhaustion, and distance during exercise and decreases in resting and exercise heart rates) (Meamarbashi et al., 2013).

Epilepsy

See Seizure: Epilepsy

Epstein-Barr

See Mono; see also Antiviral: Epstein-Barr Virus

Estrogen

Estrogens are hormones produced by the ovaries that regulate the development of female characteristics and the menstrual cycle in females.

Oils: 🖐ᵉClaryCalm, 🖐ᵉclary sage

Other Products: ᴼPhytoestrogen Lifetime Complex

🖐: Apply on the lower abdomen. Dilute 1–2 drops in 1 Tbs. (15 ml) fractionated coconut oil, and use as massage oil.

🌑: Take capsules as directed on package.

🔄: Diffuse into the air. Inhale directly from bottle. Apply oil to hands, tissue, or cotton wick, and inhale.

✛: **Body System(s) Affected:** Reproductive System.

Exhaustion

See Energy: Exhaustion

Expectorant

See Congestion: Expectorant

Eyes

Eyes are the organs of the body responsible for detecting and adjusting to light and focusing images of the surrounding environment onto the optical nerve for transfer to the brain for processing.

Oils: ᵉlemongrass, ᵉsandalwood, ᵉcypress, ᵉlemon, ᵉfennel, ᵉeucalyptus, ᵉlavender, ᵉOn Guard

Other Products: ᴼMicroplex VMz for nutrients that help support healthy eye cell function.

—Blocked Tear Ducts:

Tears from the eye normally drain through small tubes called tear ducts. The tear ducts carry tears from the surface of the eye into the nose where they are reabsorbed or evaporate. When these tear ducts are blocked, the eyes become watery and irritated. Blocked tear ducts are most common in babies and in older adults.

Oils: ᵉlavender

—Cataracts:

A cataract is a clouding of the normally transparent lens of the eye. This clouding results in blurry vision, seemingly faded colors, double vision, glare, and difficulty seeing at night. Over time, the clouding can increase and lead to severe vision problems.

Oils: ᵉclove, ᵉlavender

Blend 1: Combine 8 drops lemongrass, 6 drops cypress, and 3 drops eucalyptus. Apply around the eye area twice a day. Do not get oil in the eyes.

—Dry/Itchy Eyes:

Oils: ᵉmelaleuca (in humidifier)

—Eye Lid Drop/Drooping Eyelid:

A drooping eyelid is characterized by an excessive sagging of the upper eyelid. Drooping can be present at birth as a result of underdeveloped eyelid muscles, or it can occur with aging. Drooping eyelids can cause visual impairment if they droop enough to partially cover the eye.

Blend 2: Combine equal parts helichrysum and peppermint, and apply 1–2 drops on the eyelid. Do not get oil in the eyes.

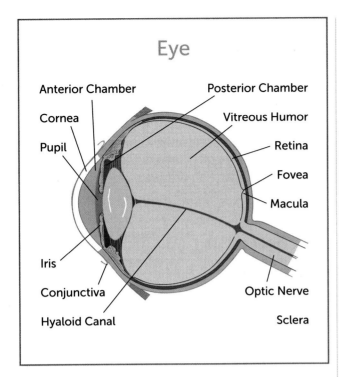

Eye

- Anterior Chamber
- Cornea
- Pupil
- Iris
- Conjunctiva
- Hyaloid Canal
- Posterior Chamber
- Vitreous Humor
- Retina
- Fovea
- Macula
- Optic Nerve
- Sclera

—**Improve Vision:**

Oils: frankincense, lemongrass, juniper berry, On Guard, sandalwood, lavender

Blend 3: Combine 10 drops lemongrass, 5 drops cypress, and 3 drops eucalyptus with 2 Tbs. (25 ml) fractionated coconut oil. Apply around the eyes morning and night, or apply on reflex points on the feet or on the ears.

—**Iris Inflammation:**

The iris is the colored part of the eye that regulates the amount of light entering the eye through the pupil. When the iris becomes inflamed, it results in a condition called iritis. Iritis is normally related to a disease or infection in another part of the body, but it can also be caused by injury to the eye. Symptoms of iritis include blurred vision, pain, tearing, light sensitivity, red eye, and a small pupil size.

Oils: eucalyptus

—**Macular Degeneration:**

Macular degeneration is an eye disease common in individuals 65 and older. It is marked by degeneration of a small, oval-shaped part of the retina called the macula. Because the macula is responsible for capturing the light from the central part of images coming into the eye, macular degeneration causes blurring or a blind spot in the central

vision, making it difficult to drive, recognize faces, read, or do any kind of detail work.

Oils: clove

—**Pink Eye:**

Pink eye, also known as conjunctivitis, is an inflammation or infection of the membranes covering the whites of the eyes (conjunctiva) and the inner part of the eyelids. Swelling, redness, itching, discharge, and burning of the eyes are common symptoms of pink eye. Frequent causes include allergies, bacterial or viral infection, contact lenses, and eye drops.

Oils: melaleuca, lavender

—**Retina (strengthen):**

The retina is a layer of nerves lining the back of the eye. The retina is responsible for sensing light and then sending impulses (via the optic nerve) back to the brain so that visual images can be formed.

Oils: cypress, lemongrass, helichrysum, juniper berry, peppermint, lavender, sandalwood

—**Swollen Eyes:**

Oils: cypress, helichrysum, peppermint (allergies), lavender

: Caution: Never put essential oils directly in the eyes! Be careful when applying oils near the eyes. Be sure to have some fractionated coconut oil handy for additional dilution if irritation occurs. Never use water to wash off an oil that irritates. Dilute as recommended, and apply 1–2 drops around eyes or to feet, thumbs, ankles, pelvis, base of neck, or reflex points on the feet.

: Diffuse into the air.

: Take capsules as directed on package.

: **Body System(s) Affected:** Muscles, Nervous System, and Immune System.

Facial Oils

See Skin

See the *Quick Usage Chart* inside the back cover for recommended dilutions.

298

Fainting

See also **Shock**

> *Simple Solutions—Fainting:* Place an open bottle of peppermint under the victim's nose, and allow the victim to inhale the aroma until he or she recovers.

Fainting is a temporary loss of consciousness caused by a momentary disruption of blood flow to the brain. Fainting can result from standing in one place too long, coughing very hard, fear, emotional trauma, heavy bleeding, or severe dehydration. Fainting can sometimes be a symptom of a more serious condition.

Oils: peppermint, rosemary, basil, lavender

: Inhale directly from bottle.

: **Body System(s) Affected:** Nervous System.

Fatigue

See **Energy: Fatigue**

Fear

See also **Anxiety, Calming**

> *Simple Solutions—Fear:* Diffuse Peace in an aromatherapy diffuser.

> *Simple Solutions—Fear:* Add 3 drops lavender and 2 drops ylang ylang to 2 Tbs. (25 ml) of water in a small misting spray bottle. Allow children to spray into the air to help spray away fears.

Fear causes the blood vessels to tighten, restricting the amount of oxygen and nutrients that can reach the cells.

Oils: Peace, Balance, Steady, ylang ylang, orange, sandalwood, clary sage, geranium, juniper berry, myrrh, bergamot, fir, cypress, marjoram

: Diffuse into the air. Inhale directly from bottle. Apply oil to hands, tissue, or cotton wick, and inhale.

: Dilute as recommended, and apply 1–2 drops to temples, back of neck, or bottoms of feet.

: **Body System(s) Affected:** Nervous System.

: **Additional Research:**

Ylang ylang: Subjects who had ylang ylang oil applied to their skin had decreased blood pressure, increased skin temperature, and reported feeling more calm and relaxed compared to subjects in a control group (Hongratanaworakit et al., 2006).

Orange: Female patients waiting for dental treatment were found to be less anxious, more positive, and more calm when exposed to orange oil odor than were patients who were not exposed to the orange oil odor (Lehrner et al., 2000).

Feet

See **Foot**

Female-Specific Conditions

See also **Endometriosis, Pregnancy/Motherhood**

—Hemorrhaging: *See* **Blood: Hemorrhaging**

—Hot Flashes:

A hot flash is a sudden, intense feeling of heat in the face and upper body, often accompanied by an increased heart rate, sweating, dizziness, headache, weakness, or anxiety. Hot flashes are generally associated with the symptoms of menopause and premenopause.

> *Simple Solutions—Hot Flash:* Add 5 drops clary sage to 1 Tbs. (15 ml) jojoba oil, and add to bathwater as a bath oil.

Oils: ClaryCalm, Balance, peppermint, clary sage

Other Products: Phytoestrogen Lifetime Complex, Daily Supplements Pack (contains Alpha CRS+, xEO Mega or vEO Mega, IQ Mega, and Microplex VMz)

Recipe 1: Both morning and evening, apply 1–2 drops each of Balance and peppermint to back of neck; then apply 1–2 drops clary sage to forearms in the morning and to ankles in the evening. The Daily Supplements Pack may also be taken to help regulate the hormonal system.

—Hormones (balancing):

Oils: ClaryCalm, ylang ylang, clary sage

Other Products: Phytoestrogen Lifetime Complex

—Infertility:

Infertility is clinically defined as the inability to get pregnant after a year of trying. This could be due to any of several underlying causes.

A B C D E F G H I J K L M N O P Q R S T U V W X Y Z

My Usage Guide

Oils: ⊘clary sage, ⊘geranium, ⊘melissa, ⊘cypress, ⊘thyme, ⊘fennel, ⊘Roman chamomile, ⊘ylang ylang

—Menopause:

Menopause is the permanent ending of a female's menstruation and fertility. For most American women, Menopause occurs around age 51 and is often recognized by hot flashes, irregular periods, vaginal dryness, mood swings, difficulty sleeping, thinning hair, abdominal weight gain, and decreased fertility.

Oils: ⊘⊘ClaryCalm, ⊘cypress, ⊘lavender⊕, ⊘Roman chamomile, ⊘orange, ⊘clary sage, ⊘⊙fennel⊕, ⊘basil, ⊘geranium, ⊘rosemary, ⊘thyme

Other Products: ⊙Phytoestrogen Lifetime Complex, ⊙Bone Nutrient Lifetime Complex

–Premenopause:

Oils: ⊘⊘ClaryCalm, ⊘clary sage, ⊘lavender

Other Products: ⊙Phytoestrogen Lifetime Complex, ⊙Bone Nutrient Lifetime Complex

—Menstruation:

Menstruation, also known as a woman's "period," is the regular shedding of the uterus lining and vaginal discharge of blood when a woman is not pregnant. A woman's period lasts between 2 and 7 days and reoccurs on an average of every 28 days.

–Amenorrhea:

Amenorrhea is the absence of menstruation. The following oils may help induce menstrual flow (emmenagogic) and may need to be avoided during pregnancy for this reason. See Pregnancy/Motherhood for further safety data.

Oils: ⊘⊘ClaryCalm, ⊘basil, ⊘clary sage, ⊘peppermint, ⊘rosemary, ⊘juniper berry, ⊘marjoram, ⊘lavender, ⊘Roman chamomile

Other Products: ⊙Phytoestrogen Lifetime Complex

–Dysmenorrhea:

Dysmenorrhea is painful menstruation. Apply one or more of these oils to the abdomen. It may also help to use a hot compress.

Oils: ⊘⊘ClaryCalm, ⊘clary sage⊕, ⊘geranium, ⊘lavender⊕, ⊘rose⊕, ⊘cypress,

⊘peppermint, ⊘marjoram, ⊘Roman chamomile, ⊘basil, ⊘rosemary, ⊘fennel

Other Products: ⊙Phytoestrogen Lifetime Complex

–Irregular:

Oils: ⊘⊘ClaryCalm, ⊘peppermint, ⊘rosemary, ⊘Roman chamomile, ⊘clary sage, ⊘fennel, ⊘lavender, ⊘spikenard, ⊘rose

Other Products: ⊙Phytoestrogen Lifetime Complex

–Menorrhagia:

Menorrhagia is abnormally heavy or extended menstrual flow. It may also refer to irregular bleeding at any time. This situation may be a sign of a more serious condition, so please see your doctor.

Oils: ⊘⊘ClaryCalm, ⊘cypress, ⊘geranium, ⊘Roman chamomile, ⊘rose

Other Products: ⊙Phytoestrogen Lifetime Complex

–Scanty:

Oils: ⊘⊘ClaryCalm, ⊘peppermint, ⊘lavender, ⊘melissa

Other Products: ⊙Phytoestrogen Lifetime Complex

—Ovaries:

Ovaries are the female reproductive organs in which eggs are produced and stored.

Oils: ⊘⊘ClaryCalm, ⊘rosemary, ⊘geranium, ⊘DigestZen

Other Products: ⊙Phytoestrogen Lifetime Complex

–Ovarian Cyst:

Oils: ⊘basil

—PMS:

Premenstrual syndrome (PMS) is a group of symptoms such as irritability, anxiety, moodiness, bloating, breast tenderness, headaches, and cramping that occurs in the days or hours before menstruation begins and then disappear once menstruation begins. PMS is thought to be caused by the fluctuation in hormones during this time or by the way progesterone is broken down by the body. Caffeine intake from bever-

---

See the Quick Usage Chart inside the back cover for recommended dilutions.

ages or chocolate is also thought to enhance PMS symptoms.

> *Simple Solutions—PMS:* Combine 3 drops clary sage and 3 drops geranium with 1 tsp. (5 ml) almond oil. Add to warm bathwater for a soothing bath.

Oils: ClaryCalm, clary sage, geranium, fennel, lavender, bergamot, grapefruit, neroli

Other Products: Phytoestrogen Lifetime Complex, Bone Nutrient Lifetime Complex or Microplex VMz contain calcium, which has been found to help lessen PMS symptoms.

−Apathetic-Tired-Listless:

Oils: ClaryCalm, grapefruit, geranium, bergamot, fennel

Other Products: Phytoestrogen Lifetime Complex

−Irritable:

Oils: ClaryCalm, clary sage, bergamot, Roman chamomile

Other Products: Phytoestrogen Lifetime Complex

−Violent Aggressive:

Oils: ClaryCalm, geranium, bergamot

Other Products: Phytoestrogen Lifetime Complex

−Weeping-Depression:

Oils: ClaryCalm, clary sage, bergamot, geranium

Other Products: Phytoestrogen Lifetime Complex

−Postpartum Depression: *See Pregnancy/Motherhood: Postpartum Depression*

🔄: Dilute as recommended, and apply to the abdomen, lower back, shoulders, or reflex points on the feet. Add 1–2 drops to 1 Tbs. (15 ml) fractionated coconut oil, and massage into abdomen, lower back, and shoulders. Apply as a warm compress to the abdomen. Add 1–2 drops to 2 tsp. (10 ml) olive oil, insert into vagina, and retain overnight with a tampon.

🔄: Place in hands and inhale. Diffuse into the air.

🔘: Take capsules as directed on package.

⚙: **Body System(s) Affected:** Reproductive System and Endocrine System.

🕐: **Additional Research:**

Lavender: Inhalation of linalool or *Lavandula burnatii* super-derived essential oil (composed from the five main lavender oils and containing a high level of linalool) was found to aid in the recovery of ether inhalation–induced decrease in adrenaline, noradrenaline, and dopamine levels in female menopausal model rats. The researchers stated that these results suggest that lavender or linalool may contribute to relieving tension and may be applicable to the treatment of menopausal disorders (Yamada et al., 2005).

Fennel: Using a mouse model of postmenopausal bone loss researchers found that oral administration of fennel oil for six weeks had an intermediate effect on the prevention of femoral bone mineral density loss and bone mineral content loss when compared to controls. These findings suggest that fennel oil has potential in preventing bone loss in postmenopausal osteoporosis (Kim et al., 2012).

Clary Sage: In an experiment with 67 female college students, an aromatherapy massage with lavender, clary sage, and rose essential oils proved to be more effective at treating dysmenorrhea than a placebo treatment of almond oil or the control (Han et al., 2006).

Clary sage, lavender, and marjoram: Compared to a synthetic fragrance, dysmenorrhea pain decreased and shortened in duration when subjects massaged a blend of lavender, marjoram, and clary sage essential oils (in a ratio of 2:1:1) daily on the abdomen between menstruations (Ou et al., 2012).

Rose: A study with 92 university-aged female students with primary dysmenorrhea found that ingestion of a capsule containing 200 mg of *Rosa damascena* extract every 6 hours at the first 3 days of menstruation was as effective as administration of Mefenamic acid (a drug with possible adverse reactions and side effects) (Bani et al., 2014).

Thyme: A study comparing administration of thyme essential oil, ibuprofen, and placebo treatment revealed that thyme essential oil alleviates dysmenorrhea pain as well as ibuprofen and works significantly better than the placebo treatment (Salmalian et al., 2014).

Fertility

*See **Female-Specific Conditions: Infertility, Male Specific Conditions: Infertility***

Fever

*See also **Cooling Oils***

Fever is an increase of the body's core temperature, typically in response to an infection or injury. A fever is the body's natural response to help enhance the immune system's ability to fight the infection.

> *Simple Solutions—Fever:* Blend 2 drops peppermint and 2 drops eucalyptus in a bowl of cool water. Moisten washcloth with water, and use to sponge the forehead, back of neck, and feet.

Oils: peppermint, lemon, lime, eucalyptus, clove, patchouli, melaleuca, ginger, lavender, basil, fir, bergamot

—To Cool the System:

Oils: ⚪clove, ⚪◑◐peppermint, ◐eucalyptus, ◐bergamot

—To Induce Sweating:

Oils: ◐basil, ◐fennel, ◐melaleuca, ◐peppermint, ◐rosemary, ◐lavender, ◐cypress

⚪: Place 1–2 drops of oil under the tongue or place 1–2 drops of essential oil into capsule; then swallow capsule. Place 1–2 drops in 1 cup (250 ml) of rice milk or water, and sip slowly.

◐: Dilute as recommended, and apply to back or to bottoms of the feet.

◑: Diffuse into the air.

⊕: **Body System(s) Affected:** Immune System.

Fibrillation

See Cardiovascular System

Fibroids

Fibroids are noncancerous growths of muscle and connective tissue in the uterus. Fibroids can be painful and may affect fertility and pregnancy.

Oils: ◐frankincense, ◐helichrysum, ◐oregano, ◐Balance, ◐lavender

◐: Place 3 drops of oil in douche. Dilute as recommended, and apply to reflex points on the feet.

⊕: **Body System(s) Affected:** Reproductive System and Endocrine System.

Fibromyalgia

Fibromyalgia is long-term localized or generalized aches, pain, or tenderness in the muscles, ligaments, or other soft tissue that can interfere with normal movement, sleep, or other activities. There is no known cause of fibromyalgia, and many different factors may contribute to the development of this condition. Some have suggested eliminating refined sugar from the diet. Others have recommended reducing stress, stretching exercises, massage, or better sleep.

Oils: ◐Deep Blue, ◐wintergreen, ◐helichrysum, ◐lavender, ◐rosemary, ◐thyme

Other Products: ⚪Mito2Max, ⚪Alpha CRS+, ⚪a2z Chewable, ⚪xEO Mega or vEO Mega, ⚪IQ Mega, ⚪Microplex VMz for nutrients needed for healthy muscle and nerve cell function.

◐: Add 1–2 drops of oil to 1 Tbs. (15 ml) fractionated coconut oil, and massage on location. Apply as a warm compress over affected area.

⚪: Take capsules as directed on package.

⊕: **Body System(s) Affected:** Immune System and Muscles.

Finger (mashed)

Recipe 1: Apply 1 drop geranium (for bruising), 1 drop helichrysum (to stop the bleeding), 1 drop lavender, 1 drop lemongrass (for tissue repair), and 1 drop Deep Blue (for pain).

Flatulence

See Digestive System: Gas/Flatulence

Flu

See Influenza

Fluids

See Edema, Diuretic

Food Poisoning

See also Antibacterial, Antifungal, Antiviral, Digestive System, Parasites

Food poisoning refers to the effects on the digestive tract by pathogenic organisms—or the toxins they produce—that are ingested into the body in food. Symptoms of food poisoning can include stomach pain, cramps, diarrhea, nausea, and vomiting.

Oils: ⚪DigestZen⊕, ⚪On Guard, ⚪rosemary

Other Products: ⚪DigestZen Softgels, ⚪On Guard+ Softgels

⚪: Add 6 drops to 1 cup (250 ml) of water. Swish around in the mouth, and swallow. Place 1–2 drops in an empty capsule, and swallow.

⊕: **Body System(s) Affected:** Digestive System and Immune System.

See the *Quick Usage Chart* inside the back cover for recommended dilutions.

302

○: **Additional Research:**

DigestZen: Peppermint and spearmint oils inhibited resistant strains of *Staphylococcus*, *E. coli*, *Salmonella*, and *Helicobacter pylori* (Imai et al., 2001).

Foot

Oils: ⊘lemon, ⊘lavender, ⊘Roman chamomile

—**Athlete's Foot:** *See Antifungal: Athlete's Foot*

—**Blisters:**

Oils: ⊘lavender, ⊘geranium, ⊘melaleuca, ⊘Purify

—**Bunion:** *See also Bursitis*

A bunion is bursitis located at the base of the big toe. It is often caused by constrictive shoes that force the big toe to point inward and the base of the big toe to jut outward. This misplacement can irritate the bursa located at the base of the toe and cause it to become inflamed, which causes further irritation.

Oils: ⊘cypress

—**Calluses:**

A callus is a flat, thick growth of skin that develops on areas of the skin where there is constant friction or rubbing. Calluses typically form on the bottoms of the feet, but they can also form on the hands or other areas of the body exposed to constant friction.

Oils: ⊘oregano

—**Club Foot:**

Oils: ⊘ginger, ⊘rosemary, ⊘lavender, ⊘Roman chamomile

—**Corns:**

Corns are painful growths that develop on the small toes due to repetitive friction in that area (often from ill-fitting footwear). If untreated, corns can cause increased pressure on underlying tissue, causing tissue damage or ulcerations.

Oils: ⊘clove, ⊘peppermint, ⊘grapefruit, ⊘Citrus Bliss

⊖: Dilute as recommended, and apply to area. Combine 1–2 drops with fractionated coconut oil, and massage on location.

⊕: **Body System(s) Affected:** Muscles, Skeletal System, and Skin.

Forgetfulness

See Memory

Free Radicals

See Antioxidant

Frigidity

See Sexual Issues: Female Frigidity

Fungus

See Antifungal

Gallbladder

The gallbladder is a small sac that stores extra bile from the liver until it is needed to help with digestion in the small intestine. The gallbladder is located just below the liver.

Oils: ⊘geranium, ⊘rosemary, ⊘lavender, ⊘juniper berry

—**Infection:**

Oils: ⊘helichrysum

—**Stones:**

Gallstones are formed by cholesterol that has crystallized from the bile stored in the gallbladder. These stones can sometimes block the duct that comes from the gallbladder or the small opening from the common hepatic duct that allows bile to flow into the small intestine. Gallstones blocking these ducts can be painful and can lead to more serious complications, such as infections or jaundice.

Simple Solutions—Gallstones: Apply 1 drop each of grapefruit and geranium over the gallbladder area. Hold a washcloth moistened with warm water over the area for 15 minutes.

Oils: ⊘grapefruit, ⊘geranium, ⊘rosemary, ⊘juniper berry, ⊘wintergreen, ⊘lime

⊖: Dilute as recommended, and apply 1–2 drops over gallbladder area. Apply as a warm compress over the gallbladder area.

A B C D E F G H I J K L M N O P Q R S T U V W X Y Z

My Usage Guide

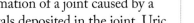: **Body System(s) Affected:** Endocrine System and Digestive System.

Gallstones

See Gallbladder: Stones

Gangrene

Gangrene is the localized decay of body tissue caused by a loss of blood to that area. Gas gangrene is caused by bacteria invading a deep wound that has lessened the blood supply or cut it off entirely. The bacteria create gases and pus in the infected area, causing severe pain and accelerating decay of the tissue.

Oils: lavender, On Guard, thyme

: Dilute as recommended, and apply 1–3 drops on location.

: **Body System(s) Affected:** Skin and Immune System.

Gas

See Digestive System: Gas/Flatulence

Gastritis

See Digestive System: Gastritis

Genitals

See Female-Specific Conditions, Male Specific Conditions/Issues

Germs

See Antibacterial, Antifungal, Antiviral

Gingivitis

See Oral Conditions: Gum Disease

Goiter

See Thyroid: Hyperthyroidism

Gout

Gout is a painful inflammation of a joint caused by a buildup of uric acid crystals deposited in the joint. Uric acid is formed during the natural breakdown of dead tissues in the body. An excess of uric acid in the bloodstream can lead to the formation of crystals in the joints or kidneys (kidney stones). Some good ways to prevent the formation of uric acid crystals include maintaining a healthy body weight (which leaves less body tissue to be broken down), exercising, and drinking plenty of water.

> *Simple Solutions—Gout:* Apply 1 drop Deep Blue on joint to help soothe pain.

Oils: lemon, geranium, Deep Blue, wintergreen, thyme

: Place 1–2 drops in 1 cup (250 ml) of water, and drink. Place 1–2 drops of oil under the tongue or place 1–2 drops in an empty capsule, and swallow.

: Dilute as recommended, and apply on location. Add 1–2 drops to 1 Tbs. (15 ml) fractionated coconut oil, and massage on location.

: **Body System(s) Affected:** Immune System.

Grave's Disease

See Thyroid: Hyperthyroidism

Grave's disease is an autoimmune disease caused by an abnormally shaped protein stimulating the thyroid to make and secrete more hormones. This can cause an enlargement of the thyroid (goiter), bulging eyes, increased heart rate, high blood pressure, and anxiety.

Oils: lemongrass, myrrh

Other Products: Microplex VMz for nutrients and minerals to help support thyroid function.

: Dilute as recommended, and apply on thyroid area or on reflex points on the feet.

: Diffuse into the air.

: Take capsules as directed on package.

: **Body System(s) Affected:** Endocrine System.

Grief/Sorrow

> *Simple Solutions—Grief:* Diffuse citrus oils in an aromatherapy diffuser.

Oils: Cheer, Console, lemon, Elevation, Balance, Steady, Forgive, lav-

See the Quick Usage Chart inside the back cover for recommended dilutions.

ender, ⊘☻bergamot⊕, ⊘☻clary sage, ⊘☻juniper berry, ⊘☻eucalyptus, ⊘☻helichrysum

⊘: Diffuse into the air. Inhale directly from bottle. Apply oil to hands, tissue, or cotton wick, and inhale. Wear 1–2 drops as perfume or cologne.

☻: Dilute as recommended, and apply 1–2 drops to the forehead, shoulders, or feet. Add 1–2 drops to 1 Tbs. (15 ml) fractionated coconut oil, and massage over whole body.

⊕: Body System(s) Affected: Emotional Balance.

🔲: Additional Research:

Lemon: Lemon odor was found to enhance the positive mood of volunteers exposed to a stressor (Kiecolt-Glaser et al., 2008).

Lemon: Lemon oil vapor was found to have strong antistress and antidepressant effects on mice subjected to several common stress tests (Komiya et al., 2006).

Lemon: Lemon oil and its component, citral, were found to decrease depressed behavior in a similar manner to antidepressant drugs in rats involved in several stress tests (Komori et al., 1995).

Lemon: In 12 patients suffering from depression, it was found that inhaling citrus aromas reduced the needed doses of antidepressants, normalized neuroendocrine hormone levels, and normalized immune function (Komori et al., 1995).

Bergamot: Lemon oil and its component, citral (also found in Bergamot), were found to decrease depressed behavior in a similar manner to antidepressant drugs in rats involved in several stress tests (Komori et al., 1995).

Gum Disease

See Oral Conditions: Gum Disease

Gums

See Oral Conditions: Gums

Habits

See Addictions

Hair

Other Products: ☻Smoothing Conditioner, ☻Protecting Shampoo, ☻Root to Tip Serum, ☻Healthy Hold Glaze.

—Beard:

Oils: ☻rosemary, ☻lemon, ☻lavender, ☻thyme, ☻cypress

—Children:

Oils: ☻lavender

—Damaged:

Other Products: ☻Smoothing Conditioner, ☻Protecting Shampoo, ☻Root to Tip Serum

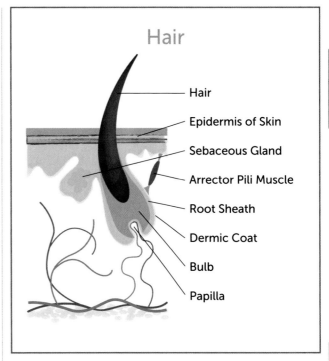

Hair

- Hair
- Epidermis of Skin
- Sebaceous Gland
- Arrector Pili Muscle
- Root Sheath
- Dermic Coat
- Bulb
- Papilla

—Dandruff: *See also Antifungal*

Dandruff is a scalp condition characterized by the excessive shedding of dead skin cells. A small amount of flaking on the scalp is normal as old skin cells die off and fall away, but dandruff results when the amount of dead skin cells becomes excessive and visible. Dandruff can be caused by many possible factors: hormonal imbalance, poor hygiene, allergies, excessive use of hair sprays and gels, excessive use of curling irons, cold weather, infrequent shampooing, etc. Many specialists believe that dandruff is caused by a tiny fungus called *Pityrosporum ovale*.

Simple Solutions—Dandruff: Combine 3 drops wintergreen with 1 tsp. (5 ml) jojoba oil, and apply to scalp in shower before washing hair.

Oils: ☻lavender, ☻wintergreen, ☻cypress, ☻rosemary, ☻cedarwood, ☻thyme, ☻manuka

—Dry:

Oils: ☻geranium, ☻sandalwood, ☻lavender, ☻rosemary, ☻wintergreen

Other Products: ☻Smoothing Conditioner, ☻Protecting Shampoo, ☻Root to Tip Serum

—Estrogen Balance:

Estrogen is a steroid hormone that causes the development of female characteristics such as breasts and larger hips, helps with calcium uptake and balance, and plays many other important roles. Estrogen also helps hair to grow faster and to stay on the head longer. If estrogen levels fall, hair loss can quickly result.

Oils: ⊘clary sage

—Fragile Hair:

Oils: ⊘clary sage, ⊘lavender, ⊘thyme, ⊘sandalwood, ⊘wintergreen, ⊘Roman chamomile

Other Products: ⊘Smoothing Conditioner, ⊘Protecting Shampoo, ⊘Root to Tip Serum

—Greasy/Oily Hair:

Oils: ⊘basil, ⊘cypress, ⊘thyme, ⊘lemon, ⊘rosemary, ⊘petitgrain

Other Products: ⊘Smoothing Conditioner, ⊘Protecting Shampoo

—Growth (stimulate):

Oils: ⊘thyme⊕, ⊘lavender⊕, ⊘rosemary⊕, ⊘ylang ylang, ⊘cedarwood, ⊘clary sage, ⊘geranium, ⊘ginger, ⊘lemon, ⊘grapefruit

—Itching:

Oils: ⊘peppermint, ⊘lavender

—Loss:

One common form of hair loss, especially in males, is androgenic alopecia (also known as male-pattern baldness in males). This condition is thought to be caused by a genetically predisposed sensitivity within the hair follicles to androgen hormones that causes them to shrink when exposed to this hormone. This shrinking of the hair follicles inhibits their ability to produce hair, leading to a receding hairline and partial baldness on the top and sides of the head in males and thinning hair in females. Another common form of baldness, especially in females, is alopecia areata, which is a condition in which hair loss occurs on all or part of the body. The most common form of alopecia areata involves the loss of round patches of hair on the scalp, leading this condition to be commonly referred to as "spot baldness."

Oils: ⊘rosemary⊕, ⊘lavender⊕, ⊘thyme⊕, ⊘ylang ylang, ⊘cedarwood⊕, ⊘wintergreen, ⊘lemon, ⊘clary sage, ⊘cypress, ⊘Roman chamomile

⊜: Apply 1–2 drops of oil to hands, and massage into hair and scalp before bath or shower; then shampoo and rinse hair as normal. Add 1–2 drops of oil to 2 Tbs. (25 ml) unscented shampoo or shower gel, and use to shampoo hair. Use shampoo and conditioner as directed on bottles.

⊕: **Body System(s) Affected:** Hair.

⊡: **Additional Research:**

Thyme, Lavender, Rosemary, Cedarwood: Patients with alopecia areata (hair loss) that massaged carrier oils containing a blend of thyme, rosemary, lavender, and cedarwood oils into their scalps were more likely to show improvement when compared to a control group that massaged carrier oils alone into their scalps (Hay et al., 1998).

Halitosis

See Oral Conditions: Halitosis

Hands

Oils: ⊘geranium, ⊘lemon, ⊘lemongrass, ⊘sandalwood, ⊘rosemary, ⊘eucalyptus

—Dry:

Oils: ⊘geranium, ⊘sandalwood

—Neglected:

Oils: ⊘geranium, ⊘lemon

—Tingling In:

Oils: ⊘lemongrass

⊜: Dilute as recommended, and apply 1–2 drops to hands. Dilute 1–2 drops in 1 Tbs. (15 ml) almond or olive oil, and use as massage oil to massage into hands.

⊕: **Body System(s) Affected:** Skin and Muscles.

Hangovers

A hangover is a set of unpleasant physical effects that comes after heavy alcohol consumption. Common symptoms of a hangover include nausea, headache, lack of energy, diarrhea, and increased sensitivity to light and noise.

> *Simple Solutions—Hangover:* Add 5 drops grapefruit, 2 drops rosemary, and 1 drop juniper berry to 1 cup (250 g) Epsom salt. Dissolve ½ cup (125 g) of the salt in warm bathwater for a soothing bath.

See the *Quick Usage Chart* inside the back cover for recommended dilutions.

Oils: ⊘⊘lemon, ⊘⊘grapefruit, ⊘⊘lavender, ⊘⊘rosemary, ⊘⊘sandalwood

◐: Add 3–4 drops to warm bathwater, and bathe. Dilute as recommended, and apply 1–2 drops to back of neck or over liver. Add 1–2 drops to 1 Tbs. (15 ml) fractionated coconut oil, and massage onto back and neck.

◐: Inhale directly from bottle. Apply oil to hands, tissue, or cotton wick, and inhale. Drop 1–2 drops in bowl of hot water, and inhale vapors. Diffuse into the air.

◐: **Body System(s) Affected:** Digestive System.

Hashimoto's Disease

See also Thyroid: Hypothyroidism

Hashimoto's disease is an autoimmune disorder where the immune system attacks the thyroid, causing it to swell up and become irritated. Hashimoto's disease does not have a unique set of symptoms, but possible symptoms include abnormal fatigue, weight gain, muscle pain and stiffness, a hoarse voice, prolonged menstrual bleeding, constipation, a feeling of tightness in the throat, sensitivity to cold, dry skin, and depression.

Oils: ⊘⊘lemongrass, ⊘⊘myrrh

Other Products: ⊙Microplex VMz, ⊙Alpha CRS+, ⊙a2z Chewable to help provide nutrients essential for thyroid cell health.

◐: Dilute as recommended, and apply 1–2 drops over thyroid area or on reflex points on the feet.

◐: Diffuse into the air. Inhale oil applied to hands.

◐: Take capsules as directed on package.

◐: **Body System(s) Affected:** Immune System and Endocrine System.

Hay Fever

See Allergies: Hay Fever

Head Lice

See Insects/Bugs: Lice

Headaches

> *Simple Solutions—Headache:* Apply 1 drop each of lavender, peppermint, and frankincense to the back of the neck and forehead.

Oils: ⊘⊘PastTense, ⊘⊘peppermint⊕, ⊘⊘rosemary, ⊘⊘Deep Blue, ⊘Rescuer, ⊘⊘cardamom, ⊘⊘eucalyptus, ⊘⊘frankincense, ⊘⊘lavender⊕, ⊘⊘patchouli, ⊘⊘basil, ⊘⊘marjoram, ⊘neroli, ⊘⊘clove

—Migraine Headache:

A migraine is a severe and painful type of headache. Symptoms of migraines include throbbing pain accompanied by nausea, vomiting, and heightened sensitivity to light. Women are much more likely than men to suffer from migraines. Migraines can be triggered by stress, anxiety, sleep or food deprivation, bright lights, loud noises, and hormonal changes.

Oils: ⊘⊘PastTense, ⊘Rescuer, ⊘⊘peppermint, ⊘⊘basil, ⊘⊘Deep Blue, ⊘⊘wintergreen, ⊘⊘spikenard, ⊘ylang ylang

—Tension Headache:

Tension headaches (also called "stress headaches") are the most common type of headache. Tension headaches are characterized by dull, constant pressure or pain (usually on both sides of the head). Tension headaches can last from 30 minutes to several days and tend to come back when a person is under stress.

Oils: ⊘⊘PastTense, ⊘Rescuer, ⊘⊘peppermint, ⊘⊘Deep Blue

—Sugar Headache (caused by low blood sugar):

Oils: ⊘⊘On Guard

◐: Dilute as recommended, and apply 1–2 drops to temples, back of neck, and forehead.

◐: Diffuse into the air. Inhale directly from bottle. Apply oil to hands, tissue, or cotton wick, and inhale.

◐: **Body System(s) Affected:** Nervous System.

◐: **Additional Research:**

Peppermint: A combination of peppermint oil and ethanol was found to have a significant analgesic effect with a reduction in sensitivity to headache, while a combination of peppermint, eucalyptus, and ethanol was found to relax muscles and to increase cognitive performance in humans (Göbel et al., 1994).

Lavender: Inhalation of lavender essential oil was found to be more effective than inhalation of a placebo for reducing the severity of headaches in subjects diagnosed with migraine headaches (Sasannejad et al., 2012).

A B C D E F G **H** I J K L M N O P Q R S T U V W X Y Z

Hearing

See Ears

Heart

See Cardiovascular System: Heart

Heartburn

See Digestive System: Heartburn

Heatstroke

Heatstroke is when the body's temperature rises dangerously high due to the body's inability to dissipate heat, typically because of high environmental temperatures and high levels of exertion. If not corrected, the body can overheat too much, causing organs and body systems to become damaged and possibly shut down—possibly leading to death. Symptoms of heatstroke include perspiration, dizziness, confusion, headaches, and nausea.

> *Simple Solutions—Heatstroke:* Get to cooler location, and remove any excess clothing. Add 2 drops peppermint to cool water in a bowl, and use to sponge down body. Seek medical attention as soon as possible.

Oils: peppermint, lavender

: Dilute as recommended, and apply 3–5 drops on neck and forehead. Cool the body as soon as possible in a cool bathtub, lake, river, or soaked linens.

Body System(s) Affected: Nervous System.

Hematoma

See also Blood: Hemorrhaging.

A hematoma is a collection of blood outside of the blood vessels. The most common form of a hematoma is a bruise. Hematomas can also form into hard, blood-filled sacs that look like welts and can move to different locations. These often dissolve on their own. Hematomas can also form in other organs as the result of injury or hemorrhaging.

> *Simple Solutions—Hematoma:* Apply 1 drop helichrysum on location, and then hold a cloth soaked in cool water on top and hold in place for 15 minutes.

Oils: helichrysum

: Dilute as recommended, and apply 1–2 drops on location.

Body System(s) Affected: Cardiovascular System.

Hemorrhaging

See Blood: Hemorrhaging

Hemorrhoids

Hemorrhoids are swollen, twisted veins that occur in the rectum or anus. They are caused by increased pressure within the veins, often due to pregnancy, frequent lifting, or constipation.

> *Simple Solutions—Hemorrhoids:* Mix 1 drop cypress with 1 drop of either helichrysum or geranium, and apply on location.

Oils: cypress, geranium, clary sage, helichrysum, patchouli, copaiba, peppermint, sandalwood, juniper berry, frankincense, myrrh

: Dilute as recommended, and apply 1–2 drops on location. Mix 1–2 drops with 1 tsp. (5 ml) fractionated coconut oil, and apply on location using a rectal syringe.

Body System(s) Affected: Cardiovascular System.

Hepatitis

See Liver: Hepatitis

Hernia

See also Back: Herniated Discs

A hernia is the protrusion of a tissue or organ through tissue or muscle outside of the body cavity in which it is normally contained. There are several different types of hernias, and the symptoms vary with each type.

—Hiatal:

A hiatal (hiatus) hernia is when a portion of the stomach protrudes through the diaphragm into the chest cavity above. This can cause pain, acid reflux, and heartburn. It can be caused by a birth defect or may be brought on by heavy lifting, stress, or being overweight.

See the *Quick Usage Chart* inside the back cover for recommended dilutions.

308

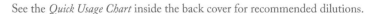

Oils: 🌿basil, 🌿peppermint, 🌿cypress, 🌿ginger, 🌿geranium, 🌿lavender, 🌿fennel, 🌿rosemary

—Incisional:

An incisional hernia is caused by a protrusion through scar tissue from an abdominal wound or incision that hasn't healed correctly.

Oils: 🌿basil, 🌿helichrysum, 🌿lemongrass, 🌿geranium, 🌿lavender, 🌿ginger, 🌿lemon, 🌿melaleuca

—Inguinal:

An inguinal hernia is when the intestines protrude into the inguinal canal (a small opening that leads from the abdominal cavity into the groin area). This can sometimes be seen as a bulge in the groin area and is usually painless, but it may become painful if the blood supply to the herniated portion of the intestine is restricted (strangulated).

Oils: 🌿lemongrass, 🌿lavender

🖐: Dilute as recommended, and apply on location, lower back, and reflex points on the feet.

➕: **Body System(s) Affected:** Muscles.

Herpes Simplex

*See also **Antiviral***

Herpes simplex type 1 and type 2 viruses are the two viruses that cause genital and oral herpes infections. These viruses cause painful outbreaks of blisters and sores to occur in the affected area when the virus is active in the skin or mucus membranes, followed by periods of latency when the virus resides in the nerve cells around the infected area.

> *Simple Solutions—Cold Sores:* Combine 4 tsp. (5 g) beeswax pellets, 1 Tbs. (10 g) cocoa butter, and 3 Tbs. (45 ml) jojoba oil, and melt in the microwave (30 seconds at a time, stirring in between) or in a double boiler. Cool slightly, and add 5 drops melissa, 5 drops peppermint, and 5 drops helichrysum essential oil. Pour into small jars or lip balm containers, and allow to cool completely. Apply a small amount of balm on cold sores as needed.

Oils: 🌿peppermint□, 🌿melaleuca□, 🌿helichrysum□, 🌿clove□, 🌿lavender, 🌿eucalyptus□, 🌿lemon, 🌿cypress, 🌿rose, 🌿bergamot

🖐: Dilute as recommended, and apply oil directly on the lesions at the first sign of outbreak.

➕: **Body System(s) Affected:** Immune System.

▭: **Additional Research:**

Peppermint: Peppermint oil demonstrated a direct virucidal activity against herpes type 1 and type 2 viruses (Schuhmacher et al., 2003).

Melaleuca: Tea tree and eucalyptus oil demonstrated ability to inhibit Herpes simplex virus (Schnitzler et al., 2001).

Helichrysum: Helichrysum was found to have significant antiviral activity against the herpes virus at non-cytotoxic concentrations (Nostro et al., 2003).

Clove: Eugenol was found to be virucidal to Herpes simplex and to delay the development of herpes-induced keratitis (inflammation of the cornea) in mice (Benencia et al., 2000).

Eucalyptus: Tea tree and eucalyptus oil demonstrated ability to inhibit Herpes simplex virus (Schnitzler et al., 2001).

Hiccups/Hiccoughs

Hiccups, or hiccoughs, are the uncontrollable spasms of the diaphragm that cause a sudden intake of breath and the closure of the glottis (the opening that stops substances from entering the trachea while swallowing). Hiccups are thought to be caused either by a lack of carbon dioxide in the blood or by something irritating the diaphragm.

> *Simple Solutions—Hiccups:* Apply 1 drop sandalwood over the diaphragm (the bottom edge of the rib cage).

Oils: 🌀🖐sandalwood

🌀: Diffuse into the air. Inhale directly from bottle. Apply oil to hands, tissue, or cotton wick, and inhale.

🖐: Dilute as recommended, and apply 1–2 drops to the diaphragm area or reflex points on the feet.

➕: **Body System(s) Affected:** Respiratory System.

High Blood Pressure

*See **Blood: Blood Pressure: High***

Hives

*See also **Allergies, Antiviral***

Hives are itchy patches of inflamed spots on the skin surrounded by redness, typically caused by an allergic reaction or a viral infection.

> *Simple Solutions—Hives:* Mix 3 drops lavender and 2 drops melaleuca with 1 tsp. (5 ml) jojoba oil in a small roll-on bottle, and apply on location.

Oils: 🌿melaleuca□, 🌿peppermint, 🌿lavender□

⬭: Dilute as recommended, and apply 1–2 drops on location. Add 1–2 drops to 1 Tbs. (15 ml) fractionated coconut oil, and massage on location.

⊕: **Body System(s) Affected:** Immune System and Skin.

⊡: **Additional Research:**

Melaleuca: Tea tree oil applied to histamine-induced weal and flare in human volunteers was found to decrease the mean weal volume when compared to a control (Koh et al., 2002).

Melaleuca: Tea tree oil applied to histamine-induced edema (swelling) in mice ears was found to significantly reduce swelling (Brand et al., 2002).

Lavender: Lavender oil was found to inhibit immediate-type allergic reactions in mice and rats by inhibiting mast cell degranulation (Kim et al., 1999).

Hodgkin's Disease

See also **Cancer**

Hodgkin's disease (or Hodgkin's lymphoma) is a type of cancer that affects lymphocytes (white blood cells). It can cause enlarged lymph nodes, fever, sweating, fatigue, and weight loss.

Oils: ⬭clove

⬭: Dilute as recommended, and apply 1–2 drops to the liver, kidney, and reflex points on the feet.

⊕: **Body System(s) Affected:** Immune System.

Hormonal System/Imbalance

See **Endocrine System**

Hot Flashes

See **Female-Specific Conditions**

Housecleaning

—**Bathrooms/Kitchens:**

Oils: ⬭lemon, ⬭fir (for cleaning and disinfecting), ⬭litsea, ⬭pink pepper

Other Products: ⬭On Guard Cleaner Concentrate to help eliminate microorganisms from household surfaces.

⬭: Place a few drops on your cleaning rag or dust cloth; or place 10 drops in a small spray bottle with distilled water, and mist on surfaces before cleaning.

—**Carpets:**

Oils: ⬭lemon, ⬭Purify

⬭: Apply on carpet stains to help remove. To freshen carpet, add 50–70 drops of these (or another favorite oil) to ½ cup (100 g) baking soda. Sprinkle over carpets, wait 15 minutes, and then vacuum.

—**Dishes:**

Oils: ⬭lemon

Other Products: ⬭On Guard Cleaner Concentrate to help purify dishes.

⬭: Add a couple of drops to dishwater for sparkling dishes and a great smelling kitchen. Can add to dishwasher as well.

—**Furniture Polish:**

Oils: ⬭lemon, ⬭fir, ⬭hinoki, ⬭Citrus Bliss, ⬭Purify

⬭: Place a few drops on a clean rag, and use to polish furniture.

—**Gum/Grease:**

Oils: ⬭lemon, ⬭lime

⬭: Place 1–2 drops on gum or grease to help dissolve.

—**Laundry:**

Oils: ⬭lemon, ⬭Purify

Other Products: ⬭On Guard Laundry Detergent to help naturally fight stains and brighten clothes.

⬭: Add a few drops of oil to the water in the washer. Add a few drops on a washcloth with clothes in the dryer. Add a few drops to a small spray bottle of water, and mist on laundry in the dryer before drying. Any of these methods can increase the antibacterial benefits and help clothes to smell fresh and clean.

—**Mold/Fungus:** *See also* **Antifungal: Mold**

Oils: ⬭⬭On Guard, ⬭Purify

⬭: Diffuse into the air.

⬭: Place a few drops on a cleaning rag, and wipe down the affected area.

—**Stains:**

Oils: ⬭lemon (has been used to remove black shoe polish from carpets)

⬭: Apply on location.

Hyperactivity

See **Calming: Hyperactivity**

See the Quick Usage Chart inside the back cover for recommended dilutions.

Hyperpnea

See Respiratory System: Hyperpnea

Hypertension

See Blood: Blood Pressure: High

Hypoglycemia

Hypoglycemia is a condition of low levels of sugar in the blood. It is most common in people with diabetes but can be caused by drugs or by a tumor in the pancreas that causes the pancreas to create too much insulin. Symptoms of hypoglycemia can include hunger, sweating, weakness, palpitations, shaking, dizziness, and confusion.

Oils: ⊘eucalyptus, ⊘On Guard, ⊘cinnamon, ⊘clove, ⊘thyme

Other Products: ⬤PB Assist+ to help maintain a healthy digestive system.

⊜: Dilute as recommended and apply 1–2 drops over pancreas and on reflex points on the feet.

⬤: Take capsules as directed on package.

⊕: **Body System(s) Affected:** Endocrine System.

Hysteria

See Calming

Immune System

See also Allergies, Antibacterial, Antifungal, Antiviral, Cancer, Lymphatic System, Parasites

The immune system is the body's defense against disease. The immune system protects the body by identifying and killing bacteria, viruses, parasites, other microorganisms, and tumor cells that would harm the body. The immune system is comprised of several different types of white blood cells (lymphocytes) that recognize, process, or destroy foreign objects, the bone marrow that creates several types of white blood cells, the thymus that creates white blood cells and teaches them to recognize foreign objects and distinguish them from the body's cells, lymphatic vessels that help transport lymph and white blood cells, and several other organs, such as the lymph nodes, tonsils, spleen, and appendix, that filter out foreign objects and serve

as a place for white blood cells to gather, interact, and share information about infections.

Oils: ⊘⊕⬤On Guard, ⊘⊕⬤oregano⊕, ⊘⊕melaleuca, ⊘⊕rosemary, ⊘⊕clove, ⊘⊕frankincense, ⊘⊕geranium, ⊘⊕lemon, ⊘⊕thyme, ⊘⊕lavender, ⊘⊕lime

Other Products: ⬤On Guard+ Softgels, ⬤Mito2Max, ⬤Alpha CRS+, ⬤a2z Chewable, ⬤xEO Mega or vEO Mega, ⬤IQ Mega, ⬤Microplex VMz to provide nutrients essential for healthy immune system function.

—Stimulates:

Oils: ⊘⊕⬤oregano⊕, ⊘cinnamon, ⊘⊕frankincense, ⊘⊕melaleuca, ⊘On Guard, ⊘⊕lavender

⊜: Dilute as recommended, and apply 1–2 drops to bottoms of feet, along spine, or under arms (around lymph nodes). Add 1–2 drops to 1 Tbs. (15 ml) fractionated coconut oil, and massage onto back, arms, and feet.

⬤: Take capsules as recommended. Place 1–2 drops of oil under the tongue or place 2–3 drops in an empty capsule, and swallow.

⊘: Diffuse into the air.

⊕: **Body System(s) Affected:** Immune System.

⊞: **Additional Research:**

Oregano: Growth-retarded pigs receiving a supplementation of oregano leaves and flowers enriched with cold-pressed oregano oil were found to have increased growth, decreased mortality, and higher numbers of immune-system cells and compounds when compared to control pigs who did not receive supplementation (Walter et al., 2004).

Impetigo

See Skin: Impetigo

Impotence

See Male Specific Conditions: Impotence

Incontinence

See Bladder: Bed Wetting and Incontinence

Indigestion

See Digestive System: Indigestion

Immune/Lymphatic System

The immune system is the body's defense against disease. The immune system protects the body by identifying and killing bacteria, viruses, parasites, other microorganisms, and tumor cells that would harm the body. The immune system is comprised of several different types of white blood cells (lymphocytes) that recognize, process, or destroy foreign objects, the bone marrow that creates several types of white blood cells, the thymus that creates white blood cells and teaches them to recognize foreign objects and distinguish them from the body's cells, lymphatic vessels that help transport lymph and white blood cells, and several other organs, such as the lymph nodes, tonsils, spleen, and appendix, that filter out foreign objects and serve as a place for white blood cells to gather, interact, and share information about infections.

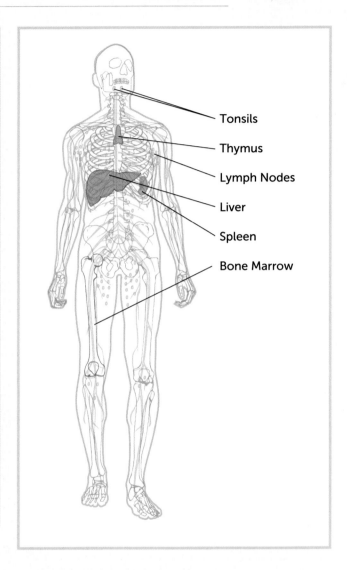

- Tonsils
- Thymus
- Lymph Nodes
- Liver
- Spleen
- Bone Marrow

Oils for Immune/Lymphatic Support

Oils: On Guard, oregano, melaleuca, rosemary, clove, frankincense, cypress, sandalwood, geranium, lemon, DigestZen, thyme, lavender, lime

Common Immune/Lymphatic Issues

Immune: Allergies, AIDS, Grave's Disease, Hashimoto's Disease, Hodgkin's Lymphoma, HIV, Leukemia, Lupus, Type I Diabetes

Lymphatic: Adenitis (Lymphatic), Lymphedema

Infection

See also Antibacterial, Antifungal, Antiviral

Oils: cinnamon, clary sage, On Guard, bergamot, myrrh (with oregano), Douglas fir (skin), basil, cypress, rosemary (with myrrh for oral infection), thyme (for urinary infection), lemongrass, lime, patchouli, lavender, oregano, juniper berry, fennel, peppermint

Other Products: On Guard+ Softgels. Microplex VMz for nutrients that help provide immune support.

—Infected Wounds:

Oils: frankincense, melaleuca, Douglas fir

Blend 1: Apply 1 drop thyme on location with hot compress daily. After infection and pus have been expelled, mix 3 drops lavender, 2 drops melaleuca, and 2 drops thyme combined with 1 tsp. (5 ml) fractionated coconut oil, and apply a little of this mixture on location twice daily.

: Dilute as recommended, and apply 1–2 drops on location. Mix 1–2 drops with 1 Tbs. (15 ml) fractionated coconut oil, and massage on location or on neck, arms, chest, or feet.

: Diffuse into the air. Add 1–2 drops to a bowl of hot water, and inhale the vapors.

: Take capsules as directed on package.

: **Body System(s) Affected:** Immune System.

Infertility

See Female-Specific Conditions: Infertility, Male Specific Conditions: Infertility

Inflammation

See also Antioxidant

Inflammation is the body's reaction to infection and injury. It is characterized by redness, swelling, warmth, and pain. Inflammation is an immune system response that allows the body to contain and fight infection or repair damaged tissue by dilating the blood vessels and allowing vascular permeability to increase blood supply to an injured or infected tissue. While a certain amount of inflammation can be beneficial in fighting disease and healing injuries, too much inflammation or chronic inflammation can actually be debilitating.

> *Simple Solutions—Inflammation from Injury:*
> Mix 3 drops frankincense and 2 drops lavender in a bowl of cold water. Dampen a washcloth with the water, and hold on location for 15–30 minutes.

Oils: frankincense, melaleuca, eucalyptus, oregano, Deep Blue, Rescuer, lavender, cardamom, patchouli, Roman chamomile, myrrh, rosemary, peppermint, wintergreen, clove, thyme, geranium, helichrysum, copaiba, Immortelle, juniper berry, cedarwood, Serenity, lemongrass, cypress

Other products: Alpha CRS+ and Microplex VMz or a2z Chewable for polyphenols and other antioxidants to help relieve oxidative stress associated with inflammation. xEO Mega or vEO Mega or IQ Mega for omega-3 fatty acids that help balance the inflammatory response.

: Dilute as recommended, and apply 1–2 drops on location and on the back of neck by the base of the skull. Add 3–4 drops to 1 Tbs. (15 ml) fractionated coconut oil, and massage on location.

: Place 1–2 drops of oil under the tongue, or place 2–3 drops of oil in an empty capsule, and swallow. Place 1–2 drops in 1 cup (250 ml) of rice or almond milk, and drink. Take supplements as directed on package.

: Diffuse into the air. Add 1–2 drops to a bowl of hot water or humidifier, and inhale the vapors to help relieve inflammation within the respiratory system.

: **Body System(s) Affected:** Immune System.

: **Additional Research:**

Frankincense: Alpha-pinene was found to block proinflammatory responses in THP-1 cells (Zhou et al., 2004).

Frankincense: *Boswellia frereana* extracts were found to inhibit proinflammatory molecules involved in joint cartilage degradation (Blain et al., 2009).

Frankincense: Compounds from *Boswellia serrata* were found to carry out anti-inflammatory activity by switching off the pro-inflammatory cytokines and mediators that initiate the inflammatory process (Gayathri et al., 2007).

Frankincense: An acetone extract of frankincense was found to decrease arthritic scores, reduce paw edema (swelling), and suppress pro-inflammatory cytokines (cellular messengers) (Fan et al., 2005).

Frankincense: Incensole acetate, isolated from frankincense resin, was found to demonstrate an anti-inflammatory and neuroprotective effect in mice with closed head injuries (Moussaieff et al., 2008).

Melaleuca: Melaleuca alternifolia oil was found to mediate the reactive oxygen species (ROS) production of leukocytes (white blood cells), indicating possible anti-inflammatory activity (Caldefie-Chézet et al., 2004).

Melaleuca: Tea tree oil applied to histamine-induced edema (swelling) in mice ears was found to significantly reduce swelling (Brand et al., 2002).

Melaleuca: Tea tree oil was found to reduce swelling during a contact hypersensitivity response in the skin of mice sensitized to the chemical hapten (Brand et al., 2002).

Melaleuca: Several water-soluble components of tea tree oil were found to suppress the production of superoxide by monocytes (a type of white blood cell involved in the immune system) (Brand et al., 2001).

Melaleuca: The water soluble terpinen-4-ol component of tea tree was found to suppress the production of pro-inflammatory mediators in human monocytes (a type of white blood cell that is part of the human immune system) (Hart et al., 2000).

Melaleuca: Inhaled tea tree oil was found to have anti-inflammatory influences on male rats with induced peritoneal inflammation (Golab et al., 2007).

Melaleuca: Tea tree oil applied to histamine-induced weal and flare in human volunteers was found to decrease the mean weal volume when compared to a control (Koh et al., 2002).

Melaleuca: Tea tree oil was found to reduce inflammation in nickel-sensitive human skin exposed to nickel (Pearce et al., 2005).

Eucalyptus: Eucalyptus oil was shown to ameliorate inflammatory processes by interacting with oxygen radicals and interfering with leukocyte activation (Grassmann et al., 2000).

Eucalyptus: 1,8 cineole (eucalyptol) was found to display an anti-inflammatory effect on rats in several tests and was found to exhibit antinociceptive (pain-reducing) effects in mice, possibly by depressing the central nervous system (Santos et al., 2000).

Eucalyptus: Eucalyptus oil was found to have an anti-inflammatory and mucin-inhibitory effect in rats with lipopolysaccharide-induced bronchitis (Lu et al., 2004).

Eucalyptus: Oils of three eucalyptus species (*citriodora, tereticornis*, and *globulus*) were found to have analgesic (pain-relieving) and anti-inflammatory properties in rats (Silva et al., 2003).

Eucalyptus: Extracts from eucalyptus and thyme were found to have high nitrous oxide (NO) scavenging abilities and to inhibit NO production in macrophage cells. This could possibly explain their role in aiding respiratory inflammatory diseases (Vigo et al., 2004).

Lavender: Oil from *Lavandula angustifolia* was found to reduce writhing in induced writhing in rats and to reduce edema (swelling) in carrageenan-induced paw edema, indicating an anti-inflammatory effect (Hajhashemi et al., 2003).

Lavender: Linalool and linalyl acetate (from lavender and other essential oils) were found to exhibit anti-inflammatory activity in rats subjected to carrageenin-induced edema (inflammation) (Peana et al., 2002).

Cardamom: Cardamom essential oil reduced rat paw edema by 76% of the control value, illustrating significant anti-inflammatory activity (al-Zuhair et al., 1996).

Roman Chamomile: Chamazulene, a chemical in chamomile oil, was found to block formation of leukotriene (a signaling chemical involved in the inflammation process) in neutrophilic (immune system) granulocytes (white blood cells containing granules). It also demonstrated an antioxidant effect (Safayhi et al., 1994).

Myrrh: At subtoxic levels, myrrh oil was found to reduce interleukin (chemical signals believed to play a role in the inflammation response) by fibroblast cells in the gums (Tipton et al., 2003).

Myrrh: Subtoxic levels of myrrh oil were found to inhibit interleukin (chemical messenger involved in inflammation), in part by inhibiting PGE(2) (Prostaglandin E, a lipid compound that has several messenger functions in the body, including in the inflammatory response) (Tipton et al., 2006).

Rosemary: An ethanol extract of rosemary was found to have an antiproliferative effect on human leukemia and breast carcinoma cells as well as an antioxidant effect (Cheung et al., 2007).

Rosemary: An ethanol extract of rosemary was found to demonstrate antinociceptive (pain blocking) and anti-inflammatory activity in mice and rats (González-Trujano et al., 2007).

Rosemary: Rosemary oil was found to have anti-inflammatory and peripheral-antinociceptive (pain sensitivity blocking) properties in mice (Takaki et al., 2008).

Peppermint: A combination of peppermint and caraway oil was found to reduce visceral hyperalgesia (pain hypersensitivity in the gastrointestinal tract) after induced inflammation in rats (Adam et al., 2006).

Peppermint: L-menthol was found to inhibit production of inflammation mediators in human monocytes (a type of white blood cell involved in the immune response) (Juergens et al., 1998).

Wintergreen: Methyl salicylate (found in wintergreen or birch oils) was found to inhibit leukotriene C4 (a chemical messenger involved in inflammatory response), while also demonstrating a gastroprotective effect against ethanol-induced gastric injury in rats (Trautmann et al., 1991).

Clove: Eugenol (found in clove EO) was found to increase the anti-inflammatory activity of cod liver oil (lowered inflammation by 30%) (Reddy et al., 1994).

Clove: Clove oil was found to increase humoral immunity and decrease cell-mediated immunity in rats, illustrating that clove oil can modulate the immune response and overall acts as an anti-inflammatory agent (Halder et al., 2011).

Thyme: Extracts from eucalyptus and thyme were found to have high nitrous oxide (NO) scavenging abilities and to inhibit NO production in macrophage cells. This could possibly explain their role in aiding respiratory inflammatory diseases (Vigo et al., 2004).

Geranium: Topical application of geranium oil was found to reduce the inflammatory response of neutrophil (white blood cell) accumulation in mice (Maruyama et al., 2005).

Helichrysum: Arzanol, extracted from helichrysum, inhibited HIV-1 replication in T cells and also inhibited the release of pro-inflammatory cytokines (chemical messengers) in monocytes (Appendino et al., 2007).

Cedarwood: *Juniperus virginiana* oil was found to have anti-inflammatory activity in mice (Tumen et al., 2013).

Dill: Oil-based dill extract displayed greater anti-inflammatory activity when topically applied to inflamed rat paws than the anti-inflammatory drug diclofenac (Naseri et al., 2012).

Influenza

See also **Antiviral**

Influenza, commonly referred to as "the flu," is a highly contagious viral infection of the respiratory system. Influenza is marked by a sudden onset of high fever, dry cough, sore throat, muscle aches and pains, headache, fatigue, loss of appetite, nausea, and nasal congestion.

> *Simple Solutions—Influenza:* Diffuse Breathe in a misting aromatherapy diffuser.

Oils: ⊘⊜Breathe, ⊘⊜melaleuca⊕, ⊘⊜◯peppermint, ⊘⊜rosemary, ⊘⊜eucalyptus, ⊘⊜Douglas fir, ⊜⊘On Guard, ⊘⊜fir (aches/pains), ⊘⊜lavender, ⊘⊜oregano, ⊘⊜thyme, ⊘orange, ⊘◯copaiba, ⊘⊜clove, ◯⊜ginger

Other Products: ◯On Guard+ Softgels. ⊜On Guard Foaming Hand Wash to help prevent the spread of influenza viruses. ◯Microplex VMz for nutrients to help support immune function.

⊘: Diffuse into the air.

⊜: Dilute as recommended, and apply to thymus area, chest, back, sinuses, or reflex points on the feet. Add 1–2 drops to hot bathwater, and bathe. Dilute 1–2

See the *Quick Usage Chart* inside the back cover for recommended dilutions.

drops in 1 Tbs. (15 ml) fractionated coconut oil, and massage on chest, back, and feet.

🌑: Place 1–2 drops of ginger or peppermint oil in an empty capsule, and swallow to help reduce feelings of nausea. Take supplements as directed on package.

⊕: **Body System(s) Affected:** Immune System and Respiratory System.

🔲: **Additional Research:**

Melaleuca: In vitro research has found that *Melaleuca alternifolia* concentrate can disturb the normal viral membrane fusion of the influenza virus and inhibit entry of influenza virus into the host cell (Li et al., 2013).

Injuries

See Skeletal System, Bruises, Cuts, Inflammation, Joints, Muscles, Pain, Skin: Scarring, Tissue: Scarring, Wounds

Insects/Bugs

See also Bites/Stings

> *Simple Solutions—Bugs:* Avoid bug bites and stings by repelling the bugs. Diffuse TerraShield, or apply TerraShield to exposed skin.

—Bees, Wasps, and Hornet Stings:

Oils: ⬙Roman chamomile, ⬙basil, ⬙Purify, ⬙Stronger, ⬙lavender, ⬙lemongrass, ⬙lemon, ⬙peppermint, ⬙thyme.

Recipe 1: Remove the stinger, and apply a cold compress of Roman chamomile to the area for several hours or as long as possible.

🔄: Dilute as recommended, and apply 1–2 drops on location after making certain that the stinger is removed.

—Gnats and Midges:

Oils: ⬙lavender, ⬙⬙TerraShield

Recipe 2: Mix 3 drops thyme in 1 tsp. (5 ml) cider vinegar or lemon juice. Apply to bites to stop irritation.

🔄: Dilute as recommended, and apply 1–2 drops to bite area.

🌀: Diffuse into the air. Place 1–2 drops on small ribbons, strings, or cloth, and hang around area to help repel mosquitoes.

—Itching:

Oils: ⬙lavender

🔄: Dilute as recommended, and apply 1–2 drops to affected area.

—Lice:

Oils: ⬙eucalyptus🔲, ⬙⬙TerraShield, ⬙rosemary, ⬙melaleuca🔲, ⬙geranium, ⬙lemon, ⬙lavender

🔄: Dilute as recommended, and rub 1–2 drops into the scalp three times a day, and apply to feet.

—Mosquitoes:

Oils: ⬙⬙TerraShield, ⬙⬙patchouli🔲, ⬙lavender, ⬙Stronger, ⬙helichrysum

🔄: Dilute as recommended, and apply 1–2 drops to feet and exposed skin. Add 3–5 drops to 1 Tbs. (15 ml) fractionated coconut oil, and apply to exposed skin. Add 2–3 drops to 2–4 Tbs. (25–50 ml) distilled water in a small spray bottle; shake well, and mist onto the skin or into small openings where bugs may come through.

🌀: Diffuse into the air. Place 1–2 drops on small ribbons, strings, or cloth, and hang around area to help repel mosquitoes.

—Repellent:

Oils: ⬙⬙TerraShield, ⬙⬙patchouli, ⬙⬙basil, ⬙⬙lavender🔲, ⬙⬙lemongrass, ⬙⬙cedarwood🔲, ⬙⬙eucalyptus, ⬙⬙arborvitae, ⬙⬙thyme, ⬙⬙Purify

Blend 1: Combine 5 drops lavender, 5 drops lemongrass, 3 drops peppermint, and 1 drop thyme. Place neat on feet. Add to 1 cup (250 ml) of water, and spray on using a fine-mist spray bottle. Or place drops of this blend on ribbons or strings and tie near windows or around picnic or camping area.

Blend 2: Combine equal parts clove, lemon, and orange, and apply 2–3 drops on skin.

Blend 3: Place 5 drops lemon and 5 drops Purify in a small spray bottle with distilled water. Shake well, and mist on your skin to help protect against insects, flies, and mosquitoes.

🔄: Dilute as recommended, and apply 1–2 drops to feet and exposed skin. Add 3–5 drops to 1 Tbs. (15 ml) fractionated coconut oil, and apply to exposed skin. Add 20–30 drops to 2–4 Tbs. (25–50 ml) distilled water in a small spray bottle; shake well, and mist onto the skin or into small openings where bugs may come through.

A B C D E F G H I J K L M N O P Q R S T U V W X Y Z

⊘: Diffuse into the air. Place 1–2 drops on small ribbons, strings, or cloth, and hang around area to help repel insects.

—Spiders:

Oils: ◎basil, ◎Purify (with melaleuca), ◎lavender, ◎lemongrass, ◎lemon, ◎peppermint, ◎thyme

⊜: Dilute as recommended, and apply 1–2 drops to affected area. Apply oil as a cold compress.

—Termites:

Oils: ◎◎patchouli⊕, ◎◎vetiver⊕ (repels), ◎◎clove⊕ (kills)

⊜: Apply oils around foundation and to soil around wood structures to help repel termites.

⊘: Diffuse into the air.

—Ticks:

Oils: ◎◎TerraShield, ◎lavender⊕, ◎◎Stronger,

Removing Ticks:

Do not apply mineral oil, Vaseline, or anything else to remove the tick as this may cause it to inject the spirochetes into the wound.

Be sure to remove the entire tick. Get as close to the mouth as possible, and firmly tug on the tick until it releases its grip. Don't twist. If available, use a magnifying glass to make sure that you have removed the entire tick.

Save the tick in a jar, and label it with the date, where you were bitten on your body, and the location or address where you were bitten for proper identification by your doctor, especially if you develop any symptoms.

Do not handle the tick.

Wash hands immediately.

Check the site of the bite occasionally to see if any rash develops. If it does, seek medical advice promptly.

⊜: After getting the tick out, apply 1 drop lavender every 5 minutes for 30 minutes.

◉: **Body System(s) Affected:** Skin.

⊕: **Additional Research:**

Melaleuca: Tea tree oil was found to be effective against both lice and dust mites in a mite chamber assay (Williamson et al., 2007).

Melaleuca: Tea tree oil was found to prevent some blood feeding by lice on treated skin; and while not highly effective at the studied dosages, tea tree oil was found to be more effective than DEET at repelling head lice (Canyon et al., 2007).

Patchouli: Clove, citronella, and patchouli oils were found to effectively repel 3 species of mosquitoes (Trongtokit et al., 2005).

Lavender: An infestation of the red bud borer pest was reduced by more than 95% in the grafted buds of apple trees by application of the essential oil of *Lavandula angustifolia* (van Tol et al., 2007).

Lavender: Lavender oil was found to be comparable to DEET in its ability to repel ticks (Hyalomma marginatum) (Mkolo et al., 2007).

Eucalyptus: Researchers found that an 8% eucalyptus oil spray was the most effective treatment (when compared against other concentrations of eucalyptus and clove oil sprays) against lice and insecticide-resistant head lice (Choi et al., 2010).

Eucalyptus: Researchers found that eucalyptus oil was an effective treatment for head lice in school-aged children (Greive et al., 2017).

Patchouli: Both patchouli oil and its constituent patchouli alcohol (patchoulol), were found to be repellent and insecticidal to Formosan termites when applied topically (Zhu et al., 2003).

Vetiver: Vetiver oil was found to repel termites and to prevent tunneling (with long-lasting effects), while clove oil was found to be highly termiticidal (Zhu et al., 2001).

Clove: Vetiver oil was found to repel termites and to prevent tunneling (with long-lasting effects), while clove oil was found to be highly termiticidal (Zhu et al., 2001).

Cedarwood: Cedarwood was found to possess highly insecticidal activity against adult mosquitoes and other household insects (Singh et al., 1984).

Cassia: Cassia oil and its components were found to repel adult female mosquitoes for about 50 minutes post-application when applied to human subjects (Chang et al., 2006).

Geranium: A sesquiterpene alcohol from geranium essential oil proved to be an effective repellant of the lone star tick (*Amblyomma americanum*) and at concentrations greater than 0.052 mg the oil was comparable to the repellant capability of DEET (Tabanca et al., 2013).

Grapefruit: Nootkatone, found in grapefruit essential oil, was found to be toxic to four tick species (Flor-Weiler et al., 2011).

Insomnia

Insomnia is difficulty falling or staying asleep. It can be triggered by stress, medications, drug or alcohol use, anxiety, or depression.

Simple Solutions—Insomnia: Add 5 drops lavender and 3 drops Roman chamomile to 2 Tbs. (25 ml) water in a small spray bottle. Spray on kids' pillows and sheets at bedtime.

Oils: ◎◎Serenity, ◎◎Calmer, ◎◎lavender⊕, ◎◎orange⊕, ◎◎Roman chamomile, ◎◎spikenard, ◎◎cypress, ◎◎ylang ylang, ◎◎Citrus Bliss, ◎◎marjoram, ◎◎petitgrain, ◎◎lemon, ◎◎rosemary, ◎◎sandalwood, ◎◎clary sage, ◎◎bergamot

Blend 1: Combine 6 drops Citrus Bliss with 6 drops lavender. Apply blend to big toes, bottoms of the feet, 2 drops around the navel, and 3 drops on the back of the neck.

Recipe 1: Combine 2 drops Roman chamomile, 6 drops geranium, 3 drops lemon, and 4 drops sandalwood. Add 6 drops of this blend to your bath at bedtime, and combine 5 drops with 2 tsp. (10 ml) fractionated coconut oil for a massage after the bath.

See the Quick Usage Chart inside the back cover for recommended dilutions.

—For Children:

–1–5 years:

Oils: ⊘⊜Calmer, ⊘lavender, ⊘Roman chamomile

–5+ years:

Oils: ⊘⊜Calmer, ⊘⊜clary sage, ⊘⊜geranium, ⊘⊜ylang ylang

⊘: Diffuse into the air. Dissolve 3 drops essential oil in 1 tsp. (5 ml) pure grain alcohol (such as vodka) or perfumer's alcohol, and combine with distilled water in a 2 oz. spray bottle; shake well, and spray into the air before sleep. Place 1–2 drops on bottom of pillow or stuffed animal.

⊜: Dilute as recommended, and apply 1–2 drops on feet and back of neck. Combine 1–2 drops essential oil with 1 Tbs. (15 ml) fractionated coconut oil, and massage onto back, legs, feet, and arms.

⊕: **Body System(s) Affected:** Nervous System.

⊕: **Additional Research:**

Lavender: Female students suffering from insomnia were found to sleep better and to have a lower level of depression during weeks they used a lavender fragrance when compared to weeks they did not use a lavender fragrance (Lee et al., 2006).

Lavender: Twenty-four sessions of lavender essential oil aromatherapy was found to improve sleep quality in midlife women with insomnia up to one week after the end of the intervention when compared to the control group (Chien et al., 2012).

Lavender: Sixty nurses with shifting sleep schedules were found to have better quality sleep after inhaling lavender essential oil (Kim et al., 2016).

Orange: Bitter orange peel oil taken orally by mice was found to reduce anxiety, increase sleeping time, and increase the time before a chemically induced seizure started (Carvalho-Freitas et al., 2002).

Intestinal Problems

See Digestive System

Invigorating

Oils: ⊘⊜wintergreen, ⊘⊜eucalyptus, ⊘⊜peppermint

⊜: Dilute as recommended, and apply 1–2 drops to back of neck or temples.

⊘: Diffuse into the air. Inhale directly from bottle. Apply oil to hands, tissue, or cotton wick, and inhale.

⊕: **Body System(s) Affected:** Emotional Balance.

Irritability

See Calming

Irritable Bowel Syndrome

See Digestive System

Itching

Itching is a tingling or irritation of the skin that produces a desire to scratch. Itching can be brought on by many factors including stress, bug bites, sunburns, allergic reactions, infections, and dry skin.

> *Simple Solutions—Itching:* Combine 10 drops lavender with 1 tsp. (5 ml) jojoba oil in a small roll-on bottle, and apply on location.

Oils: ⊜lavender, ⊜Serenity, ⊜peppermint, ⊜blue tansy

⊜: Dilute as recommended, and apply 1–2 drops on location and on ears. Add 2–3 drops to 1 Tbs. (15 ml) fractionated coconut oil, and apply a small amount on location.

⊕: **Body System(s) Affected:** Skin.

Jaundice

Jaundice is a condition characterized by a yellow appearance of the skin and the whites of the eyes. Jaundice is a result of excessive levels in the blood of a chemical called bilirubin. Bilirubin is a pigment that is made when hemoglobin from old or dead red blood cells is broken down. Jaundice occurs when the liver is unable to pass bilirubin from the body as fast as it is being produced. Jaundice is often a symptom of other diseases or conditions.

Oils: ⊘⊜geranium, ⊘⊜lemon, ⊘⊜rosemary

⊜: Dilute as recommended, and apply 1–2 drops to liver area, abdomen, and reflex points on the feet.

⊘: Diffuse into the air.

⊕: **Body System(s) Affected:** Cardiovascular System.

Jet Lag

See also Insomnia

Jet lag is the disruption of normal sleep patterns experienced while the body's internal clock adjusts to rapid changes in daylight and nighttime hours when flying to different areas of the world. Jet lag can cause tiredness, fatigue, and insomnia during normal sleeping hours. It is recommended to drink lots of fluids and to avoid alcohol or caffeine while flying to help prevent jet lag. Avoiding naps and forcing yourself to stay awake until your normal bedtime the first day can also help the body recover more quickly.

Oils: ⊘Balance, ⊘⊘Steady, ⊘peppermint, ⊘eucalyptus, ⊘geranium, ⊘lavender, ⊘grapefruit, ⊘lemongrass

⊘: Use invigorating oils such as peppermint and eucalyptus in the morning and calming oils such as lavender and geranium at night. Dilute as recommended, and apply 1–2 drops to temples, thymus, lower back, and bottoms of feet. Add 2–3 drops to 1 Tbs. (15 ml) fractionated coconut oil, and massage onto back, legs, shoulders, and feet. Add 1–2 drops to warm bathwater, and bathe.

⊕: **Body System(s) Affected:** Emotional Balance.

Joints

See also Arthritis, Skeletal System, Inflammation, Muscles

A joint is an area where two bones come together. Joints can offer limited or no movement between the bones (such as in the skull) or can offer a wide range of motion (such as in the shoulders, hands, and knees).

> *Simple Solutions—Joint Soreness:* Combine 3 drops eucalyptus, 3 drops peppermint, and 3 drops rosemary with 1 tsp. (5 ml) fractionated coconut oil in a small roll-on bottle. Apply on location, and then apply an ice pack on top.

Oils: ⊘Deep Blue, ⊘Rescuer, ⊘wintergreen, ⊘Roman chamomile (inflammation)

Other Products: ⊘Deep Blue Rub and ODeep Blue Polyphenol Complex to help comfort joint stiffness and soreness.

—Rotator Cuff (sore):

The rotator cuff is the group of muscles and tendons that connect and hold the upper arm in the shoulder joint. The rotator cuff can become sore due to repetitive stressful shoulder motions or injury.

Oils: ⊘wintergreen, ⊘Deep Blue, ⊘Rescuer, ⊘lemongrass, ⊘peppermint, ⊘fir

Other Products: ⊘Deep Blue Rub and ODeep Blue Polyphenol Complex to help comfort joint stiffness and soreness.

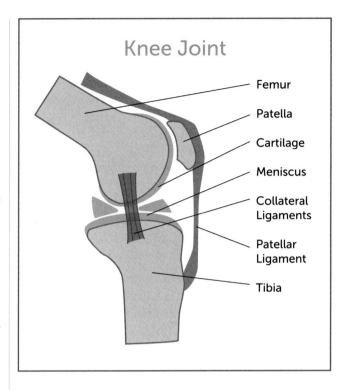

Knee Joint

- Femur
- Patella
- Cartilage
- Meniscus
- Collateral Ligaments
- Patellar Ligament
- Tibia

—Shoulder (frozen): *See also Inflammation*

A frozen shoulder refers to a condition where the range of motion of the shoulder is severely limited and painful. This can be caused by inflammation, stiffness, abnormal tissue growth within the joint capsule (connective tissue that helps cushion, lubricate, and protect the joint) around the shoulder, arthritis, or inflammation of the bursa (small fluid-filled sacs that cushions muscle, ligament, and tendon tissue from the bones as they move across them). These conditions can be extremely painful and can take a long time to heal.

Oils: ⊘Deep Blue, ⊘fir, ⊘lemongrass, ⊘basil, ⊘wintergreen, ⊘Rescuer, ⊘oregano, ⊘peppermint

Other Products: ⊘Deep Blue Rub and ODeep Blue Polyphenol Complex to help comfort joint stiffness and soreness.

Regimen 1: Begin by applying 1–2 drops of fir to the shoulder reflex point on the foot on the same side as the frozen shoulder to help with any inflammation. Check for any improvement in pain and/or range of motion. Repeat these steps using lemongrass (for torn or pulled ligaments), basil (for muscle spasms), and wintergreen (for bone problems). After determining which of these oils gets the best results for improving pain and/or

See the *Quick Usage Chart* inside the back cover for recommended dilutions.

318

range of motion, apply 1–2 drops of the oil (or oils) to the shoulder. Then apply 1–2 drops of peppermint (to help soothe the nerves) and 1–2 drops oregano (to help enhance muscle flexibility). Finally, apply fir to the opposite shoulder to create balance as it compensates for the sore one. Drink lots of water.

—Tennis Elbow:

Tennis elbow (epicondylitis) is an injury to the tendons that connect the humerus bone near the elbow to the muscles that pull the hand backwards (lateral) and forward (medial) at the wrist. This type of injury is often associated with the repetitive forehand and backhand motions of playing tennis but can be caused by other activities that stress these tendons as well.

Oils: ⊘Deep Blue, ⊘Rescuer, ⊘eucalyptus, ⊘peppermint, ⊘helichrysum, ⊘wintergreen, ⊘rosemary, ⊘lemongrass

Other Products: ⊘Deep Blue Rub and ⍥Deep Blue Polyphenol Complex to help comfort joint stiffness and soreness.

Blend 1: Combine 1 drop each of lemongrass, helichrysum, marjoram, and peppermint. Apply on location; then apply an ice pack.

⊘: Dilute as recommended, and apply 1–2 drops on location or on reflex points on the feet. Combine 5–10 drops with 1 Tbs. (15 ml) fractionated coconut oil, and massage on location.

⊕: **Body System(s) Affected:** Skeletal System.

Kidneys

The kidneys are paired organs located just below the rib cage on either side of the spine that function to filter waste and extra water from the blood. The kidneys convert the waste and extra water into urine that is then excreted through urination. The kidneys also play an important role in hormone production.

> *Simple Solutions—Kidney Stones:* Drink a glass of water with 1 tsp. (5 ml) lemon juice daily to help prevent kidney stones.

Oils: ⊘lemongrass, ⍥thyme⊕, ⍥Zendocrine, ⍥bergamot⊕, ⊘juniper berry, ⊘grapefruit, ⊘geranium, ⊘clary sage

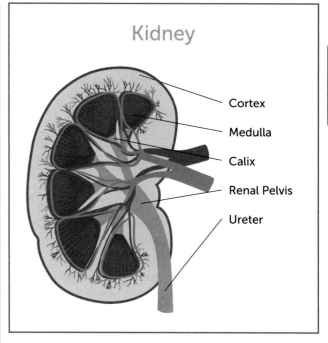

Kidney

- Cortex
- Medulla
- Calix
- Renal Pelvis
- Ureter

Other Products: ⍥xEO Mega or vEO Mega or ⍥IQ Mega to provide omega-3 fatty acids that help support kidney function. ⍥Zendocrine Zendocrine Detoxification Complex to help support healthy kidney functioning.

⊘: Dilute as recommended, and apply to kidneys and reflex points on the feet. Apply as a hot compress.

⍥: Take capsules as directed on package. Add 1–2 drops of essential oil to an empty capsule; swallow capsule.

—Diuretic: *See Diuretic*

—Infection:

Kidney infections occur when bacteria enters the urinary tract. They are marked by fever, abdominal pain, chills, painful urination, dull kidney pain, nausea, vomiting, and a general feeling of discomfort.

Oils: ⊘rosemary

⊘: Dilute as recommended, and apply to kidneys and reflex points on the feet.

⍥: Drink 1 gallon (4 L) of distilled water and ½ gallon (2 L) cranberry juice in 1 day.

—Inflammation (nephritis):

⍥: Drink 1 gallon (4 L) of distilled water and ½ gallon (2 L) cranberry juice in 1 day.

—Kidney Stones:

A kidney stone is a solid piece of material that forms as chemicals in the urine crystallize and adhere together in the kidney. Small stones may pass through urination without causing pain. Larger stones with sharp edges and corners, however, can cause an extreme amount of pain as they are passed out of the body through the urinary tract.

Oils: ⊙lemon, ⊙eucalyptus, ⊙juniper berry

⊖: Apply as a hot compress over kidneys. Dilute as recommended, and apply 1–2 drops on location.

○: Add 1–2 drops oil to 1 cup (250 ml) of water, and drink. To help pass a stone, drink ½ cup (125 ml) distilled water with juice from ½ lemon every 30 minutes for 6 hours; then take 2 Tbs. (25 ml) light extra-virgin olive oil with the juice from 1 full lemon, and repeat daily until stone passes. Drinking plenty of water can help prevent the formation of kidney stones.

●: **Body System(s) Affected:** Digestive System and Endocrine System.

▭: **Additional Research:**

Thyme: Older rats whose diets were supplemented with thyme oil were found to have a higher level of the antioxidant enzymes superoxide dismutase and glutathione peroxidase in the heart, liver, and kidneys than did older rats without this supplementation (Youdim et al., 1999).

Bergamot: The antioxidant activity of bergamot juice was found to have protective action against renal (kidney) injury of diet-induced hypercholesterolemia in rats (Trovato et al., 2010).

Knee Cartilage Injury

See Muscles: Cartilage Injury

Labor

See Pregnancy/Motherhood: Labor

Lactation

See Pregnancy/Motherhood: Lactation

Lactose Intolerance

Lactose intolerance is the inability of the body to fully digest lactose, a sugar found in milk and in other dairy products. Symptoms of lactose intolerance include abdominal pain and bloating, diarrhea, nausea, and gas.

Oils: ⊙lemongrass

○: Add 1–2 drops to 1 tsp. (5 ml) honey, and swallow; or add 1–2 drops to ½ cup (125 ml) rice or

almond milk, and drink. Place 1–2 drops in an empty capsule, and swallow.

⊖: Dilute as recommended, and apply 1–2 drops on abdomen or reflex points on the feet.

●: **Body System(s) Affected:** Digestive System.

Laryngitis

See also Allergies, Antiviral

Laryngitis is an inflammation and swelling of the voice box (called the larynx) that causes the voice to sound hoarse or raspy. Laryngitis is most commonly caused by viruses, allergies, or overuse of the voice and will generally go away by itself within two weeks.

> *Simple Solutions—Laryngitis:* Apply 1 drop sandalwood to throat. Add 1 drop lemon to 1 tsp. (5 ml) honey, dissolve in a small cup of warm water, and sip.

Oils: ⊙⊙sandalwood, ⊙frankincense, ⊙thyme, ⊙lavender

⊘: Diffuse into the air.

⊖: Dilute as recommended, and apply to neck and reflex points on the feet.

●: **Body System(s) Affected:** Immune System.

Laundry

See Housecleaning: Laundry

Leukemia

See Cancer: Leukemia

Libido

See Sexual Issues: Libido

Lice

See Insects/Bugs: Lice

Ligaments

See Muscles: Ligaments

Lipoma

See Tumor: Lipoma

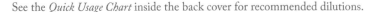

See the *Quick Usage Chart* inside the back cover for recommended dilutions.

Lips

> *Simple Solutions—Chapped Lips:* Combine 4 tsp. (5 g) beeswax pellets, 1 Tbs. (10 g) cocoa butter, and 3 Tbs. (45 ml) jojoba oil, and melt in the microwave (30 seconds at a time, stirring in between) or in a double boiler. Cool slightly, and add 15 drops myrrh. Pour into small jars or lip balm containers, and allow to cool completely. Apply a small amount of lip balm as desired.

Oils: ⊜lavender, ⊜melaleuca, ⊜lemon

Other Products: ⊜Lip Balm

—Dry lips:

Blend 1: Combine 2–5 drops geranium with 2–5 drops lavender. Apply 1–2 drops on lips.

⊜: Dilute as recommended, and apply 1 drop on lips. Combine 1–2 drops essential oil with 1 Tbs. (15 ml) fractionated coconut oil, and apply a small amount to lips.

⊕: **Body System(s) Affected:** Skin.

Liver

The liver is the largest internal organ of the body. It is located in the upper abdomen and helps with digestion, produces cholesterol used to make several hormones and cellular membranes, removes waste products and old cells from the blood, and metabolizes harmful substances and toxins into harmless chemicals. The liver also has amazing regenerative abilities. Left with as little as 25% of its original mass, the liver can regrow what was lost and return to normal size.

Oils: ⊜⊘geranium, ⊜helichrysum, ⊜⊙DigestZen, ⊙cilantro⊕, ⊙rosemary⊕, ⊙ginger⊕, ⊜cypress⊕, ⊜⊘⊙grapefruit, ⊙Zendocrine, ⊜⊙myrrh, ⊜⊘Serenity, ⊜⊘Roman chamomile

Other Products: ⊙xEO Mega or vEO Mega, ⊙IQ Mega, ⊙Alpha CRS+, ⊙Microplex VMz, ⊙a2z Chewable for omega-3 fatty acids and other nutrients that help support healthy liver cell functions. ⊙Zendocrine Detoxification Complex to help support healthy liver functioning.

—Cirrhosis:

Cirrhosis is scarring of the liver that occurs as the liver tries to repair damage done to itself. When extensive liver damage occurs, the massive scar tissue buildup makes it impossible for the liver to function. The most common causes of cirrhosis are fatty liver (resulting from obesity or diabetes) and alcohol abuse; but any damage done to the liver can cause cirrhosis.

Oils: ⊜⊘frankincense, ⊜⊘myrrh, ⊜⊘geranium, ⊜⊘rosemary⊕, ⊜⊘juniper berry, ⊜⊘rose, ⊜⊘Roman chamomile

—Cleansing:

Oils: ⊜⊘clove, ⊜⊘geranium, ⊜⊘helichrysum, ⊜⊘myrrh

—Hepatitis: *See also Antiviral.*

Hepatitis is any swelling or inflammation of the liver. This can interfere with normal liver functioning and can possibly lead to cirrhosis or cancer over time. The most common cause of hepatitis is from one of the five different forms of hepatitis viruses, but it can also be caused by alcohol consumption, other viruses, or medications. Possible symptoms of hepatitis include diarrhea, jaundice, stomach pain, loss of appetite, dark-colored urine, pale bowel movements, nausea, and vomiting.

Oils: ⊜⊘myrrh, ⊜⊘melaleuca, ⊜⊘frankincense⊕, ⊜cypress⊕, ⊜⊘rosemary, ⊜⊘oregano, ⊜⊘thyme, ⊜⊘basil, ⊜⊘cinnamon, ⊜⊘eucalyptus, ⊜⊘peppermint

–Viral:

Oils: ⊙⊜myrrh, ⊜⊘rosemary, ⊜⊘basil

Other Products: ⊙PB Assist+ or ⊙PB Assist Jr to help maintain friendly intestinal flora that help prevent toxins from pathogenic bacteria and viruses.

—Jaundice: *See Jaundice.*

—Stimulant:

Oils: ⊜⊘helichrysum

⊜: Dilute as recommended, and apply 1–2 drops over liver area and on reflex points on the feet. Apply 1–2 drops on spine and liver area for viral infections. Apply as a warm compress over the liver area.

⊘: Diffuse into the air. Inhale directly from bottle. Apply oil to hands, tissue, or cotton wick, and inhale.

⊙: Take capsules as directed on package. Add 1–2 drops essential oil to an empty capsule; swallow capsule.

⊕: Body System(s) Affected: Digestive System and Endocrine System.

⊞: Additional Research:

Frankincense: A methanol extract of Boswellia carterii was found to have a high inhibition rate of hepatitis C virus protease (Hussein et al., 2000).

Cypress: Oral administration of cypress methanolic extract displayed preventive action against CCl4-induced hepatotoxicity in rats. These results suggest that the antioxidant activity of the flavonoid content of cypress could have potential use as a treatment for liver diseases (Ali et al., 2010).

Cilantro: Ethanolic extract of the cilantro leaf was found to protect against carbon tetrachloride induced liver injury in rats, validating its use as a liver protective agent (Pandey et al., 2011).

Cilantro: In rat livers, the antioxidant activity of cilantro leaves improved the adverse effect of the repeated administration of a potent liver toxin (Moustafa et al., 2012).

Rosemary: Daily administration of rosemary essential oil displayed a protective effect against chemical-induced liver injury in rats (Ra Kovi et al., 2014).

Ginger: Daily oral administration of ginger (*Z. officinale R.*) essential oil and isolated citral (the main constituent of ginger essential oil) displayed preventative effects on the formation of alcohol fatty liver disease in mice administered an alcoholic liquid diet for four weeks (Liu et al., 2013).

Loss of Smell

See Nose: Olfactory Loss

Lou Gehrig's Disease

Lou Gehrig's disease (also known as amyotrophic lateral sclerosis) is a progressive and fatal neurological disease that affects nerve cells in the brain and spinal cord. As the disease progresses, motor neurons die and the brain loses its ability to control muscle movement. Later stages of the disease can lead to complete paralysis. Eventually, control of the muscles needed to breathe, to speak, and to eat is lost.

Oils: ⃝cypress, ⃝Balance, ⃝⃝frankincense, ⃝⃝sandalwood, ⃝Serenity, ⃝⃝geranium, ⃝⃝rosemary, ⃝⃝thyme

Other Products: ᴼxEO Mega or vEO Mega or ᴼIQ Mega for omega fatty acids essential for nerve cell function.

◐: Dilute as recommended, and apply 1–2 drops on brain stem, neck, spine, and reflex points on the feet. Add 1–2 drops to 1 Tbs. (15 ml) fractionated coconut oil, and apply on back, neck, and feet.

⟳: Diffuse into the air. Inhale directly from bottle. Apply oil to hands, tissue, or cotton wick, and inhale.

◖: Take capsules as directed on package.

⊕: Body System(s) Affected: Nervous System.

Lumbago

See Back: Lumbago/Lower Back Pain

Lungs

See Respiratory System: Lungs

Lupus

Lupus is an autoimmune disease that occurs when the immune system begins attacking its own tissues and organs. Lupus can cause pain, damage, and inflammation in the joints, blood vessels, skin, and organs. Common symptoms include joint pain or swelling, fever, muscle pain, and red rashes (often on the face). Lupus is more common in women than in men.

Oils: ⃝clove, ⃝⃝Elevation, ⃝On Guard, ⃝Balance, ⃝⃝melissa

◐: Dilute as recommended, and apply 1–2 drops on adrenal glands, under the arms, on neck, or on bottoms of the feet.

⟳: Diffuse into the air. Inhale directly from bottle. Apply oil to hands, tissue, or cotton wick, and inhale.

⊕: Body System(s) Affected: Immune System.

Lyme Disease

See also Antibacterial, Insects/Bugs: Ticks

Lyme disease is a bacterial infection that comes from the bite of an infected tick. The first symptom is usually a red rash, which may look like a bullseye. As the infection spreads to other parts of the body, flu-like symptoms will occur, such as fever, chills, headache, body aches, stiff neck, and fatigue. If untreated, serious neurological and joint problems may develop after months or even years after the initial infection. Prevention of tick bites and quick removal of ticks reduce the chances of developing Lyme disease.

Oils: ⃝⃝oregano⁺, ⃝⃝cinnamon⁺, ⃝⃝clove⁺, ⃝⃝TerraShield (prevent), ⃝⃝lavender (prevent)

◐: Dilute as recommended, and apply 1–2 drops over location or on bottoms of the feet.

⟳: Diffuse into the air. Inhale directly from bottle. Apply oil to hands, tissue, or cotton wick, and inhale.

⊕: Body System(s) Affected: Immune System.

See the *Quick Usage Chart* inside the back cover for recommended dilutions.

322

⬚: Additional Research:

Oregano, Cinnamon, Clove: Oregano, cinnamon, and clove oils were found to eradicate biofilm structures of *Borrelia burgdorferi*—the bacteria that causes Lyme disease—in laboratory tests (Feng et al., 2017).

Lymphatic System

See also Immune System

The lymphatic system is made up of the tissues and organs (bone marrow, thymus, spleen, lymph nodes, etc.) that produce and store the cells used to fight infection and disease. The lymphatic system transports immune cells through a fluid called lymph.

Oils: cypress, sandalwood, DigestZen

Blend 1: Combine 5 drops Roman chamomile, 5 drops lavender, and 5 drops orange with 2 Tbs. (25 ml) fractionated coconut oil, and massage onto the skin over lymph nodes.

Other Products: Alpha CRS+, a2z Chewable, xEO Mega or vEO Mega or IQ Mega, and Microplex VMz for nutrients that help support healthy immune function.

—Cleansing:

Oils: lemon, lime

—Decongestant For:

Oils: cypress, grapefruit, Citrus Bliss, lemongrass, helichrysum, orange, rosemary, thyme

—Drainage Of:

Oils: helichrysum, lemongrass

—Eliminates Waste Through:

Oils: lavender

—Increase Function of:

Oils: lemon

⚫: Diffuse into the air. Inhale directly from bottle. Apply oil to hands, tissue, or cotton wick, and inhale.

⬚: Dilute as recommended, and apply 1–2 drops on neck, arms, thyroid area, and reflex points on the feet. Add 1–2 drops to warm bathwater, and bathe.

⬚: Take capsules as directed on package.

Malaria

Malaria is a disease caused by single-celled *Plasmodium* parasites. These parasites are spread by mosquitoes from one infected person to another. Symptoms of malaria include light-headedness, shortness of breath, fever, chills, nausea, and, in some cases, coma and death. The best way to prevent malaria is to avoid being bit by using mosquito repellent and mosquito nets, especially between dusk and dawn, in areas of the world where malaria is common.

> *Simple Solutions—Malaria:* To keep mosquitoes at bay, add 2–3 drops TerraShield to 2–4 Tbs. (25–50 ml) distilled water in a small spray bottle; shake well, and mist onto exposed skin or into small openings where bugs may come through.

> *Simple Solutions—Malaria:* Mix 1 drop lemon with 1 tsp. (5 ml) honey and 1 cup (250 ml) warm water, and drink slowly.

Oils: TerraShield, eucalyptus, lemongrass, lavender, lemon

⬚: Dilute as recommended, and apply 1–2 drops to feet and exposed skin. Add 3–5 drops to 1 Tbs. (15 ml) fractionated coconut oil, and apply to exposed skin. Add 2–3 drops to 2–4 Tbs. (25–50 ml) distilled water in a small spray bottle; shake well, and mist onto the skin or into small openings where bugs may come through.

⚫: Diffuse into the air. Place 1–2 drops on small ribbons, strings, or cloth, and hang around area to help repel mosquitoes.

⬚: Mix 1–2 drops lemon with 1 tsp. (5 ml) honey and 1 cup (250 ml) distilled water, and drink.

⬚: **Body System(s) Affected:** Immune System.

⬚: **Additional Research:**

Eucalyptus: A eucalyptus-based repellent containing p-menthane-3,8-diol as the active ingredient was found to be as effective as DEET in repelling the mosquito commonly known to carry a deadly malaria disease (complete protection for 6–7.75 hours) (Trigg, 1996).

Male-Specific Conditions/Issues

> *Simple Solutions—Jock Itch:* Combine 15 drops melaleuca with 2 Tbs. (15 g) cornstarch. Sprinkle a small amount on location once or twice a day as needed.

—**Genital Area**

  –**Infection:**

  Oils: ⊘melaleuca, ⊘oregano, ⊘eucalyptus, ⊘lavender

  –**Inflammation:**

  Oils: ⊘lavender, ⊘Roman chamomile

  –**Swelling:**

  Oils: ⊘cypress, ⊘lavender, ⊘rosemary, ⊘eucalyptus

—**Impotence:**

  Impotence, also known as erectile dysfunction, is the frequent inability to have or sustain an erection. This may be caused by circulation problems, nerve problems, low levels of testosterone, medications, or psychological stresses.

  Oils: ⊘Oclary sage, ⊘Ocassia⊕, ⊘Oclove, ⊘Oginger, ⊘Odill⊕, ⊘Osandalwood

—**Infertility:**

  Infertility is clinically defined as the inability to achieve pregnancy after a year of trying.

  Oils: ⊘⊘basil, ⊘⊘clary sage, ⊘thyme, ⊘Ogeranium⊕, ⊘Ocinnamon⊕

—**Jock Itch:** *See also Antifungal: Ringworm*

  Jock itch is a type of fungal infection that infects the skin of the genital area, causing itching or painful red patches of skin. It occurs more often during warm weather.

  Oils: ⊘melaleuca, ⊘lavender, ⊘cypress

  Recipe 1: Place 2 drops of any of the above oils in 1 tsp. (5 ml) fractionated coconut oil, and apply to area morning and night. Alternately, place 2 drops oil in a small bowl of water, and wash the area with the water and then dry well each morning and night.

  ⊘: Dilute as recommended, and apply 1–2 drops on location or on reflex points on the feet. Dilute 1–2 drops in 1 Tbs. (15 ml) fractionated coconut oil, and massage on location. Add 1–2 drops essential oil to warm water, and bathe.

  ◯: Place 1–2 drops in an empty capsule, and swallow.

  ⊘: Diffuse into the air. Inhale directly from bottle. Apply oil to hands, tissue, or cotton wick, and inhale.

  ⊕: **Body System(s) Affected:** Reproductive System.

⊡ **Additional Research:**

Cassia: Methanol extract of cassia was found to effectively manage sexual dysfunction in aged rats (Goswami et al., 2013).

Dill: Male mice internally administered low doses of dill extracts displayed a short-term increase in mounting frequency and an enhanced protein phosphorylation level in testicular lysate, suggesting that low doses of dill enhances aphrodisiac activity in males and may be beneficial in treating male sexual dysfunction (Iamsaard et al., 2013). (It should be noted that high doses of dill extract have been shown to decrease fertility in male rats, but no significant difference in sperm count, sperm motility, or testosterone concentrations occur (Monsefi et al., 2011).)

Geranium: Male mice exposed to a harmful insecticide, known to cause sperm damage, were successfully treated with geranium essential oil through its antioxidant effects. Compared to the control group, the oral administration of geranium oil prevented testicular oxidative damage, reduced lipid peroxidation, and improved total sperm motility, viability, and morphology in mice spermatozoa (Slima et al., 2013).

Cinnamon: Cinnamon bark essential oil was found to have a protective effect against damages in male rat reproductive organs and cells induced by carbon tetrachloride (a common toxic substance) (Yüce et al., 2014).

Cassia: Methanol extract of Cinnamomum cassia was found to increase the sexual function of young male rats (Goswami et al., 2014).

Massage

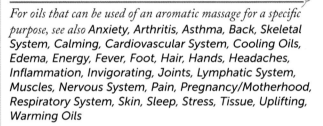

*For oils that can be used of an aromatic massage for a specific purpose, see also **Anxiety, Arthritis, Asthma, Back, Skeletal System, Calming, Cardiovascular System, Cooling Oils, Edema, Energy, Fever, Foot, Hair, Hands, Headaches, Inflammation, Invigorating, Joints, Lymphatic System, Muscles, Nervous System, Pain, Pregnancy/Motherhood, Respiratory System, Skin, Sleep, Stress, Tissue, Uplifting, Warming Oils***

Massage is the manipulation of the soft tissues in the body through holding, moving, compressing, or stroking. Massage can be done to help aid circulation, relax muscles, relieve pain, reduce swelling, speed healing after strains and sprains, restore function to the body, and release tension and stress.

> *Simple Solutions—Massage:* Add 10 drops of your favorite essential oil or blend to 1 Tbs. (15 ml) fractionated coconut oil or another carrier oil such as almond, olive, jojoba, sesame seed, or flaxseed to create your own personal massage oil.

Oils: ⊘AromaTouch—a blend specifically created to aid in therapeutic massage to relax and soothe muscles, to increase circulation, and to stimulate tissues. See other conditions for specific oils that can be used to create a massage oil for that condition.

Other Products: ⊘Deep Blue Rub and ODeep Blue Polyphenol Complex to help soothe tired, achy, and sore muscles and improve circulation within the tissue.

Blend 1: Combine 5 drops Roman chamomile, 5 drops lavender, and 5 drops orange with 2 Tbs.

See the *Quick Usage Chart* inside the back cover for recommended dilutions.

324

(25 ml) fractionated coconut oil, and use as massage oil for a relaxing massage.

⟐: Add 1–10 drops of essential oil to 1 Tbs. (15 ml) fractionated coconut oil or another carrier oil such as almond, olive, jojoba, sesame seed, or flaxseed to create a massage oil. *See also the section on the Aroma Massage Technique in the Science and Application of Essential Oils section of this book.*

✛: **Body System(s) Affected:** Muscles and Skin.

Measles

See Childhood Diseases: Measles

Melanoma

See Cancer: Skin/Melanoma

Memory

See also Alzheimer's Disease

Memory is the mental capacity to retain and recall facts, events, past experiences, and impressions. Memory retention can be enhanced by memory exercises, adequate sleep, and associations with previous knowledge. Aroma also plays a role in memory. At least one study has indicated that individuals exposed to an aroma while learning had an easier time remembering what they had learned when exposed to the same aroma, while those who were exposed to a differing aroma had a more difficult time remembering what they had learned⌐.

> *Simple Solutions—Memory:* Place 5 drops of rosemary on a natural stone or unglazed clay pendant, and wear while studying and again while taking a test to help recall facts.

Oils: rosemary⌐, peppermint⌐, Thinker, frankincense, basil⌐, Citrus Bliss, clove⌐, lemon, juniper berry, cedarwood, ginger, grapefruit, lime, bergamot, rose⌐, dill⌐, lavender, lemongrass, petitgrain

Other Products: ○xEO Mega or vEO Mega, ○IQ Mega, ○Microplex VMz for omega-3 fatty acids and other nutrients essential to brain cell health.

—Improve:

Oils: clove, clary sage

—Stimulate:

Oils: rosemary

⟐ Diffuse into the air. Inhale directly from bottle. Apply oil to hands, tissue, or cotton wick, and inhale. Wear as a perfume or cologne.

⟐ Dilute as recommended, and apply 1–2 drops on temples or back of neck.

○ Take capsules as directed on package.

✛ **Body System(s) Affected:** Nervous System.

▦ **Additional Research:**

Subjects who had learned a list of 24 words when exposed to an odor had an easier time relearning the list when exposed to the same odor compared to those who were exposed to an alternate odor (Smith et al., 1992).

Rosemary: Volunteers completing a battery of tests were found to be more content when exposed to lavender and rosemary aromas. Rosemary aroma also was found to enhance quality of memory compared to control (Moss et al., 2003).

Peppermint: In human trials, the aroma of peppermint was found to enhance memory and to increase alertness (Moss et al., 2008).

Basil: A study evaluating memory retention and retrieval of mice revealed that the hydroalcoholic extract of Ocimum basilicum significantly increased memory retention and retrieval. The memory enhancing effects were attributed to the antioxidant activity of flavonoids, tannins and terpenoids in the basil extract (Sarahroodi et al., 2012).

Clove: Administration of clove essential oil for three weeks before treatment with scopolamine (a known agent causing memory impairment) was shown to significantly reverse the scopolamine-induced memory deficit, when compared to pretreatment with saline only (Halder et al., 2011).

Rose: Oral administration of Rosa damascena extract for one month was found to enhance adult neurogenesis, hippocampal volume, and synaptic plasticity, as well as reverse the amyloid-β-associated memory abnormalities in a rat model of amyloid-β-induced Alzheimer's disease. These results indicate that rose extract may have memory-enhancing ability (Esfandiary et al., 2014).

Dill: A combined extract of *Cissampelos pareira* and *Anethum graveolens* was found to produce cognitive-enhancing and neuroprotective effects on spatial memory in memory deficit induced rats (Thukham-Mee et al., 2012).

Menopause

See Female-Specific Conditions: Menopause

Menstruation

See Female-Specific Conditions: Menstruation

Mental

See Alertness, Brain, Energy, Memory, Stress

Metabolism

Metabolism refers to the processes involved in converting ingested nutrients into substances that can be used within the cells of the body for energy or to create needed cellular structures. This process is car-

---

Primary Recommendations • Secondary Recommendations • Other Recommendations / ⟐=Aromatic, ⟐=Topical, ○=Internal

ried out by various chemical reactions facilitated by enzymes within the body.

—**Balance:**

Oils: ◐clove, ◐◐Balance, ◐◐Steady, ◐◐oregano

◐ Diffuse into the air. Inhale oil applied to tissue or cotton wick.

◐ Dilute as recommended, and apply 1–2 drops on neck or on bottoms of the feet.

◐: **Body System(s) Affected:** Digestive System and Endocrine System.

Metals

See **Detoxification**

Mice (Repel)

Oils: ◐◐Purify

◐ Apply 1–2 drops in small openings or crevices where mice are likely to appear. Add 1–5 drops to small cotton balls, and place in openings where mice may come in.

◐ Diffuse into the air.

Migraines

See **Headaches: Migraine Headache**

Mildew

See also **Antifungal**

Mildew is a whitish fungus that forms a flat growth on plants and organic material. Mildew attacks clothing, leather, paper, ceilings, walls, floors, shower walls, windowsills, and other places with high moisture levels. Mildew can produce a strong musty odor, especially in places with poor air circulation.

> *Simple Solutions—Mildew:* Add 25 drops Purify to ¼ cup (50 ml) water in a small spray bottle, and spray on surface to help neutralize mildew.

Oils: ◐Purify

◐: Place a few drops in a small spray bottle with distilled water, and spray into air or on surface to help neutralize mildew.

Mind

See **Alertness, Brain, Energy: Fatigue: Mental Fatigue, Memory**

Minerals (Deficiency)

Minerals are naturally occurring, inorganic substances with a chemical composition and structure. Some minerals are essential to the human body. A person is considered to have a mineral deficiency when the concentration level of any mineral needed to maintain optimal health is abnormally low in the body.

Other Products: ◐Microplex VMz contains a balanced blend of minerals essential for optimal cellular health, including calcium, magnesium, zinc, selenium, copper, manganese, chromium, and molybdenum; ◐TerraGreens for a whole food source of essential nutrients.

◐: Take capsules as directed on package.

◐: **Body System(s) Affected:** Digestive System.

Miscarriage

See **Pregnancy/Motherhood: Miscarriage**

Moles

See **Skin: Moles**

Mono (Mononucleosis)

See also **Antiviral**

Mononucleosis is a viral disease caused by the Epstein-Barr virus that usually spreads through contact with infected saliva, tears, and mucus. Most adults have been exposed to this virus sometime in their lives, but many display no symptoms or only very mild flu-like symptoms. Mononucleosis symptoms are most often seen in adolescents and young adults. Symptoms of this disease include fatigue, weakness, severe sore throat, fever, swollen lymph nodes, swollen tonsils, headache, loss of appetite, and a soft or swollen spleen. Once individuals are exposed to the Epstein-Barr virus, they carry the virus for the rest of their lives. The virus sporadically becomes active, but the symptoms do not appear again. Whenever the virus is active, however, it can be spread to others—even if the person carrying it shows no symptoms.

See the Quick Usage Chart inside the back cover for recommended dilutions.

Simple Solutions—Mono: Combine 3 drops oregano, 3 drops On Guard, and 3 drops thyme. Rub 3 drops of this blend on the feet.

Oils: Breathe, On Guard

Other Products: On Guard+ Softgels

: Dilute as recommended, and apply 1–3 drops on throat and feet.

: Diffuse into the air. Inhale oil directly from bottle, or inhale oil that is applied to the hands.

: **Body System(s) Affected:** Immune System.

Mood Swings

A mood swing is a rapid change of mood caused by fatigue or by a sudden shift in the body's hormonal balance.

Simple Solutions—Mood Swing: Diffuse Balance to help balance emotions.

Oils: clary sage, Serenity, Calmer, lavender, Balance, Steady, rosemary, Elevation, geranium, rose, ylang ylang, sandalwood, lemon, peppermint, bergamot, fennel

: Diffuse into the air. Inhale oil directly or applied to the hands.

: **Body System(s) Affected:** Emotional Balance.

Morning Sickness

See Pregnancy/Motherhood: Morning Sickness

Mosquitoes

See Insects/Bugs: Mosquitoes

Motion Sickness

See Nausea: Motion Sickness

MRSA

See Antibacterial

Mucus

See Congestion

Multiple Sclerosis

See also Brain: Myelin Sheath

Multiple sclerosis (MS) is an autoimmune disease in which the immune system attacks and gradually destroys the myelin sheath (which covers and insulates the nerves) and the underlying nerve fibers of the central nervous system. This destruction of the myelin sheath interferes with communication between the brain and the rest of the body. Symptoms of MS include partial or complete loss of vision, tingling, burning, pain in parts of the body, tremors, loss of coordination, unsteady gait, dizziness, and memory problems.

Oils: frankincense, sandalwood, peppermint, clove, cypress, juniper berry, Serenity, oregano, thyme, birch, rosemary, wintergreen

Other Products: xEO Mega or vEO Mega or IQ Mega for omega-3 fatty acids that help support nerve and brain function.

: Dilute as recommended, and apply 1–2 drops to spine, back of neck, and feet. Dilute 1–3 drops in 1 Tbs. (15 ml) fractionated coconut oil, and massage on back and neck.

: Take capsules as directed on package.

: Diffuse into the air. Inhale directly from bottle. Apply oil to hands, tissue, or cotton wick, and inhale.

: **Body System(s) Affected:** Nervous System and Immune System.

: **Additional Research:**

Multiple Sclerosis: Beta caryophyllene (found in clove oil) was found to help protect against neuroinflammation and the demyelinating processes in the central nervous system in a murine model of multiple sclerosis (Alberti et al., 2017).

Mumps

See Childhood Diseases: Mumps

Muscles

See also Cardiovascular System: Heart Tissue

Muscle is the tissue in the body that has the ability to contract, making movement possible. The three main types of muscle in the body are smooth muscle (such as that in the stomach, intestines, and blood vessels), cardiac muscle (found in the heart), and skeletal muscle (attached to the bones). Skeletal muscles are connected to the bones with tough fibrous tissue called tendons and allow for coordinated, controlled movement of the body, such as walking, pointing, or eye movement. Smooth muscles and cardiac muscles move automatically without conscious control to perform their functions.

Oils: ⊙marjoram, ⊙Deep Blue, ⊙Rescuer, ⊙peppermint⊕, ⊙AromaTouch, ⊙copaiba⊕, ⊙birch, ⊙cypress, ⊙wintergreen, ⊙lemongrass, ⊙lavender

Other Products: ⊙Deep Blue Rub and ⊙Deep Blue Polyphenol Complex to help relieve sore muscles, ⊙Mito2Max, ⊙Alpha CRS+, ⊙a2z Chewable, ⊙xEO Mega or vEO Mega, ⊙IQ Mega, ⊙Microplex VMz for coenzyme Q10 and other nutrients to support muscle cell energy and function.

—Aches and Pains: *See also Pain*

Muscle pain usually results from overuse, tension, stress, strain, or injury. However, muscle pain can also be caused by a disease or infection affecting the whole body, such as the flu, fibromyalgia, or a connective tissue disorder.

> *Simple Solutions—Muscle Aches/Pains:* Blend 10 drops Deep Blue in 1 Tbs. (15 ml) fractionated coconut oil. Gently massage oil into aching muscles.

Oils: ⊙marjoram, ⊙Deep Blue, ⊙Rescuer, ⊙copaiba⊕, ⊙birch, ⊙clove, ⊙AromaTouch, ⊙oregano, ⊙peppermint, ⊙wintergreen, ⊙fir (with inflammation), ⊙vetiver, ⊙Roman chamomile, ⊙helichrysum, ⊙ginger, ⊙lavender, ⊙rosemary, ⊙thyme

Other Products: ⊙Deep Blue Rub and ⊙Deep Blue Polyphenol Complex to help relieve sore muscles.

—Bruised: *See Bruises*

—Cardiac Muscle: *See also Cardiovascular System: Heart*

Cardiac muscle is the type of muscle found in the walls of the heart.

Oils: ⊙⊘marjoram, ⊙⊘lavender, ⊙⊘peppermint, ⊙⊘rosemary, ⊙cinnamon

—Cartilage Injury:

Cartilage is a type of connective tissue in the body. It is firmer than other tissues and is used to provide structure and support without being as hard or as rigid as bone. Types of cartilage include hyaline cartilage, elastic cartilage, and fibrocartilage. Hyaline cartilage lines the bones and joints,

helping them move smoothly. Elastic cartilage is found in the ear and larynx and is used to keep other tubular structures, such as the nose and trachea, open. Fibrocartilage is the strongest and most rigid cartilage. It is found in the intervertebral discs and other high-stress areas and serves to connect tendons and ligaments to bones. The hyaline cartilage surrounding bones and joints can become torn or injured if the joint is bent or twisted in a traumatic way. This can cause pain, swelling, tenderness, popping, or clicking within the joint and can limit movement.

Oils: ⊙birch, ⊙wintergreen, ⊙marjoram, ⊙Rescuer, ⊙lemongrass, ⊙fir, ⊙peppermint

—Cramps/Charley Horses:

A muscle cramp or charley horse is the sudden, involuntary contraction of a muscle. Muscle cramps can occur in any muscle in the body, but they usually occur in the thigh, calf, or arch of the foot. Cramps can be caused by excessive strain to the muscle, injury, overuse, dehydration, or lack of blood flow to the muscle. Muscle cramps can happen during or after a physical activity and while lying in bed.

> *Simple Solutions—Charley Horse:* Blend 5 drops lemongrass and 5 drops peppermint in 1 Tbs. (15 ml) fractionated coconut oil. Gently massage oil into cramping muscles.

Oils: ⊙lemongrass with ⊙peppermint, ⊙marjoram, ⊙Deep Blue, ⊙Rescuer, ⊙rosemary, ⊙basil, ⊙thyme, ⊙vetiver, ⊙Roman chamomile, ⊙cypress, ⊙grapefruit, ⊙clary sage, ⊘lavender

—Development:

When muscles are stretched or used during exercise, they produce a substance that activates stem cells already present in the tissue. Once these cells are activated, they begin to divide—creating new muscle fiber and thereby increasing the size and strength of the muscles.

Oils: ⊙birch, ⊙wintergreen, ⊙Deep Blue

—Fatigue:

Muscle fatigue is the muscle's temporary reduction in strength, power, and endurance. This happens when there is an increase in lactic acid and blood flow to the muscle, a depletion of glycogen, or a deprivation of oxygen to the tissue.

See the *Quick Usage Chart* inside the back cover for recommended dilutions.

Oils: ⊜marjoram, ⊜fir, ⊜cypress, ⊜peppermint, ⊜eucalyptus, ⊜grapefruit, ⊜rosemary, ⊜thyme

Other Products: ⊜Deep Blue Rub and ⵔDeep Blue Polyphenol Complex

—Inflammation: *See Inflammation*

—Ligaments:

A ligament is a sheet or band of tough connective tissue and fibers that connects bones together or helps bind and support a joint.

> *Simple Solutions—Ligament Injury:* Add 10 drops lemongrass to 1 tsp. (5 ml) fractionated coconut oil in a small roll-on bottle. Apply on location, and then apply an ice pack on top.

Oils: ⊜lemongrass

—Over Exercised:

When a person overexercises, his or her muscles do not get sufficient rest or time to heal. This continued muscle strain can cause muscle sprains, strain, and even tears to soft tissue. It may also cause stiffness and soreness to the neck, upper or lower back, shoulder, arm, or joint.

Oils: ⊜fir, ⊜eucalyptus, ⊜copaiba⊕, ⊜Rescuer, ⊜lavender, ⊜thyme, ⊜ginger

Other Products: ⊜Deep Blue Rub and ⵔDeep Blue Polyphenol Complex to help provide comfort to tired and sore muscles.

Recipe 1: Add 3 drops marjoram and 2 drops lemon to warm bathwater, and soak.

Blend 1: Combine 2 drops eucalyptus, 2 drops peppermint, and 2 drops ginger with 1 Tbs. (15 ml) fractionated coconut oil, and massage into muscles.

—Rheumatism (Muscular): *See Fibromyalgia*

—Smooth Muscle:

Oils: ⊜marjoram, ⊜rosemary⊕, ⊜ⵔpeppermint, ⊜fennel, ⊜cypress, ⊜juniper berry, ⊜clary sage, ⊜melissa, ⊜lavender, ⊜sandalwood, ⊜bergamot

—Spasms:

A muscle spasm is a sudden, involuntary contraction or twitching of a muscle. This may or may not cause pain.

Oils: ⊜basil, ⊜marjoram, ⊜Deep Blue, ⊜Rescuer, ⊜Roman chamomile, ⊜peppermint, ⊜cypress, ⊜clary sage, ⊜lavender

—Sprains:

A sprain is an injury to a ligament caused by excessive stretching. The ligament can have little tears in it or it can be completely torn apart to be considered a sprain. The most common areas to receive a sprain are the ankle, knee, and wrist. After a person receives a sprain, the area will swell rapidly and be quite painful. If the ligament is torn apart, surgery may be required.

Oils: ⊜marjoram, ⊜lemongrass, ⊜fir, ⊜Rescuer, ⊜helichrysum, ⊜rosemary, ⊜thyme, ⊜copaiba⊕, ⊜vetiver, ⊜eucalyptus, ⊜clove, ⊜ginger, ⊜lavender

—Strain:

A strain is a tear of the muscle tissue due to excessive strain or overstretching. Strains can cause inflammation, pain, and discoloration of the skin around the injured area.

Oils: ⊜lemongrass, ⊜Deep Blue, ⊜Rescuer, ⊜ginger (circulation), ⊜helichrysum (pain)

—Stiffness:

Oils: ⊜Deep Blue

Other Products: ⊜Deep Blue Rub and ⵔDeep Blue Polyphenol Complex

—Tendinitis:

Tendinitis is the inflammation of a tendon due to injury, repetitive exercise or strain, or diseases such as arthritis, gout, and gonorrhea. This can cause swelling and pain in the affected tendon.

> *Simple Solutions—Tendinitis:* Apply 1 drop marjoram on location, and cover with a cool pack for 15 minutes.

Oils: ⊜marjoram, ⊜lavender

—Tension (especially in shoulders and neck):

Muscle tension is a condition in which the muscle remains in a semi-contracted state for an extended period of time. This is usually due to physical or emotional stress.

Muscles

Muscle is the tissue in the body that has the ability to contract, making movement possible. The three main types of muscle in the body are smooth muscle (such as that in the stomach, intestines, and blood vessels), cardiac muscle (found in the heart), and skeletal muscle (attached to the bones). Skeletal muscles are connected to the bones with tough fibrous tissue called tendons and allow for coordinated, controlled movement of the body, such as walking, pointing, or eye movement. Smooth muscles and cardiac muscles move automatically without conscious control to perform their functions.

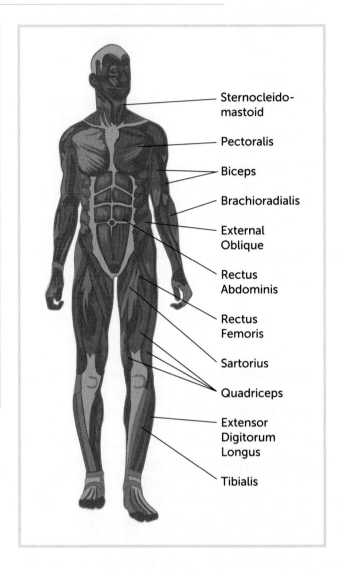

- Sternocleido-mastoid
- Pectoralis
- Biceps
- Brachioradialis
- External Oblique
- Rectus Abdominis
- Rectus Femoris
- Sartorius
- Quadriceps
- Extensor Digitorum Longus
- Tibialis

Oils for Muscle Support

Oils: marjoram, Deep Blue, peppermint, AromaTouch, birch, clove, cypress, wintergreen, fir (with inflammation), vetiver, Roman chamomile, lemongrass, lavender, helichrysum, ginger, rosemary, thyme

Common Muscle Issues

Skeletal Muscle: Aches/Pains, Bruises, Cramps/Charley Horses, Fatigue, Inflammation, Muscular Dystrophy, Spasms, Strain, Stiffness, Tension

Cardiac Muscle: Angina, Arrhythmia, Palpitations, Tachycardia

Smooth Muscle: Cramps (Abdominal)

Oils: ⊘marjoram, ⊘Deep Blue, ⊘Rescuer, ⊘peppermint⊕, ⊘helichrysum, ⊘juniper berry, ⊘lavender, ⊘Roman chamomile, ⊘spikenard

Other Products: ⊘Deep Blue Rub and ⊙Deep Blue Polyphenol Complex

—Tone:

Apply these oils before exercise to help tone muscles.

Oils: ⊘birch, ⊘cypress, ⊘wintergreen, ⊘marjoram, ⊘basil, ⊘peppermint, ⊘orange, ⊘thyme, ⊘rosemary, ⊘juniper berry, ⊘grapefruit, ⊘lavender

⊖: Dilute as recommended, and apply 1–2 drops on location. Add 2–4 drops to 1 Tbs. (15 ml) fractionated coconut oil, and massage into desired muscles or joints. Add 1–2 drops to warm bathwater, and bathe. Apply as hot or cold (for strains or sprains) compress.

⊙: Take capsules as directed on package. Place 1–2 drops of oil under the tongue or add 1–2 drops essential oil to empty capsule, and swallow.

⊘: Diffuse into the air.

⊕: **Body System(s) Affected:** Muscles.

⊡: **Additional Research:**

Peppermint: A combination of peppermint oil and ethanol was found to have a significant analgesic effect with a reduction in sensitivity to headache; while a combination of peppermint, eucalyptus, and ethanol were found to relax muscles, and increase cognitive performance in humans (Göbel et al., 1994).

Rosemary: Rosemary oil demonstrated a relaxant effect on smooth muscle from the trachea of rabbits and guinea pigs (Aqel, 1991).

Muscular Dystrophy

Muscular dystrophy is any of several genetic diseases that cause gradual weakening of the skeletal muscles. The most common forms, Duchenne and Becker muscular dystrophies, are caused by a gene defect that inhibits or alters the production of dystrophin, a protein necessary for proper muscle cell structure.

Oils: ⊘marjoram, ⊘lemongrass, ⊘basil, ⊘rosemary, ⊘AromaTouch, ⊘Deep Blue, ⊘geranium, ⊘lavender, ⊘lemon, ⊘orange, ⊘ginger

Other Products: ⊘Deep Blue Rub and ⊙Deep Blue Polyphenol Complex to help relieve and relax tense and aching muscles.

⊖: Dilute as recommended, and apply 1–2 drops on location. Add 2–4 drops to 1 Tbs. (15 ml) fractionated coconut oil, and massage into desired

muscles. Add 1–2 drops to warm bathwater and bathe. Apply as cold compress.

⊕: **Body System(s) Affected:** Nervous System and Muscles.

Myelin Sheath

See Brain: Myelin Sheath

Nails

Oils: ⊘lemon, ⊘frankincense, ⊘myrrh, ⊘Citrus Bliss, ⊘melaleuca (infection⊕), ⊘eucalyptus, ⊘lavender, ⊘grapefruit, ⊘rosemary, ⊘cypress, ⊘oregano, ⊘thyme

Blend 1: Combine 2 drops frankincense, 2 drops lemon, and 2 drops myrrh with 2 drops wheat germ oil. Apply 2–3 times per week.

Other Products: ⊙Microplex VMz for nutrients essential to healthy nail growth.

⊖: Dilute as recommended, and apply 1–2 drops to nails. Add 1–2 drops to 1 tsp. (5 ml) fractionated coconut oil, and apply to nails.

⊙: Take capsules as directed on package.

⊕: **Body System(s) Affected:** Skin.

⊡: **Additional Research:**

Melaleuca: Topical application of 100% tea tree oil was found to have results similar to topical application of 1% clotrimazole (antifungal drug) solution on onychomycosis (also known as tinea, or fungal nail infection) (Buck et al., 1994).

Nasal

See Nose

Nausea

Nausea is a sick feeling in the stomach producing an urge to vomit.

> *Simple Solutions—Motion Sickness:* Inhale the aroma of peppermint.

> *Simple Solutions—Nausea:* Add 2 drops ginger to a bowl of hot water, and inhale the warm vapor coming from the water.

Oils: ⊙⊘⊖ginger⊕, ⊘peppermint⊕, ⊘⊖lavender, ⊙⊘⊖cardamom, ⊘⊖DigestZen, ⊙⊘⊖green mandarin, ◐◉patchouli, ◐◉juniper berry, ◐◉clove, ◐◉spikenard

Other Products: ○DigestZen Softgels

—Morning Sickness: *See Pregnancy/Motherhood: Morning Sickness*

—Motion Sickness:

Motion sickness is a feeling of illness that occurs as a result of repeated movement, such as that experienced in a car, on a boat, or on a plane. These motions interfere with the body's sense of balance and equilibrium. The most common symptoms of motion sickness include dizziness, fatigue, and nausea.

Oils: ◉peppermint, ◉DigestZen, ◉ginger

—Vomiting:

Oils: ○◉ginger⊕, ◉peppermint, ◐◉patchouli, ◐○fennel, ◐rose, ◐Roman chamomile

◐: Place 1–2 drops essential oil in an empty capsule, and swallow. Take supplements as directed.

◉: Diffuse into the air. Inhale directly from bottle. Apply oil to hands, tissue, or cotton wick, and inhale.

◐: Dilute as recommended, and apply 1–2 drops to the feet, temples and wrists. Dilute 1–2 drops essential oil in 1 Tbs. (15 ml) fractionated coconut oil, and massage on stomach. Apply oil as a warm compress.

◐: **Body System(s) Affected:** Digestive System.

◐: **Additional Research:**

Ginger: Ginger root given orally to pregnant women was found to decrease the severity of nausea and frequency of vomiting compared to control (Vutyavanich et al., 2001).

Ginger: Ginger root given one hour before major gynecological surgery resulted in lower nausea and fewer incidences of vomiting compared to control (Nanthakomon et al., 2006).

Ginger: In a trial of women receiving gynecological surgery, women receiving ginger root had less incidences of nausea compared to a placebo. Ginger root has similar results to the antiemetic drug (a drug effective against vomiting and nausea) metoclopramide (Bone et al., 1990).

Peppermint: Oral administration of capsules containing two drops of either spearmint or peppermint oil to cancer patients during chemotherapy cycles was found to reduce the intensity of nausea when compared to the control (Tayarani-Najaran et al., 2013).

Neck

Oils: ◐lemon, ◐geranium, ◐clary sage, ◐orange, ◐basil, ◐helichrysum

◐: Dilute 1–5 drops oil in 1 Tbs. (15 ml) fractionated coconut oil, and massage on neck.

◐: **Body System(s) Affected:** Skeletal System and Muscles.

Nervous System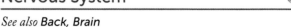

*See also **Back, Brain***

> *Simple Solutions—Neuralgia:* Blend 5 drops marjoram and 5 drops eucalyptus with 1 tsp. (5 ml) carrier oil in a small roll-on bottle, and apply along nerve.

The nervous system is a network of nerve cells that regulates the body's reaction to external and internal stimuli. The nervous system sends nerve impulses to organs and muscles throughout the body. The body relies on these impulses to function. The nervous system is comprised of the central nervous system (the brain and spinal cord) and the peripheral nervous system (all other nerves). The peripheral nervous system is comprised of the somatic nervous system (nerves that connect to the skeletal muscles and sensory nerve receptors in the skin) and the autonomic nervous system (nerves that connect to the cardiac and smooth muscles and other organs, tissues, and systems that don't require conscious effort to control). The autonomic system is divided further into two main parts: the sympathetic and parasympathetic nervous systems. The sympathetic nervous system functions to accelerate heart rate, increase blood pressure, slow digestion, and constrict blood vessels. It activates the "fight or flight" response in order to deal with threatening or stressful situations. The parasympathetic nervous system functions to slow heart rate, store energy, stimulate digestive activity, and relax specific muscles. It allows the body to return to a normal and calm state after experiencing pain or stress.

Oils: ◐◉peppermint⊕ (soothes and strengthens damaged nerves), ◐◉basil (stimulates), ◐◉lavender⊕, ◐◉lemon⊕, ◐◉grapefruit⊕, ◐◉frankincense⊕, ○◐◉turmeric⊕, ◐◉bergamot, ◐◉cedarwood (nervous tension), ◐◉lemongrass (for nerve damage), ◐◉marjoram (soothing), ◐◉geranium (regenerates), ◐◉Serenity, ◐◉Roman chamomile, ◐◉juniper berry, ◐◉vetiver, ◐◉cinnamon, ◐◉neroli, ◐◉ginger, ◐◉orange, ◐◉sandalwood

Other Products: ○Mito2Max to help support healthy nerve function. ○xEO Mega or vEO Mega or ○IQ Mega for essential omega fatty acids that help support nerve cell health. ○Microplex VMz,

See the *Quick Usage Chart* inside the back cover for recommended dilutions.

332

ⓞa2z Chewable for nutrients and minerals necessary for proper nerve cell function. ⓞAlpha CRS+ for nutrients that help support nerve cell health and energy.

—Bell's Palsy:

Bell's palsy is a weakness or paralysis of muscles on one side of the face. Bell's palsy tends to set in quickly, normally in a single day. Symptoms include numbness of one side of the face, loss of ability to taste, drooling, pain in or behind the ear, facial droop, headache, and change in the amount of saliva or tears produced. In most cases Bell's palsy symptoms will begin to improve within a few weeks. But in some few cases the symptoms continue for life.

Oils: ⓐⓑpeppermint, ⓐⓑrosemary, ⓐⓑthyme

—Carpal Tunnel Syndrome: *See Carpal Tunnel Syndrome*

—Huntington's Disease:

Huntington's disease (HD) is a progressive neurodegenerative disorder passed genetically from one generation to the next. As the disease develops, it causes nerve cells in the brain to waste away, resulting in a loss of control over body movement, emotions, and mental reasoning. Early symptoms include unsteady walking and decreased coordination. Later symptoms include sudden involuntary jerking body movements, slurred speech, decreased mental capacity, and psychological and emotional problems. Those carrying the HD gene have a 50% chance of passing it on to each of their children.

Oils: ⓐⓑpeppermint, ⓞⓐⓑturmeric⊕, ⓐⓑbasil

Other Products: Oils: ⓞMito2Max to help support healthy nerve function. ⓞxEO Mega or vEO Mega

—Lou Gehrig's Disease (ALS): *See Lou Gehrig's Disease*

—Multiple Sclerosis (MS): *See Multiple Sclerosis*

—Neuralgia:

Neuralgia is intense pain felt along the path of a nerve. Neuralgia results from damage or irritation to a nerve. Causes can include certain drugs, diabetes, infections, inflammation, trauma, and chemical irritation.

Oils: ⓑmarjoram, ⓑeucalyptus⊕, ⓑRoman chamomile, ⓑlavender, ⓑjuniper berry, ⓑhelichrysum, ⓑcedarwood

—Neuritis:

Neuritis is the inflammation of a nerve or of a group of nerves. Neuritis causes pain, poor reflexes, and muscle atrophy.

Oils: ⓑeucalyptus⊕, ⓑRoman chamomile, ⓑlavender, ⓑjuniper berry, ⓑclove, ⓑcedarwood

—Neurotonic:

Oils: ⓑmelaleuca, ⓑthyme

—Paralysis:

Paralysis is the loss of one's ability to move and control one or more specific sets of muscles. Paralysis generally occurs as a result of damage to the nervous system, especially damage to the spinal cord. Primary causes include injury, stroke, multiple sclerosis, amyotrophic lateral sclerosis (Lou Gehrig's disease), botulism, spina bifida, and Guillain-Barré syndrome.

Oils: ⓐⓑpeppermint, ⓐⓑlemongrass, ⓐⓑgeranium, ⓐⓑBalance, ⓐⓑPurify, ⓐⓑcypress, ⓐⓑjuniper berry, ⓐⓑginger, ⓐⓑhelichrysum

—Parasympathetic Nervous System:

The parasympathetic nervous system functions to slow heart rate, store energy, stimulate digestive activity, and relax specific muscles. It allows the body to return to a normal and calm state after experiencing pain or stress.

Oils: ⓐⓑlavender⊕ (stimulates), ⓐⓑlemongrass (regulates), ⓐⓑmarjoram (tones), ⓐⓑSerenity, ⓐⓑBalance

—Parkinson's Disease: *See Parkinson's Disease*

—Sympathetic Nervous System:

The sympathetic nervous system functions to accelerate heart rate, increase blood pressure, slow digestion, and constrict blood vessels in most tissues and organs, while dilating arterioles in the skeletal muscles where increased blood flow is needed. It activates the "fight or flight" response in order to deal with threatening or stressful situations.

Oils: ⓐⓑgrapefruit⊕ (stimulates), ⓐⓑeucalyptus, ⓐⓑpeppermint, ⓐⓑginger

A B C D E F G H I J K L M **N** O P Q R S T U V W X Y Z

Primary Recommendations • Secondary Recommendations • Other Recommendations / ⓐ=Aromatic, ⓑ=Topical, ⓞ=Internal

The nervous system is a network of nerve cells that regulates the body's reaction to external and internal stimuli. The nervous system sends nerve impulses to organs and muscles throughout the body. The body relies on these impulses to function. The nervous system is comprised of the central nervous system (the brain and spinal cord) and the peripheral nervous system (all other nerves). The peripheral nervous system is comprised of the somatic nervous system (nerves that connect to the skeletal muscles and sensory nerve receptors in the skin) and the autonomic nervous system (nerves that connect to the cardiac and smooth muscles and other organs, tissues, and systems that don't require conscious effort to control). The autonomic system is divided further into two main parts: the sympathetic and parasympathetic nervous systems. The sympathetic nervous system functions to accelerate heart rate, increase blood pressure, slow digestion, and constrict blood vessels. It activates the "fight or flight" response in order to deal with threatening or stressful situations. The parasympathetic nervous system functions to slow heart rate, store energy, stimulate digestive activity, and relax specific muscles. It allows the body to return to a normal and calm state after experiencing pain or stress.

Common Nervous System Issues

Nervous: Alzheimer's Disease, Bell's Palsy, Carpal Tunnel Syndrome, Concussion, Dementia, Dizziness, Headache, Huntington's Disease, Lou Gehrig's Disease, Multiple Sclerosis, Neuralgia, Neuritis, Paralysis, Parkinson's Disease, Seizures, Stroke

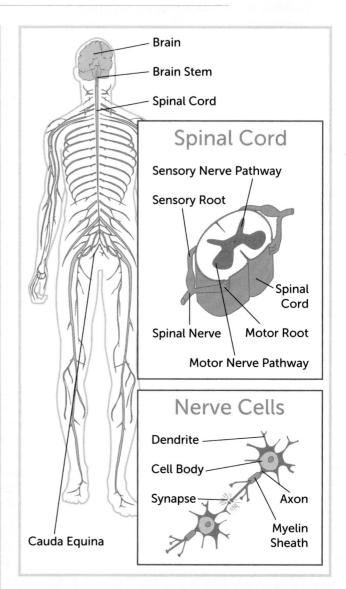

Oils for Nervous System Support

Oils: peppermint (soothes and strengthens damaged nerves), basil (stimulates), lavender, lemon, grapefruit, frankincense, bergamot, cedarwood (nervous tension), lemongrass (for nerve damage), marjoram (soothing), geranium (regenerates), Serenity, Roman chamomile, juniper berry, vetiver, cinnamon, ginger, orange, sandalwood

—Virus of Nerves: *See also Antiviral*

Oils: ⊘frankincense, ⊘clove

⊜: Dilute as recommended, and apply 1–3 drops on location, spine, back of neck, and reflex points on the feet. Add 2–4 drops to 1 Tbs. (15 ml) fractionated coconut oil, and massage on location. Add 1–2 drops to warm bathwater, and bathe.

⊘: Diffuse into the air. Inhale directly from bottle. Apply oil to hands, tissue, or cotton wick, and inhale.

◐: Take 1–2 drops of oil in a capsule or in a beverage. Take capsules as directed on package.

⊕: **Body System(s) Affected:** Nervous System.

▥: **Additional Research:**

Peppermint: Pretreatment of human and rat astrocyte cells (cells found in the nerve and brain that support the blood-brain barrier and help repair the brain and spinal cord following injuries) with peppermint oil was found to inhibit heat-shock induced apoptosis of these cells (Koo et al., 2001).

Lavender: Lavender oil scent was found to lower sympathetic nerve activity and blood pressure, while elevating parasympathetic nerve activity in rats. It was further found that applying an anosmia-inducing agent (something that causes a loss of smell) eliminated the effects of the lavender oil scent (Tanida et al., 2006).

Lavender: Lavender oil was found to inhibit sympathetic nerve activity, while exciting parasympathetic nerve activity in rats. Linalool, a component of lavender, was shown to have similar effects (Shen et al., 2005).

Lemon: Inhaling the aroma of lemon essential oil was found to decrease pain response in rats and was also found to modulate the neuronal response to formalin-induced pain (Aloisi et al., 2002).

Lemon: Several constituents of lemon oil and their metabolites (chemicals made by these chemicals in the body) were found to increase the release of monoamines (various chemicals responsible for neurotransmission and neuro-modulation) in rat brain tissue, indicating a possible effect on brain nerve cell behavior (Fukumoto et al., 2006).

Lemon: Pretreatment of human and rat astrocyte cells (cells found in the nerve and brain that support the blood-brain barrier and help repair the brain and spinal cord following injuries) with lemon oil was found to inhibit heat-shock induced apoptosis of these cells (Koo et al., 2002).

Grapefruit: The scent of grapefruit oil and its component, limonene, was found to affect the autonomic nerves and reduce appetite and body weight in rats exposed to the oil for 15 minutes three times per week (Shen et al., 2005).

Grapefruit: Inhalation of essential oils such as pepper, estragon, fennel, and grapefruit was found to have a stimulating effect on sympathetic activity; while inhalation of essential oils of rose or patchouli caused a decrease in sympathetic activity in healthy adults (Haze et al., 2002).

Frankincense: Incensole acetate, isolated from frankincense resin, was found to demonstrate an anti-inflammatory and neuroprotective effect in mice with a closed head injury (Moussaieff et al., 2008).

Turmeric: *Curcuma longa* essential oil was found to increase the survival rate of neurons in a mouse model of ischemic stroke (Preeti et al., 2008).

Turmeric: Aromatic turmerone (ar-turmerone) from turmeric essential oil was found to protect neurons in the brain from damage by inhibiting inflammation in a mouse model (Chen et al., 2018).

Eucalyptus: 1,8 cineole (eucalyptol) was found to display an anti-inflammatory effect on rats in several tests and was found to exhibit antinociceptive (pain-reducing) effects in mice, possibly by depressing the central nervous system (Santos et al., 2000).

Nervousness

Nervousness is a state of high anxiety, distress, agitation, or psychological uneasiness.

Simple Solutions—Nervousness: Diffuse orange oil in an aromatherapy diffuser.

Oils: ⊘⊘orange, ⊘⊘spikenard, ⊘⊘neroli

⊘: Diffuse into the air. Inhale directly from bottle. Apply oil to hands, tissue, or cotton wick, and inhale.

⊜: Dilute as recommended, and apply 1–2 drops to temples.

⊕: **Body System(s) Affected:** Emotional Balance.

Nose

Oils: ⊘⊘melaleuca, ⊘⊘rosemary

Simple Solutions—Nosebleed: Combine 2 drops cypress, 1 drop helichrysum, and 2 drops lemon in 1 cup (250 ml) ice water. Soak a cloth in the water, and apply the cloth to nose and back of neck.

—Bleeding:

A nosebleed (medically called *epistaxis*) is the loss of blood through the nose. Nosebleeds are fairly common and can be caused by many factors. The most common causes of nosebleed are dry air that causes the nasal membrane to dry out and crack, allergies, nose trauma/injury, and colds and other viruses.

Oils: ⊘helichrysum, ⊘cypress, ⊘lemon, ⊘frankincense, ⊘lavender

—Nasal Nasopharynx:

The nasopharynx is the upper part of the throat (pharynx) situated behind the nose. The nasopharynx is responsible for carrying air from the nasal chamber into the trachea.

Oils: ⊘⊘eucalyptus

—Nasal Polyp:

A nasal polyp is an abnormal tissue growth inside the nose. Since nasal polyps are not cancerous, very small polyps generally do not cause any problems. But larger polyps can obstruct the nasal passage and make it difficult to breath or smell and can cause frequent sinus infections. Possible symptoms of polyps include runny nose, decreased sense of smell, decreased sense of taste, snoring, facial pain or headache, itching around the eyes, and persistent congestion.

A B C D E F G H I J K L M **N** O P Q R S T U V W X Y Z

Oils: ⊘⊘frankincense, ⊘⊘oregano, ⊘⊘Breathe, ⊘⊘peppermint, ⊘⊘Purify, ⊘⊘basil

—Olfactory Loss:

Olfactory loss (or anosmia) is the loss of one's ability to smell. The most common causes for olfactory loss are sinonasal disease, head injury, and infection of the upper respiratory tract.

Oils: ⊘⊘peppermint, ⊘⊘basil

—Rhinitis: *See also Allergies, Antiviral, Colds*

Rhinitis is an inflammation of the nasal mucous membrane (the moist lining inside the nasal cavity where mucus is produced that acts as an air filtration system by trapping incoming dirt particles and moving them away for disposal). Rhinitis can cause runny nose, nasal congestion, sneezing, ear problems, and phlegm in the throat. Rhinitis is commonly caused by viral infections and allergies and can be acute (short-term) or chronic (long-term).

Oils: ⊘⊘eucalyptus, ⊘⊘peppermint, ⊘⊘lemon⊕, ⊘⊘lavender, ⊘⊘basil

Other Products: ⊙TriEase Softgels

⊜: Dilute as recommended, and apply 1–2 drops on nose (use extreme caution to avoid getting oil in the eye). Dilute as recommended, and apply 1 drop to a cotton swab, and swab the inside of the nose.

⊘: Diffuse into the air, and inhale the vapors through the nose. Inhale directly from bottle. Apply oil to hands, tissue, or cotton wick, and inhale.

⊕: **Body System(s) Affected:** Respiratory System.

⊞: **Additional Research:**

Lemon: A study including 100 patients (ages 3–79) suffering from vasomotor allergic rhinopathy, showed that topical application of a citrus lemon based spray resulted in a total reduction of eosinophils granulocytes and mast cells. These results suggest that the lemon-based nasal spray is a good alternative to conventional medicine for the treatment of perennial and seasonal allergic and vasomotor rhinopathy (Ferrara et al., 2012).

Nursing

See Pregnancy/Motherhood: Lactation

Obesity

See Weight: Obesity

Odors

See Deodorant, Deodorizing

Oral Conditions

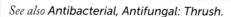

*See also **Antibacterial, Antifungal: Thrush**.*

—Abscess:

A tooth abscess is a collection of pus at the root of an infected tooth. The main symptom of a tooth abscess is a painful, persistent, throbbing toothache. The infected tooth may be sensitive to heat, cold, and pressure caused by chewing. Later symptoms may include swelling in the face, swollen lymph nodes in the neck or jaw, and a fever. Abscesses may eventually rupture, leaving a foul-tasting fluid in the mouth. If left untreated, an abscess can spread to other areas of the head and neck.

Oils: ⊘clove, ⊘On Guard, ⊘Purify, ⊘helichrysum, ⊘melaleuca, ⊘frankincense, ⊘Roman chamomile, ⊘wintergreen

Other Products: ⊘On Guard Natural Whitening Toothpaste, ⊘On Guard Mouthwash

Blend 1: Blend 1 drop each of clove, wintergreen, myrrh, and helichrysum to help with infection.

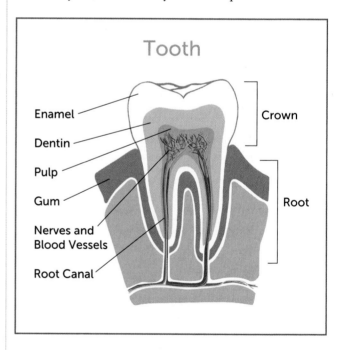

Tooth

Enamel
Dentin
Pulp
Gum
Nerves and Blood Vessels
Root Canal

Crown
Root

—Cavities:

A cavity is a decayed area or hole in a tooth caused by bacteria in the mouth. A cavity that is allowed to progress without treatment can result in pain, infection, and loss of the tooth. Good oral hygiene and eating less sugar can help to reduce the risk of cavities.

See the *Quick Usage Chart* inside the back cover for recommended dilutions.

Simple Solutions—Cavity: Apply 1 drop clove on location to help soothe pain.

Oils: ⊘On Guard, ⊘melaleuca⊕, ⊘peppermint⊕, ⊘eucalyptus⊕, ⊘cinnamon⊕

Other Products: ⊘On Guard Natural Whitening Toothpaste, ⊘On Guard Mouthwash

—Gums:

The gums (also called "gingiva") are the soft pink tissue surrounding the teeth. The gums form a seal around the teeth and are snugly attached to the bone underneath to withstand the friction of food passing over them in chewing.

Oils: ⊘myrrh, ⊘lavender, ⊘melaleuca, ⊘helichrysum, ⊘Roman chamomile

Other Products: ⊘On Guard Natural Whitening Toothpaste, ⊘On Guard Mouthwash

—Gum Disease:

Gum disease is an infection of the tissue and bones surrounding the teeth and is caused by a buildup of plaque. Gum disease consists of two parts: first gingivitis and then periodontal disease. Gingivitis is an inflammation of the gums because of bacteria associated with plaque buildup. When infected with gingivitis, the gums become red and swollen and often bleed during teeth brushing. Periodontal disease occurs when gingivitis is left untreated and becomes progressively worse. The inflamed gums begin pulling away from the teeth and leave empty pockets where food particles can easily collect and become infected. As the disease progresses, the gums pull farther away from the teeth and the bacteria eats away at the tissue and bone. As this occurs, the teeth lose their anchoring and can fall out.

Simple Solutions—Gingivitis/Gum Disease: Add 2 drops myrrh to ¼ tsp. (2 g) baking soda. Apply on gum lines, and leave for 60 seconds. Rinse mouth with water, and spit out.

Oils: ⊘melaleuca⊕, ⊘On Guard, ⊘myrrh, ⊘helichrysum, ⊘rose

Other Products: ⊘On Guard Natural Whitening Toothpaste, ⊘On Guard Mouthwash

—Halitosis (Bad Breath):

Halitosis is the technical term for "bad breath." Common causes of halitosis include smoking, drinking, poor oral hygiene, gum disease, dry mouth, tooth decay, and certain foods.

Simple Solutions—Halitosis: Add 10–15 drops peppermint or spearmint to 1 tsp. (5 ml) water in a small spray bottle. Shake, and spray 1–2 sprays in mouth as needed.

Oils: ⊘peppermint⊕, ⊘On Guard, ⊘patchouli, ⊘lavender

Other Products: ⊘On Guard Natural Whitening Toothpaste, ⊘On Guard Mouthwash

—Mouth Ulcers:

Mouth ulcers are open, often painful, sores that occur in the mouth. Common mouth ulcers include canker sores and cold sores. Stress, anxiety, fatigue, injury, illness, hormonal changes, and food allergies can often trigger mouth ulcers.

Oils: ⊘basil, ⊘myrrh, ⊘orange

Other Products: ⊘On Guard Natural Whitening Toothpaste, ⊘On Guard Mouthwash

—Teeth Grinding:

Teeth grinding (also called bruxism) is the habit of clenching the teeth and rubbing them against one another. Teeth grinding often occurs unconsciously while a person is asleep. If teeth grinding is frequent, it can lead to tooth damage, jaw pain, and headaches.

Oils: ⊘⊘Serenity

—Teething Pain:

Around ages 4–7 months, a baby will get his or her first teeth. Some infants teethe without discomfort; but for other infants, teething can be a painful process. Common symptoms of teething include irritability or fussiness, drooling, chin rash, biting, difficulty sleeping, and low-grade fever.

Oils: ⊘lavender

—Toothache:

A toothache is a pain around a tooth. Toothaches can result from many factors, including infection, injury, decay, jaw problems, cavities, damaged fillings, and gum disease. Common symptoms of a toothache include sharp or

A B C D E F G H I J K L M N O P Q R S T U V W X Y Z

throbbing pain, swelling around the tooth, fever, headache, and foul-tasting drainage from the infected tooth.

Oils: ⊘clove, ⊘melaleuca, ⊘Purify, ⊘Roman chamomile

Other Products: ⊘On Guard Natural Whitening Toothpaste, ⊘On Guard Mouthwash

—**Toothpaste:**

Oils: ⊘On Guard

Other Products: ⊘On Guard Natural Whitening Toothpaste

Recipe 1: Mix 1–2 drops On Guard with ½ tsp. (3 g) baking soda to form a paste, and use as toothpaste to brush onto the teeth.

⊘: Dilute as recommended, and apply 1–2 drops on location or along jawbone. Apply the oils with a hot compress on the face. Use On Guard Natural Whitening Toothpaste as directed. Dilute as recommended, and apply 1–2 drops to a small cotton ball or cotton swab; swab on location. Mix 1–2 drops with ½ cup (125 ml) of water, and use as mouth-rinse. Add 1–2 drops to toothpaste. Place 5–6 drops with 2 Tbs. (25 ml) distilled water in a small spray bottle, and mist into the mouth.

⊘: Diffuse into the air.

⊕: **Body System(s) Affected:** Skeletal System and Skin.

⊞: **Additional Research:**

Melaleuca: Among several oils tested, tea tree (melaleuca), manuka, and eucalyptus demonstrated strong antibacterial activity against detrimental oral bacteria (Takarada et al., 2004).

Melaleuca: Tea tree, peppermint, and sage oils were found to inhibit oral bacteria, with thymol and eugenol being the most active components of these oils (Shapiro et al., 1994).

Melaleuca: Cinnamon oil exhibited a strong antimicrobial activity against two detrimental oral bacteria. Manuka, tea tree, and the component thymol also exhibited antimicrobial potency (Filoche et al., 2005).

Melaleuca: In 34 patients with fixed orthodontic appliances, a dental gel containing 5% melaleuca essential oil performed better than Colgate Total gel when comparing microbial biofilm and quantification of *Streptococcus mutans* in the patients' saliva (Santamaria et al., 2014).

Peppermint: Peppermint oil blended with toothpaste was found to be more effective at lower concentrations in inhibiting the formation of dental plaque than chlorhexidine (an antiseptic) in human volunteers (Shayegh et al., 2008).

Peppermint: Peppermint and rosemary oils were each found to be more effective at preventing dental biofilm (plaque) formation than chlorhexidine (an antiseptic) (Rasooli et al., 2008).

Eucalyptus: Among several oils tested, tea tree (melaleuca), manuka, and eucalyptus demonstrated strong antibacterial activity against detrimental oral bacteria (Takarada et al., 2004).

Eucalyptus: Subjects using a mouthwash containing thymol, menthol, methyl salicylate, and eucalyptol for 6 months were found to not have developed oral bacteria that were resistant to the oils (Charles et al., 2000).

Cinnamon: Cinnamon oil exhibited a strong antimicrobial activity against two detrimental oral bacteria. Manuka, tea tree, and the component thymol also exhibited antimicrobial potency (Filoche et al., 2005).

Osteomyelitis

See Skeletal System: Osteomyelitis

Osteoporosis

See Skeletal System: Osteoporosis

Ovaries

Ovaries are the female reproductive organs in which eggs are produced and stored.

Oils: ⊘⊘rosemary (regulates), ⊘⊘geranium, ⊘⊘Whisper, ⊘⊘DigestZen

—**Ovarian Cyst:**

An ovarian cyst is a fluid-filled sac within the ovary. While ovarian cysts are common, and most cause no problems, they may cause feelings of aching or pressure and can cause pain, bleeding, and other problems if they become too large or become twisted or rupture.

Oils: ⊘⊘basil

⊘: Dilute as recommended, and apply 1–2 drops on abdomen and reflex points on the feet. Add 1–2 drops to 1 Tbs. (15 ml) fractionated coconut oil, and massage into abdomen and lower back. Apply as a warm compress to the abdomen. Add 1–2 drops to 2 tsp. (10 ml) olive oil, insert into vagina, and retain overnight with a tampon.

⊘: Diffuse into the air. Inhale directly from bottle. Apply oil to hands, tissue, or cotton wick, and inhale.

⊕: **Body System(s) Affected:** Reproductive Systems.

Overeating

See Eating Disorders: Overeating

Overweight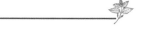

See Weight

See the *Quick Usage Chart* inside the back cover for recommended dilutions.

338

Oxygenating

The term "oxygenate" means to supply, to treat, or to infuse with oxygen. All of the cells in the body require oxygen to create the energy necessary to live and function correctly. The brain consumes 20% of the oxygen we inhale.

Oils: 🜋🜊sandalwood, 🜋🜊frankincense, 🜋🜊oregano, 🜋🜊fennel

🌀: Diffuse into the air. Inhale directly from bottle. Apply oil to hands, tissue, or cotton wick, and inhale.

🜊: Dilute as recommended, and apply 1–2 drops to forehead, chest, and sinuses.

Pain

> *Simple Solutions—Pain:* Add 25 drops Deep Blue to 1 Tbs. (15 ml) fractionated coconut oil to make a soothing massage oil for sore muscles.

> *Simple Solutions—Pain:* Combine 15 drops lavender with 1 tsp. (5 ml) jojoba oil in a small roll-on bottle, and apply on small cuts or scrapes to help soothe pain.

Oils: 🜋🜋lavender🜊, 🜊eucalyptus🜊, 🜊Deep Blue, 🜊Rescuer, 🜋lemon🜊, 🜊rosemary🜊, 🜊clove🜊, 🜊cypress, 🜊fir, 🜊helichrysum, 🜊geranium, 🜊frankincense, 🜊lemongrass, 🜊marjoram, 🜊melaleuca, 🜊peppermint, 🜊rosemary, 🜊wintergreen, 🜊blue tansy

Other Products: 🜊Deep Blue Rub and ⭕Deep Blue Polyphenol Complex to help soothe muscles and joints. ⭕Alpha CRS+, ⭕a2z Chewable to help relieve oxidation associated with inflammation that contributes to pain.

—Bone:

Bone pain is a gnawing, throbbing sensation in the bones and has many possible causes, including fractures, cancer, infection, injury, leukemia, and osteoporosis.

Oils: 🜊Deep Blue, 🜊Rescuer, 🜊wintergreen, 🜊lavender, 🜊cypress, 🜊juniper berry, 🜊fir, 🜊cedarwood, 🜊helichrysum, 🜊peppermint, 🜊sandalwood

—Chronic:

Chronic pain is generally defined as pain that lasts three months or longer.

Oils: 🜊Deep Blue, 🜊Rescuer, 🜊wintergreen, 🜊cypress, 🜊fir, 🜊juniper berry, 🜊helichrysum, 🜊cedarwood, 🜊ginger ⭕, 🜊peppermint, 🜊sandalwood

—General:

Oils: 🜊Deep Blue, 🜊Rescuer, 🜊wintergreen, 🜊lavender, 🜊cypress, 🜊marjoram, 🜊fir, 🜊helichrysum, 🜊peppermint, 🜊sandalwood

—Inflammation: *See also Inflammation*

Oils: 🜊rosemary⭕, 🜊eucalyptus⭕, 🜊lavender⭕, 🜊Deep Blue, 🜊Rescuer,

Other Products: 🜊Deep Blue Rub and ⭕Deep Blue Polyphenol Complex

—Joints:

Oils: 🜊Deep Blue, 🜊Rescuer, 🜊wintergreen, 🜊Roman chamomile

Other Products: 🜊Deep Blue Rub and ⭕Deep Blue Polyphenol Complex

—Muscle:

Oils: 🜊Deep Blue, 🜊Rescuer, 🜊fir, 🜊clove, 🜊lavender, 🜊lemongrass (ligaments), 🜊cypress, 🜊marjoram, 🜊helichrysum, 🜊peppermint, 🜊sandalwood, 🜊wintergreen

Other Products: 🜊Deep Blue Rub and ⭕Deep Blue Polyphenol Complex

—Tissue:

Oils: 🜊Deep Blue, 🜊Rescuer, 🜊helichrysum

Other Products: 🜊Deep Blue Rub and ⭕Deep Blue Polyphenol Complex

🜊: Dilute as recommended, and apply 1–2 drops on location. Combine with carrier oil, and massage into affected muscles and joints. Apply as a warm compress over affected areas.

⭕: Take capsules as directed on package.

🌀: Diffuse into the air. Inhale oil that is applied to a tissue or cotton wick.

✦: **Body System(s) Affected:** Nervous System, Skeletal System, Muscles, and Skin.

📖: **Additional Research:**

Lavender: Lavender oil was found to work as an anaesthetic (reducing pain) in a rabbit reflex test (Ghelardini et al., 1999).

Lavender: Oil from *Lavandula angustifolia* was found to reduce writhing in induced writhing in rats and to reduce edema (swelling) in carrageenan-induced paw edema, indicating an anti-inflammatory effect (Hajhashemi et al., 2003).

Lavender: The odor of lavender combined with relaxing music was found to lessen the intensity of pain following a vascular wound dressing change (Kane et al., 2004).

Lavender: In patients suffering from arthritis, it was found that a blend of lavender, marjoram, eucalyptus, rosemary, peppermint, and carrier oils reduced perceived pain and depression compared to a control (Kim et al., 2005).

Eucalyptus: A combination of peppermint oil and ethanol was found to have a significant analgesic effect with a reduction in sensitivity to headache; while a combination of peppermint, eucalyptus, and ethanol was found to relax muscles and to increase cognitive performance in humans (Göbel et al., 1994).

Eucalyptus: 1,8 cineole (eucalyptol) was found to have antinociceptive (pain-reducing) properties similar to morphine. Beta-pinene was found to reverse the effects of morphine in a degree similar to naloxone (a drug used to counter the effects of morphine overdose) (Liapi et al., 2007).

Eucalyptus: 1,8 cineole (eucalyptol) was found to display an anti-inflammatory effect on rats in several tests and was found to exhibit antinociceptive (pain-reducing) effects in mice, possibly by depressing the central nervous system (Santos et al., 2000).

Lemon: Inhaling the aroma of lemon essential oil was found to decrease pain response in rats and was also found to modulate the neuronal response to formalin-induced pain (Aloisi et al., 2002).

Lemon: Rats exposed long-term to lemon essential oil were found to demonstrate different anxiety and pain threshold levels than untreated rats. It was also found that exposure to lemon oil induced chemical changes in the neuronal circuits involved in anxiety and pain (Ceccarelli et al., 2004).

Rosemary: In patients suffering from arthritis, it was found that a blend of lavender, marjoram, eucalyptus, rosemary, peppermint, and carrier oils reduced perceived pain and depression compared to a control (Kim et al., 2005).

Rosemary: A combination of peppermint oil and ethanol was found to have a significant analgesic effect with a reduction in sensitivity to headache; while a combination of peppermint, eucalyptus, and ethanol was found to relax muscles and to increase cognitive performance in humans (Göbel et al., 1994).

Rosemary: 1,8 cineole (eucalyptol) was found to have antinociceptive (pain-reducing) properties similar to morphine. Beta-pinene was found to reverse the effects of morphine in a degree similar to naloxone (a drug used to counter the effects of morphine overdose) (Liapi et al., 2007).

Rosemary: An ethanol extract of rosemary was found to demonstrate antinociceptive (pain-blocking) and anti-inflammatory activity in mice and rats (González-Trujano et al., 2007).

Rosemary: Rosemary oil was found to have anti-inflammatory and peripheral antinociceptive (pain sensitivity–blocking) properties in mice (Takaki et al., 2008).

Clove: Beta-caryophyllene (found in clove oil) demonstrated anaesthetic (pain-reducing) activity in rats and rabbits (Ghelardini et al., 2001).

Rosemary: 1,8 cineole (eucalyptol) was found to display an anti-inflammatory effect on rats in several tests and was found to exhibit antinociceptive (pain-reducing) effects in mice, possibly by depressing the central nervous system (Santos et al., 2000).

Rosemary: An ethanol extract of rosemary was found to demonstrate antinociceptive (pain-blocking) and anti-inflammatory activity in mice and rats (González-Trujano et al., 2007).

Rosemary: Rosemary oil was found to have anti-inflammatory and peripheral antinociceptive (pain sensitivity–blocking) properties in mice (Takaki et al., 2008).

Coriander: Injection of coriander extract in mice was found to have a greater analgesic effect than dexamethasone (an anti-inflammatory drug) or stress, when mice were subjected to acute and chronic pain tests (Taherian et al., 2012).

Ginger: A double-blind, placebo-controlled study demonstrated that aroma massage with ginger and orange essential oils relieved knee joint pain in elderly subjects more than the placebo (massage with olive oil) or the control (conventional treatment without massage) (Yip et al., 2008).

Painting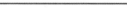

Add one 15 ml bottle of your favorite essential oil (or oil blend) to any 5-gallon bucket of paint. Stir vigorously, mixing well, and then either spray paint or paint by hand. This should eliminate the paint fumes and after-smell.

Palpitations

See Cardiovascular System: Palpitations

Pancreas

The pancreas is a gland organ located behind the stomach. The pancreas is responsible for producing insulin and other hormones and for producing "pancreatic juices" that aid in digestion.

Oils: ⊘cypress, ⊘rosemary, ⊘⊘Breathe, ⊘⊘lemon, ⊘⊘On Guard

—Pancreatitis:

Pancreatitis is the term used to describe pancreas inflammation. Pancreatitis occurs when the pancreatic juices that are designed to aid in digestion in the small intestine become active while still inside the pancreas. When this occurs, the pancreas literally begins to digest itself. Acute pancreatitis lasts for only a short time and then resolves itself. Chronic pancreatitis does not resolve itself but instead gradually destroys the pancreas.

Oils: ⊘⊘lemon, ⊘⊘marjoram

—Stimulant For:

Oils: ⊘helichrysum

—Support:

Oils: ⊘⊘cinnamon, ⊘⊘geranium, ⊘⊘fennel

⊜: Dilute as recommended, and apply 1–2 drops over pancreas area or on reflex points on the feet.

⊘: Diffuse into the air. Inhale directly from bottle. Apply oil to hands, tissue, or cotton wick, and inhale.

⊕: **Body System(s) Affected:** Endocrine System and Digestive System.

Panic

See Anxiety

Paralysis

See Nervous System: Paralysis

See the *Quick Usage Chart* inside the back cover for recommended dilutions.

340

Parasites

A parasite is an organism that grows on or in another organism at the host organism's expense. A parasite cannot live independently and is fed and sheltered by the host organism without making any helpful contribution itself.

Oils: oregano, thyme, fennel, Roman chamomile, DigestZen, lavender, melaleuca, clove

Other Products: DigestZen Softgels

—Intestinal:

Intestinal parasites are parasites that infect the intestinal tract. These parasites enter the intestinal tract through the mouth by unwashed or uncooked food, contaminated water, and unclean hands. Symptoms of intestinal parasites include diarrhea, abdominal pain, weight loss, fatigue, gas or bloating, nausea or vomiting, stomach pain, passing a worm in a stool, stools containing blood and mucus, and rash or itching around the rectum or vulva.

Oils: lemon, oregano, Roman chamomile

—Worms:

Parasitic worms are worm-like organisms that live inside another living organism and feed off their host organism at the host organism's expense, causing weakness and disease. Parasitic worms can live inside of animals as well as humans.

Oils: DigestZen, lavender, rosemary, thyme, peppermint, Roman chamomile, bergamot, melaleuca

Blend 1: Combine 6 drops Roman chamomile, 6 drops eucalyptus, 6 drops lavender, and 6 drops lemon with 2 Tbs. (25 ml) fractionated coconut oil. Apply 10–15 drops over abdomen with a hot compress, and apply 1–2 drops on intestine and colon reflex points on the feet.

○: Place 2–4 drops essential oil in empty capsule, and swallow. Add 1–2 drops to ½ cup (125 ml) rice or almond milk; drink.

◒: Apply as warm compress over abdomen. Add 2–3 drops to 1 Tbs. (15 ml) fractionated coconut oil, and apply as rectal retention enema for 15 minutes or more. Dilute as recommended, and apply to abdomen and reflex points on the feet.

⊕: **Body System(s) Affected:** Immune System and Skin.

⊞: **Additional Research:**

Oregano: Oregano oil administered orally was found to improve gastrointestinal symptoms in 7 of 11 patients who had tested positive for the parasite Blastocystis hominis and was found to cause disappearance of this parasite in 8 cases (Force et al., 2000).

Lavender: Essential oil from *Lavandula angustifolia* demonstrated ability to eliminate protozoal pathogens Giardia duodenalis, Trichomonas vaginalis, and Hexamita inflata at concentrations of 1% or less (Moon et al., 2006).

Melaleuca: Melaleuca oil was effective at killing *Anisakis simplex* larva in vitro. Data suggests that the mechanism of action against anisakis involves inhibition of acetylcholinesterase (Gómez-Rincón et al., 2014).

Parasympathetic Nervous System

See **Nervous System: Parasympathetic Nervous System**

Parkinson's Disease

Parkinson's disease is a progressive neurodegenerative disease marked by impairment of muscle movement and speech. Symptoms of Parkinson's disease include slowed motion, muscle stiffness, difficulty maintaining balance, impaired speech, loss of automatic movements (such as blinking, smiling, and swinging the arms while walking), and hand tremors.

Oils: cinnamon, marjoram, lavender, clary sage, frankincense, Balance, sandalwood, Serenity, vetiver, cypress (circulation), bergamot, geranium, helichrysum, juniper berry, lemon, orange, peppermint, rosemary, thyme

Other Products: Mito2Max to help support healthy nerve function. Alpha CRS+, a2z Chewable contain Coenzyme Q10, which has been studied for its potential benefits in alleviating Parkinson's disease. xEO Mega or vEO Mega for essential omega fatty acids that help support healthy nerve cell function.

◒: Add 5–10 drops essential oil to 1 Tbs. (15 ml) fractionated coconut oil and massage on affected muscles, back, legs, and neck. Dilute as recommended and apply 1–2 drops to base of neck or reflex points on the feet. Add 3–5 drops to warm bathwater, and bathe.

○: Take capsules as directed on package.

◐: Diffuse into the air. Inhale directly from bottle. Apply oil to hands, tissue, or cotton wick, and inhale.

⊕: **Body System(s) Affected:** Nervous System and Muscles.

ⓘ: Additional Research:

Cinnamon: The process of α-syn protein aggregation is a major component of Parkinson's disease. Preventing α-syn aggregation may help in the treatment of Parkinson's disease. Researchers have discovered that an aqueous cinnamon extract precipitation has a curative effect on α-syn aggregation in a Drosophila model of Parkinson's disease. Furthermore, in vitro tests have revealed that the cinnamon extract has an inhibitory effect on the process of α-syn fibrillation (Shaltiel-Karyo et al., 2012).

Eugenol (found in cassia, cinnamon, and clove): Eugenol administration was found to prevent induced dopamine depression and lipid peroxidation inductivity in the mouse striatum model, suggesting that eugenol may be useful in the treatment of Parkinson's disease (Kabuto et al., 2007).

Coenzyme Q10: A study of Parkinson's disease patients found that CoQ10 was significantly lower in the cortex region of their brains than in the brains of healthy patients (Hargreaves et al., 2008).

Coenzyme Q10: Pretreatment of mice with CoQ10 was found to protect dopaminergic neurons from iron-induced oxidative stress that has been theorized to play a role in the development of Parkinson's disease (Kooncumchoo et al., 2006).

Coenzyme Q10: A mitochondrial defect in fibroblast cells cultivated from 18 Parkinson's disease patients was found to be ameliorated in 50% of these cells treated with CoQ10 (Winkler-Stuck, 2004).

Pelvic Pain Syndrome

Pelvic pain syndrome is characterized by pain in the pelvis area that continues for several months. Symptoms include severe and steady pain, dull aching, a feeling of pressure deep in the pelvis, painful bowel movements, pain during intercourse, and pain when sitting down.

> *Simple Solutions—Pelvic Pain Syndrome:* Add 3 drops ginger and 2 drops geranium to 1 tsp. (5 ml) jojoba oil. Place oil mixture in warm bathwater as a soothing bath oil.

Oils: ⬡ginger, ⬡geranium, ⬡clove, ⬡bergamot, ⬡thyme, ⬡rose

●: Place 2–3 drops in warm bathwater, and soak for 10 minutes. Add 5–10 drops to 1 Tbs. (15 ml) fractionated coconut oil, and massage on pelvis and upper legs.

Periodontal Disease

See Oral Conditions: Gum Disease

Pests

See Insects/Bugs, Mice

Phlebitis

See Cardiovascular System: Phlebitis

Pimples

See Acne

Pink Eye

See Eyes: Pink Eye

Pineal Gland

The pineal gland is a tiny endocrine gland located close to the center of the brain. It is responsible for producing the hormone melatonin that regulates the sleep/wake cycle. The pineal gland also serves to regulate blood pressure, sexual development, growth, body temperature, and motor function.

Oils: ⬡frankincense, ⬡sandalwood, ⬡vetiver, ⬡ginger, ⬡cedarwood

●: Diffuse into the air. Inhale oil directly from bottle. Apply oil to hands, tissue, or cotton wick, and inhale.

●: **Body System(s) Affected:** Endocrine System.

Pituitary Gland

The pituitary gland is a small endocrine gland located at the base of the brain that secretes hormones directly into the bloodstream. It is composed of three different lobes, each responsible for producing a different set of hormones. The anterior lobe secretes the human growth hormone (stimulates overall body growth), adrenocorticotropic hormone (controls hormone secretion by the adrenal cortex), thyrotropic hormone (stimulates activity of the thyroid gland), and the gonadotropic hormones (control growth and reproductive activity of the ovaries and testes). The intermediate lobe stimulates melanocytes (control pigmentation such as skin color) The posterior lobe secretes antidiuretic hormone (causes water retention by the kidneys) and oxytocin (stimulates the mammary glands to release milk and causes uterine contractions). The pituitary gland is often referred to as the "master" endocrine gland because it controls the functioning of the other endocrine glands.

Oils: ⬡frankincense, ⬡sandalwood, ⬡vetiver, ⬡ginger

—Balances:

Oils: ⬡⬡ylang ylang, ⬡⬡geranium

—Increases Oxygen:

Oils: ⬡⬡frankincense, ⬡⬡sandalwood

See the *Quick Usage Chart* inside the back cover for recommended dilutions.

⊘: Diffuse into the air. Inhale oil directly from bottle. Apply oil to hands, tissue, or cotton wick, and inhale.

⊜: Dilute as recommended, and apply 1–2 drops to forehead, back of neck, and reflex points on big toes.

⊕: **Body System(s) Affected:** Endocrine System.

Plague

See also Antibacterial

Plague is a potentially deadly bacterial disease that is caused by the *Yersinia pestis* bacteria, which is transmitted to humans and animals through close contact or through bites from fleas that have previously bitten infected animals. Symptoms include fever, headaches, and extremely swollen and hot lymph nodes. If left untreated, plague can quickly invade the lungs—causing severe pneumonia, high fever, bloody coughing, and death.

Oils: ⊘⊜clove, ⊘⊜On Guard, ⊘⊜frankincense, ⊘⊜oregano

⊜: Dilute as recommended, and apply to neck, chest, and reflex points on the feet.

⊘: Diffuse into the air.

⊕: **Body System(s) Affected:** Immune System.

Plaque

See Antibacterial, Oral Conditions

Pleurisy

See Antibacterial, Respiratory System: Pleurisy

PMS

See Female-Specific Conditions: PMS

Pneumonia

See also Respiratory System, Antibacterial, Antifungal, Antiviral

Pneumonia is an illness characterized by lung inflammation in which the lungs are infected by a bacteria, fungus, or virus. The result is a cough, chest pain, difficulty breathing, fever, shaking chills, headache, muscle pain, and fatigue. Pneumonia is a special concern for young children and individuals over the age of 65. Pneumonia ranges in seriousness from mild to life threatening.

> *Simple Solutions—Pneumonia:* Diffuse Breathe in a misting aromatherapy diffuser for 15 minutes every hour throughout the day.

Oils: ⊘⊜Breathe, ⊘⊜On Guard, ⊘⊜thyme⊕, ⊘cinnamon⊕, ⊘⊜oregano⊕, ⊘⊜eucalyptus, ⊘⊜melaleuca, ⊘⊜lavender, ⊘lemon, ⊘⊜tangerine⊕, ⊘⊜frankincense, ⊘⊜myrrh

Other Products: ⊙On Guard+ Softgels

⊘: Diffuse into the air. Place 4 drops in ½ cup (125 ml) hot water, and inhale steam deeply.

⊙: Take capsules as directed on package.

⊜: Dilute as recommended, and apply to chest, back, and reflex points on the feet. Apply as warm compress to the chest. Place 2–3 drops in 1 tsp. (5 ml) fractionated coconut oil; place oil in rectum, and retain overnight.

⊕: **Body System(s) Affected:** Immune System and Respiratory System.

⊡: **Additional Research:**

Thyme: Oils with aldehyde or phenol as major components demonstrated a high level of antibacterial activity (Inouye et al., 2001).

Thyme: Cinnamon, thyme, and clove essential oils demonstrated an antibacterial effect on several respiratory tract pathogens (Fabio et al., 2007).

Cinnamon: Oils with aldehyde or phenol as major components demonstrated a high level of antibacterial activity (Inouye et al., 2001).

Cinnamon: Cinnamon, thyme, and clove essential oils demonstrated an antibacterial effect on several respiratory tract pathogens (Fabio et al., 2007).

Oregano: Oregano oil was found to kill antibiotic resistant strains of Staph, *E. coli*, Klebsiella pneumoniae, *Helicobacter pylori*, and Mycobacterium terrae (Preuss et al., 2005).

Tangerine: In rats with induced pulmonary fibrosis oral treatment of hydrodistilled tangerine essential oil suppressed body weight loss and significantly improved scores of alveolitis and fibrosis of lung tissue. The effects of tangerine essential oil on lung fibrosis were associated with free radical scavenging and antioxidant activity (Zhou et al., 2012).

Poison Ivy/Oak

Poison oak and poison ivy are plants with an oily sap called urushiol that causes an itchy rash when it comes into contact with the skin. Infection by poison oak or poison ivy is recognized by redness and itching of the skin, a rash, red bumps, and later oozing blisters. A rash caused by poison oak or by poison ivy usually lasts from 5 to12 days.

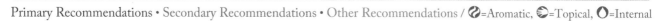

Primary Recommendations • Secondary Recommendations • Other Recommendations / ⊘=Aromatic, ⊜=Topical, ⊙=Internal

Simple Solutions—Poison Oak/Ivy: Wash skin
with soap and water as soon as possible after
contact. If rash and itching develop, add 10
drops lavender and 10 drops Roman chamomile
to ½ cup (125 ml) calamine lotion. Apply a
small amount on affected areas up to twice per
day as needed.

Oils: rose, lavender, Elevation, Roman chamomile

: Dilute as recommended, and apply 1–2 drops on location. Add 2–3 drops to 1 tsp. (5 ml) fractionated coconut oil, and apply on location.

: **Body System(s) Affected:** Skin.

Pollution

See Purification

Polyps

See Colon: Polyps, Nose: Nasal Polyp

Pregnancy/Motherhood

Pregnancy is the period of time (generally 9 months) in which a woman carries a developing fetus in her uterus.

Oils: geranium, ylang ylang, lavender, grapefruit, Roman chamomile

Other Products: Alpha CRS+, a2z Chewable, xEO Mega or vEO Mega, Microplex VMz for nutrients essential to support cellular health and body function.

—**Anxiety/Tension:** *See Calming*

—**Baby (Newborn):**

Oils: frankincense (1 drop on crown), myrrh (1 drop on umbilical cord and navel), Balance (1 drop on feet and spine)

: Apply as indicated above.

—**Breasts:**

In the first trimester of pregnancy, a woman's breasts become sore and tender as the body begins to prepare itself for breast-feeding. During pregnancy the breasts enlarge, the nipples grow larger and become darker, and the breasts may

begin to leak colostrum—the first milk the body makes in preparation for the developing baby.

Oils: lavender (soothes), geranium (soothes), Roman chamomile (sore nipples), fennel (tones)

: Add 3–5 drops to 1 Tbs. (15 ml) fractionated coconut oil, and massage on location.

—**Delivery:**

Delivery is the act or process of giving birth.

Oils: lavender (stimulates circulation, calming, antiseptic), clary sage, Balance

: Dilute as recommended, and apply 1–2 drops on hips, bottoms of feet, or abdomen. Add 3–5 drops to 1 Tbs. (15 ml) fractionated coconut oil, and massage on hips, bottoms of feet, or abdomen.

: Diffuse into the air. Inhale directly from bottle. Apply oil to hands, tissue, or cotton wick, and inhale.

—**Avoid Episiotomy:**

Oils: geranium

: Add 5–10 drops to ½ tsp. (2 ml) olive oil, and massage perineum.

—**Diffuse:**

Oils: Serenity, Elevation

: Diffuse into the air.

—**Uterus:**

Oils: clary sage

: Apply 1–3 drops around the ankles to help tone uterus.

—**Transition:**

Oils: basil

: Dilute as recommended, and apply 1–2 drops to temples or abdomen.

—**Early Labor:**

Preterm labor is labor that begins before the 37th week of pregnancy. Babies born before the 37th week are considered premature. Signs of preterm labor include contractions every 10 minutes or more often, cramps, low backache, pelvic pressure, and change in vaginal discharge (fluid or blood).

Oils: lavender

: Gently apply 1–3 drops on stomach or on heart area to help stop.

See the *Quick Usage Chart* inside the back cover for recommended dilutions.

344

−**Energy:**

Blend 1: Combine 2 drops Roman chamomile, 2 drops geranium, and 2 drops lavender in 2 tsp. (10 ml) fractionated coconut oil, and massage into the skin.

—**Hemorrhaging:**

Postpartum hemorrhaging is excessive bleeding following childbirth. It is commonly defined as losing 500 ml of blood after vaginal birth and 1000 ml of blood after a cesarean birth. Postpartum hemorrhaging generally occurs within 24 hours following the birth and can be life threatening if not stopped.

Oils: ⊜helichrysum

⊜: Apply 1–3 drops on lower back to help prevent hemorrhaging.

—**High Blood Pressure:**

High blood pressure can potentially be dangerous in pregnancy. High blood pressure can cause a decreased flow of blood to the placenta, slowing down the baby's growth; premature placenta separation from the uterus, taking away the baby's oxygen and nutrients and causing heavy bleeding in the mother; premature birth; and the risk of future disease. Pregnancy can in some cases actually cause a woman's blood pressure to increase.

Oils: ⊘⊜ylang ylang⊕, ⊘⊜eucalyptus⊕, ⊘⊜lavender, ⊘⊜clove, ⊘⊜clary sage, ⊘⊜lemon. **Note:** Avoid rosemary, thyme, and possibly peppermint.

Bath 1: Place 3 drops ylang ylang in bathwater, and bathe in the evening twice a week.

Blend 2: Combine 5 drops geranium, 8 drops lemongrass, and 3 drops lavender in 2 Tbs. (25 ml) fractionated coconut oil. Rub over heart and on reflex points on left foot and hand.

⊜: Dilute as recommended, and apply on location, on reflex points on feet and hands, and over heart.

⊘: Diffuse into the air. Apply oils to hands, and inhale oils from hands cupped over the nose. Inhale oil applied to a tissue or cotton wick.

—**Labor (during):**

Oils: ⊜clary sage (may combine with fennel), ⊜lavender⊕

⊜: Apply 3 drops around ankles or on abdomen.

—**Labor (post):**

Oils: ⊜lavender, ⊜geranium

⊜: Dilute as recommended, and apply 1–3 drops on abdomen, ankles, or bottoms of feet.

—**Lactation (Milk Production):**

Lactation is the production and secretion of milk from the mammary glands of females for the nourishment of their young offspring. Lactation is commonly referred to as "breast-feeding."

Simple Solutions—Nursing: Blend 3 drops lavender, 2 drops geranium, and 1 drop Roman chamomile with 1 Tbs. (15 ml) almond oil. Apply a small amount on breasts to help soothe. Wash off before feeding the baby.

Oils: ⊜clary sage (start production), ⊜fennel or ⊜basil (increase production), ⊜peppermint (decrease production), ⊜Whisper (contains jasmine⊕ that may help decrease production)

⊜: Dilute as recommended, and apply 1–2 drops on breasts. Apply peppermint with cold compress to help reduce production. *Caution: Fennel should not be used for more than 10 days, as it will excessively increase flow through the urinary tract.*

—**Mastitis:** *See also* **Antibacterial.**

Mastitis is a breast infection occurring in women who are breast-feeding. Mastitis causes the breast to become red, swollen, and very painful. Symptoms of mastitis include breast tenderness, fever, general lack of well-being, skin redness, and a breast that feels warm to the touch. Mastitis generally occurs in just one breast, not in both.

Oils: ⊜lavender, ⊜Citrus Bliss (combine with lavender), ⊜patchouli⊕

⊜: Dilute as recommended, and apply 1–2 drops on breasts.

—**Miscarriage (after):**

A miscarriage is a pregnancy that ends on its own within the first 20 weeks. Signs of a miscarriage include vaginal bleeding, fluid or tissue being ejected from the vagina, and pain and cramping in the abdomen or lower back. Miscarriages occur before the baby is developed enough to survive. About half of all pregnancies end in miscarriage, but most happen too early for the mother to be aware that it has occurred. Women who miscarry after about 8 weeks of pregnancy should consult their doctor as soon as possible afterwards to prevent any future complications.

Oils: frankincense, grapefruit, geranium, lavender, Roman chamomile

: Dilute 5–6 drops in 1 Tbs. (15 ml) fractionated coconut oil, and massage on back, legs, and arms. Add 3–4 drops to warm bathwater, and bathe.

—Morning Sickness:

Morning sickness is the nauseated feeling accompanying the first trimester of pregnancy for many women. Morning sickness can often include vomiting. For most women, morning sickness begins around the sixth week of pregnancy and ends around the twelfth week. Although it is called "morning" sickness, the symptoms can occur at any time during the day.

Simple Solutions—Morning Sickness: Add 2 drops ginger to a bowl of hot water, and inhale the warm vapor coming from the water.

Oils: ginger, peppermint, lemon

: Dilute as recommended, and apply 1–3 drops on ears, down jaw bone, and on reflex points on the feet.

: Place 1–3 drops in empty capsule; swallow capsule.

: Diffuse into the air. Inhale directly from bottle. Apply oil to hands, tissue, or cotton wick, and inhale. Apply 1 drop on pillow to inhale at night.

—Placenta:

The placenta is the organ responsible for sustaining life in an unborn baby. The placenta attaches to the uterus wall and connects to the mother's blood supply to provide nutrients and oxygen for the fetus. The placenta plays other essential roles as well: It removes waste created by the fetus, triggers labor and delivery, and protects the fetus against infection.

Oils: basil (to help retain)

: Dilute as recommended, and apply 1–2 drops on lower abdomen and reflex points on the feet.

—Postpartum Depression:

Postpartum depression is depression sometimes experienced by mothers shortly after giving birth. New mothers may experience symptoms such as irritableness, sadness, uncontrollable emotions, fatigue, anxiety, difficulty sleeping, thoughts of suicide, hopelessness, and guilt. Postpartum depression is typically thought to result from a hormonal imbalance caused by the pregnancy and childbirth.

Oils: Elevation, lemon, lavender, frankincense, clary sage, geranium, grapefruit, bergamot, Balance, myrrh, orange

: Diffuse into the air. Inhale directly from bottle. Apply oil to hands, tissue, or cotton wick, and inhale.

: Dilute as recommended, and apply 1–2 drops to temple or forehead. Add 5–10 drops to 1 Tbs. (15 ml) fractionated coconut oil, and use as massage oil. Add 1–3 drops to warm bathwater, and bathe.

—Preeclampsia: *See also Pregnancy/Motherhood: High Blood Pressure*

Preeclampsia, also known as toxemia, is pregnancy-induced high blood pressure. Symptoms include protein in the urine, elevated blood pressure levels, sudden weight gain, blurred vision, abdominal pains in the upper-right side, and swelling in the hands and face. Women suffering from preeclampsia are often put on bed rest for the remainder of the pregnancy to ensure the safety of the mother and baby.

Oils: cypress

: Dilute 1:1 in fractionated coconut oil, and apply 1–2 drops on bottoms of feet and on abdomen.

: Diffuse into the air. Inhale directly from bottle. Apply oil to hands, tissue, or cotton wick, and inhale.

—Self Love:

Oils: Elevation

: Diffuse into the air. Wear as perfume.

—Stretch Marks: *See Skin: Stretch Marks*

: **Body System(s) Affected:** Reproductive System and Endocrine System.

: **Additional Research:**

Lavender: A triple blind randomized placebo-controlled trial, consisting of 60 subjects and evaluating the use of lavender oil for Cesarean postoperative pain management, found that inhalation of lavender (when compared to inhalation of a placebo) decreased postoperative pain and increased patient satisfaction. Furthermore, patients inhaling lavender oil required significantly lower dosages of Diclofenac suppository as a supplemental analgesic drug than the placebo group. The researchers state that lavender essential oil is not recommended as the sole analgesic treatment (Olapour et al., 2013).

See the Quick Usage Chart inside the back cover for recommended dilutions.

Ylang ylang: Subjects who had ylang ylang oil applied to their skin had decreased blood pressure, increased skin temperature, and reported feeling more calm and relaxed compared to subjects in a control group (Hongratanaworakit et al., 2006).

Ylang ylang: Inhaled ylang ylang oil was found to decrease blood pressure and pulse rate and to enhance attentiveness and alertness in volunteers compared to an odorless control (Hongratanaworakit et al., 2004).

Eucalyptus: Treatment of rats with 1,8-cineole (or eucalyptol—found in eucalyptus, rosemary, and marjoram) demonstrated an ability to lower mean aortic pressure (blood pressure), without decreasing heart rate, through vascular wall relaxation (Lahlou et al., 2002).

Jasmine: Jasmine flowers applied to the breast were found to be as effective as the antilactation drug bromocriptine in reducing breast engorgement, milk production, and analgesic (pain-relieving drug) intake in women after giving birth. (Shrivastav et al., 1988).

Ginger: Ginger root given orally to pregnant women was found to decrease the severity of nausea and frequency of vomiting compared to control (Vutyavanich et al., 2001).

Lemon: A randomized clinical trial carried out on 100 pregnant women suffering from mild to moderate nausea found inhalation of lemon essential oil to be more effective at preventing nausea than inhalation of a carrier oil on days two and four of a four day trial (Yavari kia et al., 2014).

Patchouli: Patchouli alcohol (a tricyclic sesquiterpene and an essential oil of *Pogostemon cablin*) was found to inhibit chemically induced mastitis in a mouse model by inhibiting inflammation, suggesting patchouli may prevent mastitis (Li et al., 2014).

Lemon: Lemon oil vapor was found to have a strong antistress and antidepressant effects on mice subjected to several common stress tests (Komiya et al., 2006).

Lemon: Lemon oil and its component, citral, were found to decrease depressed behavior in a similar manner to antidepressant drugs in rats involved in several stress tests (Komori et al., 1995).

Lemon: In 12 patients suffering from depression, it was found that inhaling citrus aromas reduced the needed doses of antidepressants, normalized neuroendocrine hormone levels, and normalized immune function (Komori et al., 1995).

Lavender: Female students suffering from insomnia were found to sleep better and to have a lower level of depression during weeks they used a lavender fragrance when compared to weeks they did not use a lavender fragrance (Lee et al., 2006).

Lavender: Incensole acetate was found to open TRPV receptor in mice brain, a possible channel for emotional regulation (Moussaieff et al., 2008).

Lavender: Inhaling lavender oil was found to decrease the severity of labor pains in a small study of women giving birth for the first time (Yazdkhasti et al., 2016).

Prostate

The prostate gland is a small organ just beneath that bladder that is part of the male reproductive system. Its primary function is to create and store fluid that helps nourish and protect the sperm.

Oils: ☻helichrysum, ☻frankincense, ☻juniper berry

—Benign Prostatic Hyperplasia:

The size of the prostate begins at about the same size as a walnut but increases in size as a male ages. If the prostate grows too large, it can block passage of urine from the bladder through the urethra. This blockage can lead to increased risk for developing urinary tract stones, infections, or damaged kidneys.

Oils: ☻fennel

—Prostate Cancer: *See Cancer: Prostate*

—Prostatitis:

Prostatitis is an inflamed prostate, typically due to infection. This can cause pain in the lower back and groin area, painful urination, and the need to urinate frequently.

Oils: ☻thyme, ☻cypress, ☻lavender

☻: Dilute as recommended, and apply to the posterior, scrotum, ankles, lower back, or bottoms of feet.

◐: Add 5 drops to 1 Tbs. (15 ml) fractionated coconut oil, insert into rectum, and retain throughout the night.

✚: **Body System(s) Affected:** Reproductive System.

Psoriasis

Psoriasis is a skin condition characterized by patches of red, scaly skin that may itch or burn. The most commonly affected areas are the elbows, knees, scalp, back, face, palms, and feet. But other areas can be affected as well. Psoriasis doesn't have a known cure or cause, but it is thought an auto-immune disorder may play a role. Psoriasis tends to be less severe in the warmer months.

> *Simple Solutions—Psoriasis:* Combine 2 drops Roman chamomile with 2 drops lavender, and apply on location.

Oils: ☻helichrysum, ☻thyme, ☻lavender, ☻melaleuca, ☻Roman chamomile, ☻cedarwood, ☻bergamot

☻: Dilute as recommended, and apply 1–2 drops on location.

✚: **Body System(s) Affected:** Skin.

Pulmonary

See Respiratory System: Lungs

Purification

Oils: ☻Purify, ☻lemon, ☻lemongrass, ☻eucalyptus, ☻melaleuca, ☻cedarwood, ☻orange, ☻fennel

—Air:

Oils: ☻lemon, ☻peppermint, ☻Purify

—Cigarette Smoke:

   Oils: *Purify

—Dishes:

   Oils: lemon

—Water:

   Oils: lemon, Purify, peppermint

⊘: Diffuse into the air. Add 10–15 drops to 2 Tbs. (25 ml) distilled water in a small spray bottle; shake well, and mist into the air.

⊜: Add 1–2 drops to dishwater for sparkling dishes and a great smelling kitchen. Add 1–2 drops to warm bathwater, and bathe. Add 1–2 drops to bowl of water, and use to clean the outside of fruit and vegetables.

◐: Add 1 drop oil to 1½–2 cups (375–500 ml) of drinking water to help purify.

Pus

See Infection

Radiation

Radiation is energy emitted from a source and sent through space or matter. Different forms of radiation can include light, heat, sound, radio, micro-waves, gamma rays, or X-rays, among others. While many forms of radiation are around us every day and are perfectly safe (such as light, sound, and heat), frequent or prolonged exposure to high-energy forms of radiation can be detrimental to the body, possibly causing DNA mutation, damaged cellular structures, burns, cancer, or other damage.

Oils: peppermint, sandalwood

—Gamma Radiation:

   Oils: peppermint

—Radiation Therapy:

   Radiation treatments can produce tremendous toxicity within the liver. Cut down on the use of oils with high phenol content to prevent increasing liver toxicity. Oils with high phenol content include wintergreen, birch, clove, basil, fennel, oregano, thyme, melaleuca, and cinnamon.

—Ultraviolet Radiation:

   Oils: sandalwood, frankincense, melaleuca, thyme, clove

—Weeping Wounds From:

   Oils: melaleuca, thyme, oregano

◐: Place 1–2 drops under the tongue or place 2–3 drops in an empty capsule, and swallow.

⊜: Dilute as recommended, and apply 1–2 drops on location.

⊕: **Additional Research:**

Peppermint: In mice exposed to whole-body gamma irradiation, only 17% of mice who had been fed peppermint oil died; while 100% of mice who did not receive peppermint oil died. It was also found that the mice pre-fed peppermint oil were able to return blood cell levels to normal after 30 days, while control mice were not (and consequently died)—suggesting a protective or stimulating effect of the oil on blood stem cells (Samarth et al., 2004).

Peppermint: Peppermint extract fed orally to mice demonstrated the ability to protect the testes from gamma radiation damage (Samarth et al., 2009).

Peppermint: Peppermint oil fed to mice prior to exposure to gamma radiation was found to decrease levels of damage from oxidation, as compared to mice not pretreated with peppermint (Samarth et al., 2006).

Peppermint: Mice treated with oral administration of peppermint extract demonstrated a higher ability to tolerate gamma radiation than non-treated mice (Samarth et al., 2003).

Peppermint: Mice pretreated with peppermint leaf extract demonstrated less bone marrow cell loss than mice not pretreated with peppermint when exposed to gamma radiation (Samarth et al., 2007).

Sandalwood: Pretreatment with alpha-santalol before UVB (ultraviolet-b) radiation significantly reduced skin tumor development and multiplicity and induced proapoptotic and tumor-suppressing proteins (Arasada et al., 2008)

Sandalwood: A solution of 5% alpha-santalol (from sandalwood) was found to prevent skin-tumor formation caused by ultraviolet-b (UVB) radiation in mice (Dwivedi et al., 2006).

Melaleuca: Melaleuca alternifolia oil was found to mediate the reactive oxygen species (ROS) production of leukocytes (white blood cells), indicating a possible anti-inflammatory activity (Caldefie-Chézet et al., 2004).

Thyme: Various essential oils demonstrated an antioxidant effect toward skin lipid squalene oxidized by UV irradiation, with a blend of thyme and clove oil demonstrating the highest inhibitory effect (Wei et al., 2007).

Clove: Various essential oils demonstrated an antioxidant effect toward skin lipid squalene oxidized by UV irradiation, with a blend of thyme and clove oil demonstrating the highest inhibitory effect (Wei et al., 2007).

Rashes

See Skin: Rashes

Raynaud's Disease

See also Arteries, Cardiovascular System: Circulation

Raynaud's disease is a condition that causes the arteries supplying blood to the skin to suddenly narrow and inhibit blood circulation. As a result, specific areas of the body feel numb and cool. The most commonly affected areas are the toes, fingers, nose, and ears. During an attack, the skin turns white and then blue.

See the *Quick Usage Chart* inside the back cover for recommended dilutions.

348

As circulation returns and warms the affected areas, a prickling, throbbing, stinging, or swelling sensation often accompanies it. These attacks are often triggered by cold temperatures and by stress.

Oils: cypress, rosemary, geranium, helichrysum, fennel, clove, lavender

⊜: Dilute as recommended, and apply 1–2 drops on the affected area, to carotid arteries, and on reflex points on the feet.

⊘: Diffuse into the air. Inhale oil directly from bottle, or inhale oil that is applied to hands, tissue, or cotton wick.

⊕: **Body System(s) Affected:** Cardiovascular System.

Relaxation

Relaxation is a state of rest and tranquility, free from tension and anxiety.

> *Simple Solutions—Relaxing:* Combine 3 drops lavender and 3 drops Roman chamomile with 1 cup (250 g) Epsom salt. Add ½ cup (125 g) of salt to warm bathwater for a relaxing bath.

Oils: lavender, ylang ylang, lemon, AromaTouch, neroli, star anise, Roman chamomile, geranium, frankincense, fir, sandalwood, clary sage

⊘: Diffuse into the air. Inhale directly from bottle. Apply oil to hands, tissue, or cotton wick, and inhale.

⊜: Add 5–10 drops to 1 Tbs. (15 ml) fractionated coconut oil (or another carrier oil), and use as massage oil. Place 1–2 drops in warm bathwater, and bathe.

⊕: **Body System(s) Affected:** Emotional Balance.

⊞: **Additional Research:**

Lavender: Nurses working in an ICU setting demonstrated decreased perception of stress when receiving a topical application of *Lavandula angustifolia* and Salvia sclarea essential oils (Pemberton et al., 2008).

Lavender: Subjects who smelled a cleansing gel with lavender aroma were more relaxed and able to complete math computations faster (Field et al., 2005).

Lavender: Subjects exposed to 3 minutes of lavender aroma were more relaxed and able to perform math computations faster and more accurately (Diego et al., 1998).

Lavender: Mice who inhaled lavender were found to have a decreased motility (natural movement) dependent on exposure time. Additionally, mice injected with caffeine (causing a hyperactivity) were found to reduce their movement to near normal levels after inhaling lavender (Buchbauer et al., 1991).

Ylang ylang: Subjects who had ylang ylang oil applied to their skin had decreased blood pressure, increased skin temperature, and reported feeling more calm and relaxed compared to subjects in a control group (Hongratanaworakit et al., 2006).

Lemon: Lemon oil was found to have an antistress effect in mice involved in several behavioral tasks (Komiya et al., 2006).

Respiratory System

The respiratory system's primary purposes are to supply the blood with oxygen that is then delivered to all parts of the body and to remove waste carbon dioxide from the blood and eliminate it from the body. The respiratory system consists of the mouth, nose, and pharynx (through which air is first taken in), larynx (voice box), trachea (airway leading from the larynx to the lungs), bronchi (which branch off from the trachea and into the lungs), bronchioles (smaller tubes that branch off from the bronchi), alveoli (tiny sacs filled with capillaries that allow inhaled oxygen to be transferred into the blood and carbon dioxide to be expelled from the blood into the air in the lungs), pleura (which covers the outside of the lungs and the inside of the chest wall), and diaphragm (a large muscle at the bottom of the chest cavity that moves to pull air into the lungs (inhale) and to push air out of the lungs (exhale)).

Oils: Breathe, eucalyptus, peppermint, Douglas fir, cinnamon, manuka, On Guard, cardamom, melaleuca, fir, clary sage, fennel, helichrysum, marjoram, oregano, bergamot, clove, frankincense, lemon, rosemary, lime

Blend 1: Combine 5 drops eucalyptus, 8 drops frankincense, and 6 drops lemon. Apply to bottoms of feet; or add to 2 Tbs. (25 ml) fractionated coconut oil, and apply as a hot compress on chest.

Recipe 1: Combine 10 drops eucalyptus and 10 drops myrrh with 1 Tbs. (15 ml) fractionated coconut oil. Insert rectally for overnight retention enema.

Other Products: Breathe Respiratory Drops, Breathe Vapor Stick, TriEase Softgels

—**Asthma:** *See Asthma*

—**Breathing:**

Oils: Breathe, cinnamon, frankincense, rosemary, Douglas fir, thyme, marjoram, juniper berry, ginger

Other Products: Breathe Vapor Stick, Breathe Respiratory Drops

—**Bronchitis:** *See Bronchitis*

—**Congestion:** *See Congestion*

—**Cough:** *See Cough*

Respiratory System

The respiratory system's primary purposes are to supply the blood with oxygen that is then delivered to all parts of the body and to remove waste carbon dioxide from the blood and eliminate it from the body. The respiratory system consists of the mouth, nose, and pharynx (through which air is first taken in), larynx (voice box), trachea (airway leading from the larynx to the lungs), bronchi (which branch off from the trachea and into the lungs), bronchioles (smaller tubes that branch off from the bronchi), alveoli (tiny sacs filled with capillaries that allow inhaled oxygen to be transferred into the blood and carbon dioxide to be expelled from the blood into the air in the lungs), pleura (which covers the outside of the lungs and the inside of the chest wall), and diaphragm (a large muscle at the bottom of the chest cavity that moves to pull air into the lungs [inhale] and to push air out of the lungs [exhale]).

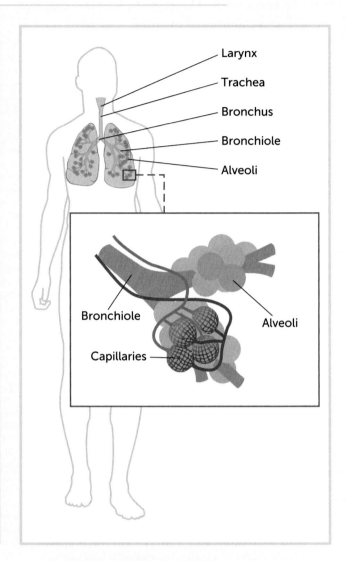

Oils for Respiratory System Support

Oils: ⊕Breathe, ⊕eucalyptus⊕, ⊕peppermint⊕, ⊕Douglas fir, ⊕cinnamon⊕, ⊕On Guard, ⊕cardamom⊕, ⊕melaleuca, ⊕fir, ⊕clary sage, ⊕fennel, ⊕helichrysum, ⊕marjoram, ⊕oregano, ⊕bergamot⊕, ⊕clove, ⊕frankincense, ⊕lemon, ⊕rosemary, ⊕lime

Common Respiratory Issues

Respiratory: Allergies, Asthma, Bronchitis, Colds, Cystic Fibrosis, Cough, Hyperpnea, Influenza (Flu), Pleurisy, Pneumonia

—**Cystic Fibrosis:**

Cystic fibrosis is an inherited genetic condition that causes glands the lungs and other organs to secrete less hydrated, more sticky secretions. The stickiness of these secretions cause blockages and inflammation, damaging the lungs and other organs over time.

Simple Solutions—Cystic Fibrosis: Diffuse bergamot in an aromatherapy diffuser.

Oils: ᵃᵗbergamot⁰

—**Hyperpnea:**

Hyperpnea is rapid or heavy breathing that occurs normally as a result of strenuous physical exertion and abnormally in conjunction with fever and disorders.

Oils: ᵃᵗylang ylang

—**Lungs:**

The lungs are paired organs located on either side of the heart. The lungs function to exchange oxygen and carbon dioxide (breathing). Oxygen passes into the blood by inhaling, and exhaling expels carbon dioxide. The lungs keep the body supplied with the oxygen necessary to keep cells alive. The lung on the right side of the body contains three lobes (sections) and is slightly larger than the lung on the left side of the body, which has two lobes.

Oils: ᵃᵗBreathe, ᵃᵗeucalyptus, ᵃᵗsandalwood, ᵃᵗfrankincense, ᵃᵗElevation, ᵃᵗOn Guard (for infections)

Other Products: ᵒZendocrine Detoxification Complex to help support healthy lung functioning.

—**Oxygen:**

Oils: ᵃfrankincense, ᵃsandalwood, ᵃcedarwood

—**Pleurisy:**

Pleurisy is an inflammation of the moist membrane (pleura) that surrounds the lungs and lines the rib cage. Pleurisy is characterized by a dry cough, chest pain, and difficulty breathing. Viral infection is the most common cause of pleurisy; but lung infections, chest injuries, and drug reactions are also possible causes. Pleurisy usually lasts between a few days and a couple weeks.

Oils: ᵃᵗcypress, ᵃᵗthyme

—**Pneumonia:** *See Pneumonia*

🌀: Diffuse into the air. Inhale directly from bottle. Apply oil to hands, tissue, or cotton wick, and inhale.

🌐: Dilute as recommended, and apply to chest, sinuses, neck, or reflex points on the feet. Add 2–3 drops to water, and gargle. Apply to chest as warm compress. Add 20 drops to 1 Tbs. (15 ml) fractionated coconut oil, and insert rectally for overnight retention enema.

⬤: Take supplements as directed on package.

⊕: **Body System(s) Affected:** Respiratory System.

▦: **Additional Research:**

Eucalyptus: Extracts from eucalyptus and thyme were found to have high nitrous oxide (NO) scavenging abilities and inhibited NO production in macrophage cells. This could possibly explain their role in aiding respiratory inflammatory diseases (Vigo et al., 2004).

Eucalyptus: Eucalyptus oil was found to have an anti-inflammatory and mucin-inhibitory effect in rats with lipopolysaccharide-induced bronchitis (Lu et al., 2004).

Eucalyptus: Therapy with 1,8 cineole (eucalyptol) in both healthy and bronchitis-afflicted humans was shown to reduce production of LTB4 and PGE2—both metabolites of arachidonic acid, a known chemical messenger involved in inflammation—in white blood cells (Juergens et al., 1998).

Peppermint: L-menthol was found to inhibit production of inflammation mediators in human monocytes (a type of white blood cell involved in the immune response) (Juergens et al., 1998).

Cinnamon: Vapor of cinnamon bark oil and cinnamic aldehyde was found to be effective against fungi involved in respiratory tract mycoses (fungal infections) (Singh et al., 1995).

Cinnamon: Cinnamon bark, lemongrass, and thyme oils were found to have the highest level of activity against common respiratory pathogens among 14 essential oils tested (Inouye et al., 2001).

Cardamom: Administration of cardamom to mice was found to have a protective effect against pan masala–induced damage in the lungs of mice (pan masala is an herbal and tobacco blend sold in India) (Kumari et al., 2013).

Bergamot: Bergamot extract was found to display inhibitory activity on IL-8 gene expression (IL-8 is involved in the inflammatory processes associated with cystic fibrosis), indicating that bergamot may possess possible anti-inflammatory properties to reduce lung inflammation in cystic fibrosis patients (Borgatti et al., 2011).

Restlessness

See Calming

Rheumatic Fever

See also Antibacterial

Rheumatic fever is the inflammation of the heart and joints in response to a strep throat or scarlet fever infection. This inflammation can cause permanent damage to the heart. Symptoms of rheumatic fever include painful and swollen joints, chest pain, fever, fatigue, the sensation of a pounding heartbeat, shortness of breath, rash, sudden jerky body movements, and unusual displays of emotion. Rheumatic fever is most common in children between ages 5 and 15.

Oils: ⊘ginger (for pain)

⊜: Dilute as recommended, and apply 1–2 drops on location.

⊕: **Body System(s) Affected:** Immune System and Cardiovascular Systems.

Rheumatism

See Arthritis: Rheumatoid Arthritis

Rhinitis

See Nose: Rhinitis

Ringworm

See Antifungal: Ringworm

Rocky Mountain Spotted Fever

See also Antibacterial, Insects/Bugs: Ticks

Rocky Mountain spotted fever is a bacterial disease that spreads through the bite of an infected tick. Symptoms include high fever, severe headache, and a red, non-itchy rash that first appears on the wrists and ankles, then spreads from there.

Oils: ⊙⊘⊘On Guard, ⊘⊘cinnamon, ⊘Purify, ⊘⊘TerraShield (prevent), ⊘⊘lavender (prevent)

⊜: Dilute as recommended, and apply 1–2 drops over location or on bottoms of the feet.

⊘: Diffuse into the air. Inhale directly from bottle. Apply oil to hands, tissue, or cotton wick, and inhale.

⊙: Place 1–2 drops of oil under the tongue, or place oils in empty capsules and swallow.

⊕: **Body System(s) Affected:** Immune System.

Sadness

See Grief/Sorrow

Salmonella

See Antibacterial, Food Poisoning

Scabies

See Skin: Scabies

Scarring

See Skin: Scarring, Tissue: Scarring

Schmidt's Syndrome

See Adrenal Glands: Schmidt's Syndrome

Sciatica

Sciatica is pain resulting from the irritation of the sciatic nerve. The sciatic nerve is the longest nerve in the body. It runs from the spinal cord through the buttock and hip area and down the back of each leg. When the sciatic nerve is pinched or irritated due to something such as a herniated disk, the pain experienced along the sciatic nerve is called "sciatica." Symptoms of sciatica include pain in the area, numbness and weakness along the sciatic nerve, tingling sensations, or a loss of bladder or bowel control.

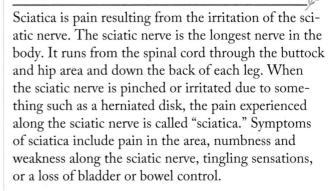

Simple Solutions—Sciatica: Mix 5 drops peppermint with 1 tsp. (5 ml) fractionated coconut oil in a small roll-on bottle. Apply on lower back every 3 hours as needed.

Oils: ⊘peppermint, ⊘Roman chamomile, ⊘helichrysum, ⊘thyme, ⊘Deep Blue (for pain), ⊘Balance, ⊘fir, ⊘sandalwood, ⊘lavender, ⊘wintergreen

⊜: Dilute as recommended, and apply 1–2 drops on lower back, buttocks, or legs. Add 5–10 drops to 1 Tbs. (15 ml) fractionated coconut oil, and massage on spine, back, legs, and bottoms of feet.

⊕: **Body System(s) Affected:** Nervous System.

Scrapes

See Wounds

Scurvy

Scurvy is a disease caused by a deficiency of ascorbic acid (vitamin C). Some results of scurvy are general weakness, anemia, gum disease (gingivitis), skin hemorrhages, spots on the skin (usually the thighs and legs), and bleeding from the mucous membranes.

Oils: ⊘ginger

Other Products: ⊙Microplex VMz contains vitamin C necessary for preventing scurvy.

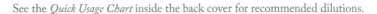

See the *Quick Usage Chart* inside the back cover for recommended dilutions.

352

◐: Dilute as recommended, and apply 1–2 drops over kidneys, liver, and reflex points on the feet.

○: Take capsules as directed on package.

⊕: **Body System(s) Affected:** Skin and Digestive System.

Sedative

See Calming: Sedative

Seizure

A seizure is an uncontrolled, abnormal electrical discharge in the brain which may produce a physical convulsion, minor physical signs, thought disturbances, or a combination of symptoms. The symptoms depend on what parts of the brain are involved.

Oils: ◐clary sage, ◐lavender⊕, ◐rose⊕, ◐○peppermint⊕, ◐Balance, ◐clove⊕, ◐Serenity, ◐Elevation

Other Products: ○Mito2Max to help support healthy nerve function. ○xEO Mega or vEO Mega, ○Microplex VMz contain omega fatty acids, minerals, and other nutrients that support healthy brain function.

—Convulsions:

A convulsion is the repeated, rapid contracting and relaxing of muscles resulting in the uncontrollable shaking of the body. Convulsions usually last about 30 seconds to 2 minutes and are often associated with seizures.

Oils: ◐lavender⊕, ◐clary sage, ◐Balance

—Epilepsy:

Epilepsy is a neurological condition where the person has recurring, unpredictable seizures. Epilepsy has many possible causes; although in many cases the cause is unknown. Possible causes may include illness, injury to the brain, or abnormal brain development.

Oils: ◐clary sage

—Grand Mal Seizure:

The grand mal seizure, also known as the tonic-clonic seizure, is the most common seizure. The tonic phase lasts about 10–20 seconds. During this stage, the person loses consciousness, and the muscles contract—causing the person to fall down. During the clonic phase, the person experiences violent convulsions. This phase usually lasts less than two minutes.

Oils: ◐Balance (on feet), ◐◑Serenity (around navel), ◐Elevation (over heart)

Other Products: ○Microplex VMz contains zinc and copper—an imbalance of zinc and copper has been theorized to play a role in grand mal seizures.

◐: Dilute as recommended, and apply 1–2 drops to back of neck, navel, heart, or reflex points on the feet.

○: Take capsules as directed on package.

◑: Diffuse into the air.

⊕: **Body System(s) Affected:** Nervous System.

⊕: **Additional Research:**

Lavender: Linalool (found in several essential oils) was found to inhibit induced convulsions in rats by directly interacting with the NMDA receptor complex (Brum et al., 2001).

Rose: Aqueous and ethanolic extracts of *Rosa damascena* were found to have potential anticonvulsant effect in drug-induced seizure model mice (Hosseini et al., 2011).

Rose: Injection of rose essential oil before induction of amygdala kindling seizures in male rats significantly retarded the development of seizure stages and possessed the ability to counteract kindling stimulation when compared to the control group (Ramezani et al., 2008).

Peppermint: Mice pretreated with an injection of peppermint essential oil demonstrated no seizures and 100% post-treatment survival after being injected with a lethal dose of pentylenetetrazol (PTZ) to cause seizures. Seven other essential oils were also tested, but peppermint was the most successful at preventing seizures and death. All tested essential oil treated mice (except oregano which caused complete fatality before administering PTZ) demonstrated increased seizure latency and intensity when compared to the control (Koutroumanidou et al., 2013).

Clove: The aqueous and ethanolic extracts of clove were found to induce an anticonvulsive effect by increasing seizure latency in drug-induced seizure model mice, when compared to control (Hosseini et al., 2012).

Dill: The aqueous extract of *Anethum graveolens* was shown to have an anticonvulsant effect in a mouse model of epilepsy (Arash et al., 2013).

Sexual Issues

Simple Solutions—Low Libido: Blend 5 drops ylang ylang and 1 drop cinnamon with 1 Tbs. (15 ml) fractionated coconut oil to make a romantic massage oil.

—Arousing Desire: *See Aphrodisiac*

—Frigidity:

Female frigidity is a female's lack of sexual drive or her inability to enjoy sexual activities. This disorder has many possible physical and psychological causes, including stress, fatigue, guilt, fear, worry, alcoholism, or drug abuse.

Oils: ◑◐clary sage, ◑◐ylang ylang, ◑◐Whisper, ◑◐rose

A
B
C
D
E
F
G
H
I
J
K
L
M
N
O
P
Q
R
S
T
U
V
W
X
Y
Z

—Impotence:

Impotence in men, also known as erectile dysfunction, is the frequent inability to have or sustain an erection. This may be caused by circulation problems, nerve problems, low levels of testosterone, medications, or psychological stresses.

Oils: ⊖Oclary sage, ⊖Oclove, ⊖Orose, ⊖Oginger, ⊖Osandalwood

—Libido (low):

Libido is a term used by Sigmund Freud to describe human sexual desire. Causes for a lack of sexual desire can be both physical and psychological. Some possible causes include anemia, alcoholism, drug abuse, stress, anxiety, past sexual abuse, and relationship problems.

Oils: ⊗⊖ylang ylang, ⊗⊖Elevation

Other Products: OMito2Max

  –Men:

    Oils: ⊗⊖cinnamon, ⊗⊖ginger, ⊗⊖myrrh

  –Women:

    Oils: ⊗⊖clary sage, ⊖geranium

🌀: Diffuse into the air. Dissolve 2–3 drops in 2 tsp. (10 ml) pure grain or perfumer's alcohol, combine with distilled water in a 1–2 oz. spray bottle, and spray into the air or on clothes or bed linens.

🔄: Dilute as recommended, and wear on temples, neck, or wrists as perfume or cologne. Combine 3–5 drops of your desired essential oil with 1 Tbs. (15 ml) fractionated coconut oil to use as a massage oil. Combine 1–2 drops with ¼ cup (50 g) Therapeutic Bath Salts, and dissolve in warm bathwater for a romantic bath.

🌑: Take capsules as directed. Place 1–2 drops oil in an empty capsule, and swallow.

⊕: **Body System(s) Affected:** Reproductive System.

Sexually Transmitted Diseases (STD)

See AIDS/HIV, Herpes Simplex

Shingles

See also Antiviral, Childhood Diseases: Chickenpox, Nervous System: Neuralgia

Shingles is a viral infection caused by the same virus that causes chickenpox. After a person has had chickenpox, the virus lies dormant in the nervous system. Years later, that virus can be reactivated by stress, immune deficiency, or disease and cause shingles. Symptoms of shingles start with tingling, pain, neuralgia, or itching of an area of skin and become visually obvious as red blisters form in that same area along the nerve path, forming a red band on the skin. Blisters most commonly appear wrapping from the middle of the back to the middle of the chest but can form on the neck, face, and scalp as well. Another name for shingles is herpes zoster.

> *Simple Solutions—Shingles:* Blend 3 drops lavender, 3 drops melaleuca, and 3 drops thyme with 1 tsp. (5 ml) fractionated coconut oil. Apply on feet and on location.

Oils: ⊖melaleuca, ⊖eucalyptus, ⊖lavender, ⊖lemon, ⊖geranium, ⊖bergamot

🔄: Dilute as recommended, and apply 1–2 drops on location. Add 5–10 drops essential oil to 1 Tbs. (15 ml) fractionated coconut oil, and massage on location and on bottoms of feet.

⊕: **Body System(s) Affected:** Skin, Nervous System, and Immune System.

Shock

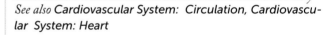

See also Cardiovascular System: Circulation, Cardiovascular System: Heart

Shock is a life-threatening condition where the body suffers from severely low blood pressure. This can be caused by low blood volume due to bleeding or dehydration, inadequate pumping of the heart, or dilation of the blood vessels due to head injury, medications, or poisons from bacterial infections. Shock can cause pale or bluish skin that feels cold or clammy to the touch, confusion, rapid breathing, and a rapid heartbeat. Without the needed oxygen being sent to the body's tissues and cells, the organs can shut down and, in severe cases, can lead to death. Shock often accompanies severe injuries or other traumatic situations. A person suffering from shock should be made to lie down with the feet elevated above the head, be kept warm, and have the head turned to the side in case of vomiting. Check breathing often, and ensure that any visible bleeding is stopped. Get emergency medical help as soon as possible.

See the Quick Usage Chart inside the back cover for recommended dilutions.

Simple Solutions—Shock: Follow the instructions outlined above, and hold an open bottle of peppermint under the victim's nose.

Oils: ⊘⊜peppermint, ⊜Roman chamomile, ⊜helichrysum (may help stop bleeding), ⊜melaleuca, ⊘Elevation, ⊘⊜ylang ylang, ⊜Balance, ⊘⊜myrrh, ⊘⊜melissa, ⊘⊜basil, ⊜rosemary

⊜: Dilute as recommended, and apply 1–2 drops on back of neck, feet, over heart, or on front of neck.

⊘: Diffuse into the air. Inhale directly from bottle. Apply oil to hands, tissue, or cotton wick, and inhale.

⊕: **Body System(s) Affected:** Cardiovascular System and Nervous System.

Shoulder

See Joints: Shoulder

Sinuses

Sinuses are several hollow cavities within the skull that allow the skull to be more lightweight without compromising strength. These cavities are connected to the nasal cavity through small channels. When the mucous membrane lining these channels becomes swollen or inflamed due to colds or allergies, these channels can become blocked—making it difficult for the sinuses to drain correctly. This can lead to infection and inflammation of the mucous membrane within the sinuses (sinusitis). There are sinus cavities behind the cheek bone and forehead and near the eyes and nasal cavity.

Simple Solutions—Sinusitis: Add 2 drops eucalyptus to a bowl of hot water, and inhale the vapor.

Oils: ⊘⊜helichrysum, ⊘⊜eucalyptus, ⊘⊜Breathe, ⊘⊜peppermint, ⊘⊜On Guard, ⊜cedarwood

—Sinusitis:

Oils: ⊘⊜eucalyptus, ⊘⊜rosemary, ⊘⊜Breathe, ⊜DigestZen, ⊘⊜peppermint, ⊘⊜melaleuca, ⊘⊜fir, ⊘⊜ginger

Recipe 1: For chronic sinusitis, apply 1–2 drops DigestZen around navel 4 times daily; apply 2 drops peppermint under tongue 2 times daily.

⊘: Diffuse into the air. Inhale directly from bottle. Apply oil to hands, tissue, or cotton wick, and inhale. Place 1–2 drops in a bowl of hot water, and inhale vapors.

⊜: Dilute as recommended, and apply 1–2 drops along the sides of the nose or forehead (often clears out sinuses immediately).

⊕: **Body System(s) Affected:** Respiratory System.

Skeletal System

In an adult individual, the skeletal system is comprised of 206 bones. These bones provide structure to the body and allow for movement, as well as provide protection for vital organs and tissues. Bones contain bone marrow where blood cells are created. Bones also act as storage reservoirs for calcium and other minerals that the body needs.

Oils: ⊜wintergreen, ⊜fir, ⊜cypress, ⊜juniper berry, ⊘⊜cedarwood, ⊜lavender, ⊜lemongrass, ⊜marjoram, ⊜peppermint, ⊜sandalwood

Other Products: ⊙Microplex VMz contains nutrients essential for bone development, such as calcium, magnesium, zinc, and vitamin D.

—Bone Spurs:

A bone spur (osteophyte) is a bony projection formed on a normal bone. Bone spurs form as the body tries to repair itself by building extra bone in response to continued pressure, stress, or rubbing. Bone spurs can cause pain if they rub against soft tissues or other bones.

Oils: ⊜wintergreen, ⊜cypress, ⊜marjoram

—Broken:

Simple Solutions—Broken Bone : Combine 1 drop each of lemongrass, clove, eucalyptus, and melaleuca. Apply gently over bone once daily until healed.

Oils: ⊜Deep Blue (for pain), ⊜⊙frankincense

Recipe 1: Apply wintergreen and cypress oils at night before bed. Apply helichrysum, oregano, and Balance in the morning.

Blend 1: Combine equal parts lemongrass, clove, eucalyptus, and melaleuca. Apply on location.

Skeletal System

In an adult individual, the skeletal system is comprised of 206 bones. These bones provide structure to the body and allow for movement, as well as provide protection for vital organs and tissues. Bones contain bone marrow where blood cells are created. Bones also act as storage reservoirs for calcium and other minerals that the body needs.

Specialized bones serve other functions, such as those in the middle ear that help transmit sound vibrations from the eardrum to the inner ear.

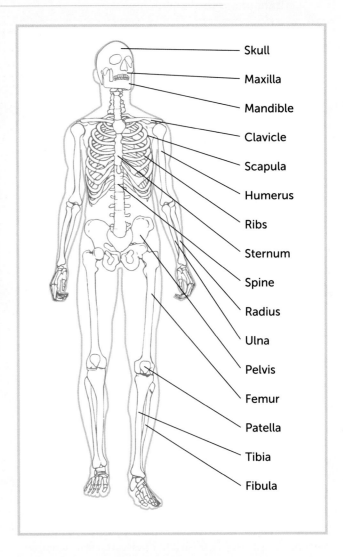

- Skull
- Maxilla
- Mandible
- Clavicle
- Scapula
- Humerus
- Ribs
- Sternum
- Spine
- Radius
- Ulna
- Pelvis
- Femur
- Patella
- Tibia
- Fibula

Oils for Skeletal System Support

Oils: wintergreen, fir, cypress, juniper berry, Deep Blue, cedarwood, lavender, lemongrass, marjoram, peppermint, sandalwood

Common Skeletal Issues

Skeletal: Arthritis, Bone Spurs, Breaks, Bruises, Calcified Spine, Fractures, Herniated Disc, Leukemia, Osteomyelitis, Osteoporosis

Other Products: ⃝Microplex VMz contains essential bone nutrients calcium, magnesium, zinc, and vitamin D.

—Bruised

Oils: ⃝Deep Blue, ⃝helichrysum

—Cartilage:

Cartilage is a type of connective tissue in the body that provides structure and support for other tissues without being hard and rigid like bone. Unlike other connective tissues, cartilage does not have blood vessels. Cartilage is found in many areas of the body, including the joints, ears, nose, bronchial tubes, and intervertebral discs.

Oils: ⃝sandalwood (helps regenerate), ⃝fir (inflammation)

—Development:

Other Products: ⃝Microplex VMz contains essential bone nutrients necessary for development, such as calcium, magnesium, zinc, and vitamin D.

—Osteomyelitis: *See also Antibacterial, Antifungal*

Osteomyelitis is a bone infection that is usually caused by bacteria. The infection often starts in another area of the body and then spreads to the bone. Symptoms include fever, pain, swelling, nausea, drainage of pus, and uneasiness. Diabetes, hemodialysis, recent trauma, and IV drug abuse are risk factors for osteomyelitis.

> *Simple Solutions—Osteomyelitis:* Combine 3 drops lemongrass, 2 drops clove, 2 drops eucalyptus, and 2 drops melaleuca with 1 tsp. (5 ml) fractionated coconut oil. Apply once or twice a day on location as needed.

Recipe 1: Apply equal parts lemongrass, clove, eucalyptus, and melaleuca, either blended together or applied individually on location.

—Osteoporosis:

Osteoporosis is a disease characterized by a loss of bone density, making the bones extremely fragile and susceptible to fractures and breaking. Osteoporosis develops when bone resorption exceeds bone formation. Osteoporosis is significantly more common in women than in men, especially after menopause; but the disease does occur in both genders.

Oils: ⃝clove, ⃝geranium, ⃝peppermint, ⃝wintergreen, ⃝fir, ⃝Deep Blue, ⃝thyme, ⃝rosemary⃝, ⃝lemon, ⃝cypress

Other Products: ⃝Bone Nutrient Lifetime Complex, ⃝Phytoestrogen Lifetime Complex

—Pain:

Oils: ⃝Deep Blue, ⃝Rescuer, ⃝wintergreen, ⃝juniper berry, ⃝fir

—Rotator Cuff: *See Joints: Rotator Cuff*

⃝: Dilute as recommended, and apply on location or on reflex points on feet.

⃝: Take capsules as directed. Place 1–2 drops of oil in an empty capsule; swallow.

⃝: **Body System(s) Affected:** Skeletal System.

⃝: **Additional Research:**

Rosemary and eucalyptus: Oral intake of rosemary or eucalyptus essential oil (as well as several monoterpenes found in other essential oils) was shown to inhibit bone resorption in rats (Mühlbauer et al., 2003).

Skin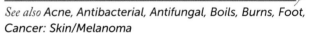

See also Acne, Antibacterial, Antifungal, Boils, Burns, Foot, Cancer: Skin/Melanoma

The skin is the organ the covers the body, offering the first layer of protection to the internal organs and tissues from exposure to the environment and fungal, bacterial, and other types of infection. It helps regulate body heat and helps prevent evaporation of water from the body. The skin also carries nerve endings that allow the body to sense touch, heat, and pain. The skin is comprised of three layers. The upper layer is the epidermis, the middle layer is the dermis, and the deeper layer is the hypodermis (or subcutis layer).

Oils: ⃝peppermint, ⃝melaleuca, ⃝HD Clear, ⃝Immortelle, ⃝sandalwood, ⃝frankincense, ⃝lavender, ⃝magnolia, ⃝neroli, ⃝⃝manuka, ⃝⃝Yarrow Pom, ⃝myrrh, ⃝geranium, ⃝rosemary, ⃝spikenard, ⃝Balance, ⃝ylang ylang, ⃝marjoram, ⃝cypress, ⃝juniper berry, ⃝green mandarin, ⃝cedarwood, ⃝Zendocrine, ⃝turmeric, ⃝vetiver, ⃝arborvitae, ⃝helichrysum, ⃝lemon, ⃝orange, ⃝lime, ⃝patchouli

Other Products: ⃝Anti-Aging Moisturizer, ⃝Baby Lotion, ⃝Baby Hair and Body Wash, ⃝Detoxifying Mud Mask, ⃝Exfoliating Body Scrub, ⃝Anti-Aging Eye Cream, ⃝Diaper Rash Cream, ⃝Facial

A B C D E F G H I J K L M N O P Q R S T U V W X Y Z

Cleanser, ✺Hydrating Cream, ✺Hydrating Body Mist with Beautiful, ✺Hydrating Serum, ✺Invigorating Scrub, ✺Refreshing Body Wash, ✺Replenishing Body Butter, ✺Bightening Gel, ✺Pore Reducing Toner, ✺Reveal Facial System, and ✺Skin Serum for vibrant, youthful-looking skin. ✺HD Clear Foaming Face Wash and ✺HD Clear Facial Lotion to help improve tone and texture of the skin. ✺On Guard Foaming Hand Wash to help protect against harmful microorganisms on the skin. ✺Citrus Bliss and ✺Serenity Bath Bars, or ✺Hand and Body Lotion to help cleanse and moisturize the skin. ✺Correct-X to help cleanse and support the skin's natural healing process. ○xEO Mega or vEO Mega, ○IQ Mega, ○Alpha CRS+, ○a2z Chewable, ○Microplex VMz contain omega fatty acids and other nutrients essential for healthy skin cell function. ○Zendocrine Detoxification Complex to help support healthy cleansing and filtering of the skin.

🜄: Dilute as recommended, and apply 1–2 drops on location. Add 5–10 drops to 2 Tbs. (25 ml) fractionated coconut oil, and use as massage oil. Add 1 drop essential oil to 1 tsp. (5 ml) unscented lotion, and apply on the skin. Add 1–2 drops to 1 Tbs. (15 ml) bath or shower gel, and apply to skin. Apply foaming hand wash to skin instead of soap, or use bath bars when washing hands or bathing.

◯: Take capsules as directed on package. Add 3–5 drops of oil to an empty capsule; swallow capsule.

—**Acne**: *See Acne*

—**Boils**: *See Boils*

—**Burns**: *See Burns*

—**Calluses**:

A callus is a flat, thick growth of skin that develops on areas of the skin where there is constant friction or rubbing. Calluses typically form on the bottoms of the feet but can also form on the hands or other areas of the body exposed to constant friction.

Simple Solutions—Callus: Combine 5 drops oregano oil with 1 Tbs. (15 ml) jojoba oil. Apply a small amount daily over calluses.

Oils: ✺oregano, ✺HD Clear, ✺Roman chamomile

🜄: Dilute as recommended, and apply 1–2 drops on area.

—**Chapped/Cracked**:

Chapped or cracked skin is the result of the depletion of natural oils (sebum) in the skin, leading to dehydration of the skin beneath it. Some common causes for chapped skin include exposure to the cold or wind, repeated contact with soap or chemicals that break down oils, or a lack of essential fatty acids in the body.

Oils: ✺myrrh, ✺HD Clear, ✺Immortelle, ✺○Yarrow Pom

Other Products: ✺Baby Lotion, ✺Diaper Rash Cream, ✺Hand and Body Lotion, ✺Hydrating Body Mist with Beautiful, ✺Hydrating Cream and ✺Hydrating Serum to help moisturize and protect. ✺Correct-X to help cleanse and support the skin's natural healing process. ○xEO Mega or vEO Mega or ○IQ Mega to help supply essential omega fatty acids necessary for healthy skin. ✺Citrus Bliss and ✺Serenity Bath Bars contain natural oils that help moisturize and soften the skin.

🜄: Dilute as recommended, and apply 1–2 drops on location. Add 5–10 drops to 1 Tbs. (15 ml) fractionated coconut oil, and massage on location.

◯: Take capsules as directed on package.

—**Corns**: *See Foot: Corns*

—**Dehydrated**:

Oils: ✺geranium, ✺lavender, ✺Immortelle

Other Products: ✺Baby Lotion, ✺Baby Hair and Body Wash, ✺Hand and Body Lotion, ✺Hydrating Body Mist with Beautiful, ✺Hydrating Cream and ✺Hydrating Serum to help moisturize and protect. ✺Citrus Bliss and ✺Serenity Bath Bars contain natural oils that help moisturize and soften.

🜄: Dilute as recommended, and apply 1–2 drops on location. Add 5–10 drops to 2 Tbs. (25 ml) fractionated coconut oil, and use as massage oil. Add 1 drop essential oil to 1 tsp. (5 ml) unscented lotion, and apply on the skin. Add 1–2 drops to 1 Tbs. (15 ml) bath or shower gel, and apply to skin.

See the *Quick Usage Chart* inside the back cover for recommended dilutions.

358

—Dermatitis/Eczema:

Dermatitis is any inflammation of the upper layers of the skin that results in redness, itching, pain, or possibly blistering. It can be caused by contact with an allergen or irritating substance, fungal infection, dehydration, or possibly another medical condition.

Simple Solutions—Dermatitis/Eczema: Blend 2 drops helichrysum and 2 drops juniper berry with 1 tsp. (5 ml) jojoba oil in a small roll-on container, and apply on affected skin.

Oils: HD Clear, helichrysum, juniper berry, thyme, geranium, arborvitae, melaleuca, lavender, patchouli, bergamot, rosemary

: Add 5–10 drops to 1 Tbs. (15 ml) fractionated coconut oil, and apply on location. Dilute as recommended, and apply 1–2 drops on location.

—Diaper Rash: *See Children and Infants: Diaper Rash*

—Dry:

Simple Solutions—Dry Skin: Blend 4 drops geranium and 1 drop sandalwood with 1 tsp. (5 ml) jojoba oil in a small roll-on container, and apply on dry skin as needed.

Oils: geranium, lavender, Roman chamomile, Immortelle, sandalwood, lemon

Other Products: Anti-Aging Moisturizer, Hydrating Body Mist with Beautiful, Hydrating Cream and Hydrating Serum to help relieve dryness and reduce the visible signs of aging. Baby Lotion, Baby Hair and Body Wash, and Hand and Body Lotion to help moisturize and protect. Reveal Facial System to help promote healthy skin matrix building and moisture retention.

: Add 5–10 drops to 1 Tbs. (15 ml) fractionated coconut oil, and use as massage oil. Add 2–3 drops essential oil to 1 tsp. (5 ml) Hand and Body Lotion, and apply on the skin.

—Energizing:

Oils: bergamot, lemon

Other Products: Invigorating Scrub to polish and exfoliate the skin. Citrus Bliss Invigorating

Bath Bar contains natural oatmeal kernels that help exfoliate.

: Dilute as recommended, and apply 1–2 drops on location. Add 5–10 drops to 2 Tbs. (25 ml) fractionated coconut oil, and use as massage oil. Add 1 drop essential oil to 1 tsp. (5 ml) Hand and Body Lotion, and apply on the skin. Add 1–2 drops to 1 Tbs. (15 ml) bath or shower gel, and apply to skin. Massage Invigorating Scrub over wet skin for up to one minute before rinsing with warm water.

—Facial Oils: *See also Dehydrated, Dry, Energizing, Oily/Greasy, and Revitalizing in this section for other oils that can be used for specific skin types/ conditions.*

Oils: myrrh, sandalwood, vetiver

: Add 5–10 drops to 1 Tbs. (15 ml) fractionated coconut oil, and apply to face. Add 1–2 drops essential oil to 1 tsp. (5 ml) unscented lotion, and apply on the skin.

—Fungal Infections: *See Antifungal: Athlete's Foot, Antifungal: Ringworm*

—Impetigo:

Impetigo is a bacterial skin infection that causes sores and blisters full of a yellowish fluid. These sores can be itchy and painful and can easily be spread to other areas of the skin or to another person.

Oils: geranium, lavender, HD Clear, myrrh

: Boil ½ cup (125 ml) of water; let cool. Add 5–10 drops essential oil. Wash sores with this water, and then cover sores for an hour. Apply oils as a hot compress on location.

—Itching:

An itch is a tingling and unpleasant sensation that evokes the desire to scratch. Itching can be caused by various skin disorders or diseases, parasites such as scabies and lice, allergic reactions to chemicals or drugs, dry skin, insect bites, etc. Scratching the itching area too hard or too often can damage the skin.

Oils: peppermint, lavender, magnolia, manuka, Serenity

Other Products: Citrus Bliss Invigorating Bath Bar contains natural oatmeal kernels that can help exfoliate skin and soothe itching.

Skin

The skin is the organ that covers the body, offering the first layer of protection to the internal organs and tissues from exposure to the environment and fungal, bacterial, and other types of infection. It helps regulate body heat and helps prevent evaporation of water from the body. The skin also carries nerve endings that allow the body to sense touch, heat, and pain. The skin is comprised of three layers. The upper layer is the epidermis, the middle layer is the dermis, and the deeper layer is the hypodermis (or subcutis layer).

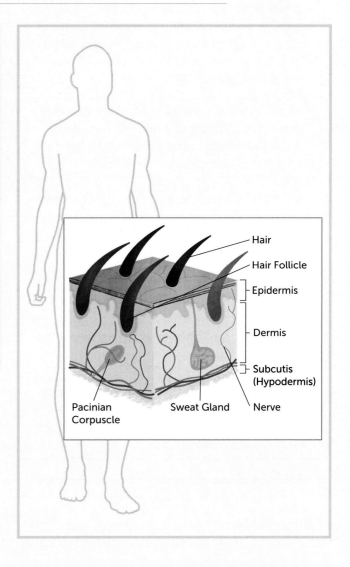

Oils for Skin Support

Oils: ⊖peppermint, ⊖melaleuca, ⊖HD Clear, ⊖Immortelle, ⊖sandalwood, ⊖frankincense, ⊖lavender, ⊖magnolia, ⊖neroli, ⊖⊖manuka, ⊖OYarrow Pom, ⊖myrrh, ⊖geranium, ⊖rosemary, ⊖spikenard, ⊖Balance, ⊖ylang ylang, ⊖marjoram, ⊖cypress, ⊖juniper berry, ⊖green mandarin, ⊖cedarwood, OZendocrine, ⊖turmeric, ⊖vetiver, ⊖arborvitae, ⊖helichrysum, ⊖lemon, ⊖orange, ⊖lime, ⊖patchouli

Common Skin Issues

Skin: Acne, Boils, Burns, Callouses, Chapped Skin, Corns, Cuts, Dehydrated Skin, Dermatitis, Dry Skin, Fungal Infections, Impetigo, Itching, Melanoma, Moles, Oily/Greasy Skin, Psoriasis, Rashes, Scabies, Scarring, Scrapes, Sensitive Skin, Stretch Marks, Sunburn, Vitiligo, Wrinkles

⊘: Dilute as recommended, and apply 1–2 drops on location and on ears. Wash body with Bath Bar.

—Melanoma: *See Cancer: Skin/Melanoma*

—Moles:

Moles are small growths on the skin of pigment-producing skin cells that usually appear brown or black in color. Moles typically appear within a person's first 20 years of life and usually stay with a person throughout his or her life. While moles are not dangerous, melanoma (a type of skin cancer that develops in pigment cells) can resemble a mole at first. Moles that vary in color or that appear to change fairly quickly in size or shape could be cancerous and should be examined.

Simple Solutions—Moles: Apply 1 drop frankincense on location. Seek medical attention if appearance or color of moles changes.

Oils: ⊘frankincense, ⊘sandalwood, ⊘geranium, ⊘lavender

⊘: Dilute as recommended, and apply 1 drop on location.

—Oily/Greasy:

Oils: ⊘lemon, ⊘HD Clear, ⊘cypress, ⊘frankincense, ⊘geranium, ⊘lavender, ⊘marjoram, ⊘orange, ⊘rosemary

Other Products: ⊘HD Clear Foaming Face Wash and ⊘HD Clear Facial Lotion to help balance skin sebum levels. ⊘Facial Cleanser to cleanse the skin and leave it feeling smooth and fresh.

⊘: Add 5–10 drops to 1 Tbs. (15 ml) fractionated coconut oil, and use as massage oil. Use Facial Cleanser as directed on package.

—Psoriasis: *See Psoriasis*

—Rashes:

A rash is an area of irritated skin, redness, or red bumps on the body. Rashes may be localized or may cover large patches of the body. A rash may be caused by a chemical or allergen irritating the skin or may occur as a symptom of another medical condition or infection.

Simple Solutions—Rashes: Combine 2 drops lavender and 2 drops Roman chamomile with 1 tsp. (5 ml) jojoba oil in a small roll-on container. Apply on affected areas once or twice a day to help soothe.

Oils: ⊘melaleuca, ⊘spikenard, ⊘OYarrow Pom, ⊘lavender, ⊘magnolia, ⊘Roman chamomile, ⊘hinoki, ⊘turmeric, ⊘spikenard

⊘: Dilute as recommended, and apply 1–2 drops on location. Add 1–5 drops to 1 Tbs. (15 ml) fractionated coconut oil, and apply on location.

—Revitalizing:

Oils: ⊘cypress, ⊘lemon, ⊘Immortelle, ⊘HD Clear, ⊘fennel, ⊘lime, OYarrow Pom, ⊘green mandarin

Other Products: ⊘Hydrating Body Mist with Beautiful. ⊘Invigorating Scrub to polish and exfoliate the skin. ⊘Reveal Facial System to help promote healthy skin matrix building and moisture retention. ⊘Citrus Bliss Invigorating Bath Bar contains natural oatmeal kernels that help exfoliate.

⊘: Add 5–10 drops to 1 Tbs. (15 ml) fractionated coconut oil, and use as massage oil. Add 2–3 drops essential oil to 1 tsp. (5 ml) unscented lotion, and apply on the skin. Massage Invigorating Scrub over wet skin for up to one minute before rinsing with warm water.

—Ringworm: *See Antifungal: Ringworm*

—Scabies:

Scabies is an infestation of the skin by mites (*Sarcoptes scabei*) that burrow into the upper layers of the skin, causing small, extremely itchy bumps.

Simple Solutions—Scabies: Blend 10 drops On Guard with 1 Tbs. (15 ml) fractionated coconut oil. Apply a small amount on location once or twice a day as needed.

Oils: ⊘On Guard, ⊘HD Clear, ⊘melaleuca, ⊘peppermint, ⊘lavender, ⊘bergamot

⊘: Add 5–10 drops to 1 Tbs. (15 ml) fractionated coconut oil, and apply a small amount on location morning and night. Dilute as recommended, and apply 1–2 drops on location.

Primary Recommendations • Secondary Recommendations • Other Recommendations / ⊘=Aromatic, ⊘=Topical, O=Internal

—Scarring:

Scars are fibrous connective tissue that is used to quickly repair a wound or injury in place of the regular skin or tissue.

Simple Solutions—Scars: Add 2 drops frankincense and 2 drops helichryum to 1 tsp. (5 ml) almond oil in a small roll-on container. Apply a small amount on scars daily as needed..

Oils: ✺lavender (burns), ✺rose (helps prevent), ✺frankincense (helps prevent), ✺❍Yarrow Pom, ✺helichrysum (reduces), ✺geranium, ✺myrrh, ✺neroli

Other Products: ✺Correct-X to help cleanse and support the skin's natural healing process.

Blend 1: Combine 5 drops helichrysum and 5 drops lavender with 1 Tbs. (15 ml) sunflower oil or with liquid lecithin (an emulsifier extracted from eggs or soy), and apply on location.

Blend 2: Combine 1 drop lavender, 1 drop lemongrass, and 1 drop geranium; apply on location to help prevent scar formation.

🔄: Dilute as recommended, and apply 1–2 drops on location.

—Sensitive:

Oils: ✺lavender, ✺neroli, ✺magnolia, ✺geranium

🔄: Dilute as recommended, and apply 1–2 drops on location.

—Skin Ulcers:

A skin ulcer is an open sore where the epidermis and possibly part or all of the dermis is missing, exposing the deeper layers of the skin. This can be caused by burns, pressure, friction, irritation, or infections damaging the upper layers of the skin.

Oils: ✺lavender, ✺myrrh, ✺HD Clear, ✺helichrysum, ✺Purify

🔄: Dilute as recommended, and apply 1–2 drops on location.

—Stretch Marks:

Stretch marks are thin purple or red areas of the skin that appear as the skin is rapidly stretched over a short period of time, stretching and tearing the dermis layer (middle layer) of the skin. Many women notice the appearance of stretch marks in the last few months of pregnancy, but stretch marks can also appear on men or women during any period of rapid weight gain. These marks most often appear on the breasts, stomach, buttocks, thighs, and hips. Stretch marks tend to fade over time, but it is difficult to eliminate them completely.

Simple Solutions—Stretch Marks: Add 2 drops lavender and 3 drops myrrh to 1 tsp. (5 ml) hazelnut oil in a small roll-on bottle. Apply on location once per day.

Oils: ✺lavender, ✺myrrh, ✺neroli

🔄: Add 5–10 drops to 1 Tbs. (15 ml) fractionated coconut oil or hazelnut oil, and apply on location.

—Sunburn: *See Burns: Sunburn*

—Tones:

Oils: ✺lemon, ✺green mandarin

🔄: Add 4–5 drops to 1 Tbs. (15 ml) fractionated coconut oil, and use as massage oil (avoid direct sunlight for 24 hours after application).

—Vitiligo:

Vitiligo is white patches of the skin caused by the death or dysfunction of pigment-producing cells in the area. While the exact cause is unknown, vitiligo may be caused by an immune or genetic disorder or may have a relationship to thyroid problems.

Oils: ✺sandalwood, ✺vetiver, ✺frankincense, ✺myrrh, ✺Purify

🔄: Dilute as recommended, and apply 1–2 drops behind ears and on back of neck or on reflex points on the feet; then cup hands together, and inhale the aroma from the hands.

—Wrinkles:

A wrinkle is a fold or crease in the skin that develops as part of the normal aging process. Wrinkles are thought to be caused by a breakdown of collagen (a protein that gives structure to cells and tissue) in the skin, causing the skin to become more fragile and loose.

Simple Solutions—Wrinkles: Blend 3 drops myrrh, 2 drops dill, and 1 drop cilantro with 1 tsp. (5 ml) jojoba oil in a small roll-on bottle. Apply on location once per day.

See the *Quick Usage Chart* inside the back cover for recommended dilutions.

Oils: 🔵Immortelle, 🔵lavender, 🔵myrrh⊕, 🔵fennel, 🔵dill⊕, 🔵geranium, 🔵frankincense, 🔵spikenard, 🔵rose, 🔵rosemary, 🔵clary sage, 🔵cypress, 🔵helichrysum, 🔵lemon, 🔵orange, 🔵oregano, 🔵sandalwood, 🔵thyme, 🔵neroli, 🔵ylang ylang

Other Products: 🔵Anti-Aging Moisturizer and 🔵Veráge Moisturizer to help relieve dryness and reduce the visible signs of aging. 🔵Tightening Serum and 🔵Veráge Toner to help tighten the skin to eliminate fine lines and wrinkles. 🔵Hydrating Body Mist with Beautiful, 🔵Hydrating Cream, and 🔵Veráge Immortelle Hydrating Serum to help promote fuller, smoother looking skin. 🔵Reveal Facial System and 🔵Veráge Cleanser to help promote healthy skin matrix building and moisture retention.

Blend 1: Combine 1 drop frankincense, 1 drop lavender, and 1 drop lemon. Rub on morning and night around the eyes (be careful not to get in eyes).

Blend 2: Combine 1 drop sandalwood, 1 drop helichrysum, 1 drop geranium, 1 drop lavender, and 1 drop frankincense. Add to 2 tsp. (10 ml) unscented lotion, and apply to skin.

🔵: Dilute as recommended, and apply 1–2 drops to skin. Add 5–10 drops to 1 Tbs. (15 ml) fractionated coconut oil or other carrier oil such as jojoba, apricot, hazelnut, or sweet almond, and apply on areas of concern. Add 3–5 drops to ½ cup (125 g) Therapeutic Bath Salts, and dissolve in warm bathwater before bathing.

⊕: **Body System(s) Affected:** Skin.

⊕: **Additional Research:**

Myrrh: Myrrh essential oil was shown to be an efficient quencher of singlet oxygen (a type of antioxidant action) by its ability to decrease formation of squalene peroxide in UV irradiated sebum on the facial skin of human subjects. These findings suggest that topical application of myrrh essential oil can help decrease sebum damage and in turn protect skin from aging (Auffray, 2007).

Dill: An in vitro study using human fibroblast cells from adult skin showed that dill extract was able to stimulate LOXL gene expression to induce elastogenesis in adult skin cells. These findings suggest that dill extract may be able to increase skin elasticity and firming (Cenizo et al., 2006).

Cilantro: Cilantro extract was found to protect human keratinocytes (epidermis cells) against H2O2-induced oxidative stress, suggesting that cilantro may be useful at protecting skin cells from oxidative damage (Park et al., 2012).

Sleep

*See also **Insomnia***

Sleep is a regular period in which the body suspends conscious motor and sensory activity. Sleep is thought to play a role in restoring and healing the body and processing the memories of the day.

Oils: 🔵🔵lavender⊕, 🔵🔵Serenity, 🔵🔵Calmer, 🔵🔵spikenard, 🔵🔵Roman chamomile⊕, 🔵marjoram

Recipe 1: Combine 5 drops geranium and 5 drops lavender with ¼ cup (50 g) Therapeutic Bath Salts; dissolve in warm bathwater, and bathe in the evening to help promote a good night's sleep.

🔵: Dilute as recommended, and apply 1–2 drops essential oil to spine, bottoms of feet, or back of neck. Add 1–2 drops to warm bathwater, and bathe before sleeping. Add 5–10 drops to 1 Tbs. (15 ml) fractionated coconut oil, and massage on back, arms, legs, and feet.

🔵: Diffuse into the air. Add 1–2 drops to bottom of pillow before sleeping. Add 2–5 drops to 2 Tbs. (25 ml) distilled water in a small spray bottle, and mist into the air or on linens before sleeping.

⊕: **Body System(s) Affected:** Nervous System, Endocrine System, and Emotional Balance.

⊕: **Additional Research:**

Lavender and Roman Chamomile: A study with 56 percutaneous coronary intervention patients in an intensive care unit found that an aromatherapy blend of lavender, Roman chamomile, and neroli decreased anxiety and improved sleep quality when compared to conventional nursing intervention (Cho et al., 2013).

Sleep: Sixty nurses with shifting sleep schedules were found to have better quality sleep after inhaling lavender essential oil (Kim et al., 2016).

Slimming and Toning Oils

*See **Weight: Slimming/Toning***

Smell (loss of)

*See **Nose: Olfactory Loss***

Smoking

*See **Addictions: Smoking, Purification: Cigarette Smoke***

Snake Bite

*See **Bites/Stings: Snakes***

A
B
C
D
E
F
G
H
I
J
K
L
M
N
O
P
Q
R
S
T
U
V
W
X
Y
Z

Sores

See Wounds, Antibacterial, Antifungal, Antiviral

Sore Throat

See Throat: Sore, Antibacterial, Antiviral, Infection

Spasms

See Muscles, Digestive System

Spina Bifida

Spina bifida is a birth defect in which the vertebrae of the lower spine do not form correctly, leaving a gap or opening between them. In the most severe cases, this can cause the meninges (the tissue surrounding the spinal cord), or even the spinal cord itself, to protrude through the gap. If the spinal cord protrudes through the gap, it can prevent the nerves from developing normally, causing numbness, paralysis, back pain, and loss of bladder and bowel control and function. This latter type often also develops with a defect in which the back part of the brain develops in the upper neck rather than within the skull, often causing a mental handicap.

Oils: eucalyptus, lavender, Roman chamomile, lemon, orange, rosemary

Other Products: Alpha CRS+ contains 400 mg of folic acid, which has been found to significantly reduce the chance of spina bifida developing in infants if taken as a daily supplement by their mothers before conception (Centers for Disease Control and Prevention, 2004).

○: Take capsules as directed on package

◑: Dilute as recommended, and apply 1–2 drops to bottoms of feet, along spine, on forehead, and on back of neck.

✺: Diffuse into the air.

⊕: Body System(s) Affected: Skeletal and Nervous Systems.

Spine

See Back

Spleen

See also Lymphatic System

The spleen is a fist-sized spongy tissue that is part of the lymphatic system. Its purpose is to filter bacteria, viruses, fungi, and other unwanted substances out of the blood and to create lymphocytes (white blood cells that create antibodies).

Oils: marjoram

◑: Dilute as recommended and apply 1–2 drops over spleen or on reflex points on the feet. Apply as a warm compress over upper abdomen.

⊕: Body System(s) Affected: Cardiovascular System and Immune System.

Sprains

See Muscles: Sprains

Spurs

See Skeletal System: Bone Spurs

Stains

See Housecleaning: Stains

Staph Infection

See Antibacterial: Staph Infection

Sterility

See Female-Specific Conditions: Infertility, Male Specific Conditions: Infertility

Stimulating

Oils: peppermint, Elevation, eucalyptus⊕, orange, ginger, grapefruit, rose, rosemary⊕, basil

✺: Diffuse into the air. Inhale directly from bottle. Apply oil to hands, tissue, or cotton wick, and inhale.

◑: Dilute as recommended, and apply 1–2 drops to forehead, neck, or bottoms of feet. Add 1–2 drops to an unscented bath gel, and add to warm bathwater while filling; bathe. Add 5–10 drops to

1 Tbs. (15 ml) fractionated coconut oil, and use as massage oil.

⊕: Body System(s) Affected: Emotional Balance.

▢: Additional Research:

Eucalyptus: Imaging of the brain demonstrated that inhalation of 1,8-cineol (eucalyptol—a constituent of many essential oils, especially eucalyptus, rosemary, and marjoram) increased global cerebral blood flow after an inhalation time of 20 minutes (Nasel et al., 1994).

Rosemary: Imaging of the brain demonstrated that inhalation of 1,8-cineol (eucalyptol—a constituent of many essential oils, especially eucalyptus, rosemary, and marjoram) increased global cerebral blood flow after an inhalation time of 20 minutes (Nasel et al., 1994).

Stings

See Bites/Stings

Stomach

See Digestive System: Stomach

Strep Throat

See Throat: Strep

Stress

> *Simple Solutions—Stress:* Diffuse lavender or grapefruit oil in an aromatherapy diffuser.

> *Simple Solutions—Stress:* Add 10 drops lavender to 1 cup (250 g) Epsom salt. Dissolve ½ cup (125 g) of the salt in warm bathwater for a relaxing bath.

Stress is the body's response to difficult, pressured, or worrisome circumstances. Stress can cause both physical and emotional tension. Symptoms of stress include headaches, muscle soreness, fatigue, insomnia, nervousness, anxiety, and irritability.

Oils: lavender, InTune, Thinker, lemon, ylang ylang, bergamot, petitgrain, neroli, Elevation, Serenity, Calmer, grapefruit, Rescuer, AromaTouch, Roman chamomile, geranium, spikenard, Balance, frankincense, marjoram

—Chemical:

Oils: lavender, rosemary, grapefruit, geranium, clary sage, lemon

—Emotional Stress:

Oils: Elevation, clary sage, Peace, bergamot, Console, petitgrain, geranium, Roman chamomile, sandalwood

—Environmental Stress:

Oils: bergamot, cypress, geranium, cedarwood

—Mental Stress:

Oils: lavender, InTune, Thinker, grapefruit, bergamot, petitgrain, sandalwood, geranium

—Performance Stress:

Oils: grapefruit, bergamot, ginger, rosemary

—Physical Stress:

Oils: Serenity, lavender, bergamot, geranium, marjoram, Rescuer, Roman chamomile, rosemary, thyme

—Stress Due to Tiredness or Insomnia:

Blend 1: Add 15 drops clary sage, 10 drops lemon, and 5 drops lavender to 2 Tbs. (25 ml) fractionated coconut oil. Massage on skin.

⊘: Diffuse into the air. Inhale directly from bottle. Apply oil to hands, tissue, or cotton wick, and inhale. Wear as perfume or cologne.

⊜: Add 5–10 drops to 1 Tbs. (15 ml) fractionated coconut oil, and massage on skin. Add 1–2 drops to ¼ cup (50 g) Therapeutic Bath Salts, and dissolve in warm bathwater before bathing. Dilute as recommended, and apply 1–2 drops on neck, back, or bottoms of feet.

⊕: Body System(s) Affected: Emotional Balance and Nervous System.

▢: Additional Research:

Lavender: Nurses working in an ICU setting demonstrated decreased perception of stress when receiving a topical application of *Lavandula angustifolia* and Salvia sclarea essential oils (Pemberton et al., 2008).

Lavender: Subjects placed in a small, soundproof room for 20 minutes were found to have reduced mental stress and increased arousal rate when exposed to the scent of lavender (Motomura et al., 2001).

A B C D E F G H I J K L M N O P Q R **S** T U V W X Y Z

My Usage Guide

Lemon: Lemon oil vapor was found to have strong antistress and antidepressant effects on mice subjected to several common behavioral stress tests (Komiya et al., 2006).

Ylang ylang: Subjects who had ylang ylang oil applied to their skin had decreased blood pressure, increased skin temperature, and reported feeling more calm and relaxed compared to subjects in a control group (Hongratanaworakit et al., 2006).

Stretch Marks

See Skin: Stretch Marks

Stroke

See also Brain, Blood: Clots, Cardiovascular System

A stroke occurs when the blood supply to the brain is interrupted. Within a few minutes, brain cells begin to die. The affected area of the brain is unable to function, and one or more limbs on one side of the body become weak and unable to move. Strokes can cause serious disabilities, including paralysis and speech problems.

Oils: cypress, helichrysum, fennel, cedarwood, basil

—Muscular Paralysis:

  Oils: lavender

  Blend 1: Combine 1 drop basil, 1 drop lavender, and 1 drop rosemary, and apply to spinal column and paralyzed area.

: Inhale oil directly or applied to hands, tissue, or cotton wick. Diffuse into the air.

: Dilute as directed, and apply 1–2 drops to the back of the neck and the forehead.

: **Body System(s) Affected:** Cardiovascular System and Nervous System.

: **Additional Research:**

Fennel: Both fennel oil and its constituent, anethole, were found to significantly reduce thrombosis (blood clots) in mice. They were also found to be free from the prohemorrhagic (increased bleeding) side effect that aspirin (acetylsalicylic acid) has (Tognolini et al., 2007).

Cedarwood: A chemical constituent, α-eudesmol, found in cedarwood oil demonstrated the ability to protect against brain injury after cerebral ischemia (stroke) in rats. Specifically, α-eudesmol was found to attenuate cerebral edema formation, reduce cerebral infarct size, and inhibit calcium-dependent glutamate release from synaptosomes (Asakura et al., 2000).

Basil: Oral pretreatment of basil extract was found to protect against brain damage induced by bilateral carotid artery occlusion in mice by reducing tissue death size and the oxidative degradation of lipids and restoring antioxidant content and motor functions. The researchers state that these results suggest that basil could be useful clinically in the prevention of stroke (Bora et al., 2011).

Sudorific

A sudorific is a substance that induces sweating.

Oils: thyme, rosemary, lavender, Roman chamomile, juniper berry

: Add 5–10 drops to 1 Tbs. (15 ml) fractionated coconut oil, and apply to skin.

: **Body System(s) Affected:** Endocrine System.

Suicidal Feelings

See Depression

Sunburn

See Burns: Sunburn

Sunscreen

Oils: helichrysum, arborvitae, sandalwood

: Add 5–10 drops to 1 Tbs. (15 ml) fractionated coconut oil, and apply to the skin.

: **Body System(s) Affected:** Skin.

: **Additional Research:**

Arborvitae: Application of β-thujaplicin on mouse ear skin decreased sunburn cell formation by 40% as compared to untreated skin, suggesting that β-thujaplicin can inhibit ultraviolet B-induced apoptosis and skin damage (Baba et al., 1998).

Swelling

See Edema, Inflammation

Sympathetic Nervous System

See Nervous System: Sympathetic Nervous System

Tachycardia

See Cardiovascular System: Tachycardia

Taste (Impaired)

See also Nose: Olfactory Loss

Taste is the sensation of sweet, sour, salty, or bitter by taste buds on the tongue when a substance enters the mouth. This sensation, combined with the smell of the food, helps create the unique flavors we experience in food.

Oils: helichrysum, peppermint

: Dilute as recommended, and apply 1 drop on the tongue or reflex points on the feet.

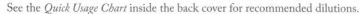

See the *Quick Usage Chart* inside the back cover for recommended dilutions.

Teeth

See Oral Conditions

Temperature

See Cooling Oils, Warming Oils

Tendinitis

See Muscles: Tendinitis

Tennis Elbow

See Joints: Tennis Elbow

Tension

Oils: ⚬Serenity, ⚬Calmer, ⚬lavender, ⚬Aroma-Touch, ⚬Rescuer, ⚬cedarwood, ⚬ylang ylang, ⚬Roman chamomile, ⚬frankincense, ⚬basil (nervous), ⚬bergamot (nervous), ⚬grapefruit

⚬: Inhale oil applied to hands. Diffuse into the air.

⚬: Add 3–5 drops to ½ cup (125 g) Therapeutic Bath Salts, and dissolve in warm bathwater before bathing. Add 5–10 drops to 1 Tbs. (15 ml) fractionated coconut oil, and use as massage oil.

⚬: **Body System(s) Affected:** Emotional Balance.

Testes

Testes are the male reproductive organs. The testes are responsible for producing and storing sperm and male hormones such as testosterone. Hormones produced in the testes are responsible for the development of male characteristics: facial hair, wide shoulders, low voice, and reproductive organs.

Oils: ⚬rosemary

—Regulation:

Oils: ⚬clary sage, ⚬sandalwood, ⚬geranium

⚬: Dilute as recommended, and apply 1–2 drops on location or on reflex points on the feet.

⚬: Diffuse into the air. Inhale directly from bottle. Apply oil to hands, tissue, or cotton wick, and inhale.

⚬: **Body System(s) Affected:** Reproductive System.

Throat

See also Respiratory System, Neck

Oils: ⚬cypress, ⚬oregano

—Congestion:

Oils: ⚬peppermint, ⚬myrrh

—Cough: *See Respiratory System*

—Dry:

Oils: ⚬lemon, ⚬grapefruit

—Infection In:

Oils: ⚬lemon, ⚬On Guard, ⚬peppermint, ⚬oregano, ⚬clary sage

Other Products: ⚬On Guard+ Softgels

—Laryngitis: *See Laryngitis*

—Sore:

Oils: ⚬melaleuca, ⚬On Guard, ⚬oregano, ⚬sandalwood, ⚬lime, ⚬bergamot, ⚬geranium, ⚬ginger, ⚬myrrh

> *Simple Solutions—Sore Throat:* Add 4 drops On Guard and 1 tsp. (5 g) salt to ¼ cup (50 ml) warm water, and stir until salt is dissolved. Gargle with the solution for 30 seconds, then spit out. Repeat up to 2 times a day until sore throat is gone.

> *Simple Solutions—Sore Throat:* Add 3 drops eucalyptus and 2 drops lemon to 1 tsp. (5 ml) honey, and dissolve in 2 Tbs. (25 ml) of water. Place in a small spray bottle. Shake well, and mist 3–4 sprays into throat as needed to help soothe.

Other Products: ⚬On Guard Protecting Throat Drops to soothe irritated and sore throats.

—Strep:

Strep throat is a throat infection caused by streptococci bacteria. This infection causes the throat and tonsils to become inflamed and swollen, resulting in a severe sore throat. Symptoms of strep throat include a sudden severe sore throat, pain when swallowing, high fever, swollen tonsils and lymph nodes, white spots on the back of the throat, skin rash, and sometimes vomiting. Strep throat should be closely monitored so that it doesn't develop into a more serious condition such as rheumatic fever or kidney inflammation.

Oils: ⚫☀♻On Guard▢, ♻melaleuca, ♻ginger, ♻geranium, ♻oregano

—Tonsillitis:

Tonsillitis is inflammation of the tonsils, typically due to infection. Tonsillitis causes the tonsils to become swollen and painful. Symptoms of tonsillitis include sore throat, red and swollen tonsils, painful swallowing, loss of voice, fever, chills, headache, and white patches on the tonsils.

Oils: ♻melaleuca, ♻On Guard, ☀ginger, ♻lavender, ♻lemon, ♻bergamot, ♻clove, ☀thyme, ♻Roman chamomile

💧: Add 1 drop to 1 cup (250 ml) water (4 cups (1 L) for On Guard), and drink. Place 1 drop oil under the tongue. Take supplement as directed.

🖐: Dilute as recommended, and apply 1–2 drops on throat or reflex points on the feet. Add 1–2 drops to ½ cup (125 ml) water, and gargle.

🌀: Diffuse into the air. Inhale directly from bottle. Apply oil to hands, tissue, or cotton wick, and inhale.

♻: **Body System(s) Affected:** Respiratory System and Immune System.

📖: **Additional Research:**

On Guard: Cinnamon, thyme, and clove essential oils demonstrated an antibacterial effect on several respiratory tract pathogens including streptococci (Fabio et al., 2007).

On Guard: Eucalyptus globulus oil was found to inhibit several bacteria types, including strep (Cermelli et al., 2008).

Thrush

*See **Antifungal: Candida, Antifungal: Thrush, Children and Infants: Thrush***

Thymus

*See also **Immune System, Lymphatic System***

The thymus is an organ responsible for the development of T cells needed for immune system functioning. The thymus is located just behind the sternum in the upper part of the chest.

Oils: ☀On Guard

🖐: Dilute as recommended, and apply over thymus or on bottoms of feet.

♻: **Body System(s) Affected:** Immune System.

Thyroid

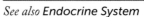

*See also **Endocrine System***

The thyroid is a gland located in the front of the neck that plays a key role in regulating metabolism. The thyroid produces and secretes the hormones needed to regulate blood pressure, heart rate, body temperature, and energy production.

—Dysfunction:

Oils: ♻clove

—Hyperthyroidism: *See also Grave's Disease*

Hyperthyroidism is when the thyroid gland produces too much of its hormones, typically due to the thyroid becoming enlarged. This can result in a noticeably enlarged thyroid gland (goiter), sudden weight loss, sweating, a rapid or irregular heartbeat, shortness of breath, muscle weakness, nervousness, and irritability.

Oils: ♻myrrh, ♻lemongrass

Blend 1: Combine 1 drop myrrh and 1 drop lemongrass, and apply on base of throat and on reflex points on the feet.

—Hypothyroidism: *See also Hashimoto's Disease*

Hypothyroidism is the result of an underactive thyroid. Consequently, the thyroid gland doesn't produce enough of necessary hormones. Symptoms include fatigue, a puffy face, a hoarse voice, unexplained weight gain, higher blood cholesterol levels, muscle weakness and aches, depression, heavy menstrual periods, memory problems, and low tolerance for the cold.

Oils: ♻peppermint, ♻clove, ♻lemongrass

Blend 2: Combine 1 drop lemongrass with 1 drop of either peppermint or clove, and apply on base of throat and on reflex points on the feet.

—Supports:

Oils: ☀myrrh

🖐: Dilute as recommended, and apply 1–2 drops on base of throat, hands, or reflex points on the feet.

🌀: Diffuse into the air. Inhale oils applied to hands.

♻: **Body System(s) Affected:** Endocrine System.

Tinnitus

*See **Ears: Tinnitus***

See the *Quick Usage Chart* inside the back cover for recommended dilutions.

Tired

See Energy

Tissue

Tissue refers to any group of similar cells that work together to perform a specific function in an organ or in the body. Some types of tissue include muscle tissue, connective tissue, nervous tissue, or epithelial tissue (tissue that lines or covers a surface, such as the skin or the lining of the blood vessels).

Oils: lemongrass, helichrysum, basil, marjoram, sandalwood, Roman chamomile, lavender

Other Products: Deep Blue Rub and Deep Blue Polyphenol Complex to help soothe muscle and connective tissues.

—Cleanses Toxins From:

Oils: fennel

—Connective Tissue: *See Muscles*

—Deep Tissue Pain: *See Pain: Tissue*

—Repair:

Oils: lemongrass, helichrysum, orange

—Regenerate:

Oils: lemongrass, helichrysum, geranium, patchouli

—Scarring:

Scar tissue is the dense and fibrous tissue that forms over a healed cut or wound. The scar tissue serves as a protective barrier but is still inferior to the healthy, normal tissue. In an area of scar tissue, sweat glands are nonfunctional, hair does not grow, and the skin is not as protected against ultraviolet radiation. Scars fade and become less noticeable over time but cannot be completely removed.

Oils: lavender (burns), rose (helps prevent), frankincense (helps prevent), helichrysum (reduces), geranium, myrrh

Blend 1: Combine 5 drops helichrysum and 5 drops lavender with 1 Tbs. (15 ml) sunflower oil or with liquid lecithin (an emulsifier extracted from eggs or soy), and apply on location.

Blend 2: Combine 1 drop lavender, 1 drop lemongrass, and 1 drop geranium, and apply on location to help prevent scar formation.

: Dilute as recommended, and apply 1–2 drops on location or on reflex points on the feet. Apply as warm compress. Add 5–10 drops to 1 Tbs. (15 ml) fractionated coconut oil, and massage on location.

Tonic

A tonic is a substance given to invigorate or strengthen an organ, tissue, or system or to stimulate physical, emotional, or mental energy and strength.

—General:

Oils: lemongrass, cinnamon, sandalwood, clary sage, grapefruit, ginger, geranium, marjoram, myrrh, orange, Roman chamomile, ylang ylang

—Heart:

Oils: thyme, lavender

—Nerve:

Oils: clary sage, melaleuca, thyme

—Skin:

Oils: lemon

—Uterine:

Oils: thyme

: Add 5–10 drops to 1 Tbs. (15 ml) fractionated coconut oil, and massage on location. Dilute as recommended, and apply 1–2 drops to area or to reflex points on the feet. Add 1–2 drops to warm bathwater before bathing.

: Diffuse into the air. Inhale directly from bottle. Apply oil to hands, tissue, or cotton wick, and inhale.

Tonsillitis

See Throat: Tonsillitis

Toothache

See Oral Conditions: Toothache

Toxemia

See also Antibacterial, Pregnancy/Motherhood: Preeclampsia

Toxemia is the general term for toxic substances in the bloodstream. This is typically caused by a bacterial infection in which bacteria release toxins into the blood.

Oils: cypress

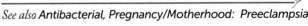

🔘: Dilute as recommended, and apply 1–2 drops on neck, over heart, or on bottoms of feet. Add 5–10 drops to 1 Tbs. (15 ml) fractionated coconut oil, and massage on neck, back, chest, and legs.

🌀: Diffuse into the air.

☯: **Body System(s) Affected:** Immune System and Cardiovascular System.

Toxins

See **Detoxification**

Travel Sickness

See **Nausea: Motion Sickness**

Tuberculosis (T.B.)

See also **Antibacterial, Respiratory System**

Tuberculosis is a bacterial disease spread through the air (via coughing, spitting, sneezing, etc.). Tuberculosis most commonly infects the lungs, but it can infect other bodily systems as well. Symptoms of tuberculosis include a chronic cough (often with blood), fever, chills, weakness and fatigue, weight loss, and night sweats. Tuberculosis is contagious and sometimes deadly.

Oils: eucalyptus, cypress, Breathe, thyme, cedarwood, On Guard, lemon, melissa, vetiver, peppermint, sandalwood

Other Products: Breathe Respiratory Drops, Breathe Vapor Stick

—**Airborne Bacteria:**

   Oils: On Guard, lemongrass, geranium, Purify, Breathe

—**Pulmonary:**

   Oils: oregano, cypress, eucalyptus, frankincense

🌀: Diffuse into the air. Inhale directly from bottle. Apply oil to hands, tissue, or cotton wick, and inhale. Add 2–3 drops to bowl of hot water, and inhale vapors.

🔘: Dilute as recommended, and apply 1–2 drops on chest, back, or reflex points on the feet. Add 1–2 drops to 1 tsp. (5 ml) fractionated coconut oil, and apply as rectal implant. Add 5–10 drops to 1 Tbs.

(15 ml) fractionated coconut oil, and massage on chest, back, and feet.

☯: **Body System(s) Affected:** Respiratory System and Immune System.

📖: **Additional Research:**

Vetiver: The ethanolic extract of vetiver root was found to inhibit both virulent and avirulent strains of *M. tuberculosis*, suggesting that vetiver could be useful in treating tubercular infections (Saikia et al., 2012).

Lemongrass: A formulation of lemongrass and geranium oil was found to reduce airborne bacteria by 89% in an office environment after diffusion for 15 hours (Doran et al., 2009).

Geranium: A formulation of lemongrass and geranium oil was found to reduce airborne bacteria by 89% in an office environment after diffusion for 15 hours (Doran et al., 2009).

Tumor

See also **Cancer**

A tumor is an abnormal growth of cells in a lump or mass. Some tumors are malignant (cancerous) and some are benign (noncancerous). Benign tumors in most parts of the body do not create health problems. *For information on cancerous (malignant) tumors, see Cancer.*

Oils: frankincense, DDR Prime, clove, sandalwood

—**Lipoma:**

   Lipoma is a benign tumor of the fatty tissues that most commonly forms just below the surface of the skin; but it can also form in any other area of the body where fatty tissue is present.

   Oils: frankincense, clove, DDR Prime, grapefruit, ginger

🔘: Dilute as recommended, and apply 1–2 drops on location.

💧: Take 3–5 drops in an empty capsule, or with food and beverage. Take up to twice per day as needed.

🌀: Diffuse into the air. Inhale directly from bottle. Apply oil to hands, tissue, or cotton wick, and inhale.

Typhoid

See also **Antibacterial**

Typhoid fever is a bacterial infection caused by the bacteria *Salmonella typhi*. Typhoid is spread through food and water infected with the feces of typhoid carriers. Possible symptoms of typhoid include abdominal pain, severe diarrhea, bloody stools, chills, severe fatigue, weakness, chills, delirium, hallucinations, confusion, agitation, and fluctuating mood.

See the *Quick Usage Chart* inside the back cover for recommended dilutions.

370

Oils: 🜂cinnamon, 🜂peppermint, 🜂Purify, 🜂lemon, 🜂Breathe

🜍: Dilute as recommended, and apply over intestines or on reflex points on the feet.

🜁: Diffuse into the air.

✛: **Body System(s) Affected:** Immune System and Digestive System.

Ulcers

See also **Digestive System**

An ulcer is an open sore either on the skin or on an internal mucous membrane (such as that lining the stomach).

> *Simple Solutions—Ulcers:* Mix 1 drop lemon in 1 tsp. (5 ml) honey. Dissolve in 1 cup (250 ml) of warm water, and drink.

Oils: 🜔frankincense, 🜔myrrh, 🜔marjoram🜔, 🜔lemon🜔, 🜔dill🜔, 🜔oregano, 🜔rose, 🜔thyme, 🜔clove, 🜔bergamot

—Duodenal:

A duodenal ulcer is an ulcer in the upper part of the small intestine.

Oils: 🜔frankincense, 🜔myrrh, 🜔lemon, 🜔oregano, 🜔rose, 🜔thyme, 🜔clove, 🜔bergamot

—Gastric: *See also* **Digestive System: Gastritis.**

A gastric ulcer is an ulcer in the stomach.

Oils: 🜔geranium, 🜔peppermint, 🜔marjoram🜔, 🜔lemon🜔, 🜔dill🜔, 🜔frankincense, 🜔orange, 🜔bergamot

—Leg:

An ulcer on the leg may be due to a lack of circulation in the lower extremities or possibly due to a bacterial, fungal, or viral infection. *See also* **Cardiovascular System: Circulation, Antibacterial, Antifungal, Antiviral.**

Oils: 🜍Purify, 🜍lavender, 🜍Roman chamomile, 🜍geranium

—Mouth: *See* **Canker Sores**

—Peptic:

A peptic ulcer is an ulcer that forms in an area of the digestive system where acid is present, such as in the stomach (gastric), esophagus, or upper part of the small intestine (duodenal). *See also* **Duodenal, Gastric** in this section.

Recipe 1: Flavor 4 cups (1 L) of water with 1 drop cinnamon, and sip all day.

—Varicose Ulcer:

A varicose ulcer is an ulcer on the lower leg where varicose (swollen) veins are located.

Oils: 🜍melaleuca, 🜍geranium, 🜍lavender, 🜍eucalyptus, 🜍thyme

🜔: Add 1 drop oil to rice or almond milk, and drink. Place oil in an empty capsule and swallow. Add 1 drop or less as flavoring to food after cooking.

🜍: Dilute as recommended, and apply 1–2 drops over area. Apply as warm compress.

✛: **Body System(s) Affected:** Skin and Digestive System.

⊟: **Additional Research:**

Marjoram: Oral administration of marjoram extract was shown to significantly decrease the incidence of ulcers, basal gastric secretion, and acid output in rats (Al-Howiriny et al., 2009).

Lemon: Lemon essential oil and its majority compound (limonene) exhibited a gastroprotective effect against induced gastric ulcers in rats (Rozza et al., 2011).

Dill: Oral administration of dill seed extract was found to have effective antisecretory and anti-ulcer activity against HCl- and ethanol-induced stomach lesions in mice (Hosseinzadeh et al., 2002).

Unwind

See **Calming**

Uplifting

Oils: 🜁Cheer, 🜁lemon🜁, 🜁orange, 🜁petitgrain, 🜁Elevation, 🜁Brave, 🜁Console, 🜁Passion, 🜁Citrus Bliss, 🜁Forgive, 🜁bergamot, 🜁grapefruit, 🜁yarrow, 🜁Whisper, 🜁myrrh, 🜁wintergreen, 🜁lavender

🜁: Diffuse into the air. Inhale directly from bottle. Apply oil to hands, tissue, or cotton wick; inhale. Wear as perfume or cologne.

✛: **Body System(s) Affected:** Emotional Balance.

⊟: **Additional Research:**

Lemon: Lemon odor was found to enhance the positive mood of volunteers exposed to a stressor (Kiecolt-Glaser et al., 2008).

Lemon: Lemon oil and its component, citral, were found to decrease depressed behavior in a similar manner to antidepressant drugs in rats involved in several stress tests (Komori et al., 1995).

Ureter

See Urinary Tract

Urinary Tract

The urinary tract is the collection of organs and tubes responsible for producing and excreting urine. The urinary tract is comprised of the kidneys, bladder, ureters, and urethra.

Oils: sandalwood, thyme, melaleuca, bergamot, lavender, rosemary

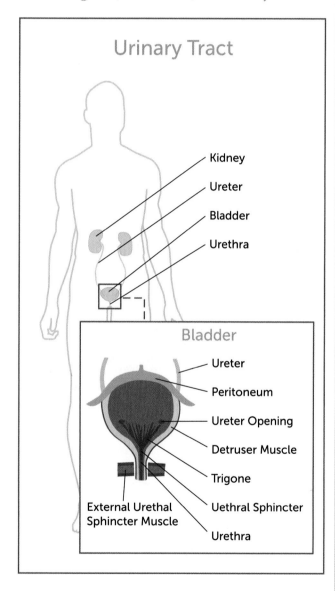

Urinary Tract

Kidney
Ureter
Bladder
Urethra

Bladder

Ureter
Peritoneum
Ureter Opening
Detruser Muscle
Trigone
External Urethal Sphincter Muscle
Uethral Sphincter
Urethra

—General Stimulant:

Oils: eucalyptus, bergamot

—Infection: *See also Bladder: Cystitis/Infection*

Oils: Purify, lemongrass, cedarwood, geranium, bergamot, juniper berry

Blend 1: Combine 1 drop On Guard with 1 drop oregano; apply as a hot compress over abdomen and pubic area.

Other Products: On Guard+ Softgels

—Stones In: *See also Kidneys: Kidney Stones*

Stones are solid masses that form as minerals and other chemicals crystallize and adhere together. They can form in the bladder or kidneys. While small stones generally cause no problems, larger stones may block the ureters or urethra, causing intense pain and possibly injury.

Oils: fennel, geranium

—Support:

Oils: geranium, cypress, melaleuca

⊜: Dilute as recommended, and apply 1–2 drops over lower abdomen, lower back, or pubic area. Add 5–10 drops to 1 Tbs. (15 ml) fractionated coconut oil, and massage on abdomen, lower, back, or pubic area. Apply as a warm compress.

◐: Take supplement as directed.

◉: Diffuse into the air.

⊕: **Body System(s) Affected:** Endocrine System and Digestive System.

Uterus

See also Endometriosis, Female-Specific Conditions

The uterus is the female reproductive organ in which a fetus is formed and develops until birth.

Oils: frankincense, lemon, myrrh, cedarwood, geranium

—Regeneration of Tissue:

Oils: frankincense

—Uterotonic:

An uterotonic is a medication used to stimulate contractions of the uterus. Uterotonics should be avoided or used with extreme caution during pregnancy as they may be abortive. Uterotonics are used to start or speed up labor, to reduce hemorrhaging, and to cause contractions after a miscarriage.

See the *Quick Usage Chart* inside the back cover for recommended dilutions.

Oils: ⊘thyme

—Uterine Cancer: *See Cancer: Uterine*

⊜: Dilute as recommended, and apply 1–2 drops on lower abdomen or on reflex points on the feet and ankles. Add 2–5 drops essential oil to 1 tsp. (5 ml) fractionated coconut oil, and insert into vagina for overnight retention (a tampon may be used if necessary to help retain the oil). Apply as a warm compress.

✛: **Body System(s) Affected:** Reproductive System.

Vaginal

—Candida: *See also Antifungal: Candida*

Candida refers to a genus of yeast that are normally found in the digestive tract and on the skin of humans. These yeast are typically symbiotically beneficial to humans. However, several species of *Candida*, such as *Candida albicans*, can cause infections, such as vaginal candidiasis, that cause localized itching, soreness, and redness.

Oils: ⊘melaleuca⊕, ⊘⊘oregano⊕, ⊘clove⊕, ⊘On Guard, ⊘bergamot, ⊘peppermint⊕, ⊘thyme⊕, ⊘lavender⊕, ⊘eucalyptus, ⊘rosemary, ⊘⊘DigestZen

—Infection: *See also Candida (above), Antibacterial, Antifungal, Antiviral*

Vaginal infections occur when there is a disruption in the normal balance of vaginal organisms, such as the sudden presence of yeast, bacteria, or viruses. Common signs of vaginal infection include redness, swelling, itching, pain, odor, change in discharge color or amount, a burning sensation when urinating, and pain or bleeding during intercourse. The most common vaginal infections are yeast infection, trichomoniasis, and bacterial vaginosis.

Oils: ⊘rosemary, ⊘cinnamon (dilute heavily), ⊘melaleuca, ⊘oregano, ⊘thyme, ⊘myrrh, ⊘clary sage, ⊘cypress, ⊘juniper berry, ⊘eucalyptus, ⊘lavender

—Vaginitis:

Vaginitis is vaginal inflammation, typically due to infection, characterized by redness, swelling, itching, irritation, discharge, and pain of the vaginal area.

Oils: ⊘rosemary, ⊘cinnamon (dilute heavily), ⊘eucalyptus, ⊘melaleuca, ⊘lavender

Recipe 1: Valerie Worwood suggests combining 1 drop lavender, 1 drop melaleuca, 1 tsp. (5 ml) vinegar, ½ tsp. (2 ml) lemon juice, and 2½ cups (625 ml) of warm water for a douche that can be used 3 days a week.

⊜: Dilute oils as recommended, and apply 1–2 drops on location. Add 2–3 drops to 1 tsp. (5 ml) fractionated coconut oil, insert using vaginal syringe, and retain using tampon overnight. Add 2–3 drops to 1 tsp. (5 ml) fractionated coconut oil, soak tampon in mixture, insert, and leave in all day or overnight. Add 1–2 drops to warm water, and use in a douche. Add 1–2 drops to warm bathwater, and bathe.

⊘: Place 1–2 drops under the tongue, or place 2–3 drops in an empty capsule, and swallow.

✛: **Body System(s) Affected:** Reproductive System.

⊞: **Additional Research:**

Melaleuca: Tea tree oil was found to inhibit 301 different types of yeasts isolated from the mouths of cancer patients suffering from advanced cancer, including 41 strains that are known to be resistant to antifungal drugs (Bagg et al., 2006).

Melaleuca: Eleven types of Candida were found to be highly inhibited by tea tree oil (Banes-Marshall et al., 2001).

Melaleuca: Tea tree oil was found to disrupt the cellular membrane and to inhibit respiration in *Candida albicans* (Cox et al., 2000).

Melaleuca: Melaleuca oil at concentrations of .16% was found to inhibit the transformation of C. albicans from single-cell yeast to the pathogenic mycelial (multi-cellular strands) form (D'Auria et al., 2001).

Melaleuca: Tea Tree oil was found to alter the membrane properties and functions of *Candida albicans* cells, leading to cell inhibition or death (Hammer et al., 2004).

Melaleuca: Terpinen-4-ol, a constituent of tea tree oil, and tea tree oil were found to be effective against several forms of vaginal Candida infections in rats, including azole-resistant forms (Mondello et al., 2006).

Melaleuca: Melaleuca oil inhibited several Candida species in vitro (Vazquez et al., 2000).

Oregano: Mice infected with *Candida albicans* who were fed origanum oil or carvacrol diluted in olive oil had an 80% survival rate after 30 days, while infected mice fed olive oil alone all died after 10 days (Manohar et al., 2001).

Clove: Clove oil was found to have very strong radical scavenging activity (antioxidant). It was also found to display an antifungal effect against tested Candida strains (Chaieb et al., 2007).

Peppermint: Peppermint oil was found to have a higher fungistatic and fungicidal activity against various fungi (including Candida) than the commercial fungicide bifonazole (Mimica-Dukić et al., 2003).

Thyme: Thyme oil was found to inhibit Candida species by causing lesions in the cell membrane and inhibiting germ tube (an outgrowth that develops when the fungi is preparing to replicate) formation (Pina-Vaz et al., 2004).

Lavender: Lavender oil demonstrated both fungistatic (stopped growth) and fungicidal (killed) activity against *Candida albicans* (D'Auria et al., 2005).

Varicose Ulcers

See Ulcers: Varicose Ulcer

Varicose Veins

Varicose veins are twisted, enlarged, blue and purple veins most often found on the legs and ankles. They have several possible causes, including weakened valves causing blood to pool around the vein. In some cases, varicose veins are merely a cosmetic problem because of their appearance, but in other cases they can be quite painful. *See also Hemorrhoids for varicose veins of the anus or rectum.*

> *Simple Solutions—Varicose Veins:* Add 3 drops cypress and 1 drop lemongrass to 1 Tbs. (15 ml) fractionated coconut oil. Gently massage a small amount on location daily.

Oils: cypress, lemongrass, lemon, peppermint, helichrysum, Citrus Bliss, geranium, lavender, rosemary, juniper berry, orange

: Dilute as recommended, and apply oils gently from ankles up the legs. *Consistent application of oils for an extended period of time is the key.* Add 3–5 drops to 1 Tbs. (15 ml) fractionated coconut oil, and massage above the veins towards the heart. Wearing support hose and elevating the feet can also help keep blood from pooling in the legs.

: **Body System(s) Affected:** Cardiovascular System and Skin.

Vascular System

See Cardiovascular System; see also Arteries, Capillaries, Veins

Vasodilator

See Arteries: Arterial Vasodilator

Veins

A vein is a blood vessel that carries blood from the capillaries back to the heart. Veins may also have one-way valves on the inside that help keep blood from flowing backwards and pooling in the lower extremities due to gravity.

Oils: lemongrass, cypress, lemon, helichrysum

—**Blood Clot in Vein:**

Blend 1: Apply 1 drop cypress and 1 drop helichrysum on location of clot to help dissolve.

: Dilute as recommended, and apply 1–2 drops on location. Add 5–10 drops to 1 Tbs. (15 ml) fractionated coconut oil, and massage on location.

: **Body System(s) Affected:** Cardiovascular System.

Vertigo

See also Ears, Nausea: Motion Sickness

Vertigo refers to the sensation that the environment and objects around an individual are moving or spinning, usually causing a loss of balance or feelings of nausea. Vertigo may be caused by ear infections, ear disorders, or motion sickness.

Oils: ginger, helichrysum, geranium, basil, lavender

Recipe 1: Apply 1–2 drops each of helichrysum, geranium, and lavender to the tops of each ear (massaging slightly); then apply the oils behind each ear, pulling your hands down behind the jaw bone to just below the jaw. Finish by applying 1–2 drops of basil behind and down each ear. This can be performed multiple times a day until symptoms decrease.

: Dilute as recommended, and apply 1–2 drops around ears and on reflex points on the feet.

: Inhale oil directly from bottle. Apply oil to hands, tissue, or cotton wick, and inhale.

: **Body System(s) Affected:** Nervous, Respiratory, and Digestive Systems.

Viral Disease/Viruses

See Antiviral

Vitiligo

See Skin: Vitiligo

Voice (Hoarse)

See also Laryngitis

A hoarse voice is typically caused by laryngitis (inflammation of the larynx due to infection), but it can also be caused by other problems such as an ulcer, sore, polyp, or tumor on or near the vocal cords.

Oils: bergamot

See the *Quick Usage Chart* inside the back cover for recommended dilutions.

374

Recipe 1: Add 1 drop melaleuca, 1 drop rosemary, 1 drop clove, and 1 drop lemon to 1 tsp. (5 ml) honey. Swish around in the mouth for a couple of minutes to liquefy with saliva; then swallow.

◯: Add 1 drop to 1 tsp. (5 ml) honey, and swallow.

✿: **Body System(s) Affected:** Respiratory System.

Vomiting

See Nausea: Vomiting

Warming Oils

Oils: ♨cinnamon, ♨oregano, ♨yuzu, ♨thyme, ♨marjoram, ♨rosemary, ♨juniper berry

◌: Add 5–10 drops to 1 tsp. (5 ml) fractionated coconut oil, and massage briskly into skin.

✿: **Body System(s) Affected:** Skin.

Warts

A wart is a small, firm, hard growth on the skin, usually located on the hands and feet, that is typically caused by a virus.

> *Simple Solutions—Wart:* Combine 5 drops cypress, 10 drops lemon, and 2 Tbs. (25 ml) apple cider vinegar. Apply on location twice daily; bandage. Keep a bandage on until wart is gone.

Oils: ♨frankincense, ♨On Guard, ♨melaleuca, ♨oregano (layer with On Guard), ♨clove, ♨cypress, ♨arborvitae, ♨cinnamon, ♨lemon, ♨lavender

Recipe 1: Combine 5 drops cypress, 10 drops lemon, and 2 Tbs. (25 ml) apple cider vinegar. Apply on location twice daily; bandage. Keep a bandage on until wart is gone.

—Genital:

A genital wart is a small, painful wart or cluster of warts located in the genital area or in the mouth or throat. This type of wart is typically spread by contact with the skin through sexual activity.

Oils: ♨frankincense, ♨On Guard, ♨melaleuca, ♨oregano, ♨thyme

—Plantar:

Plantar warts are painful warts that grow on the bottoms of the feet. They are usually flattened and embedded into the skin due to the pressure caused by walking on them.

Oils: ♨oregano

◌: Dilute as recommended, or dilute 1–2 drops of oil in a few drops fractionated coconut oil; then apply 1–2 drops on location daily.

✿: **Body System(s) Affected:** Skin and Immune System.

Water Purification

Oils: ◯◌lemon, ◯◌Purify, ◯peppermint, ◯orange

◯: Add 1 drop of oil to 1½–2 cups (375–500 ml) of drinking water to help purify.

◌: Add 1–2 drops to dishwater for sparkling dishes and a great smelling kitchen. Add 1–2 drops to warm bathwater, and bathe. Add 1–2 drops to a bowl of water, and use the water to clean the outsides of fruits and vegetables.

Water Retention

See Edema, Diuretic

Weakness

See Energy

Weight

Proper exercise and nutrition are the most critical factors for maintaining a healthy weight. Other factors that may influence weight include an individual's metabolism, level of stress, hormonal imbalances, low or high thyroid function, or the level of insulin being produced by the body.

> *Simple Solutions—Overeating:* Diffuse Slim & Sassy to help reduce cravings during the day.

—Obesity:

Obesity is the condition of being overweight to the extent that it affects health and lifestyle. By definition, obesity is considered as a body mass index (BMI) of 30 kg/m² or greater.

Oils: ♨◯grapefruit◌ ♨◯Slim & Sassy, ♨◯oregano◌, ◯Yarrow Pom, ♨◯thyme◌, ♨◯orange◌, ♨rosemary, ♨◌juniper berry, ♨fennel

Other Products: ○Slim & Sassy TrimShakes, ○Slim & Sassy Contrōl Instant Drink Mix, ○Slim & Sassy Contrōl Bars, ○Mito2Max for enhanced cellular energy. ○TerraGreens for a whole food source of essential nutrients and antioxidants. ○Alpha CRS+ contains polyphenols resveratrol and epigallocatechin-3-gallate (EGCG), which have been studied for their abilities to help prevent obesity.

—Slimming/Toning:

Oils: ⊘○grapefruit▭, ○⊘Slim & Sassy, ○Yarrow Pom, ⊘○orange, ⊘lemongrass, ⊘rosemary, ⊘thyme, ⊘lavender

Other Products: ○Slim & Sassy TrimShakes.

—Weight Loss:

Oils: ⊘○Slim & Sassy, ⊘Elevation, ○Yarrow Pom, ⊘⊘patchouli

Other Products: ○Slim & Sassy TrimShakes, ○Slim & Sassy Contrōl Instant Drink Mix, ○Slim & Sassy Contrōl Bars. ○TerraGreens for a whole food source of essential nutrients.

Recipe 1: Add 5 drops lemon and 5 drops grapefruit to 1 gallon (4 L) of water, and drink throughout the day.

⊘: Diffuse oil into the air. Inhale oil directly from bottle; or inhale oil that is applied to hands, tissue, or cotton wick.

○: Add 8 drops of Slim & Sassy to 2 cups (500 ml) of water, and drink throughout the day between meals. Add 1 drop of oil to 1½–2 cups (375–500 ml) of water, and drink. Drink Trim or V Shake 1–2 times per day as a meal alternative. Take capsules as directed on package.

⊕: **Body System(s) Affected:** Digestive System.

▭: **Additional Research:**

Grapefruit: The scent of grapefruit oil and its component, limonene, was found to affect the autonomic nerves and to reduce appetite and body weight in rats exposed to the oil for 15 minutes three times per week (Shen et al., 2005).

Grapefruit: Grapefruit essential oil was found to directly inhibit adipogenesis of adipocytes, indicating that grapefruit has an antiobesity effect (Haze et al., 2010).

Carvacrol (found in oregano and thyme essential oils): After 10 weeks of feeding, the body weight gain, visceral fat-pad weights, and final body weights of mice fed a high-fat diet and carvacrol were significantly lower than that of mice fed a high-fat diet without carvacrol (specifically a 24% decrease in final body weight, a 43% decrease in body weight gain, and a 36% decrease in total visceral fat-pad weight was observed when carvacrol was ingested)(Cho et al., 2012). Interestingly, the food intake during the 10-week feeding period did not differ among the groups and mRNA expressions were different among the two groups (Cho et al., 2012).

D-Limonene (found in lime, lemon, bergamot, dill, grapefruit, lavender, lemongrass, Roman chamomile, tangerine, and wild orange essential oils): Oral intake of D-limonene effectively protects against the development of hyperglycemia and dyslipidemia in mice fed a high-fat diet (Jing et al., 2013). This study also found evidence suggesting that D-limonene may prevent lipid accumulation in the livers of mice fed a high-fat diet and improve metabolic dysfunctions by ameliorating glucose tolerance in obese mice (Jing et al., 2013).

Lime: Injection of lime essential oil prevented weight gain by suppressing the appetite of mice even when administered ketotifen, an antihistamine with the undesirable side effects of decreased metabolism and increased appetite (Asnaashari et al., 2010).

Cinnamon: When compared to six other plant extracts, cinnamon and apple polyphenolic plant extracts were found to be anti-obesogenic due to their body fat–lowering effect in diet-induced obesity model rats (Boque et al., 2013).

Whiplash

Whiplash is the over-stretching or tearing of the muscles, ligaments, and/or tendons in the neck and head. This is typically caused by a sudden collision or force pushing the body in one direction, while the head's tendency to remain in the same place causes the head to quickly rock in the opposite direction the body is going.

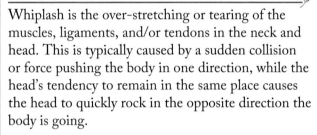

Simple Solutions—Whiplash: Blend 3 drops lemongrass and 2 drops marjoram with 1 Tbs. (15 ml) fractionated coconut oil. Gently massage a small amount into the neck and shoulders daily.

Oils: ⊘Deep Blue, ⊘Rescuer, ⊘lemongrass (ligaments), ⊘marjoram (muscles), ⊘birch, ⊘basil, ⊘juniper berry, ⊘helichrysum, ⊘vetiver, ⊘clove, ⊘peppermint, ⊘Roman chamomile

⊘: Dilute as recommended, and apply 1–2 drops on back of neck. Add 5–10 drops to 1 Tbs. (15 ml) fractionated coconut oil, and massage on back of neck, on shoulders, and on upper back.

⊕: **Body System(s) Affected:** Skeletal System and Muscles.

Whooping Cough

*See **Childhood Diseases: Whooping Cough***

Withdrawal

*See **Addictions: Withdrawal***

Women

*See **Female-Specific Conditions***

See the *Quick Usage Chart* inside the back cover for recommended dilutions.

376

Workaholic

See Addictions: Work

Worms

See Antifungal: Ringworm, Parasites: Worms

Wounds

See also Antibacterial, Blood: Bleeding

A wound is a general term for an injury that involves tissue (typically the skin or underlying skeletal muscles) being torn, cut, punctured, scraped, or crushed.

> *Simple Solutions—Wounds:* Apply 1 drop helichrysum on area to help stop bleeding. Add 1 drop each lavender, melaleuca, and basil to a bowl of warm water. Use water to wash wound.

Oils: clove, melaleuca, helichrysum, lavender, lemongrass, Purify, Stronger, basil, yarrow, cypress, eucalyptus, frankincense, Roman chamomile, copaiba, peppermint (after wound has closed), myrrh, rose, blue tansy, sandalwood, thyme, juniper berry, bergamot

Recipe 1: Place 1–3 drops of helichrysum on fresh wound to help stop bleeding. Add 1 drop clove to help reduce pain. Once bleeding has stopped, apply a drop of lavender (to help start healing), a drop of melaleuca (to help fight infection), and a drop of lemongrass (for possible ligament damage). Bandage the wound. When changing the bandage, apply 1 drop basil or sandalwood to help promote further healing. Add 1 drop Purify or On Guard to help prevent infection.

Other Products: Correct-X to help cleanse and support the skin's natural healing process.

Blend 1: Add 1 drop lavender to 1 drop Purify and apply to wound.

—**Children/Infants:**

   Oils: Roman chamomile, Stronger

   Recipe 2: Add 1–3 drops each of helichrysum and lavender to 1 tsp. (5 ml) fractionated coconut oil, and apply a small amount to wound.

—**Bleeding:**

   Oils: helichrysum, rose, lavender, lemon

Blend 2: Combine 1 drop Roman chamomile, 1 drop geranium, and 1 drop lemon, and apply with a warm compress 2–3 times a day for 3–4 days, then reduce to once a day until healed.

—**Disinfect:**

   Oils: melaleuca, Stronger, thyme, lavender

—**Healing:**

   Oils: basil, helichrysum, Stronger, melaleuca, lavender, myrrh, sandalwood

—**Inflammation:** *See Inflammation*

—**Scarring:** *See Skin: Scarring, Tissue: Scarring*

—**Surgical:**

   Oils: peppermint, melaleuca

   Blend 2: Add 3 drops helichrysum, 3 drops frankincense, and 4 drops lavender to 2 tsp. (10 ml) fractionated coconut oil. Apply a few drops when changing bandages.

—**Weeping:**

   Oils: myrrh, patchouli

: Dilute as recommended, and apply 1–2 drops on location.

: **Body System(s) Affected:** Skin and Immune System.

: **Additional Research:**

> **Basil:** Basil (*Ocimum gratissimum*) oil was found to facilitate the healing process of wounds in rabbits to a greater extent than two antibacterial preparations, Cicatrin and Cetavlex (Orafidiya et al., 2003)
>
> **Clove:** Beta-caryophyllene (found in clove and copal oils) demonstrated anaesthetic (pain reducing) activity in rats and rabbits (Ghelardini et al., 2001).
>
> **Cinnamon:** A topically applied cinnamon oil based microemulsion showed increased wound healing ability in rats by preventing sepsis of the excised wound (Ghosh et al., 2013).

Wrinkles

See Skin: Wrinkles

Yeast

See Antifungal: Candida

Yoga

Oils: Arise, Align, Anchor, sandalwood, cedarwood, litsea

: Diffuse into the air.

: **Body System(s) Affected:** Emotional Balance.

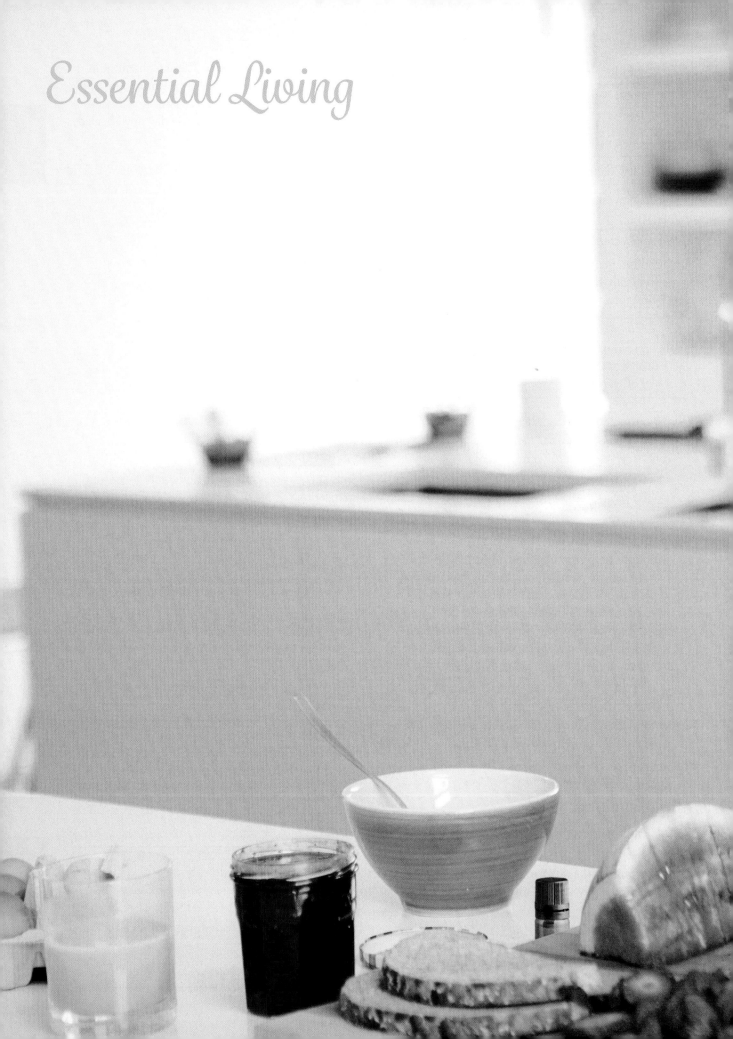

Essential Living

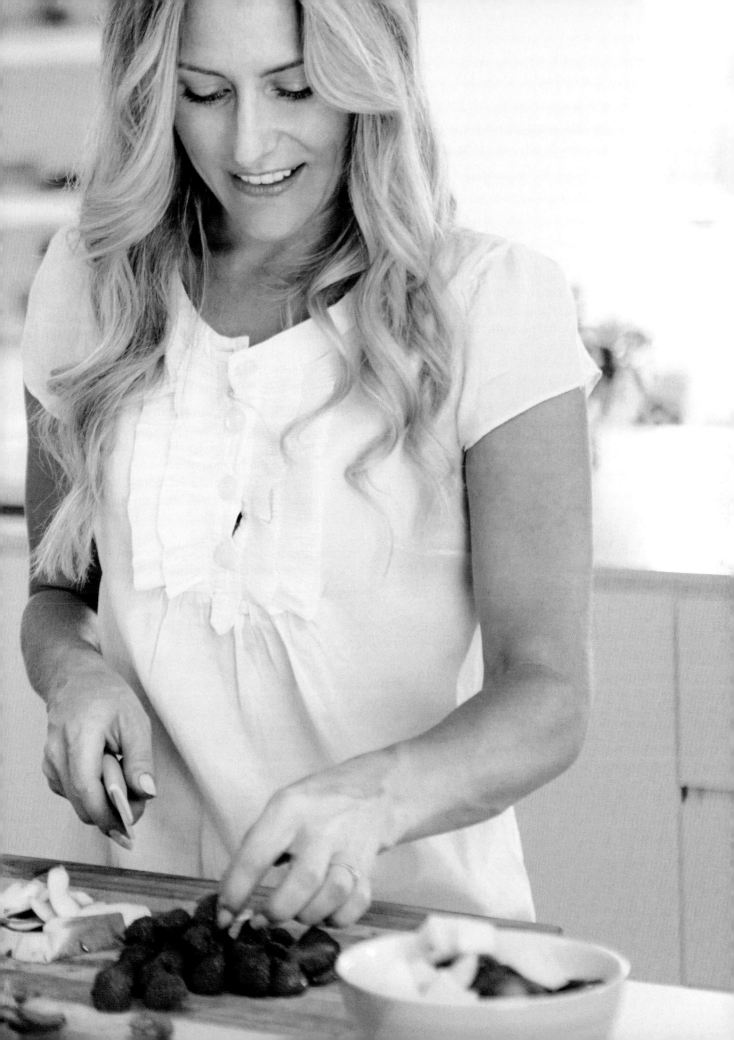

Bath & Shower Tips

Using essential oils in the bath or shower instead of products with artificial perfumes and fragrances allows one to simultaneously enjoy the topical and aromatic benefits of an essential oil or blend.

Bath and Shower Tips

Bathwater: Add 3–6 drops of oil to the bathwater while the tub is filling. Because the individual oils will separate as the water calms down, the skin will quickly draw the oils from the top of the water. Some people have commented that they were unable to endure more than 6 drops of oil. Such individuals may benefit from adding the oils to a bath and shower gel base first. Soak in the tub for 15 minutes.

Bath and Shower Gel: Add 3–6 drops of oil to 1 Tbs. (15 ml) of a natural bath and shower gel base; add to the water while the tub is filling. Adding the oils to a bath and shower gel base first allows one to obtain the greatest benefit from the oils, as they are more evenly dispersed throughout the water and not allowed to immediately separate.

Washcloth: When showering, add 3–6 drops of oil to a bath and shower gel base before applying to a washcloth and using to wash the body.

Body Sprays: Fill a small spray bottle with distilled water, and add 10–15 drops of your favorite essential oil or blend. Shake well, and spray onto the entire body just after taking a bath or shower.

Footbath: Add enough hot water to a basin to cover the ankles. Add 1–3 drops of your desired essential oil. Soak feet for 5–10 minutes, inhaling the aroma of the oils.

Hand Bath: Pour enough hot water in a basin to cover hands up to the wrists. Add 1–3 drops of your desired essential oil. Soak hands for 5–10 minutes while bending, pulling, and massaging the fingers and hands to stimulate. Try combining essential oils with 1 Tbs. (15 ml) honey in a hand bath or regular bath to help moisturize the skin.

Shower: With the water turned on, drop peppermint, rosemary, or Breathe on the shower floor as you enter to help invigorate and open the nasal passages. Use soothing oils at night to help promote a feeling of calmness and relaxation. Alternately, fill a tub/shower combo with about an inch or two of water; then place oils in the water before turning on the shower. This will allow the oils to more easily be drawn into the feet during the shower and also allow the aroma to be inhaled.

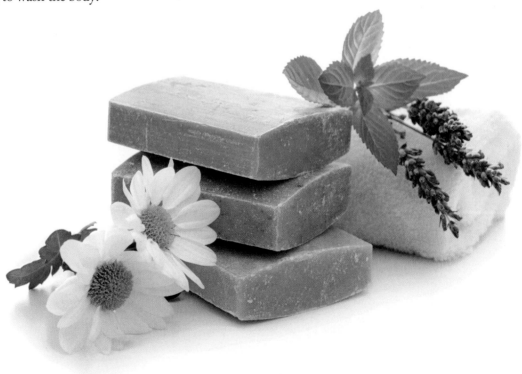

Bath & Shower Recipes

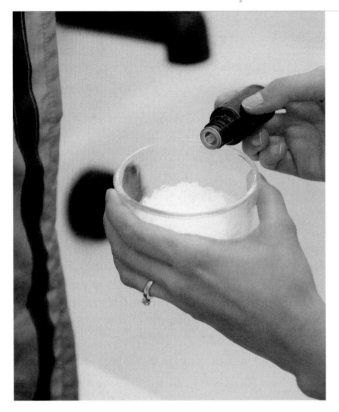

Bath Salts Base

1 c. (250 g) Epsom salt (or sea salt)

15 drops EO *(see blend ideas below)*

Combine essential oils with salt in a container. Dissolve ¼–½ cup (50–125 g) of this bath salt mixture in warm bathwater before bathing.

Bath Oils Base

2 T. (25 ml) fractionated coconut oil
(or jojoba or sweet almond oil)

15 drops EO *(see blend ideas below)*

Blend vegetable oil with essential oils in a small container. Add 1 tsp. (5 ml) of this bath oil to warm bathwater before bathing.

Relaxing Bliss

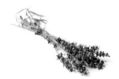 + + +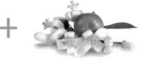

| 5 drops lavender | 5 drops petitgrain | 3 drops fennel | 2 drops orange |

Soothe Your Troubles

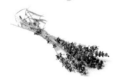 + 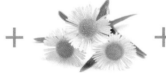 + +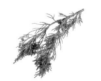

| 4 drops lavender | 4 drops R. chamomile | 4 drops cedarwood | 3 drops lemongrass |

Refreshed and Ready to Go

 + 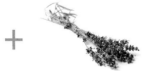 + +

| 5 drops peppermint | 4 drops lavender | 3 drops grapefruit | 3 drops lemongrass |

Fizzing Bath Bombs

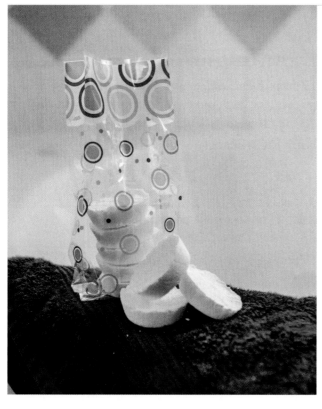

Fizzing Bath Bomb Base

⅔ c. (125 g) baking soda   ½ c. (75 g) cornstarch

⅓ c. (75 g) Epsom salt   2 t. (10 ml) water

2 t. (10 g) coconut oil   Spray bottle with water

15 drops EO *(see blend ideas below)*

Combine the dry ingredients in one bowl and the wet ingredients in another. Add the wet ingredients to the dry ingredients slowly while stirring with a whisk. Knead the mixture until it has the texture of mildly wet sand and clumps together when pressed. If it is too dry, moisten it slightly with a mist from the spray bottle, one spritz at a time, just until it holds together. Form into balls, or mold in small soap or candy molds or a mini muffin tin (lined with paper muffin cups). Allow to dry for 1–2 hours, then remove from molds or tins, and allow to dry overnight.

To use, place a bath bomb in warm bathwater, and enjoy!

Sweet Dreams

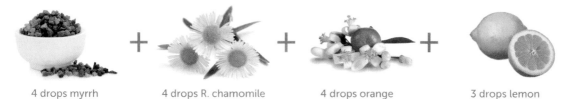

8 drops lavender   +   4 drops orange   +   2 drops R. chamomile   +   1 drop sandalwood

Calm Seas

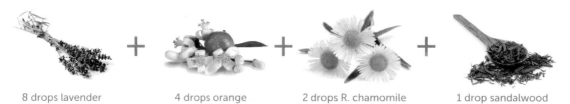

4 drops myrrh   +   4 drops R. chamomile   +   4 drops orange   +   3 drops lemon

Up and At 'em

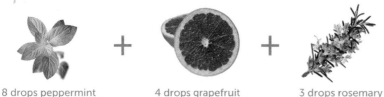

8 drops peppermint   +   4 drops grapefruit   +   3 drops rosemary

Sugar Scrub (Exfoliating)

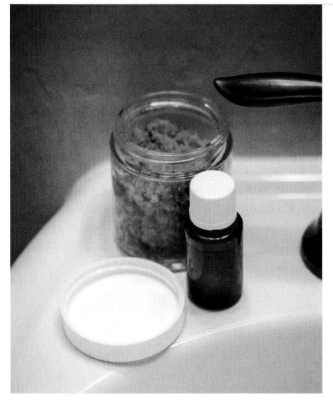

Simple Sugar Scrub Base

¼ c. (50 g) raw sugar   ¼ c. (50 ml) sweet almond oil

8 drops vitamin E oil (optional natural preservative)

15 drops EO *(see blend ideas below)*

Mix all ingredients together in a glass bowl. Store in airtight containers. To use, place a small amount of the scrub in the palm, and scrub over moistened skin. Rinse off in a shower or tub. (Note: The oils in this scrub can make the floor of the bathtub or shower slippery, so use caution when rinsing off.)

Try using different coarsenesses of sugar to create progressively smoother scubs (e.g., a course raw sugar "buffing" scrub followed by a fine white sugar "polishing" scrub.

Lemon Rosemary Scrub

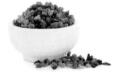 +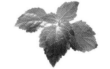

10 drops lemon   5 drops rosemary

Skin-Toning Scrub

 +

9 drops myrrh   4 drops patchouli   2 drops geranium

Invigorating Scrub

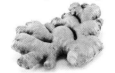 + 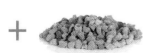 +

5 drops ginger   5 drops frankincense   5 drops grapefruit

Deodorant

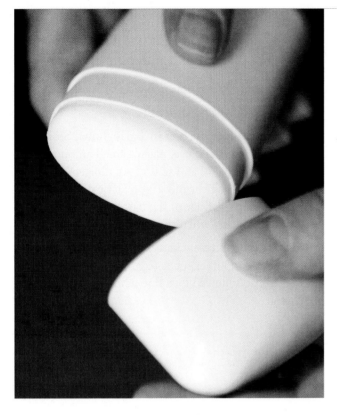

Deodorant Base

3 T. (35 g) coconut oil	1 T. (5 g) beeswax pellets
¼ c. (30 g) cornstarch	¼ c. (50 g) baking soda
6 drops vitamin E oil	Deodorant container

15 drops EO *(see blend ideas below)*

Melt beeswax and coconut oil in a double boiler or in the microwave (stirring every 30 seconds until just melted). Stir in cornstarch, baking soda, and vitamin E oil. Allow to cool slightly; then add essential oils. Pour into an empty deodorant container. Allow to cool and harden completely. Apply deodorant as needed.

Purifying Lavender Melaleuca

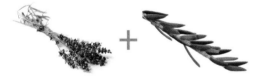

8 drops lavender   +   7 drops melaleuca

Flower Power

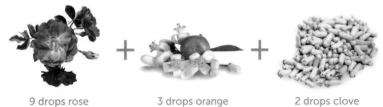

9 drops rose   +   3 drops orange   +   2 drops clove

Spicy Fresh

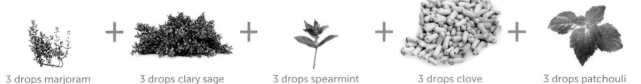

3 drops marjoram   +   3 drops clary sage   +   3 drops spearmint   +   3 drops clove   +   3 drops patchouli

Shaving

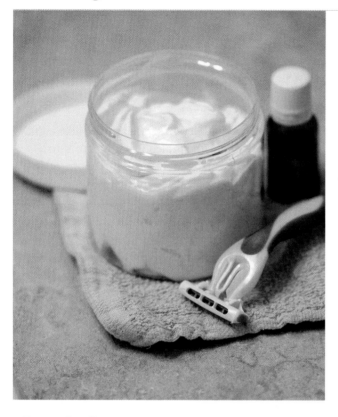

Aftershave Lotion

4 t. (5 g) beeswax pellets	⅓ c. (65 g) coconut oil
30 drops vitamin E oil	7 T. (100 ml) aloe vera gel
½ t. (2 ml) glycerin	¼ c. (50 ml) witch hazel

15 drops EO *(see blend ideas below)*

Melt beeswax and coconut oil in a double boiler or in the microwave (stirring every 30 seconds until just melted). In a separate bowl, mix together the aloe vera gel, witch hazel, and vegetable glycerin. Using a handheld mixer, whip the oil mixture for a few seconds, then start slowly pouring in the aloe vera mixture while still whipping. Add in the essential oils, and whip for a few minutes until thickened like lotion. Store in an airtight container, and use a small amount just after shaving.

Ease the Burn

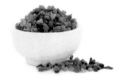 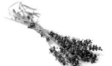

9 drops lavender + 6 drops R. chamomile

Skin-Toning

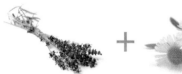 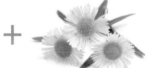 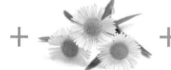

6 drops myrrh + 6 drops R. chamomile + 3 drops lavender

Sensitive Skin

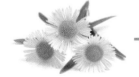 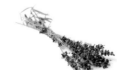 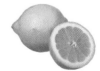

8 drops R. chamomile + 3 drops lavender + 1 drop peppermint + 1 drop lemon

Essential Living

Natural Perfumes

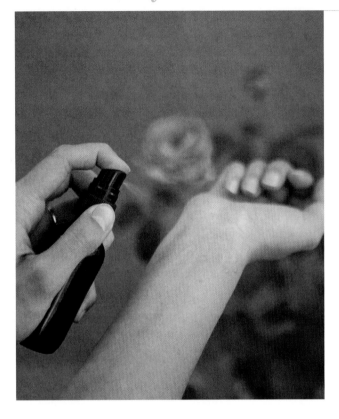

Simple Perfume Base

1 t. (5 ml) pure grain or perfumer's alcohol
OR 1 t. (5 ml) jojoba oil

15 drops EO *(see blend ideas below)*

Mix essential oils with a pure grain alcohol (like vodka or Everclear) or perfumer's alcohol, and pour into a small spray bottle. Alternately, mix with jojoba oil in a small roll-on bottle for an alcohol-free perfume. Apply a small amount on wrists, neck, or other desired points.

Solid Perfume Base

1 t. (2 g) beeswax pellets   1 T. (15 ml) jojoba oil

15 drops EO *(see blend ideas below)*

Combine beeswax and jojoba oil, and melt in the microwave (stirring every 30 seconds until just melted) or in a double boiler. Let cool slightly, and add essential oils and vitamin E oil. Pour into a small jar or lockets. Apply a small amount on the wrists, neck, or other points on the skin as desired.

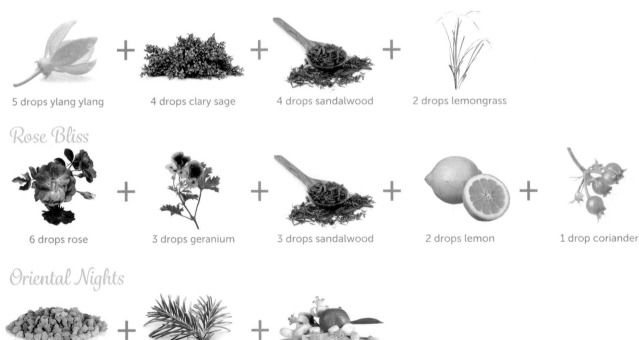

Romance

5 drops ylang ylang + 4 drops clary sage + 4 drops sandalwood + 2 drops lemongrass

Rose Bliss

6 drops rose + 3 drops geranium + 3 drops sandalwood + 2 drops lemon + 1 drop coriander

Oriental Nights

7 drops frankincense + 5 drops white fir + 3 drops orange

Tip: Combine your alcohol-based perfume with 2 tsp. (10 ml) water for a lighter eau de toilette, or ¼ cup (50 ml) water for a room or body spray.

Lotions

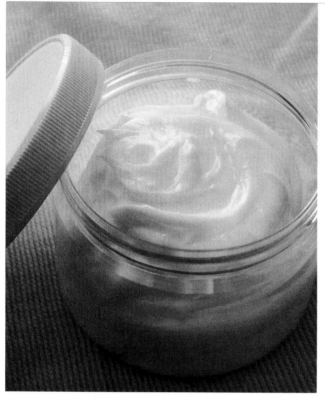

Simple Lotion Base

¼ c. (20 g) beeswax pellets

½ c. (100 g) coconut oil

½ c. (125 ml) aloe vera gel

15 drops EO *(see blend ideas below)*

Combine beeswax and coconut oil, and melt in the microwave (stirring every 30 seconds until just melted) or in a double boiler. Allow mixture to cool to room temperature (about an hour). Using a handheld mixer, whip the mixture, and slowly add in the aloe vera gel and essential oils. Whip together until well incorporated and fluffy. Store in an airtight jar or lotion dispenser in a cool location. Apply a small amount on the skin as desired. This lotion is great when feeling warm on a hot summer day!

Cool Mint

 +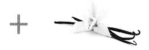

12 drops peppermint   3 drops vanilla extract

Skin-Soothing

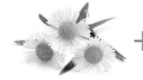 + 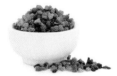 +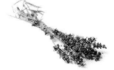

6 drops R. chamomile   6 drops myrrh   3 drops lavender

Lavender Fields

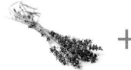 +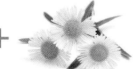

10 drops lavender   5 drops R. chamomile

Lip Balms

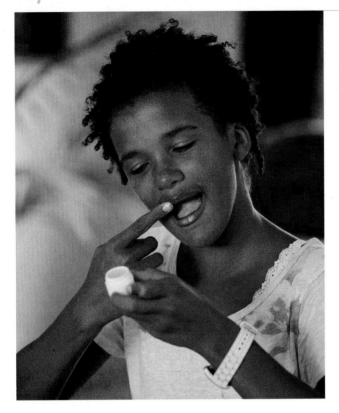

Lip Balm Base

4 t. (5 g) beeswax pellets

1 T. (15 g) cocoa butter

3 T. (45 ml) jojoba oil

15 drops EO *(see blend ideas below)*

Combine beeswax and cocoa butter, and melt in the microwave (stirring every 30 seconds until just melted) or in a double boiler. Mix in jojoba oil until incorporated. Let cool slightly, and add essential oils. Pour into small jars or lip balm dispensers. Allow to cool and solidify completely. Apply a small amount on the lips as desired.

Minty Fresh

 +

10 drops peppermint   5 drops spearmint

Creamsicle

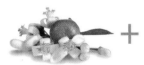 + +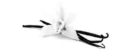

10 drops orange   3 drops grapefruit   2 drops vanilla extract

Lemon Thyme

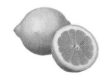 +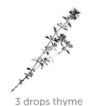

12 drops lemon   3 drops thyme

Lip Stain & Lip Scrub

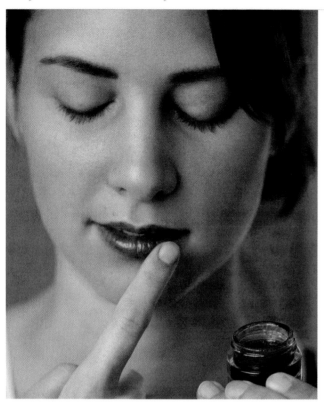

Berry Mint Lip Stain

3 blackberries

3 raspberries

1 small strawberry (no stem)

½ t. (3 ml) sweet almond oil

1 drop peppermint essential oil OR 1 drop of a blend from the previous page

Heat the berries in the microwave or over a double boiler until soft. Mash the berries with a fork until well blended. Allow to cool slightly, and mix in the sweet almond oil and essential oil. Strain the mixture through a coffee filter or cheesecloth to remove pulp and seeds. Place in a small salve or lip gloss jar, and store in the refrigerator. To use, dip your finger into the stain and apply to the lips. Wash finger immediately after application to avoid staining the finger.

Brown Sugar Mint Lip Scrub

3 T. (40 g) brown sugar

1 T. (15 g) coconut oil

2 drops peppermint essential oil OR 2 drops of a blend from the previous page

Mix together all of the ingredients. Store in a small glass jar. To use, place a small amount on the lips, and rub lips together for a couple minutes to help exfoliate. Rinse lips with water.

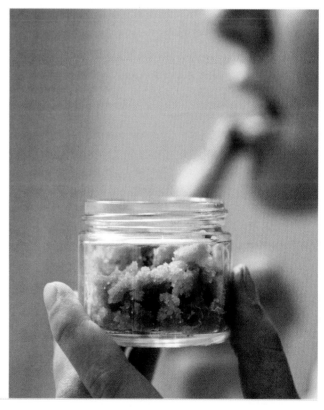

Essential Living

Sleeping/Relaxing

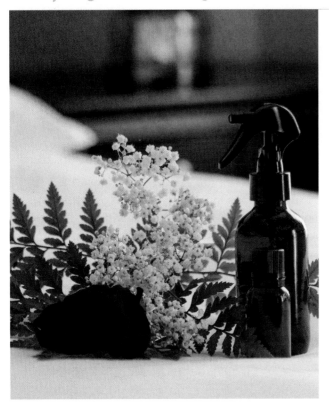

"Time to Sleep" Linen Spray

1 t. (5 ml) pure grain or perfumer's alcohol

¼ c. (50 ml) water

Small misting spray bottle

15 drops Serenity or another soothing essential oil *(see below)*

Mix essential oils with a pure grain alcohol (like vodka or Everclear) or perfumer's alcohol in a small spray bottle. Add water. To use this spray, shake well, then mist a few spritzes on pillows, sheets, or other linens before bed time.

Soothing Essential Oils:

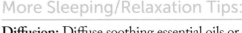

Serenity	lavender	ylang ylang	R. chamomile
clary sage	orange	vetiver	geranium
melissa	sandalwood	bergamot	rose
spikenard	petitgrain		

More Sleeping/Relaxation Tips:

Diffusion: Diffuse soothing essential oils or blends to help you feel calm and relaxed before going to sleep.

Pillow: Place 1–2 drops of a soothing essential oil or blend on a pillow or stuffed animal before you sleep to help calm your mind and body.

Relaxing Bath: Mix 1–3 drops of a soothing essential oil with bath salts or directly in warm bathwater for a relaxing bath.

Waking Up/Energizing

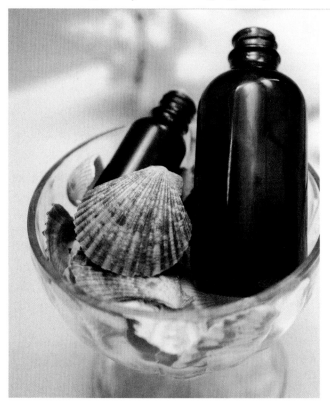

Invigorating Shower

3 drops Elevation or another invigorating essential oil *(see below)*

Place 3 drops of the essential oil or blend on the floor of a shower just before entering for an invigorating morning shower.

Invigorating Essential Oils:

 Passion

 Elevation

 peppermint

 eucalyptus

 white fir

 lemon

 basil

 wintergreen

 thyme

More Energizing/Invigorating Tips:

Diffusion: Diffuse an invigorating oil in the morning. Some individuals like to use a timer to start their diffuser a few minutes before their alarm clock goes off to help the body begin to wake up naturally.

Morning Beverage: Add a few drops of peppermint, lemon, or orange to water, a fresh fruit/vegetable smoothie, or another healthy beverage.

Essential Living

Kitchen

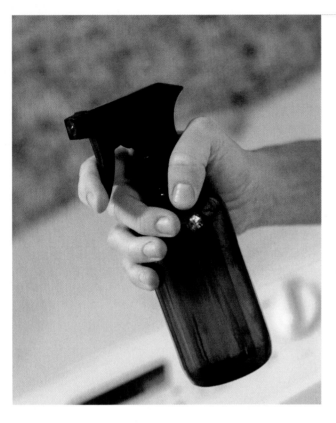

Disinfecting Spray

½ c. (125 ml) white vinegar

½ c. (125 ml) water

Small spray bottle

15 drops On Guard or another disinfecting essential oil *(see below)*

Combine all ingredients in a small spray bottle. Shake well, and spray on counters, cutting boards, microwave, refrigerator, garbage cans, or other desired surfaces; use a rag to wipe off.

Other Kitchen Cleaning Tips:

Counter Cleaning: Add 1–2 drops of lemon, On Guard, or another disinfecting oil to a damp rag. Use to wipe down counters, tables, or stoves.

Trash Can Deodorizer: Add 3–5 drops of a deodorizing essential oil or blend *(see bottom right)* to 1 Tbs. (15 g) baking powder. Sprinkle into trash can.

Dishes: Add a few drops of lemon to dishwater for sparkling dishes and a great-smelling kitchen. You can add the essential oil to a dishwasher as well.

Disinfecting Essential Oils:

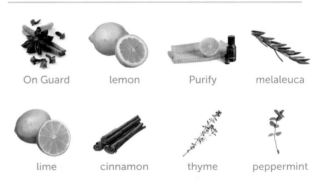

On Guard   lemon   Purify   melaleuca

lime   cinnamon   thyme   peppermint

Deodorizing Essential Oils:

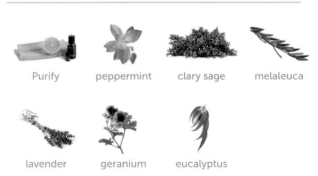

Purify   peppermint   clary sage   melaleuca

lavender   geranium   eucalyptus

Kitchen

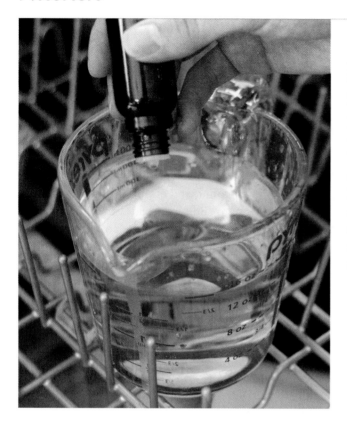

Dishwasher Cleaner

2 c. (500 ml) white vinegar

10 drops lemon essential oil

Remove the lower rack from your dishwasher. Using a rag soaked in warm, soapy water, wipe down the bottom of the dishwasher to remove any loose food or dirt. Replace the bottom rack. Place the vinegar and lemon oil in a dishwasher-safe bowl or cup. Place this on the top rack of the dishwasher. Run your dishwasher on the hottest setting without any other dishes for a full cycle. Open and enjoy a clean, great-smelling dishwasher!

Streak-Free Glass & Mirror Spray

2 T. (25 ml) white vinegar

2 T. (25 ml) rubbing alcohol

1½ t. (5 g) cornstarch

¾ c. (175 ml) water

5 drops lemon and 5 drops lime essential oil

Small spray bottle

Combine vinegar, alcohol, cornstarch, and essential oils in the spray bottle. Screw on the spray top, and shake to combine. Unscrew the top, and add water. Screw on the spray top, and shake again to combine. To use, shake, then spray on glass or mirror. Wipe glass or mirror with a rag.

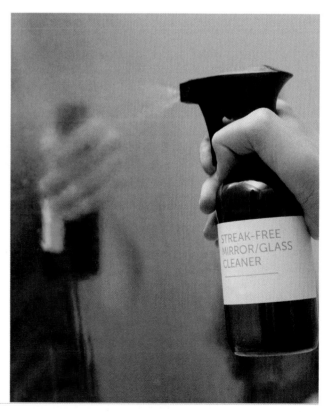

Bathroom

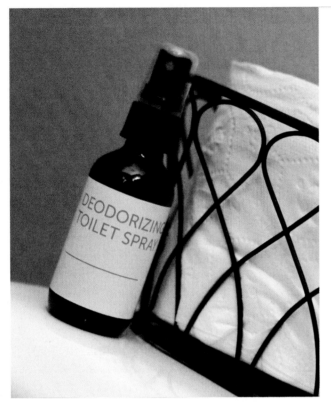

Toilet Spray

1 t. (5 ml) vegetable glycerin

1 t. (5 ml) rubbing alcohol

¼ c. (50 ml) water

Small spray bottle

15 drops EO *(see blend ideas below)*

Blend glycerin, alcohol, and essential oils in spray bottle, and shake to combine. Add water, and shake again to combine. To use, shake the bottle, then spray a few times in the toilet before you do your business.

Sweet Citrus

 + +

5 drops lemongrass   5 drops bergamot   5 drops grapefruit

Ocean Breeze

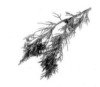 + +

7 drops cedarwood   5 drops lemon   3 drops rosemary

Herbal Bliss

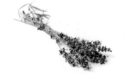 + + 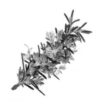 +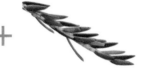

4 drops lavender   4 drops peppermint   4 drops rosemary   2 drops melaleuca

Other Household Tips

Other Bathroom Cleaning Tips:

Mildew Spray: Mix 5 drops lemon and 5 drops white fir with ¼ cup (50 ml) water in a small spray bottle. Spray on areas with mildew.

Deodorizing Spray: Place 5–8 drops of a deodorizing essential oil (try 5 drops grapefruit and 1 drop peppermint) in a 1 oz. spray bottle, and fill the remainder of the bottle with water. Shake well, and spray into the air.

Mold: Diffuse On Guard into the air to help eliminate mold.

Laundry Tips:

Gum/Grease: Use lemon or Citrus Bliss to help take gum or grease out of clothes (test in a small, inconspicuous area first to ensure that the oil won't affect delicate dyes or fabrics).

Washing: Add a few drops of Purify to the wash water to help kill bacteria and germs in clothes.

Drying: Put Purify, Elevation, lemongrass, or another favorite oil or blend on a wet rag, and then place the rag in the dryer with clothing. Or mist oils from a spray bottle directly into the dryer to keep clothes smelling great—without artificial perfumes or fragrances.

Furniture Tips:

Polish: For a simple furniture polish, put a few drops of lemon, Purify, or white fir oil on a dust cloth, and use to wipe down wood.

Clothes/Closets:

Clothing Deodorizer: Place a tissue or cotton ball with several drops of Purify, lavender, lemongrass, melaleuca, peppermint, Citrus Bliss, or another favorite oil in a perforated wood, glass, or stone container. Place container in a closet, shoe cupboard, or drawer to keep clothes naturally smelling great.

Painting Tips:

Paint Fumes: To effectively remove paint fumes and after smell, add one 15 ml bottle of oil to any 5-gallon bucket of paint. Purify and citrus single oils have been favorites, but Citrus Bliss and Elevation would work just as well. Either a paint sprayer or brush and roller can be used to apply the paint after mixing the oils into the paint by stirring vigorously. Oils may eventually rise to the top if using a water-based paint. Occasional stirring may be necessary to keep the oils mixed.

Carpet Care Tips:

Carpet Cleaner/Deodorizer: Mix 1 cup (200 g) baking soda and 20–50 drops melaleuca, lemon, Purify, or another favorite oil in a glass jar. Close jar, shake together, and let stand overnight. Sprinkle lightly over carpets, let sit for 15 minutes, and then vacuum.

Grease/Gum Remover: Try lemon or lime oil on stubborn greasy stains, or use to help dissolve gum stuck to the carpet (be certain to test oil in a small, inconspicuous area of the carpet first to ensure it won't affect any delicate dyes in the carpet).

Bug/Pest Repellent Tips:

Bug-Repelling Oils: TerraShield, lavender, lemongrass, patchouli, basil, Purify.

Mice-Repelling Oil: Purify.

Personal Bug Repellent: Apply repelling oils directly on the skin (dilute with fractionated coconut oil if you are covering a large area).

Bug Spray: Add 10–15 drops of repelling oil to 2 Tbs. (25 ml) water in a small misting spray bottle. Shake well, and mist over exposed skin and clothing.

Diffusion: Diffuse repelling oils in a room.

Pest Repellent: Place repelling oils on a string, ribbon, or cotton ball, and hang near air vents or windows, or place in cracks and other areas where bugs or pests come through.

Wipes

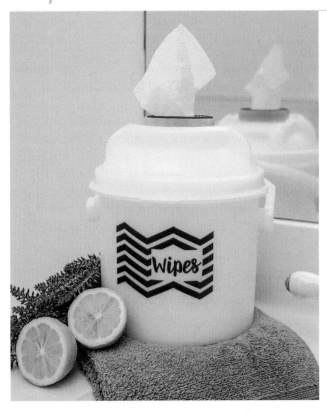

Wipe Base

2 T. (25 ml) Castile soap (or other unscented soap)

2 T. (25 ml) jojoba oil

2 c. (500 ml) water

8 drops vitamin E oil

1 roll paper towels (heavy-duty work best) OR dry bamboo wipes

2 round plastic storage containers

15 drops EO *(see blend ideas below)*

Cut the roll of paper towels in half with a serrated knife, remove the cardboard tube from the center, and place each half in one of the round plastic storage containers. Combine the soap, jojoba oil, water, vitamin E oil, and essential oils together. Pour half of the liquid over each of the paper towel halves, and allow liquid to soak into the paper towels. To use, pull wipes from the center of the roll. Seal the storage container afterwards to keep wipes moist. Use within 1–2 weeks.

Baby Wipes

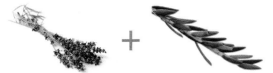

10 drops lavender + 5 drops melaleuca

Facial Cleansing Wipes

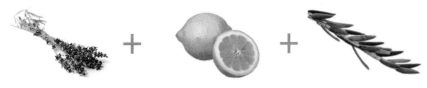

5 drops lavender + 5 drops lemon + 5 drops melaleuca

Disinfecting Wipes

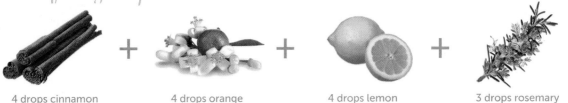

4 drops cinnamon + 4 drops orange + 4 drops lemon + 3 drops rosemary

Kids

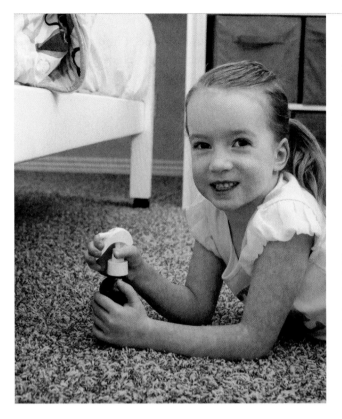

Kid's Room Spray Base

½ c. (125 ml) water

Small spray bottle

15 drops EO *(see blend ideas below)*

Combine water and essential oils in a small spray bottle (the kind with a trigger spray is easiest for kids to use). Give to older children to spray into the air as needed or desired.

Kid's Diffuser Blends

Diffuser

15 drops EO *(see blend ideas below)*

Diffuse one of the blends below in a water misting home or car diffuser.

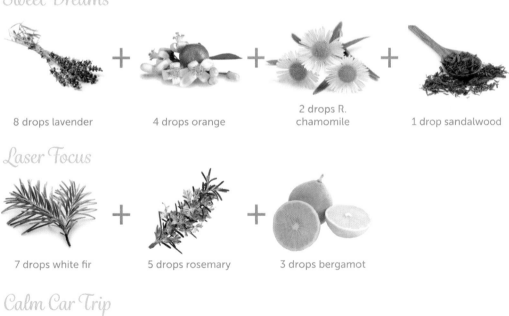

Sweet Dreams

8 drops lavender + 4 drops orange + 2 drops R. chamomile + 1 drop sandalwood

Laser Focus

7 drops white fir + 5 drops rosemary + 3 drops bergamot

Calm Car Trip

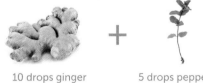

10 drops ginger + 5 drops peppermint

Diffuser Blends

The aroma of essential oils can be a major contributor to helping create the right atmosphere at home. Studies have shown that certain aromas can help a space feel warm and inviting, while other aromas, like orange, can help relax and reduce anxiety. Here are a few ideas to get you started, but try experimenting with other oils to see what kind of mood they contribute to.

CALMING SCENT

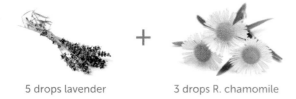

5 drops lavender   +   3 drops R. chamomile

FLOWERS APLENTY

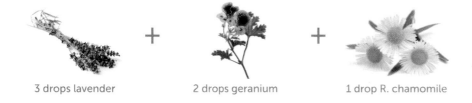

3 drops lavender   +   2 drops geranium   +   1 drop R. chamomile

ENERGIZING BLEND

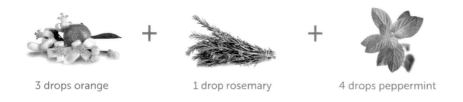

3 drops orange   +   1 drop rosemary   +   4 drops peppermint

REFRESHING BLEND

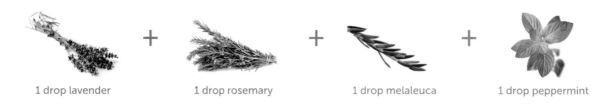

1 drop lavender   +   1 drop rosemary   +   1 drop melaleuca   +   1 drop peppermint

DEEP BREATH

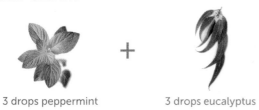

3 drops peppermint   +   3 drops eucalyptus

RELAXING BREATH

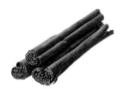 +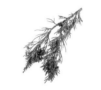

3 drops lavender   3 drops bergamot

CITRUS SPICE

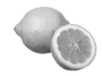 + 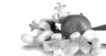 + 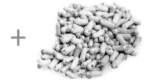 +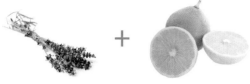

3 drops lemon   4 drops orange   2 drops grapefruit   1 drop clove

STRESS LESS

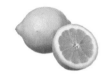 + 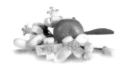 + +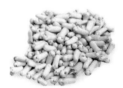

2 drops lemon   2 drops orange   2 drops clove   2 drops cedarwood

SPRINGTIME BLISS

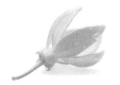 + 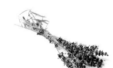 +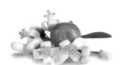

1 drop ylang ylang   2 drops lavender   5 drops orange

HOLIDAY GLOW

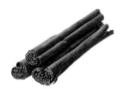 + 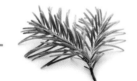 +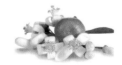

3 drops cinnamon   7 drops white fir   5 drops orange

WINTER WONDERLAND

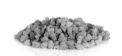 + 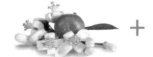 +

1 drop frankincense   2 drops orange   1 drop peppermint

First Aid Oils

Clove	Use as an analgesic (for topical pain relief) and a drawing salve (to pull toxins/infection from the body). Good for acne, constipation, headaches, nausea, and toothaches.
Frankincense	Enhances effect of any other oil. It facilitates clarity of mind, accelerates all skin recovery issues, and reduces anxiety and mental and physical fatigue. Reduces hyperactivity, impatience, irritability, and restlessness. Helps with focus and concentration.
Lavender	Use for agitation, bruises, burns (can mix with melaleuca), leg cramps, herpes, heart irregularities, hives, insect bites, neuropathy, pain (inside and out), bee stings, sprains, sunburn (combine with frankincense), and sunstroke. Relieves insomnia, depression, and PMS and is a natural antihistamine (asthma or allergies).
Lemon	Use for arthritis, colds, constipation, coughs, cuts, sluggishness, sore throats, sunburn, and wounds. It lifts the spirits and reduces stress and fatigue. Internally it counteracts acidity, calms an upset stomach, and encourages elimination.
Lemongrass	Use for sore and cramping muscles and charley horses (with peppermint; drink lots of water). Apply to bottoms of feet in winter to warm them.
Melaleuca	Use for bug bites, colds, coughs, cuts, body odor, eczema, fungus, infections (ear, nose, or throat), microbes (internally), psoriasis, rough hands, slivers (combine with clove to draw them out), sore throats, and wounds.
Oregano	Use as heavy-duty antibiotic (internally with olive oil or coconut oil in capsules or topically on bottoms of feet—follow up with lavender and peppermint). Also for fungal infections and for reducing pain and inflammation of arthritis, backache, bursitis, carpal tunnel syndrome, rheumatism, and sciatica. Always dilute.
Peppermint	Use as an analgesic (for topical pain relief, bumps, and bruises). Can also be used for circulation, fever, headache, indigestion, motion sickness, nausea, nerve problems, or vomiting.

First Aid Blends

Purify	Use for airborne pathogens, cuts, germs (on any surface), insect bites, itches (all types and varieties), and wounds. Also boosts the immune system.
DigestZen	Use for all digestion issues such as bloating, congestion, constipation, diarrhea, food poisoning (internal), heartburn, indigestion, motion sickness, nausea, and stomachache. Also works well on diaper rash.
AromaTouch	Use for relaxation and stress relief. It is soothing and anti-inflammatory and enhances massage.
On Guard	Use to disinfect all surfaces. It eliminates mold and viruses and helps to boost the immune system (bottoms of feet or internally; use daily).
TerraShield	Deters all flying insects and ticks from human bodies and pets.
Breathe	Use for allergies, anxiety, asthma, bronchitis, congestion, colds, coughs, flu, and respiratory distress.
Deep Blue	Use for pain relief. Works well in cases of arthritis, bruises, carpal tunnel, headaches, inflammation, joint pain, migraines, muscle pain, sprains, and rheumatism. Follow with peppermint to enhance effects.

Essential Oils and Cooking

Essential oils are great for adding flavor or spice to your favorite meal. Essential oils can impart the natural, fresh taste of fresh herbs and spices but are more concentrated and can easily be used year-round when fresh herbs are not available. Essential oils are also a great substitute for dried or powdered spices, since dried spices have lost many of the liquid essential oils that impart much of the flavor and aroma found in the natural plant. Additionally, while many commercially available flavoring extracts use artificial flavors or are diluted in alcohol or propylene glycol, essential oils provide a concentrated, pure flavor that is extracted naturally from the plant.

Many great essential oil cookbooks are available that can help you get started using essential oils in cooking. But it is fairly easy (and a lot of fun) to substitute essential oils into your own favorite recipes in place of spices, flavoring extracts, and fresh or dried herbs.

Essential Oils Commonly Used in Cooking

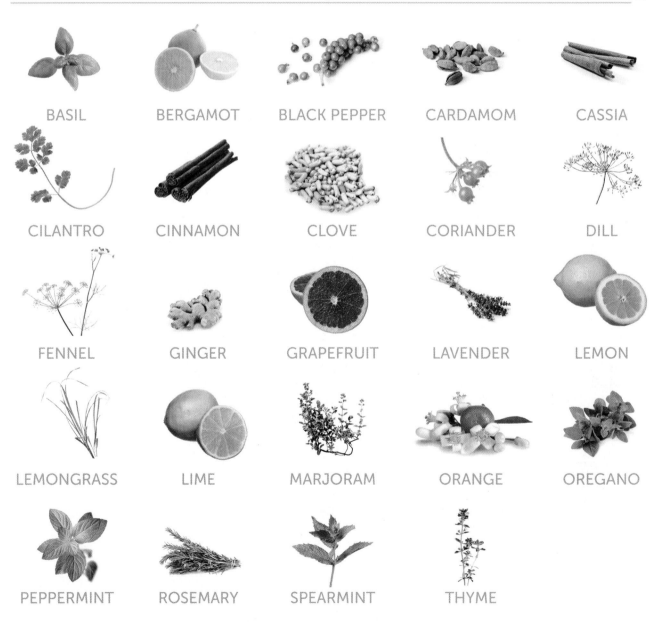

BASIL   BERGAMOT   BLACK PEPPER   CARDAMOM   CASSIA

CILANTRO   CINNAMON   CLOVE   CORIANDER   DILL

FENNEL   GINGER   GRAPEFRUIT   LAVENDER   LEMON

LEMONGRASS   LIME   MARJORAM   ORANGE   OREGANO

PEPPERMINT   ROSEMARY   SPEARMINT   THYME

Essential Oil Cooking Tips

1. Know what part of the plant the oil came from. Citrus oils are pressed from the peel, so they can substitute for the zest but not the juice.

2. Getting the exact amount of oil drops can be tricky due to the different viscosity levels of the oils. If using the regular bottle with the orifice reducer, place your drops on a spoon; then stir into your mixture to ensure you have the right amount.

3. Putting your cooking oils in dropper bottles allows you to easily control the number of drops used and provides sufficient space to dip a toothpick into the oil when needed.

4. A little goes a long way. Start with only a drop of oil, taste, and repeat until you are satisfied with the flavor. Some oils are really strong, and a toothpick dipped in the oil, then stirred into your mixture, may be sufficient.

5. Use glass or stainless steel mixing bowls. Try to avoid plastic cookware, as the oils can damage certain types of plastic.

6. Always keep your oils away from heat, light, and humid conditions to maintain a long shelf life. Refrigerator storage is fine.

7. Make sure to recap your bottles so the oils don't evaporate out.

8. Because oils are altered by heat and may evaporate, it is always best to add the oils at the end of cooking if possible.

9. Give a subtle hint of herbs to your savory baked goods by creating a spray in a 4 oz. glass trigger spray bottle. Add a few drops of essential oil and 2 Tbs. (25 ml) olive oil to the spray bottle, and then fill the bottle the rest of the way with distilled water. Use this mixture to spray items like empanadas, tortilla chips, baked french fries, egg rolls, etc.

10. If you are cooking with kids, make sure to keep the oils out of their reach.

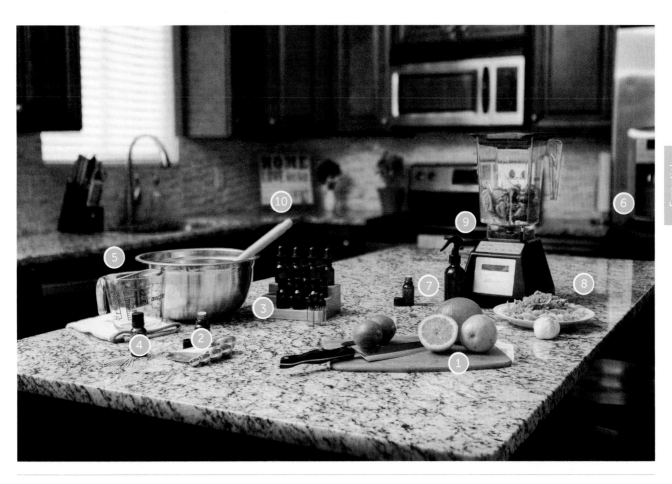

Oil Substitution Guidelines

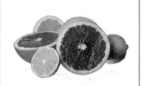 Typically, 1 drop of a citrus oil can substitute for 1 tsp. (2 g) of citrus zest. If the recipe calls for the zest from 1 citrus fruit, you can use 3–10 drops of the citrus essential oil instead.

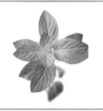 For minty oils such as peppermint and spearmint, try substituting 1 drop of essential oil for 1 tsp. (500 mg) dried mint leaves or 1 Tbs. (3 g) fresh mint leaves.

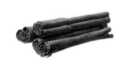 Cinnamon and cassia are pretty similar, and typically what we know as ground cinnamon is really ground cassia; however, the strength of their flavor is quite a bit different. You will want to start by substituting 1 drop of cinnamon for 1–2 Tbs. (8–15 g) ground cinnamon and 1 drop of cassia for 1 tsp. (2 g) ground cinnamon or cassia.

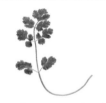 For herbaceous oils like basil, marjoram, oregano, rosemary, cilantro, dill, etc., start with a toothpick dipped in the oil and stirred into the mixture, and then add more to taste as needed.

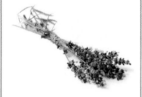 Floral herbs like lavender can be used in cooking; but because floral flavors are uncommon, you want just a hint of this flavor. Start with a toothpick, and add more if needed.

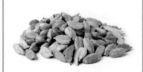 For other flavors, a good rule of thumb is to substitute 1 drop of oil for 1–2 tsp. (500 mg–1 g) of dried spice or herb and 1 drop of oil for 1–2 Tbs. (3–5 g) of fresh herb. If you think the oil is strong or if the recipe calls for less than the above quantities, start with a toothpick dip instead. Taste, and add more if needed.

Recipes

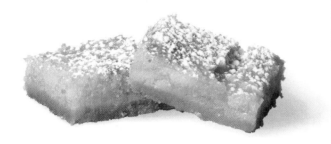

Luscious Lemon Bars

2 c. (240 g) flour	1 t. (4 g) baking powder
½ c. (100 g) sugar	Dash of salt
1 c. (225 g) butter	½ c. (125 ml) water
¼ t. (2 g) salt	½ c. (125 ml) lemon juice
4 eggs	3 drops lemon EO
6 T. (45 g) flour	1 T. (8 g) powdered sugar
1½ c. (300 g) sugar	Lemon zest (optional)

Preheat oven to 350°F (175°C). Mix together flour, sugar, and salt. Cut in the butter until the dough reaches a fine crumb consistency. Press the dough into the bottom of a 9" × 13" pan. Bake for 20 minutes till golden. While crust is baking, beat eggs in a large mixing bowl. In a separate dish, stir together flour, sugar, baking powder, and salt. Add flour mixture to eggs, and stir till smooth. Gradually stir in lemon juice, water, and lemon oil. Pour mixture over baked crust, and return to the oven. Bake 30 minutes or until set. Allow to cool completely, and sift powdered sugar over the top. Garnish with zest if desired. *Substitute orange oil and orange juice to make orange bars.

Rosemary Roasted Red Potatoes

16–24 red potatoes, washed and dried
½–¾ c. (125–175 ml) all-natural ranch dressing
1 drop ea. rosemary and oregano essential oils
2 T. (20 g) garlic powder
1–2 t. (2–5 g) smoked paprika
Sea salt and black pepper to taste

Preheat oven to 450°F (230°C). Dice potatoes into 1" (2.5 cm) pieces, and place in 9" × 13" (23 × 33 cm) pan. Blend essential oils with ranch dressing, and toss with potatoes to coat. Sprinkle potato mixture with garlic,

paprika, salt, and pepper. Cover with aluminum foil, and bake for 25–40 minutes. Remove foil, stir potatoes, and bake uncovered for 15–20 minutes, stirring once more, until golden.

Lemon Tarragon Dressing

1 t. (500 mg) dried tarragon
1 t. (500 mg) dried basil leaves
1 c. (250 ml) organic, cold-pressed olive oil
Dash of black pepper
Dash of red pepper
6 drops lemon essential oil

Mix well, and drizzle on salad or fish or anything! Keep unused portion in the fridge.

Strawberry Citrus Breakfast Ice Cream*

¼ ripe avocado
1 c. (150 g) frozen strawberries
2 T. (25 ml) plain yogurt
1 T. (15 ml) honey or agave
1 drop ea. orange and lime essential oils

Place all ingredients minus oils into a food processor, and purée on high. Remove from food processor, and stir in oils. Serve immediately. *Prepare the night before and freeze in ice-pop molds for a quick, on-the-go breakfast.

Creamy, Creamless, Raw Tomato Soup*

6 ripe tomatoes, seeded and chopped
½ c. (125 ml) water
1 t. minced garlic (1 clove)
½ t. (1 g) onion powder
1 t. (5 g) sea salt
1 ripe avocado, chopped
2 T. (25 ml) extra virgin olive oil
2 drops basil essential oil

Place tomatoes, water, garlic, onion powder, and salt in blender, and blend until smooth. Add the avocado

Recipes

and olive oil, and blend again until smooth. Pour soup into a ceramic or wooden bowl, and add basil oil, stirring to combine. Serve immediately. For a chilled soup, refrigerate for 2 hours. For warm soup, heat over stove.

Peppermint Healthy Fudge*

1½ c. (300 g) coconut oil
1¼ c. (300 ml) agave
1 c. (125 g) organic cocoa powder
½ t. (2 g) sea salt
⅛ scraped out vanilla bean (or 1 t. (5 ml) vanilla extract)
1–2 drops peppermint essential oil

Warm coconut oil until liquid. Combine all ingredients in blender, and blend until smooth. Pour into baking dish, and spread evenly. Place in fridge to set up; then cut and enjoy.

*These recipes were adapted from *The Slimmed and Sassed Cookbook* by Natalie Albaugh & Kristyan Williams, ©2011. Used with permission.

Basil Pesto Chicken

2 t. (10 ml) olive oil | 2 garlic cloves, minced
¼ c. (50 ml) olive oil | 2 c. (60 g) spinach leaves
¼ c. (35 g) pine nuts | 2 T. (25 ml) lemon juice
2 drops lemon EO | 1 drop basil EO
⅓ c. (25 g) parmesan cheese
Salt and pepper to taste
2–3 chicken breasts, cooked and sliced

Sauté garlic cloves in 2 tsp. (10 ml) olive oil for 2 minutes. Blend together spinach, pine nuts, sautéed garlic, ¼ cup (50 ml) olive oil, lemon juice, and essential oils in a blender, pulsing and scraping the sides as needed. Add parmesan cheese, salt, and pepper, and blend in. Serve over chicken and your choice of cooked pasta.

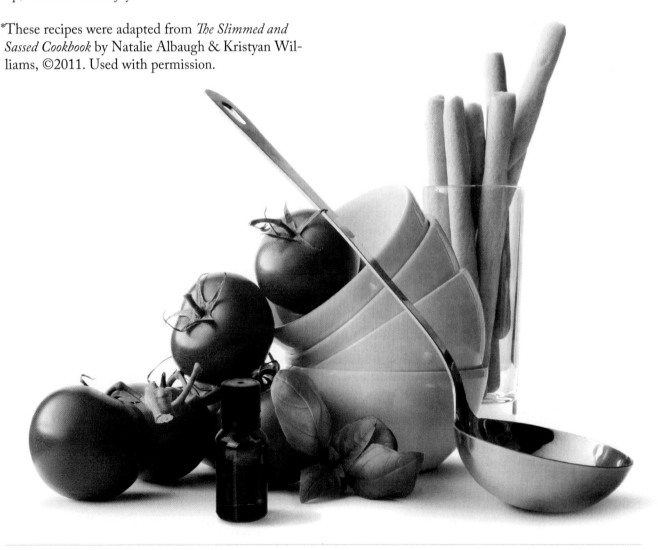

Nutrition and Essential Oils

Considering we spend so much time preparing, eating, and thinking about food, it should be no surprise that food has a great influence over our health. Eating influences us physically because the nutrients we consume are used to build the basic structures of our body and provide energy. However, consuming food also provides us with more than just nutrients. Specifically, eating also provides us with emotional comfort and is an important social, cultural, and familial activity. As food enters the mouth and is broken down by the digestive system, chemicals are sent to the brain that cause an elevation in mood (Bear et al., 2007). Food is a powerful part of human life because of the physical and emotional benefits it provides.

Modern research is finding that food may be the most basic of preventative medicines. There is no magic concoction that will guarantee that you get all the vitamins, minerals, and nutrients your body needs. Eating properly is the easiest way to control your health and ensure that your body is provided with all the nutrients it needs.

Be Nutrient Educated

Developing a healthy diet depends on daily consistency. Sprints of good eating followed by stretches of poor eating choices will lead to bad habits and will ultimately affect your health. Following the below guidelines will provide a solid foundation to a healthy diet that will quickly become second nature (Sizer & Whitney, 2014).

1. Adequacy

Six categories of nutrients are needed by the body for health and growth (Brown, 1991, p. 29). Three of the necessary nutrients—carbohydrates, proteins, and fats—provide fuel for the body. For example, carbohydrates are the leading source of fuel for the body and are vital for brain function. Glucose, found in carbohydrates, is essentially the sole fuel for the human brain. Specifically, the brain uses 60% of the body's glucose (Berg et al., 2002). Therefore, an adequate amount of glucose is needed to ensure proper brain function.

The remaining three needed nutrients—vitamins, minerals, and water—are chemicals used by the body to convert carbohydrates, proteins, and fats into energy. Sufficient amounts of water are needed to regulate the body's chemical processes, excrete waste as urine, control body temperature through sweat, and humidify the air we breathe (Singh, 2000).

Eating a nutritionally dense diet is the easiest way to guarantee the consumption of needed nutrients in adequate amounts. Consuming the recommended daily allowances of the six necessary nutrients will fulfill the need for an adequate diet. Fresh foods, rather than processed foods, are more likely to provide the proper amounts of nutrients needed by the body.

A recent study has revealed that the majority of adults in the United States fail to meet recommended daily nutrient levels (An et al., 2014; Yates, 2014). For example, only 11.3% of the people surveyed in the study met the daily recommended intake of fiber, and only 4.7% met the daily recommended intake of potassium (An et al., 2014; Yates, 2014). For those who do not consume a proper diet and fail to maintain proper enzyme and bacteria levels, dietary supplements can be used to support dietary health.

2. Balance

Our bodies are composed of countless cells that make up the tissues of our bodies. "The type and amounts of foods consumed by people affect the environment of cells and their ability to function normally" (Brown, 1991, p. 37). Cells need the right balance of nutrients to thrive. Too much of a nutrient or too little of a nutrient can cause disease. Eating nutritious foods is the best way to ensure that you are harvesting all your needed nutrients from your diet. Many nutrients are present in foods at such small levels that they are almost undetectable. Substituting nutrition supplements for food will cause you to miss out on the versatile nutrients available from food. Nutrition supplements are meant to supplement good eating, not replace it.

Fad diets that list main food groups to avoid will not help and will probably do more damage than good. The more restricted a diet is, the more likely the diet will be nutritionally deficient.

Vegetarian and vegan diets can provide all the basic nutrients but require more planning to achieve balance among the needed food groups.

3. Calorie Control

Energy intake is directly associated with energy expenditure. Active adults, growing teenagers, and pregnant women require different calorie consumption than the average adult.

Controlling the amount of calories consumed should not mean skipping meals or going for long periods of time without food. Both of these strategies often lead to binge eating once food is consumed. Instead, the most effective way to control calorie consumption is by spreading out food intake over the whole day (Maughan & Burke, 2002). Eating small, nutrient-dense snacks and well-balanced meals throughout the day will help maintain a level energy state and avoid excessive hunger.

Essential Support

Grapefruit oil and Slim & Sassy (see the Essential Oil Blends section) can be inhaled to help suppress appetite. A study conducted on lab animals found that exposure to the scent of grapefruit essential oil for 15 minutes 3 times per week can reduce appetite (Shen et al., 2005).

An easy and effective method for portion control is to serve food on small plates. Small plates will force you to limit servings. Additionally, a filled plate tricks your brain into thinking it is getting more food.

Eating due to boredom is another issue that can affect appropriate caloric intake. Instead of resorting to eating when you are bored, choose to listen to music, drink water, go for a run, read a book, or play a game. If chewing on food while watching TV or working on the computer is a habit, choose to munch on celery or carrots instead of processed snacks and desserts.

4. Nutritional Density

In the morning, you could eat a donut for breakfast or a breakfast consisting of whole wheat bread, fruit salad, eggs, and oatmeal. Surprisingly, both of these meals may consist of the same amount of calories; however, not all calories are

Start with the Basics

No matter what stage you are at in life, choosing to focus on one or more of the following recommendations will help improve your diet and health.

- Eat more whole grains.
- Prepare fresh foods.
- Fill up half your plate with fruits and vegetables.
- Drink more water.
- Choose lean meats.
- Consume more calcium.
- Eat less cholesterol, fat, salt, sugar, and other empty calories.

created equally. Filling up on the donut, although it will provide you with the same amount of energy as the more nutritionally dense option, will leave you with fewer vitamins and less calcium and iron.

In general, the more processed a food is, the less nutritionally dense it is. We are bombarded with nutritionally weak food choices that will fill us up but leave us deficient in many needed vitamins and minerals. When trying to determine which foods are nutritionally dense, remember that real foods, like fresh vegetables, fruits, whole grains, and beans, will provide more nutrition than processed foods, like potato chips, fruit juices, and white bread.

5. Moderation

Eat an assortment of grains, vegetables, fruits, protein foods, and dairy. Most people will not have a hard time eating moderate amounts of these basic food groups. However, foods rich in salt, sugar, and fat should also be eaten moderately.

Eating sweets and processed foods is perfectly acceptable, even while trying to maintain a healthy diet. As mentioned earlier, eating influences us emotionally as well as physically. Enjoying a treat on occasion will not harm your health and can be a great reward for eating well.

6. Variety

A monotonous diet is likely to produce deficiencies in certain food groups and even certain nutrients. For example, if you only ate carrots every day to fulfill your vegetable needs, you would miss out on the special vitamins and phytochemicals contained in vegetables like broccoli, sweet potatoes, and spinach. Trying new foods and recipes is an exciting and enjoyable way to add variety to your diet.

Support Digestive Health

Healthy eating is dependent on a healthy digestive system. The valuable nutrients from foods are best utilized by a properly functioning digestive system. The digestive system is responsible for breaking down nutrients, facilitating absorption of nutrients into the blood, and preventing foreign and toxic molecules from entering the bloodstream (Cencic et al., 2010). The correct composition of enzymes and good bacteria in the intestines is a measure of good digestive health.

—Enzymes

We consume food, but our bodies absorb nutrients. Enzymes located in the digestive system break down the components of food into nutrients that can be absorbed by the body. Even eating well cannot guarantee proper nutrient absorption unless your body contains appropriate amounts of enzymes. Aging, chronic stress, and inflammation can cause digestive enzyme deficiency. Dietary changes, dietary supplements, and managing chronic stress can help correct digestive enzyme deficiency.

Essential Support

To support organ cleansing and healthy tissue function, take 3–5 drops of Zendocrine in a capsule daily.

Many of the dietary supplements listed in the Essential Oil–Inspired Wellness Supplements section contain key ingredients that aid enzyme function to promote overall digestive health.

For example, DigestZen Terrazyme and Zendocrine Detoxification Complex are wellness supplements that blend food-derived enzymes and mineral cofactors that can aid in the digestion and absorption of critical nutrients that are lacking in many of today's diets. Specifically, DigestZen Terrazyme provides hydrochloric acid (helps alle-

viate stomach problems, like heartburn, associated with too little stomach acid), lactase (assists in the digestion of dairy products), and many other enzymes that support the breakdown of proteins, carbohydrates, starches, sugars, fats, oils, fiber, and gluten. These supplements can help support the digestive system by providing digestive enzymes and by providing an environment where digestive enzymes can function better.

—Intestinal Bacteria

Scientists estimate that for every human cell in the body, there are at least 10 bacterial cells (Morowitz et al., 2011). The healthy bacteria naturally present in your digestive tract are important for digestion, nutrient absorption, and supporting the immune system. The metabolic functions of these healthy bacteria provide energy, vitamins, and protection against harmful pathogens (Cencic et al., 2010). Furthermore, the composition of the bacteria located in the intestines is known to affect the digestion and absorption of food (Brussow, 2013). The intestinal bacteria also have an effect on the immune system, infection, drug metabolism, and weight gain (Brussow, 2013).

Essential Support

The oils in DigestZen (see the Essential Oil Blends section) have been studied for their abilities in balancing the digestive system and in soothing many of that system's ailments. To support digestive health, take this essential oil blend internally as a dietary supplement by adding 1 drop to your glass of water.

Along with supporting the digestive system's enzymes, Essential Oil–Inspired Wellness Supplements can also support intestinal bacteria. Supplementing your diet with PB Assist+ provides 6 strains of probiotic intestinal flora that can help support healthy colonies of friendly microflora in the digestive tract. The probiotics can also prevent the adhesion and growth of harmful bacteria in the intestines and can support immune system health. Furthermore, GX Assist can support the gastrointestinal tract by eliminating harmful pathogens that can damage healthy intestinal bacteria.

Make Goals

A one-size-fits-all diet is not appropriate nor recommended by nutritionists. For example, the athlete should eat differently than someone looking to shed some extra weight. While reading the next section, focus on molding your diet to best fit your current life goals, whether that be preparing healthy meals for your family or staying healthy during pregnancy.

—Chronic Disease Prevention

Although a poor diet can cause disease (vitamin C deficiency, for example, causes scurvy), the majority of chronic illnesses, such as diabetes and heart disease, are not caused by diet (Brown, 1991, p. 8). Instead, diet is associated with the development of the disease.

Essential Support

One of the reasons fruits and vegetables are beneficial for supporting good health is because they are packed with vitamins, minerals, and antioxidants. Antioxidants are also found in essential oils.

Some risk factors associated with chronic disease are out of our hands, including genetics, age, and environment. However, an unhealthy diet, tobacco use, and physical inactivity are examples of risk factors that are controllable. Several studies have shown that altering one's diet can help reduce the risk of chronic diseases, such as cancer, heart disease, and diabetes. In general, increasing consumption of fruits and vegetables is the easiest way to prevent chronic disease. Researchers have found that "people who eat abundant and varied fruits and vegetables each day may cut their risk for many diseases by as much as half" (Sizer & Whitney, 2014).

Cancer: The antioxidants, vitamins, and other nutrients in fruits and vegetables may reduce the risk of developing certain cancers (Kraak et al., 2005, p. 97). Limiting tobacco and alcohol intake can also reduce the risk factors for many forms of cancer (Amine et al., 2002).

Type 2 Diabetes: The World Health Organization has concluded that exercising more and cutting down on excess calories from sugar, starches, and fats will help prevent unhealthy weight gain associated with the development of type 2 diabetes (Amine et al., 2002).

Heart Disease: Reducing the consumption of salt has been shown to prevent high blood pressure, a major cause of cardiovascular disease (Kraak et al., 2005, p. 97; Amine et al., 2002). Furthermore, the potassium found in fruits and vegetables can also reduce blood pressure (Bendick & Deckelbaum, 2010). Fruits and vegetables are also powerful combatants against cholesterol. The fiber supplied by fruits and vegetables bind to lipids, like cholesterol, and decrease lipid concentration in the blood, thus lowering cholesterol levels that could cause heart disease (Kraak et al., 2005, p. 97).

Osteoporosis: Ensuring that you are consuming enough calcium (500 mg per day or more) and vitamin D will help reduce the risk of osteoporosis (Amine et al., 2002). Sun exposure and physical activity will also help strengthen bones and muscles against bone fractures (Amine et al., 2002).

Key Goal: Eat more fruits and vegetables, which contain important nutrients that can protect our bodies from chronic disease.

—Weight Loss

One of the first steps to weight management is determining what you are currently eating and how much you are eating. For a week, keep a record of all the foods and drinks you consume. Also track your daily exercise. You probably do not realize that your energy intake is surpassing your energy expenditure. Allowing energy intake to equal energy expenditure will slow weight gain. Decreasing energy intake and increasing energy expenditure will allow for weight loss.

Essential Support

Slim & Sassy (see the Essential Oil Blends section) contains oils that are often used to help control hunger and to help limit excessive calorie intake. The aroma of this blend is also uplifting and invigorating and may help increase physical energy..

Decreasing energy intake can be achieved by reducing portion size, cooking homemade meals with fresh ingredients, and eating slowly. In addition, replacing sugar-loaded, calorie-dense snacks with fruits and vegetables will help you consume needed nutrients and avoid empty calories.

Do not skip meals, especially breakfast. Instead of relying on skipping meals or enduring long periods without food intake (which will generally lead to overeating when you do finally eat a meal), spread out food intake over the whole day (Maughan & Burke, 2002). Eating throughout the day will help you remain optimistic and feel more energized. This method will also help you lose weight at a constant state. It will be easier to keep weight off if you lose it slowly over time, instead of in a short period of time.

Key Goal: Decrease energy intake by controlling portion size and consuming nutritious foods instead of empty calories.

—Meal Preparation for the Family

Eating meals together as a family has been shown to "protect against unhealthy eating and obesity during childhood and adolescence" (Dwyer et al., 2015). The more often a family eats together, the more likely children will have healthy eating habits (Dwyer et al., 2015; Lee et al., 2014). The emotional benefits are also great, as "family meals can contribute to reductions in substance use, violence, sexual activity, mental health issues, and self-harm among children and adolescents" (Dwyer et al., 2015). Family meals provide more than just physical nourishment and can establish healthy life choices throughout a child's life.

Essential Support

Cooking with essential oils can increase flavor and be a fun experience for the whole family. You can substitute essential oils for herbs in many recipes. Essential oils are strong, so only a small amount needs to be used in a recipe. See the Essential Oil Cooking Tips (page 403) and Recipes (page 405) sections for great tips and recipes using essential oils.

Researchers have also discovered that sharing meals with others could contribute to increasing happiness (Yiengprugsawan et al., 2015). In fact, the presence of other individuals during mealtime "has a greater influence on food consumption than the basic physiological functions of hunger" (Yiengprugsawan et al., 2015; see also Herman et al., 2003).

If you are eating together as a family, you are already providing a healthy environment and instilling lifelong lessons of health into your family. While preparing a healthy meal for your family, focus on filling the majority of the plate with whole grains and vegetables. Additionally, plan a variety of different foods for meals throughout the week to make sure your family is getting all the vitamins and nutrients they need. Including children in meal planning and teaching them about purchasing food can help children be more excited about a meal.

Key Goal: Add variety to your family meals, and follow the recommended serving suggestions given by ChooseMyPlate.gov.

—Athletic Training

Athletic training requires an increased amount of nutrients and energy. Therefore, athletes are vulnerable to deficiencies (Wierniuk et al., 2013). Studies show that an athlete's diet is frequently deficient in protein, carbohydrates, vitamins, minerals, and calories (Wierniuk et al., 2013). Inadequacies in diet can result in declined sports performance and an increased risk of injury.

During athletic training, you can benefit from some of the following ideas in order to ensure that your diet is not deficient. First, eat more nutrient-dense carbohydrates, like whole-grain breads, rice, pasta, fruits, starchy vegetables, beans, and dairy (Maughan & Burke, 2002). Carbohydrates provide energy and allow for muscle gain, both of which are vital during exercise. Second, to ensure proper consumption of vitamins and minerals, prepare a casserole or stir fry to easily get a variety of food types in one meal (Maughan & Burke, 2002). Lastly, spread protein intake throughout the day, rather than concentrating protein intake all in one meal (Maughan & Burke, 2002).

Key Goal: Consume an adequate amount of carbohydrates from a variety of different foods, especially 2–3 days before athletic events.

—Pregnancy

During a woman's reproductive years, health professionals advise supplementing a healthy diet with folic acid and iron. Folic acid, a B vitamin, is especially important because it is used to form the neural tube (the structure from which the brain and spinal cord form) during fetal development. Folic acid can be found in broccoli, citrus fruits, beans, avocados, nuts, and fortified cereals.

The added energy it takes to grow a baby will require additional calories during pregnancy. Focus on eating nutrient-packed foods instead of foods with empty calories. Nutrient-dense foods will ensure that you are ingesting all the vitamins, minerals, and energy that your baby needs to grow. Foods that are especially beneficial during pregnancy include orange vegetables, whole grains, lean meats, beans, and nuts.

Throughout pregnancy, avoid consuming alcohol, caffeine, and harmful substances like recreational drugs. Furthermore, review any wellness supplements or medications you may be taking with your doctor to confirm that they are safe to continue to use throughout pregnancy. Essential oils can provide therapeutic benefits at a time when a pregnant woman's options for medical drugs are limited. Many oils are safe to use during pregnancy, especially when diluted with a carrier oil, and can provide relief from the uncomfortable symptoms associated with pregnancy. However, be aware of which essential oils are not recommended during pregnancy.

Key Goal: Eat foods containing folic acid, or choose a folic acid supplement.

Essential Support

Supplementing with Microplex MVp that contains folic acid and iron is recommended during pregnancy and breastfeeding. Ask your doctor at your prenatal checkup if the wellness supplements you are taking meet the recommended daily dosage. If you plan to become pregnant in the next year, taking a supplement before becoming pregnant will ensure that your body has the right nutrients to support your baby's growth.

—Eating Healthy As a Vegetarian

A well-planned vegetarian diet can provide health benefits and reduce the risk of certain diseases. With today's extensive food options, it is easier than ever to maintain a nutritious vegetarian diet. Additionally, fortified soymilk or dietary supplements can provide many of the needed nutrients that are difficult to obtain from a vegetarian diet. The more restrictive your vegetarian diet, the more closely you will need to monitor your nutrient intake. For example, if you consume dairy products, you are likely obtaining adequate levels of nutrients from your diet alone. However, a very strict vegan diet will likely require supplementation or the consumption of fortified foods.

Specifically, vegetarians should focus on consuming adequate amounts of protein, calcium, vitamin D, vitamin B12, and iron. High levels of protein can be found in beans, peas, nuts, and soy products. Calcium can be found in calcium-fortified soymilk and orange juice, dark-green leafy vegetables, and other calcium-fortified foods. Vitamin D, along with calcium, supports bone health and can be obtained from sun exposure, egg yolks, and fortified orange juice. Vitamin B12 is a nutrient found in animal products and is needed to prevent anemia. Vitamin B12 can be found in fortified cereals and soy products, nutritional yeast, eggs, and dairy products. Iron is needed for red blood cells and can be found in plants. However, the iron found in plants is not absorbed by the body as well as the iron found in meat. Consuming foods high in vitamin C (e.g., tomatoes, potatoes, citrus fruits) at the same time as iron-rich foods increases the body's iron absorption. Important sources of iron include whole grains, green vegetables, beans, and legumes.

The easiest way to guarantee adequate amounts of needed nutrients is by supplementing a nutritious diet with a wellness supplement. It is important to remember that the high fiber content of a plant-based diet can reduce the absorption of some of the above nutrients. Consult with your doctor or nutritionist to guarantee you are consuming proper nutrient levels.

Key Goal: Choose fortified foods (soymilk, cereal, orange juice) or supplementation with an a2z Chewable or Microplex MVp to get a full range of nutrients.

Exercise and Essential Oils

In today's world, with advancements in technology and modern conveniences, it has become easier and easier to live a sedentary lifestyle, free from physical exertion. While this has made life easier in many ways, the downside to today's modern lifestyle is that the body needs a regular amount of physical exertion to maintain optimal health. With many jobs demanding more and more hours sitting at a desk, it becomes increasingly difficult to find time to give the body the exercise and motion it needs to be able to function optimally.

This sedentary lifestyle, along with poor nutritional options and choices, has led to a global epidemic of obesity, diabetes, cardiovascular disease, back and joint problems, and many other life-altering health issues (McArdle et al., 2015, p. 800).

While changing nutritional choices to include more balanced, healthy options is one key to maintaining a healthy body, making time for regular physical activity is the other key. A strong argument can be made that regular, sustained exercise is even more important to maintaining a healthy body weight than just limiting the number of calories we consume (Ross et al., 2000; Thompson et al., 2004).

In addition to contributing to overall health, regular exercise can help increase energy, build muscle, promote healthy body weight, enhance cardiovascular health, increase flexibility, and contribute to better mental and emotional health.

Essential oils can support the body and mind in many different ways to help enhance success during exercise. The following sections outline some of the many ways exercise can support the body and some of the many ways essential oils can help support the body before, during, and after physical activity.

Increase Endurance/Energy

One key benefit of regular aerobic exercise is an enhanced feeling of energy and endurance (Wu et al., 2015). This benefit is commonly attributed to increased cardiovascular efficiency, as well as an increased number of mitochondria in the cells to generate energy and prevent lactate buildup in the muscle tissues (Holloszy, 1967; Steiner et al., 1985).

Suggested Exercise Examples: Long-term, regular exercise is the key to enhancing endurance and energy. Start with low-level sustained activities, such as walking, easy bicycling, slow swimming, or easy hiking, and progress to moderate- or high-level activities such as jogging, running, bicycling, fast swimming, or steep hikes.

Essential Support

Endurance: peppermint

Energizing: peppermint, white fir, Elevation, Balance

Mental Fatigue: Serenity, lemongrass, basil

Physical Fatigue: Serenity

Muscle Fatigue: marjoram, white fir, cypress, peppermint

Body Systems/Structures Affected: Cardiovascular System, Muscles and Bones, Emotional Balance.

Build Muscle

Building muscle is important for any individual wishing to maintain a healthy lifestyle. Increased muscle mass can help increase overall metabolism in the body, as muscle tissue naturally burns more calories than fat tissue (McArdle et al., 2014, p. 193). Maintaining healthy muscle mass is also important for enhancing quality of life as the body gets older. As the body ages, the level of fat tends to increase, and the level of muscle tissue and strength tends to decrease. Regular exercise, including resistance training, can help counteract this effect and help maintain muscle strength (Goodpaster et al., 2008; Frontera et al., 1985).

Suggested Exercise Types: Resistance training (where weight resists the physical movement), such as weightlifting, elastic resistance, push-ups, pull-ups, squats, and yoga.

Essential Support

Sore Muscles: ⬮marjoram, ⬮Deep Blue, ⬮birch, ⬮clove, ⬮AromaTouch, ⬮oregano, ⬮peppermint

Muscle Development: ⬮birch, ⬮wintergreen, ⬮Deep Blue

Body Systems/Structures Affected: Muscles and Bones, Emotional Balance.

Lose Weight

When losing weight is a desired outcome, it is important to remember that the true goal is to lose *excess* fat from the body and maintain a healthy body weight. Weight loss can also occur through protein breakdown from muscle fiber and dehydration—both of which can be detrimental to the body's overall health. It is also important to note that the body needs a minimum level of fat in order to properly protect vital organs, regulate body heat, create hormones, and perform other vital functions; so focusing solely on decreasing fat can lead to other health issues. The key is to maintain a healthy level of fat within the body.

While reducing the amount of calories consumed per day is one of the keys to losing excess fat, it is important to maintain a balanced diet during weight loss that supports the body with necessary nutrients. Sufficient carbohydrates (preferably from whole-grain sources) are necessary to provide the body with energy and can actually help promote fat burning and help prevent muscle loss from protein breakdown (McArdle et al., 2015, p. 14). Sufficient exercise is also important for maintaining muscle mass when eating a reduced-calorie diet.

Regular, sustained exercise is a critical key to maintaining a healthy body weight throughout life (Rosse et al., 2000; Butte et al., 2007). Regular exercise can help boost the metabolic rate of the body, burn calories, maintain healthy muscle mass, keep the body toned and fit, and prevent weight gain.

Suggested Exercise Types: Sustained (30+ minutes), low- to moderate-level activities have been found to be the most efficient burners of fat as an energy source (Romijn et al., 1993). Try activities such as walking, jogging, swimming, rowing, aerobics, basketball, and tennis.

Essential Support

Appetite Control: ⬮◯grapefruit, ⬮◯Slim & Sassy, ⬮◯oregano, ⬮◯thyme

Uplifting: ⬮lemon, ⬮orange, ⬮Elevation, ⬮◯Citrus Bliss

Weight Loss: ⬮◯grapefruit, ⬮◯Slim & Sassy, ⬮◯oregano, ⬮◯thyme

Body Systems/Structures Affected: Muscles and Bones, Cardiovascular System, Emotional Balance, Hormonal System.

Enhance Cardiovascular Health

Perhaps one of the most discussed threats of living a sedentary lifestyle is the increased risk of cardiovascular problems, such as high blood pressure, atherosclerosis, heart attack, and angina. It is estimated that those living a sedentary lifestyle have approximately twice the risk of developing coronary heart disease than those who exercise regularly (McArdle et al., 2015, p. 875). Regular exercise has been found to have beneficial effects on blood lipid levels (Stefanick et al., 1998; Leaf et al., 1997), prevention of atherosclerosis (Kwasniewska et al., 2014; Palmefors et al., 2014), high blood pressure (Leggio et al., 2014; Maruf et al., 2014), and other risk factors for coronary heart disease (Blumenthal et al., 2012).

Suggested Exercise Types: Aerobic exercises at least 3 times a week are recommended to help enhance cardiovascular health. Try activities such as aerobics, dance exercises, walking, jogging, swimming, bicycling, hiking, tennis, or basketball.

Essential Support

Endurance: ⬮◯peppermint

Atherosclerosis: ◯⬮⬮lemon, ⬮lavender, ◯⬮melissa⬮, ◯⬮dill

High Blood Pressure: ⬮⬮ylang ylang, ⬮⬮marjoram

Heart: ⬮⬮ylang ylang, ⬮⬮marjoram, ⬮⬮geranium

Body Systems/Structures Affected: Cardiovascular System, Emotional Balance, Muscles and Bones, Respiratory System.

Enhance Flexibility

Sufficient flexibility of muscles, tendons, and connective tissue is important in maintaining proper posture and helping to prevent injuries (Witvrouw et al., 2003; Cibulka et al., 1998). Stretching before and after strenuous physical activity can be a good way to help prevent injury and to keep muscles loose.

Suggested Exercise Types: A range of static (holding a stretch) and dynamic (moving) stretching exercises, in all directions, and covering all of the regions of the body are recommended for optimal flexibility (Clark et al., 2014, p. 164). Be careful to avoid stretches that place too much strain on the tendons or on the spine or neck. Try a variety of stretching exercises and activities such as yoga, calisthenics, squats, lunges, and dance exercises.

Essential Support

Tension: ⊘marjoram, ⊘Deep Blue

Strain: ⊘lemongrass, ⊘Deep Blue

Yoga: ⊘sandalwood, ⊘cedarwood, ⊘frankincense

Body Systems/Structures Affected: Muscles and Bones, Connective Tissues.

Enhance Mental Health

As the body ages, cognitive function can decline due to many different factors (McArdle et al., 2015, p. 852). Many studies have shown, however, that regular physical activity can have both short-term and long-term benefits to cognitive ability (Spirduso, 1975; Bixby et al., 2007) and can decrease the risk of dementia (Liu et al., 2012). Exercise has been linked to improved vascular health in the brain (Davenport et al., 2012), an increased number of mitochondria in brain cells (Steiner et al., 1985), and decreased levels of pro-inflammatory markers (Nascimento et al., 2014)—all of which may help sustain proper brain function and cognition.

In addition to these mental benefits, exercise has also been shown to help reduce symptoms of depression and anxiety (Blumenthal et al., 2012; Smith et al., 2013).

Suggested Exercise Types: All exercises that sustain physical activity for an extended period of time can help enhance mental health. Try walking, jogging, swimming, gardening, yoga, hiking, kayaking, canoeing, dancing, golf, tennis, or any other activity that you enjoy.

Essential Support

Focus/Concentration: ⊘⊘InTune, ⊘lavender, ⊘lemon, ⊘peppermint

Memory: ⊘⊘rosemary, ⊘⊘peppermint, ⊘⊘frankincense

Anxiety/Depression: ⊘lavender, ⊘orange, ⊘lemon, ⊘⊘InTune, ⊘⊘Serenity, ⊘AromaTouch, ⊘Elevation, ⊘Balance (on back of neck), and ⊘Breathe (on chest)

Body Systems/Structures Affected: Nervous System, Emotional Balance, Hormonal System.

Other Essential Support for Exercise

Cramps/Charley Horse: ⊘lemongrass with ⊘peppermint, ⊘marjoram, ⊘Deep Blue

Over-exercised Muscles: ⊘white fir, ⊘eucalyptus

Muscle Aches/Pains: ⊘marjoram, ⊘Deep Blue, ⊘birch, ⊘clove, ⊘AromaTouch, ⊘oregano, ⊘peppermint

Inflammation: ⊘⊘⊘frankincense, ⊘⊘melaleuca, ⊘⊘eucalyptus, ⊘oregano, ⊘Deep Blue

Cooling Oils: ⊘⊘peppermint, ⊘⊘eucalyptus

Breathing: ⊘⊘Breathe, ⊘⊘cinnamon, ⊘⊘frankincense

Essential Living for a Balanced, Healthy Life

While the focus of this book is on the amazing properties of essential oils and the benefits that many individuals gain from using them, it is also important to discuss some of the many other lifestyle choices that are involved in living a truly balanced, healthy life. The remainder of this chapter discusses some basics that help support living a balanced, healthy life and the ways essential oils can support, enhance, and enrich these areas of our lives. For even more great tips and recipes, see the book *Modern Essentials: Living.*

Nutrition and Exercise: A Foundation for a Balanced, Healthy Life

The foundation for a balanced, healthy life starts with good nutrition and adequate physical activity (exercise). These two essentials help keep the body functioning properly and at peak efficiency and help support the body in its ability to maintain healthy immune function. Much has been written in scientific literature about the association between a sedentary lifestyle and poor nutrition and the development of chronic disease.

Some risk factors associated with chronic disease are out of our hands, including genetics, age, and environment. However, an unhealthy diet, tobacco use, and physical inactivity are examples of risk factors that are controllable. Several studies have shown that altering one's diet can help reduce the risk of chronic diseases, such as cancer, heart disease, and diabetes. In general, increasing consumption of fruits and vegetables is one of the easiest lifestyle changes to make to prevent chronic disease. Researchers have found that "people who eat abundant and varied fruits and vegetables each day may cut their risk for many diseases by as much as half" (Sizer & Whitney, 2014).

Likewise, a sedentary lifestyle, along with poor nutritional options and choices, has led to a global epidemic of chronic diseases such as obesity, diabetes, cardiovascular disease, back and joint problems, and many other life-altering health issues (McArdle et al., 2015, p. 800).

While changing nutritional choices to include more balanced, healthy options is one key to maintaining a healthy body, making time for regular physical activity is the other key. A strong argument can be made that regular, sustained exercise is even more important to maintaining a healthy body weight than just limiting the number of calories we consume (Ross et al., 2000; Thompson et al., 2004).

The sections on Nutrition and Essential Oils (page 407) and Exercise and Essential Oils (page 413) go more in depth on these topics and some of the ways nutrition and exercise can help support specific health goals during different periods of life. These sections also discuss some of the many ways essential oils can help support an individual in achieving his or her health goals.

Healthy Immune Function:

Having a solid foundation of good nutrition and exercise can help support both short-term and long-term healthy immune function. As previously noted, while there are several risk factors beyond our control in contracting a disease or developing a chronic health condition, the two biggest factors that we can control are balanced, adequate nutrient intake and sufficient physical activity. Other factors that we can control include receiving routine medical checkups to catch any developing condition early on, getting adequate, quality sleep, practicing good hygiene, and maintaining a clean personal environment. See the "Essential Living" section for tips on using essential oils to help in these areas.

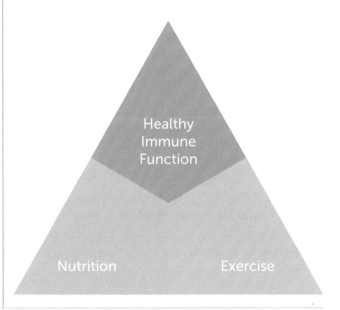

Physical Health: Providing a Core for Mental and Emotional Health

Nutrition, exercise, and healthy immune function all contribute to a solid core of good physical health. This core in turn helps support a healthy and balanced state of mental and emotional health.

Mental Health:

While there are many genetic and environmental factors that can play a role in an individual's overall state of mental health, there are many things that can be done to optimize mental health to an individual's greatest capacity.

Exercise has been linked to improved vascular health in the brain (Davenport et al., 2012), an increased number of mitochondria in brain cells (Steiner et al., 1985), and decreased levels of pro-inflammatory markers (Nascimento et al., 2014)—all of which may help sustain proper brain function and cognition.

In addition to these mental benefits, exercise has also been shown to help reduce symptoms of depression and anxiety (Blumenthal et al., 2012; Smith et al., 2013).

Essential Support

Several studies have indicated that using a specific aroma both when studying and when trying to recall that information can help boost memory recall (Smith et al., 1992; Moss et al., 2008).

Staying mentally active has also been associated with a higher level of memory recall and mental cognition throughout life (Whitehouse et al., 2006; Harvard Women's Health Watch, 2013). Ways to stay mentally active can include reading, engaging in mentally stimulating puzzles and games, discussing challenging topics with others, and staying involved in work, hobbies, or causes that require mental exertion and interaction with others.

See the topics on "Memory," "Alzheimer's Disease," "Brain," "Depression," "Anxiety," and "Nervous System" in the Personal Usage Guide section of this book for many ways that essential oils are used to help support mental health.

Emotional Health:

Just as important as maintaining mental health is maintaining a healthy state of emotions. This can mean taking care of emotional needs, maintaining an emotionally healthy outlook on life, and avoiding chronic stress.

While much is still being discovered about the complex psychological and physiological processes involved in emotions, researchers have discovered that emotions involve many different systems in the body, including the brain, the sensory system, the endocrine/hormonal system, the autonomic nervous system, the immune system, and the release or inhibition of neurotransmitters (such as dopamine) in the brain. Recent research has also begun to uncover compelling evidence that various essential oils and their components have the ability to affect each one of these systems, making the use of essential oils an intriguing tool for helping to balance emotions in the human body.

See the "Emotions" topic in the Personal Usage Guide section of this book for many ways that essential oils are used to help support emotional health.

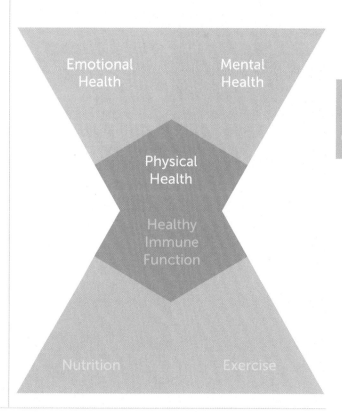

Creating Abundance in Your Life

Maintaining and strengthening a core of physical, mental, and emotional health gives an individual more freedom and ability to focus outward on the community and environment and to build abundance in his or her life.

Abundance can mean many different things to many different individuals. On its surface, abundance brings to mind the possession of financial resources, land, houses, and the many material things that make life comfortable and easy. At the heart of abundance, however, is a core of strong, solid, meaningful relationships with others—especially family and friends—and a wealth of shared and solitary experiences that enrich life and positively impact the world.

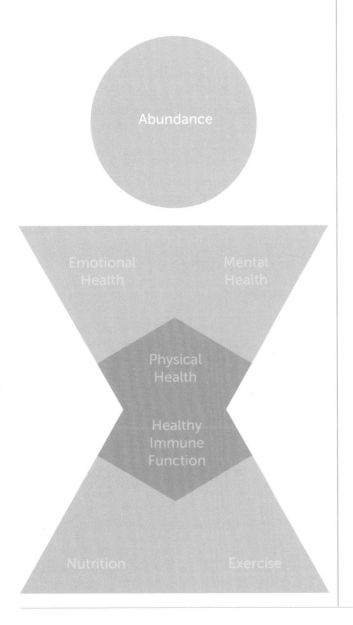

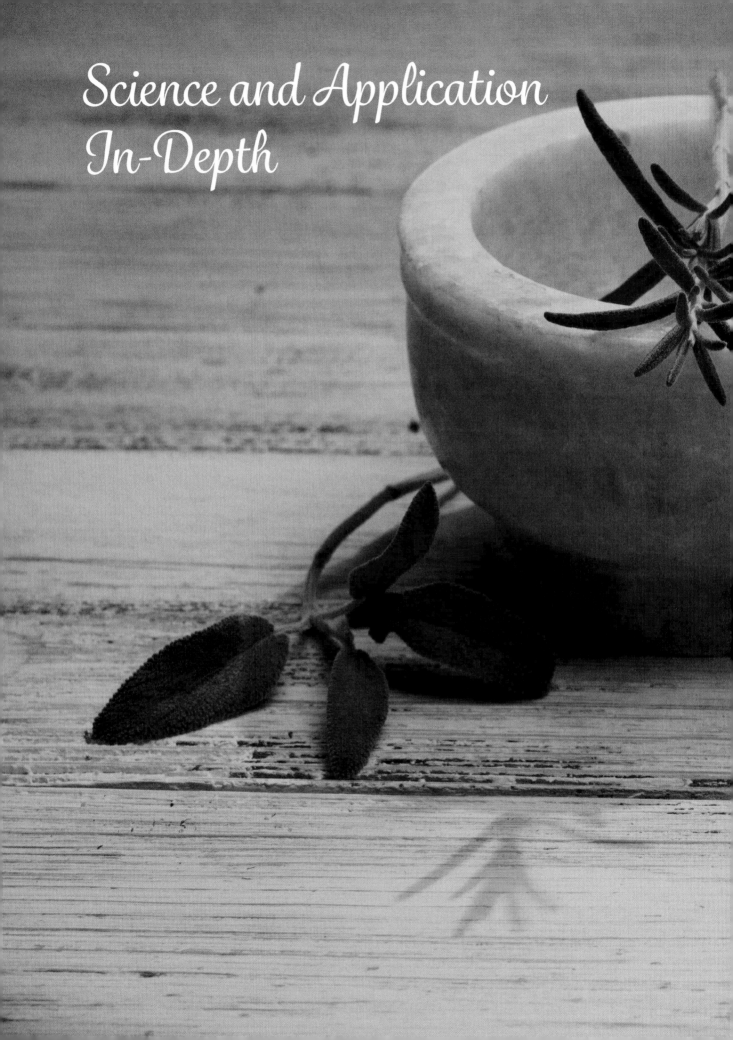

Science and Application
In-Depth

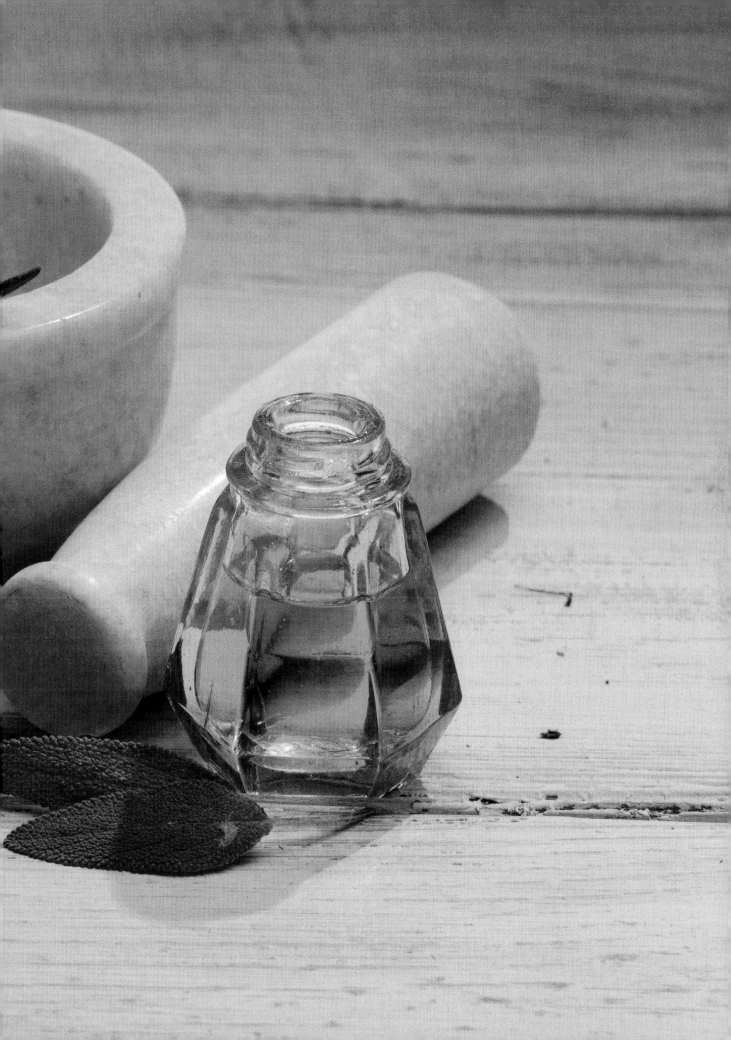

How Essential Oils Interact with the Body

With the help of key individuals like René-Maurice Gattefossé, Jean Valnet, and Robert Tisserand, essential oils have become recognized once again for their therapeutic and medicinal properties. Research on essential oils has increased exponentially since the 1990s and continues to increase each year. This section includes recent research detailing the pharmacological effects essential oils have on the body, including the following: the impact of the route of administration and chemical properties of essential oils, systemic and localized therapeutic mechanisms, and specific interactions occurring with oral administration. Understanding how an essential oil interacts with the body is crucial for interpreting its therapeutic effects and developing a personal holistic health regime.

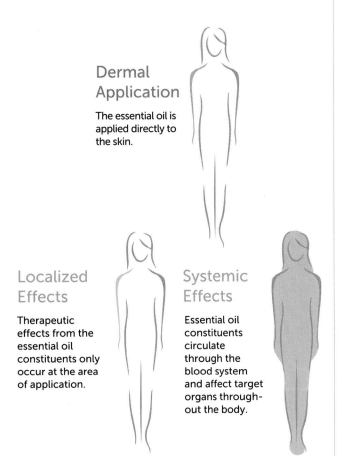

Dermal Application

The essential oil is applied directly to the skin.

Localized Effects

Therapeutic effects from the essential oil constituents only occur at the area of application.

Systemic Effects

Essential oil constituents circulate through the blood system and affect target organs throughout the body.

—Figure 1. Effects of Dermal Application
Applying essential oils to the skin can result in
localized or systemic effects.

Route of Administration and Chemical Properties Can Influence the Therapeutic Effect of an Essential Oil

Use of essential oils can elicit either systemic (whole body) therapeutic effects or localized therapeutic effects depending on the type of administration utilized (i.e., topical, aromatic, or internal) and the chemical constituents of the essential oil. Because essential oils are composed of hundreds of chemical constituents with different properties, a single essential oil has the potential to produce both systemic and localized effects simultaneously.

Application of essential oils to the skin can cause systemic or localized effects (see Figure 1). Localized effects pertain to the specific area where the essential oil was applied. Systemic effects occur when some or all of the essential oil constituents cross the epidermal layer of the skin and are absorbed into the capillaries of the tissues below (also called transdermal absorption).

Aromatic and internal applications usually result in systemic effects but can also cause localized effects. For example, an inhaled essential oil constituent can produce localized effects on lung tissue, an ingested constituent can produced localized effects on the stomach, or in both cases the constituent can be absorbed into the blood and result in systemic circulation.

Research has led to the finding that the mode of application can drastically influence the effect an essential oil has on the body. For example, when East Indian sandalwood essential oil was applied to the skin of humans, a sedative effect on the body was observed (Hongratanaworakit et al., 2004). The massage of sandalwood oil caused the subject's blood pressure and blink rate to decrease, indicating a decrease of physiological arousal (Hongratanaworakit et al., 2004). The subjects were supplied with pure air by breathing masks to prevent inhalation of the oil (Hongratanaworakit et al., 2004).

On the other hand, when the same essential oil was delivered via inhalation, a stimulatory effect occurred (Heuberger et al., 2006). Signs of increased autonomic nervous system stimulation included increased pulse rate and skin conductance level (Heuberger et al., 2006). The contradicting bioactivity of this essential oil suggests that the therapeutic properties of essential

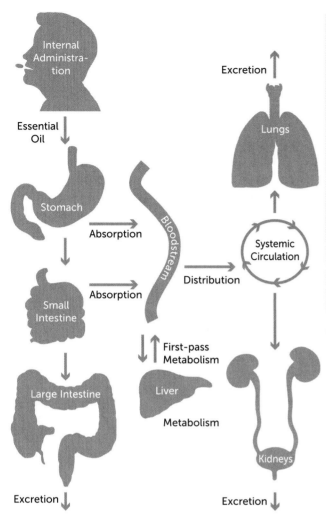

—Figure 2. Systemic Cycle
Overview of the absorption, distribution, metabolism, and excretion of
essential oils involved in whole-body therapeutic effects

Systemic and Localized Therapeutic Effects Produce Different Actions on the Body

A systemic response involves the following processes: absorption into the blood system, whole body distribution via the circulatory system, metabolism by the liver, and excretion orchestrated by the kidneys, lungs, and intestines (see Figure 2) (Turley, 2009). Contact with an essential oil can elicit a systemic response because many of the chemical constituents composing essential oils are molecularly small and have the ability to permeate cell membranes (Kohlert et al., 2000).

Systemic absorption is not required for an essential oil to be effective, and in some cases the use of an essential oil will not include absorption into the circulatory system. Instead, the essential oil will exert effects at the point of first contact. Such a localized response can occur topically or even internally.

An Overview of the Processes Involved in the Systemic Cycle

An analysis of the systemic cycle reveals the many prospective interactions an essential oil chemical constituent can have with the cells of the body. Since essential oil constituents display different actions on the body and a single essential oil can have hundreds of constituents, it is impossible to give a single mechanism to explain the therapeutic effect of all essential oils. Instead, an overview of the systemic cycle can describe the general cycle of essential oil constituents in the body.

—Absorption

Following systemic administration of an essential oil, the chemical constituents quickly dissolve in the tissue fluids of the body, pass through the walls of nearby capillaries, and are absorbed into the blood (Turley, 2009).

The most prevalent tissue fluid of the body is interstitial fluid. Interstitial fluid surrounds the outside of cells, delivers nutrients to cells, and removes cellular waste. Interstitial fluid is mainly composed of filtered water from the blood (Wiig et al., 2012). Other tissue fluids include saliva in the mouth and gastric juice in the stomach (Turley, 2009). Essential oil constituents dissolved in tissue fluid may enter cells of that tissue.

After absorption into the tissue fluids, systemic action requires absorption into nearby capillaries. Some cells, such as epidermal cells creating the

oils may depend on the administration route (Heuberger et al., 2006). This groundbreaking research suggests that using different routes of administration can expand the therapeutic potential of an essential oil.

In all cases, the chemical properties of an essential oil component influence the therapeutic action of an essential oil. There is evidence that some chemical constituents of essential oils are always systemically absorbed, independent of the route of administration used (Kohlert et al., 2000). For example, in the above studies, some East Indian sandalwood essential oil constituents were systemically absorbed when administered either through inhalation or the skin.

Diagram of Dermal Administration

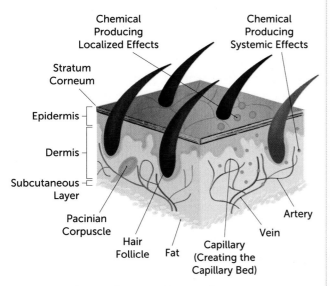

—Figure 3. Diagram of Dermal Administration
The epidermis is the area where essential oils are topically administered. Just beneath the epidermis reside veins and arteries in the dermis layer. Between these two layers, a highly lipophilic membrane, the stratum corneum, exists to act as a major barrier to drug absorption. A localized effect occurs when the essential oil dissolves into the tissue fluids of the epidermis without reaching the dermis layer. Dissolution into the dermis layer tissue fluids, housing the large capillary bed of the circulatory system, results in systemic circulation (Margetts et al., 2007).

outermost layer of the skin, do not have direct access to blood capillaries (see Figure 3). On the other hand, dermal cells located in the dermis of the skin are surrounded by capillaries. A lipophilic membrane called the stratum corneum forms a barrier between the skin surface and the capillary-rich dermis of the skin. This membrane acts as a barrier to systemic absorption. If an essential oil constituent can penetrate the stratum corneum, it will dissolve in the dermis tissue fluid, be absorbed into the capillaries, and circulate in the blood. Once an essential oil constituent enters a capillary, it has entered the circulatory system and can be distributed to other tissues in the body.

If an essential oil constituent cannot cross the stratum corneum, it will dissolve in the epidermis tissue fluids but never reach the dermis capillaries (Turley, 2009). Failure to cross the stratum corneum produces a local therapeutic effect at the site of application.

Epithelial cells also act as a barrier to systemic absorption internally. Epithelial cells line the surfaces of the body and protect the body's in-

ternal environment. The gastrointestinal barrier, the barrier lining the stomach and intestines that separates the external and internal environment of the body, is composed of a layer of epithelial cells (Johnson et al., 2012). The epithelial cell membranes are tightly joined together. Therefore, to enter the internal environment of the body, a chemical must penetrate the epithelial cells. In general, once a chemical breaches the epithelial cells, it has unimpeded access to systemic circulation (Bowen, 2006). Similarly, the lungs and other organ systems possess epithelial barriers. Properties that allow an essential oil constituent to cross the skin's stratum corneum, like small molecular size and ability to cross cell membranes, will also aid the constituent in breaching the epithelial cell barriers in the body's internal organs.

—Distribution

After absorption into the blood, the chemical constituents are distributed throughout the body via the circulatory system. The circulatory system includes the heart, vessels, and blood and is responsible for providing nutrients and oxygen to cells and removing waste from the body's tissues. Since essential oils are lipophilic (insoluble in water) and blood is primarily composed of water, essential oils must associate with and be transported by other water-soluble molecules in order to be distributed by the circulatory system (Bowles, 2003). Such molecules include plasma proteins like albumin (see below for more information).

Once the constituents are circulated in the blood, they are distributed from the blood into other body fluids and tissues (Kohlert et al., 2000).

—Plasma Proteins

Once the chemical constituents of an essential oil enter the circulatory system, some of the chemicals bind to soluble plasma proteins. The most common soluble protein is albumin. If a constituent has a high affinity for albumin, then it readily binds to albumin, displacing other bound chemicals. Bound constituents are therapeutically inactive until displaced and unbound, meaning the therapeutic effect of an essential oil will not occur if the constituent is bound to albumin. A high affinity for albumin causes an extended but low-concentration dose of the chemical. Most molecules found in essential oils have a low affinity for albumin, indicating that the essential oil stays active in the circulatory system at high unbound concentrations until the chemical is rapidly cleared from the body (K. Wang et al., 2000).

Many pharmaceutical drugs have been shown to have a high affinity for albumin. Essential oil constituents that interact with albumin may displace bound drugs (see Figure 4). Therefore, essential oils may affect pharmaceutical drugs through albumin interactions (Tisserand et al., 2014). For more information, see Table 1 on page 427, which lists possible drug interactions with essential oils. Speak to a healthcare professional if any unusual or intense side effects occur while taking drugs and essential oils simultaneously. These side effects may be due to interactions with albumin.

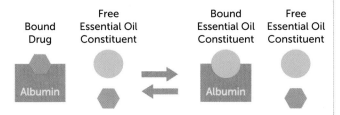

—Figure 4. Albumin
Albumin temporarily inactivates bound constituents. Free essential oil constituents can displace bound drugs and vice versa (adapted from Tisserand et al., 2014).

—Blood-Brain Barrier

Entering the circulatory system does not guarantee that a chemical will diffuse into every organ or tissue in the body. Instead, most chemicals absorb primarily into a target organ or are not able to absorb into specific organs. For example, the brain is guarded by a barrier of tightly placed cells lining its blood vessels called the blood-brain barrier. The blood-brain barrier makes it very difficult for substances to pass from the circulatory system to brain fluid and tissue. The blood-brain barrier protects the brain from foreign substances, harmful pathogens, and waste but allows nutrients (such as water, glucose, and amino acids) to pass. The blood-brain barrier is necessary for protecting the brain but diminishes the therapeutic effect of many drugs. For example, Parkinson's disease results in low neurological concentrations of a neurotransmitter called dopamine. Intake of dopamine, however, will not elevate the low

concentration because the blood-brain barrier blocks the diffusion of dopamine. Instead, doctors must administer a smaller precursor to dopamine called levodopa (which is naturally converted into dopamine once it crosses the blood-brain barrier) to increase dopamine levels in the brain. Levodopa, due to its small molecular size, is allowed to cross the blood-brain barrier. However, large dosages of levodopa must be given because most of the levodopa is broken down before it can reach brain tissue.

Chemical constituents known as sesquiterpenes—commonly found in essential oils such as frankincense and sandalwood—have demonstrated an ability to go beyond the blood-brain barrier (L. Wang et al., 2012; Zhang et al., 2009). In fact, sesquiterpenes are known to interact with neurotransmitter receptors, specifically glycine, dopamine, and serotonin receptors (L. Wang et al., 2012; Okugawa et al., 2000). These properties are very intriguing to researchers, as it means these constituents may have the potential to help with the treatment of neurological disorders such as Alzheimer's disease, Lou Gehrig's disease, Parkinson's disease, and multiple sclerosis.

—Pregnancy

Since the use of pharmaceutical drugs during pregnancy is limited due to potential negative effects, essential oils can be a relief during pregnancy. Essential oils taken during pregnancy can cross the placenta and enter fetal blood (Maickel et al., 1973; Tisserand et al., 2014). For this reason, it is typically recommended that any essential oils used during pregnancy be used in smaller amounts, often heavily diluted in a carrier oil.

—Metabolism

Essential oils are composed of many different compounds. Each compound metabolizes at a different rate. The liver metabolizes essential oils by transforming each compound of an essential oil into its metabolite form. Metabolites are formed as part of the natural process of degrading and eliminating compounds. Most metabolites have different biological actions and properties than their parent chemical constituent (Tisserand et al., 2014). For example, metabolites typically become less lipophilic than their precursors (Tisserand et

EO Science in Depth

al., 2014). Essential oil metabolites can be more, less, or equally as biologically active as their original constituents. Some metabolites, as opposed to the original chemical constituents, may be responsible for producing therapeutic effects attributed to essential oils (Muhlbauer et al., 2003). Therefore, the therapeutic effects of an essential oil may take place before or after metabolism, and the potential effects from a single oil may present at separate times.

Decreased functionality in the liver causes decreased metabolic breakdown, allowing the active compounds to remain in the circulatory system for prolonged amounts of time, thus exposing the body to more active compounds than normal. For this reason, those with liver disease and the elderly with degenerating organs should be given a reduced dose of essential oil (Turley, 2009; Tisserand et al., 2014).

—Elimination

The main orchestrators of elimination are the kidneys and the lungs. Studies using intravenous administration of terpenes (essential oil constituents) suggest that the chemical constituents can be distributed to body tissue within minutes and eliminated from the body within hours (Kohlert et al., 2000). In order to obtain the best therapeutic results, it is recommended that a small amount of oil be used regularly on a daily basis, rather than a large amount used sporadically. Due to the fast elimination of essential oils, it is unlikely that the oils accumulate in fat or other biological tissues (Kohlert et al., 2000). Furthermore, continual use will not result in toxic effects because the essential oils do not accumulate in the body.

Interactions to Consider When Using Essential Oils Orally

—First-pass Metabolism

Only essential oil constituents absorbed through the digestive system are affected by first-pass metabolism. Sublingual, transdermal, inhalation, and rectal routes of administration avoid the first-pass effect because essential oil constituents are directly absorbed into systemic circulation (Brenner et al., 2009).

Essential oils ingested orally travel through the portal vein to the liver before entering systemic blood circulation. Once a chemical enters the liver, it may be processed and altered, resulting in the formation of metabolites. This preliminary formation of metabolites is called the first-pass metabolism and results in the reduction of the concentration of a chemical available during systemic circulation. Most metabolites have different biological properties and activity than their parent chemical constituents (Tisserand et al., 2014). Therefore, oral administration of essential oils may result in a different therapeutic effect than other routes of administration because the metabolites, not the original constituents, may be circulating the blood and interacting with the body.

For example, the chemical constituent coumarin (found in the following essential oils: bergamot, black pepper, clary sage, grapefruit, lavender, lemon, lime, melissa, and peppermint) is greatly reduced by first-pass metabolism, and only 2–6% of coumarin reaches systemic circulation in its intact form (Ritschel et al., 1979). This reduction of chemical constituents occurs because a substantial proportion of essential oil constituents are chemically transformed into metabolites during first-pass metabolism (Tisserand et al., 2014).

—Fatty Meals

It is important to understand that the absorption of an essential oil into the circulatory system via the oral method can vary depending on the presence of food, rate of stomach emptying, stomach acid, and intestinal transit (Brenner et al., 2009). In particular, large or fatty meals can delay the rate of essential oil absorption (Bushra et al., 2011). Furthermore, any food in the GI tract can reduce absorption by 30–80% (Turley, 2009). However, in some cases, such as when you are trying to increase stool bulk or relieve constipation, a localized effect is preferred. In this case, eating a meal in concert with essential oil intake will help to decrease systemic absorption and cause localized therapeutic effects.

Essential Oil Constituents

An essential oil is like a toolbox, and its chemical constituents are like diverse tools with different functions and uses. Not all tools work the same, but all are necessary to build a house. Similarly, not all essential oil constituents have the same function, but they all cooperate in achieving a desired therapeutic effect. As this section shows, the possibilities of systemic or localized effect, metabolism, and plasma protein interaction of essential oil constituents create a variety of opportunities for the constituents to interact with the body. Furthermore, research has shown that different routes of administration can produce different therapeutic effects. Understanding essential oil constituent interactions with the body will help individuals interpret their own therapeutic responses to essential oils.

Table 1: Possible Drug Interactions with Essential Oils			
Drugs	Essential Oils (EO)	Route of EO Administration	Possible Interactions
Warfarin (anticoagulant)	Birch, wintergreen	All (Topical, Aromatic, Internal*)	Inhibits platelet adhesion and intensifies blood thinning
CYP2B6 (liver metabolizing enzyme) substrates	Melissa	Internal	Inhibits CYP2B6, which could enhance drug action
	Lemongrass	All (Topical, Aromatic, Internal)	
Aspirin (antiplatelet) Heparin (anticoagulant) Warfarin (anticoagulant)	Birch, cassia, cinnamon, clove, fennel (sweet), marjoram, oregano, patchouli, thyme, wintergreen	Internal*	Inhibits platelet adhesion and intensifies blood thinning
Monoamine oxidase inhibiting antidepressants (including isocarboxazid, moclobemide, phenelzine, selegiline, tranylcypromine)	Clove	Internal	Clove oil constituents inhibit monoamine oxidase enzymes, which could affect blood pressure and cause tremors or confusion
Pethidine (opioid analgesic)	Clove	Internal	Increase of serotonin, which could cause agitation, delirium, headache, convulsions, and/or hyperthermia
Selective serotonin reuptake inhibitors (including citalopram escitalopram, fluoxetine, paroxetine, sertraline)	Clove	Internal	Increase of brain serotonin levels, which could cause vomiting, nausea, increased body temperature, hallucinations, etc.
Indirect sympathomimetic drugs (including ephedrine, amphetamine)	Clove	Internal	Possible hypertension, increased heart rate, and arrhythmias
Antidiabetic drugs (including glibenclamide, tolbutamide, metformin)	Cassia, cinnamon, dill, fennel (sweet), lemongrass, marjoram, melissa, oregano	Internal	Constituents of these oils influence blood sugar levels and may cause hyperglycemia or hypoglycemia
Dermal medications (including drug patches)	Use caution with all essential oils	Topical	Essential oils can enhance skin absorption of drugs and increase blood plasma levels, resulting in a delivered dose higher than needed
The above information was adapted from *Essential Oil Safety* by Robert Tisserand and Rodney Young (2014, pp. 58–59). Only essential oils included in the Single Essential Oils section of this book are listed in this table. Other essential oils not included in this book may produce similar drug interactions. *It is not recommended to take birch or wintergreen oils internally.*			

EO Science in Depth

Essential Oil Interactions with Drugs

Essential oil interactions with drugs may be additive, synergistic, or antagonistic (Abebe 2002). For this reason, it is important to discuss with your healthcare professional possible interactions between essential oils and prescribed drugs.

One possible side effect of using essential oils with drugs is an increase in drug side effects. This would occur if an essential oil constituent were an inhibitor of the drug's metabolizing enzymes (Tisserand et al., 2014). Thus, the prescribed drug would not be metabolized or excreted, blood-drug levels would rise, and a higher concentration of the prescribed drug would be delivered to target organs.

Table 1 has been provided to give an example of some of the possible interactions that could occur with the administration of both essential oils and prescription drugs. Only essential oils included in the Single Essential Oils section of this book are listed in this table. Other essential oils not included in this book may produce similar drug interactions. Always consult with a medical professional to ensure that other drugs (not listed) will not present unwanted interactions.

Essential Oils As Enhancers

To enhance the absorption of other chemicals, pharmaceutical companies and researchers have harnessed the skin permeation capabilities of certain essential oils. Essential oils like sweet basil, eucalyptus, and peppermint can be applied to the skin in conjunction with pharmaceutical drugs to increase skin absorption of the drugs (Fang et al., 2004; Abdullah et al., 1996). For example, eucalyptus oil enhanced nicotine skin absorption in animal studies (Tisserand et al., 2014). These essential oils act as vehicles to help other drugs penetrate the stratum corneum, enter the circulatory system through dermal capillaries, and produce systemic actions. The blending or layering of these essential oils with other essential oils may also increase skin permeation and systemic effects.

Essential Oil Synergy

The tradition of combining essential oils is increasingly being supported by modern research. Essential oils have displayed interesting synergistic effects both between different oils and within the chemical constituents of a single oil. Synergy within a single oil occurs when one chemical constituent enhances the properties of other components. Furthermore, synergy between oils has led to the development of oil blends and layering techniques with increased therapeutic action.

Major components of essential oils are often praised and highlighted for maintaining the majority of the therapeutic value of an essential oil. However, increasing amounts of evidence indicate that interactions between main and minor constituents also contribute to the inherent activity of essential oils (Hyldgaard et al., 2012). For example, the minor trace components found in essential oils can enhance the antimicrobial activity of an essential oil and may produce a synergistic effect (Hyldgaard et al., 2012; Delaquis et al., 2002). This is supported by reports that crude basil essential oil has greater antimicrobial activity than blends of the oil's major individual components, linalool and methyl chavicol (Lachowicz et al., 1998).

—Antimicrobial Activity

The majority of research on essential oil synergy has been focused on antimicrobial activity. This is due to the significant interest in unlocking the synergistic antimicrobial activity of essential oils for food preservation and treatment of human pathogens. Synergy allows for the use of less essential oil without decreasing the antibacterial action (Gibriel et al., 2013). Currently, thyme essential oil can be used as a food preservative, but the concentration needed to be an efficient antimicrobial leaves a distinctive bitter flavor (Gibriel et al., 2013). Blending two or more essential oils allows for increased antibacterial potential (Gibriel et al., 2013). By combining rosemary and cumin essential oils with thyme, the antibacterial properties are increased and less essential oil is needed to properly preserve food (Gibriel et al., 2013). Using multiple essential oils as a blended food preservative will require a smaller amount of total essential oil product and will lessen the effect on food taste.

Since many interactions are possible when blending essential oils, training and experimentation are needed to achieve a synergistic blend. For example, synergistic, additive, non-interactive, and antagonistic interactions are possible when blending essential oils (see Figure 5) (Gibriel et al., 2013; de Rapper et al., 2013). Lavender essential oil was combined in a 1:1 ratio with 45 different essential oils and tested for antimicrobial properties against Gram-negative, Gram-positive, and yeast strain microorganisms (de Rapper et al., 2013). About half of the combinations produced additive

Possible Antimicrobial Activity
of Two Essential Oils

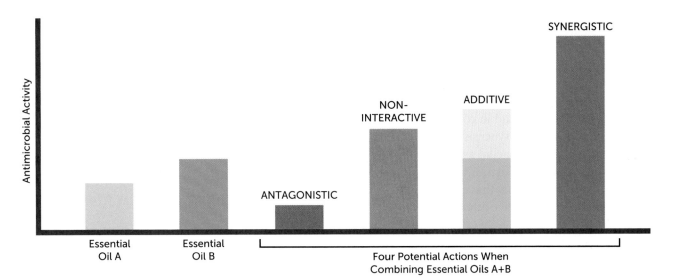

—Figure 5. This graph shows the four interactions that are possible when two essential oils are blended together. When blended, the combination of two essential oils will only display one of the following four interactions.

antimicrobial properties, while over one-fourth were synergistic and less than one fourth were non-interactive (de Rapper et al., 2013). Only one tested essential oil (*Cymbopogon citratus*, a type of lemongrass essential oil) in combination with lavender oil expressed antagonism (de Rapper et al., 2013). The most noteworthy antimicrobial synergistic blends were lavender paired with cypress, cinnamon, or orange essential oil (de Rapper et al., 2013). These findings support the use of essential oil blends in aromatherapeutic practices because over 75% of essential oil combinations investigated showed either synergistic or additive results (de Rapper et al., 2013).

Several hypotheses have attempted to explain why essential oil blends have increased antimicrobial properties when compared to single oils. A prevalent hypothesis is that some minor essential oil constituents cause damage to microbial cell membranes, allowing the antimicrobial essential oil constituents to easily enter the cell and cause direct damage (Delaquis et al., 2002; Langeveld

et al., 2014). Strong evidence suggests that no one mechanism is responsible for the antimicrobial activity of essential oil constituents and that these constituents target several different cellular functions (Tyagi et al., 2012). Furthermore, essential oils have been shown to demonstrate synergy with negative air ions, low pH, sodium chloride, and many antibiotic drugs (Tyagi et al., 2012; Lachowicz et al., 1998; Langeveld et al., 2014). The use of pure and natural essential oils will ensure the presence of all needed chemical constituents and the most efficient antimicrobial activity.

—Permeation Synergy

Synergy has also been studied with aromatic and dermal application of essential oils. Experimenters have studied essential oil organ permeation ability by testing essential oil constituents in isolation and in combination.

For example, a study conducted with mice compared organ concentrations of essential oil constituents when aromatically administered separately

EO Science in Depth

or as a mixed compound (Satou et al., 2013). Interestingly, the amount of α-pinene present in the brain and liver after mixed-compound administration was two times greater than the amount detected after isolated α-pinene administration (Satou et al., 2013). Similarly, experimenters measured the human skin permeation ability of chemical constituents commonly found in essential oils—including limonene, β-citronellol, and eugenol—alone and in concert (Schmitt et al., 2009). Limonene synergistically enhanced the permeation of β-citronellol and eugenol when used in combination (Schmitt et al., 2009). Both these experiments show that essential oil constituents produce cooperative interactions.

By testing the essential oil constituents in isolation and in combination, the researchers were able to verify the synergistic effect essential oil constituents have on one another. As research continues to progress, more synergistic interactions of essential oils will be revealed.

Plants and Essential Oils

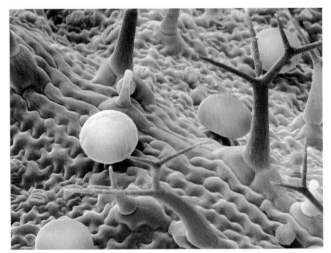
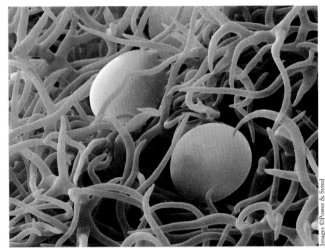

—*Scanning electron microscope images of oil trichomes in lavender (left) and rosemary (right) plants.*

Plants are ubiquitous and vital for life. Scientists have estimated that over 250,000 plant species exist in the world (Farnsworth et al., 1985). The abundant plant kingdom supports animal life by producing oxygen and playing an important role in the earth's water cycle. Humans also rely heavily on plants for food, fuel, medicine, shelter, fabric, paper, and tools.

Essential oils are another important resource originating from plants. Unlike modern drugs, which are developed and used for almost exclusively one condition, a single essential oil has the ability to treat multiple ailments. For example, lavender essential oil has been used to alleviate depression, insomnia, hay fever, wounds, and burns. Discovering why plants make essential oils can explain the expansive therapeutic properties available in a single plant's essential oil.

Plant Cell

The most basic organizational unit of a plant is the plant cell. All cells possess certain abilities, such as storage of hereditary material (DNA), synthesis of proteins and nucleic acids, and a structure separating the cell from its external environment.

Cells can be divided into two main types—prokaryotes and eukaryotes. Prokaryotes include bacteria and archaea organisms and are characterized by cells that lack a cell nucleus and membrane-encased organelles. On the other hand, plants and animals are eukaryotes

and are characterized by cells possessing a nucleus and membrane-bound organelles.

Two main characteristics set plant cells apart from animal cells: a cell wall and plastids. Plastids are organelles that manufacture and store important chemical compounds. An example of a type of plastid is chloroplasts, which possess the photosynthetic capabilities of the plant. Plants are composed of many different types of cells adapted to specific functions. These various cells work together to contribute to the survival of the plant.

Eukaryote Plant Cell

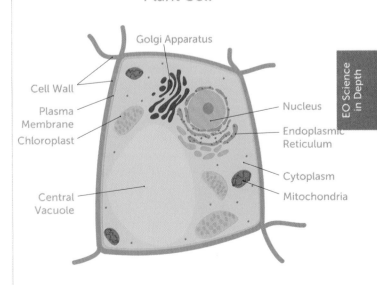

Important Plant Cell Structures and Parts

Nucleus: The nucleus houses the genetic information and regulates the functions of the cell.

Cytoplasm: The cytoplasm is composed of cytosol, a gelatinous fluid that suspends and supports the cell's organelles.

Chloroplast: The chloroplast is a plastid responsible for the photosynthetic activity of the plant. Chlorophyll pigment, located in chloroplast, harvests light energy and converts it into chemical energy (food).

Mitochondria: The mitochondria breaks down sugar molecules into energy.

Endoplasmic Reticulum: The endoplasmic reticulum manufactures, stores, and transports chemical compounds. The rough endoplasmic reticulum participates in the production of proteins, while the smooth endoplasmic reticulum makes fats or lipids.

Vacuole: The vacuole stores food, water, waste, and other chemicals and regulates the turgor pressure of the plant cell.

Cell Wall: The cell wall is the outer layer of the cell responsible for support and protection.

Primary and Secondary Metabolites

Within the cell, chemicals, or metabolites, are synthesized. These chemicals can be divided into two main classifications: primary metabolites and secondary metabolites.

Primary metabolites are chemicals synthesized by all plant cells and are vitally necessary for the cell's growth and survival. For example, nucleic acids store genetic information required for reproduction, and amino acids form proteins that are essential to all cellular functions (Svoboda et al., 2001).

On the other hand, secondary metabolites are plant chemicals that are not considered essential for cell growth and survival (Svoboda et al., 2001). Secondary metabolites are synthesized in specialized plant cells. Although not essential for cellular growth and survival, secondary metabolites are important for the survival of the organism as a whole. For example, the fitness of a plant species is attributed to the plant's secondary metabolites.

Animals, when faced with a predator, have the "fight or flight" ability; however, plants cannot run and hide from predators or dangers. Plants also lack an immune system to combat infections. Secondary metabolites

How Essential Oils Benefit Plants

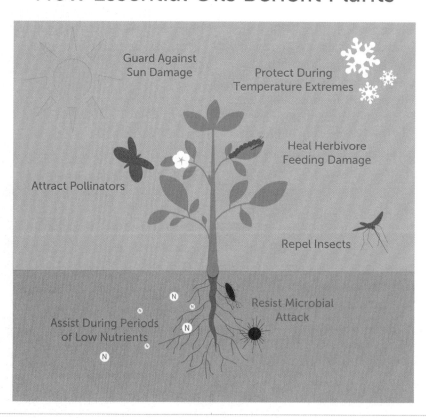

level the playing field between plants and animals by providing chemicals that protect plants from predators and infections. Specifically, secondary metabolites are used by plants for defense, self-healing, allelopathy, messaging, protection, resistance, and attraction of pollinators (Svoboda et al., 2001).

Since secondary metabolites are costly (meaning they require valuable energy for the plant to produce), plants yield secondary metabolites that possess a variety of advantages and functions. By producing a mixture of secondary metabolites that are capable of performing multiple functions for the plant, the cost of making secondary metabolites is justified and even necessary for plant survival. For example, secondary metabolites can be used to mediate ecological interactions with other organisms while also protecting the plant from harmful ultraviolet radiation damage from the sun (Shukla et al., 2009).

Essential oils are complex mixtures of secondary metabolites. Understanding the multiple protective roles that essential oils perform for the plant helps elucidate the ability of a single essential oil to produce multiple benefits for humans. The ability of an essential oil to perform protective functions for a plant parallels the therapeutic functions available when the same essential oil is applied to the human body.

The chart on the previous page lists the possible benefits an essential oil may provide for the plant. Across the plant kingdom, all these benefits have been observed; however, an essential oil rarely provides every benefit.

Essential Oil Metabolite Production, Storage, and Secretion

Researchers have estimated that only 10% of the earth's plants produce essential oils (Djilani et al., 2012). All plants have the tools necessary to produce essential oils; however, the majority of plants only produce traces of essential oils or produce other secondary metabolites for defense (Baser et al., 2009). The Australian government's Rural Industries Research and Development Corporation has

Percent of Essential Oil–Producing Plants on Earth

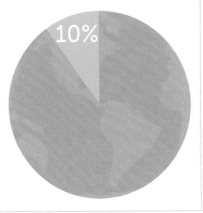

10%

stated that of the estimated 250,000–300,000 plant species, essential oils have been extracted from over 3,000 plants, of which only 200 to 300 are commonly traded on the world market (Australia Rural Industries Research and Development Corporation, n.d.).

—Production

Essential oil constituents are made within specialized plant cells. Essential oil composition varies based on many environmental factors. This variation is due to the function of essential oils. Essential oils are produced based on environmental conditions. Furthermore, essential oils are produced as a reaction to ecological events, such as leaf consumption by an insect (Prins et al., 2010). Therefore, the individual metabolites constituting an essential oil are an effect of the plant's methods for survival.

Given the complexity and sheer number of chemical constituents composing a single essential oil, it is astounding that the majority of essential oil constituents are derived from only three biosynthetic pathways. Specifically, the mevalonate pathway is responsible for the production of sesquiterpenes; the methylerythritol pathway derives mono- and diterpenes; and the shikimic acid pathway constructs phenylpropenes (Baser et al., 2009). These pathways can occur within plastids, the cytoplasm, and organelles throughout the plant cell (Cai et al., 2008). After the essential oil constituents are synthesized, the endoplasmic reticulum (an organelle in the plant cell) takes part in the transport of essential oils to storage structures within or outside of the cell (Fahn et al., 1988).

—Storage

Plants are an important step in the water cycle and, as such, maintain and hold an abundance of water in their cells and structures. Due to the hydrophobic nature of essential oils, storing oil constituents requires specialized structures. Furthermore, many essential oils are auto-toxic to the plant (Shukla et al., 2009; Prins et al., 2010). Therefore, plants must sequester essential oils in external secretory structures called glandular trichomes, in internal secretory structures, or within specialized cells. The energy cost of storing essential oils is high because complex multicellular structures are often required (Gershenzon, 1994).

EO Science in Depth

Essential oil can be found within many different plant tissues; however, they are most often found in flowers and leaves (Prins et al., 2010). Due to the extensive energy cost of making and storing essential oil, the essential oil content of a plant "rarely exceeds 1%, but in some cases, for example clove and nutmeg, it reaches more than 10%" (Djilani et al., 2012).

—Secretion

Secreting essential oils allows the oil to interact with environmental threats or send cues to other organisms. Five main anatomical structures are utilized by the plant kingdom to secrete essential oils. Only one of these five structures is used within a plant species. Furthermore, entire plant botanical families often use the same secretory structure. For example, citrus fruits of the Rutaceae family secrete essential oils through secretory cavities (Svoboda et al., 2001). On the other hand, the Labiatae family secrete essential oils through glandular trichomes (Svoboda et al., 2001).

Plant tissues capable of secreting lipophilic substances, like essential oils, can be present on the plant surface or inside the plant body (Fahn et al., 1988). Secretion can occur constantly, as in the case of epidermal cells, or only in response to physical damage, as in the case of secretory cavities. Below, more detail is provided on the five anatomical secretory structures of essential oils.

—Five Anatomical Secretory Structures of Essential Oils

—Secretory Cells

The most basic secretory anatomical structure is the secretory cell. Secretory cells, or essential oil cells, can be found within a variety of different plant tissues, including seeds, rhizomes,

Secretory Cells

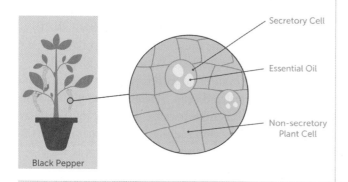

bark, and leaves (Svoboda et al., 2001). Secretory cells contain many of the same structures as the non-secretory cell illustrated at the beginning of this section; however, secretory cells are often spherical, larger than non-secretory cells, contain essential oils, and may have a thick cuticle lining (Chemical Engineering Trends, 2007; Svoboda et al., 2001). In the case of ginger, the essential oil resides as a globule within the cell membrane of the secretory cell (Svoboda et al., 2001).

Common essential oils stored in secretory cells: black pepper, cardamom, cassia, cinnamon, ginger, lemongrass, patchouli, and vetiver.

—Glandular Trichomes

Glandular trichomes are secretory anatomical structures externally present on plants. These modified epidermal hairs can cover plant flowers, leaves, and stems (Svoboda et al., 2001). Essential oils stored in glandular trichomes are usually released when the plant's outer surface is touched or brushed lightly; however, more volatile essential oil fractions may pass through the trichome cuticle (Fahn et al., 1988). Glandular trichomes are composed of secretory cells that produce the essential oil, a storage cavity to house the secreted essential oil, and a stalk cell that connects the structure to the plant.

Glandular Trichomes

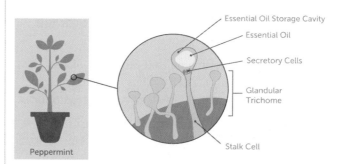

Common essential oils stored in glandular trichomes: basil, clary sage, geranium, lavender, marjoram, melissa, oregano, peppermint, rosemary, spearmint, and thyme.

—Epidermal Cells

Epidermal cells primarily function as a protective layer for the plant. Some specialized epidermal cells are also capable of producing essential oils. Epidermal cells do not store

Epidermal Cells

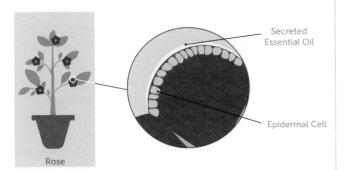

Rose

essential oils but instead continually secrete essential oils through the cell's cytoplasm, cell wall, and cuticle (Svoboda et al., 2001). Epidermal cells that secrete essential oils are mainly located in flowers. Epidermal cells constantly release essential oils and are what give rose and jasmine flowers their continual fragrance. This is also why essential oil yield from these plants is so low, since no essential oils are actually stored, just secreted.

Common essential oils secreted by epidermal cells: jasmine and rose.

–Secretory Cavities

Secretory cavities are spherical structures internally contained within a plant's fruit, leaves, flower buds, or bark (Svoboda et al., 2001). The structure is created when a cell disintegrates, leaving a cavity in the plant tissue, or it is formed by intercellular spaces between cells (Svoboda et al., 2001). The essential oil constituents contained in secretory cavities are produced by a layer of secretory cells lining the cavity. Essential oil fragrance is not released from secretory cavities until the plant tissue is damaged.

Secretory Cavities

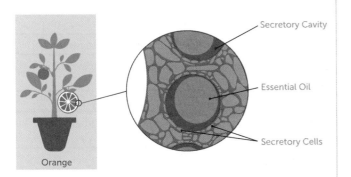

Orange

Common essential oils stored in secretory cavities: bergamot, clove, eucalyptus, frankincense, grapefruit, lemon, lime, melaleuca, myrrh, orange, and tangerine.

–Secretory Ducts

Secretory ducts can form a circuit of channels extending from the roots to the stem, leaves, and flowers (Svoboda et al., 2001). Secretory ducts are created by the joining of multiple secretory cavities throughout the plant. Like secretory cavities, the essential oil stored in secretory ducts is produced by secretory cells lining the duct.

Secretory Duct

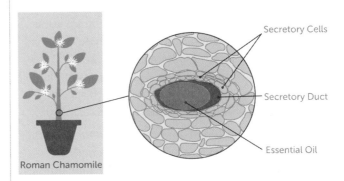

Roman Chamomile

Common essential oils stored in secretory ducts: cedarwood, cilantro, coriander, cypress, dill, fennel, helichrysum, juniper berry, Roman chamomile, and white fir.

Plants and Medicine

The use of plants for therapeutic purposes has been practiced by every culture and is the most traditional medicine. In fact, today, more than 80% of the world population uses herbal medicine to treat their daily medical needs (Gbenou et al., 2013).

Percent of World Population
Using Herbal Medicine

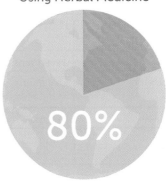

80%

EO Science in Depth

435

—Plant-Derived Medicines

Four thousand years ago, the Sumerians documented on clay tablets the use of salicylic acid, a natural substance found in the bark of the willow tree, as a painkiller (Goldberg, 2009). Today, a synthetic derivative of salicylic acid, aspirin, is still used for its analgesic properties. Furthermore, about one-fourth of prescribed drugs contain one or more active principles derived from plants (Farnsworth et al., 1985; Rates et al., 2001). Plant-based medicine is as important today as it was thousands of years ago, whether as a traditional medicine or in modern medicines. Table 2 lists common drugs descending from plants.

—Medicinal Plants

Plants have succeeded as medicines for thousands of years because of their ability to produce abundantly diverse chemicals. Many of these chemical compounds are still unknown to researchers. Remarkably, of the hundreds of thousands of plant species, it is estimated that only 5,000 species have been studied for medical use (Rates, 2001).

The coadaptation of animals and plants is another reason plants possess such strong therapeutic properties. In order to survive, plants and animals have had to adapt to one another. For example, to avoid being eaten by herbivores, plants developed chemicals, such as poisons, to deter herbivores from eating them (Pinker, 2010). In turn, herbivores developed livers to detoxify plant poisons (Pinker, 2010). This coadaptation is emphasized by the fact that many plant chemicals, including essential oils, "trigger very specific physiological responses in other organisms and, in many cases, bind to receptors with a remarkable complementarity" (Seigler, 1998). The compatibility between plant chemicals and the human body correlates with the observed therapeutic properties of essential oils.

Currently, interest in traditional plant-based medicine is expanding, and research focusing on plant chemicals is progressing at an accelerated rate. As people look to avoid the side effects of modern medicine, use of traditional plant-based medicine is increasing worldwide. Furthermore, epidemiological evidence has revealed that dietary nutrients from plants play an important role in human health and the treatment of chronic diseases (Dey et al., 2012). The health benefits offered by plants are clear. The power of medicinal plants is available in essential oils, as well as other important plant chemicals.

Common Drugs Originating from Plants		
Plant-Based Drug	**Medicinal Use**	**Plant Connection**
Aspirin	Painkiller, anti-inflammatory, and fever reducer	Aspirin is a synthetic derivative of the natural compound salicylic acid. Salicylic acid can be found in the bark of the willow tree and other plants (including cucumbers and potatoes).
Atropine	Anesthetic and anticholinergic agent (used for the treatment of extremely low heart rate [bradycardia])	Atropine is a secondary metabolite found in plants of the family Solanaceae, including nightshade, Jimson weed, and mandrake.
Digoxin	Various heart conditions (e.g. heart failure and irregular heartbeat)	Digoxin contains chemicals taken from foxglove plants.
Ephedrine	Asthma, hay fever, and colds	Ephedrine is a chemical found in plants in the genus *Ephedra*.
Morphine	Relieves intense pain	Morphine can be found in the unripe seedpods of opium poppy plants.
Paclitaxel	Treatment of solid tumor cancers	Paclitaxel is isolated from the bark of the pacific yew.
Pilocarpine	Dry mouth and glaucoma	Pilocarpine is a chemical harvested from the leaves of tropical American shrubs from the genus Pilocarpus.
Quinine	Malaria	Quinine is found naturally in cinchona tree bark.
Reserpine	Antipsychotic	Reserpine is isolated from the dried root of Indian snakeroot.

Ensuring Essential Oil Purity and Quality

Essential oils are used in the perfume, flavoring, and aromatherapy industries. The therapeutic use of essential oils, however, requires the highest quality and purity of essential oils. To ensure high standards, therapeutic-grade essential oils are tested throughout production. Tests are used to validate that an essential oil contains certain chemical constituents within an acceptable percentage range. Tests are also used to ensure that no foreign substances, such as pesticides or synthetic chemicals, are in an essential oil.

—Chemical Constituent Percentage Range

The characteristic aroma of an essential oil is the product of many different chemicals. Altering the amount of one chemical constituent in an essential oil can change the aroma and quality of an essential oil. Some chemical constituents comprise less than 1% of a total essential oil but have a significant impact on the smell and therapeutic property of the oil (Tisserand et al., 2014). Since plants—not chemists—produce essential oils, their very nature results in inconsistencies and fluctuations in chemical constituent content. Some aspects of essential oil production that influence the chemical constituent content include the following: growth environment of the plant, part of the plant distilled, age of the plant, time of harvest, distillation process, and method of storing (Tisserand et al., 2014).

To establish a standard of quality that considers the many factors affecting chemical constituent content, experts have assigned percentage ranges for each chemical constituent in an essential oil. High quality oil contains all the necessary chemical constituents within the established ranges. For example, terpinen-4-ol found in melaleuca oil is normally between 30% and 55% (Tisserand et al., 2014). Therefore, identifying the quality of an essential oil based on its chemical profile requires modern chemical analysis.

—Adulteration

Essential oil purity is a measurement of adulteration. The purity of an essential oil will affect the quality of the essential oil. A pure essential oil must be from one plant species and distillation process. Some manufacturers adulterate essential oils without consumer knowledge by blending different essential oils or different qualities, adding chemical constituents or synthetics, and diluting an essential oil. Third-party testing can evaluate the content of an essential oil, ensuring that no foreign substances have been added.

Testing

A variety of tests are used to ensure that an essential oil meets the standards of the supplier. Testing can occur during plant selection, harvesting, distillation, packaging, and storage.

—Sensory Evaluation

The simplest form of testing is performed by expert growers and distillers and involves no machinery. Instead, experts have trained their senses, particularly their olfactory senses, to detect inconsistencies in oil aroma, texture, and color. This method of testing, though useful as a preliminary assessment, cannot detect non-odorous adulterants; so physical or chemical analysis is also utilized to ensure the quality and purity of an essential oil (Tisserand, et al., 2014).

Experts performing olfactory evaluation have spent years training their noses to detect differences between pure essential oils. However, even novice essential oil users can learn to discern between pure essential oil and a synthetic fragrance. The nose can be improved through training just as any other talent. For example, try smelling pure lavender essential oil and comparing it to a known synthetic lavender product like laundry detergent or hand soap. Between inhaling each aroma, sniff your shirt in order to neutralize your senses. After comparing the fragrances, you should be able to notice a difference between the two aromas.

—Physical Analysis

Relatively inexpensive methods can be used to assess the physical characteristics of essential oils. Common physical properties used to test essential oils include specific gravity, refractive index, and optical rotation. These physical characteristics can assist in detecting non-odorous adulterants and assessing quality. Since essential oils are natural compounds produced by plants, their physical

EO Science in Depth

characteristics can vary. For example, the specific gravity of peppermint oil increases from the lower to upper leaves of the plant (Board, 2003). Furthermore, physiochemical properties of essential oils can change in the course of the plant's harvest. For example, the optical rotation of orange essential oil decreases as the fruit matures (Board, 2003). Therefore, a range of acceptable values is used to evaluate the quality of an essential oil.

Specific Gravity involves comparing the density of an essential oil to the density of water at a specific temperature. If the percentage of chemical constituents is wrong due to impurity, the density will be affected. The specific gravity of essential oil usually ranges between 0.78–0.90 g/ml (Bowles, 2003). Compared to water's specific gravity of 1.0 g/ml, essential oils are usually less dense than water and would float on top of water. However, clove bud, wintergreen, and cinnamon essential oils can be denser than water (Bowles, 2003). Along with revealing the purity of an essential oil, the specific gravity can also reveal information about the production process of an essential oil. For example, the specific gravity of clary sage oil increases during the drying process before distillation (Board, 2003).

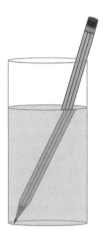

Figure 6: The different refractive indices of water and air are apparent when a pencil is placed halfway into water. The pencil looks bent because light travels slower in water than in air.

Refractive Index is a measure of the speed of light through a medium. Figure 6 shows a pencil in a container of water. Light travels slower in water than in air, causing the light to bend; so when you place a pencil in a cup of water, the pencil looks broken or bent. Similarly, light propagates differently in essential oils than it does in water or air. An instrument called a refractometer can mea-

sure the refractive index of an essential oil. The measured refractive index can then be compared to known refractive indices to identify the purity of an essential oil. The refractive index is constant for each compound, so it can easily be affected by small impurities or damage. For example, an increased refractive index in basil oil can indicate the oil has oxidized due to aging or exposure to light (Board, 2003). The increased refractive index can also indicate that the basil oil has been adulterated with the addition of cheaper reunion basil essential oil (Board, 2003).

Optical Rotation is a measurement of the rotation of polarized light as it passes through a chiral material. A chiral substance is an object with a non-superimposable mirror image. For example, hands are chiral. Hands have many similarities but have two important differences. First, hands

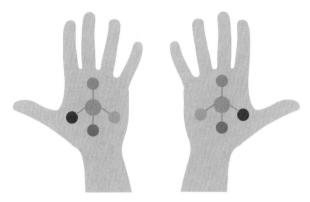

Enantiomers are defined as a chiral molecule and its mirror image. Chiral molecules are non-superimposable mirror images and can be compared to hands.

are mirror images of each other. Second, hands are not superimposable, meaning no matter how two hands are oriented they will never match up perfectly. Conversely, mittens and socks are not chiral. Mittens can fit on either hand comfortably because mittens are mirror images of each other and are superimposable.

A chiral molecule and its mirror image are collectively called enantiomers. In living organisms, only one chiral molecule of the enantiomer pair exists—a concept that has fascinated scientists since the discovery of chirality (Blackmond, 2010). However, chemical synthesis of molecules in a laboratory results in the production of an equal mixture of both enantiomers.

Enantiomers share many of the same physical characteristics, including boiling point, melting

Optical Rotation of Enantiomers Individually and Combined

Sample Tested	Polarimeter Experiment Setup	Results
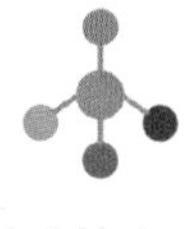 Chiral Molecule	Light Source → Light → Polarizer → Polarized Light → Sample Tube Containing Chiral Molecule	Rotated Polarized Light 30 Degrees Clockwise
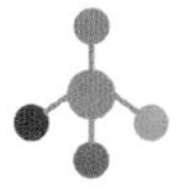 Mirror Image of Chiral Molecule	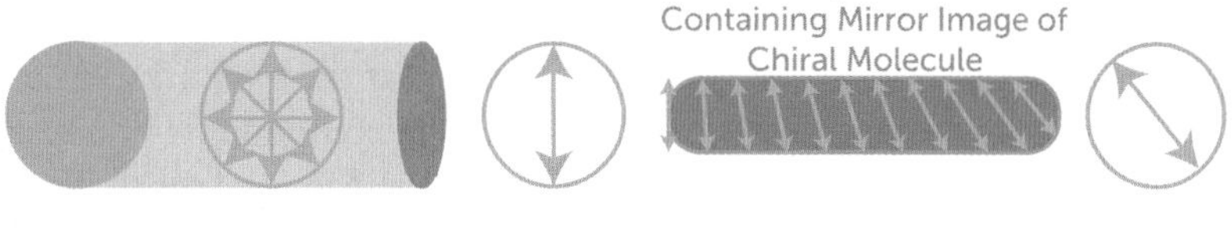 Sample Tube Containing Mirror Image of Chiral Molecule	Rotated Polarized Light 30 Degrees Counterclockwise
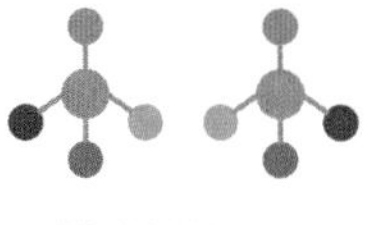 50:50 Mixture of Chiral Molecule + Mirror Image	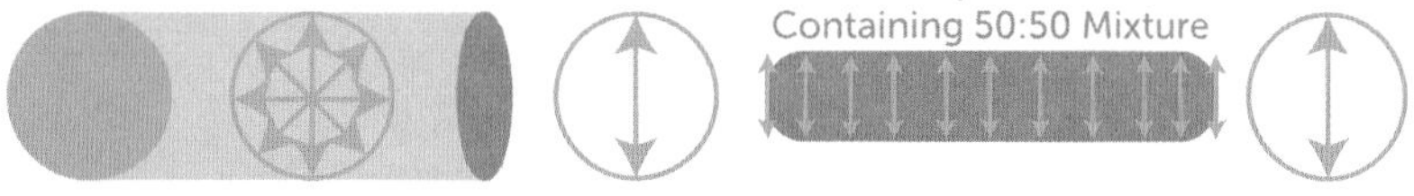 Sample Tube Containing 50:50 Mixture	Light Not Rotated

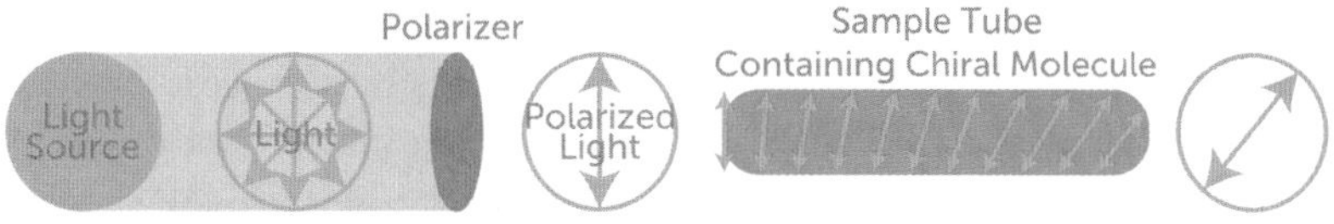

Figure 7: The optical rotation of a chiral molecule can help chemists discriminate between enantiomer molecules. Synthetic production of a chiral molecule results in an equal mixture of both enantiomers. This mixture does not rotate light because the individual rotation produced by each molecule is equal but opposite, and thus they cancel each other out.

point, specific gravity, and refractive index. On the other hand, enantiomers do differ physically when interacting with polarized light. Therefore, one of the only ways to discriminate between enantiomers is by measuring their optical rotation of polarized light. The optical rotation of enantiomers will be exactly the same except for the direction in which the molecule rotates the polarized light. For example, Figure 7 shows the optical rotation of a chiral molecule to be 30 degrees clockwise but the optical rotation of its mirror image to be 30 degrees counterclockwise.

Optical rotation can be measured by a polarimeter. A polarimeter can help identify which enantiomer is present in an essential oil, based on the direction of rotation (clockwise or counterclockwise) of an isolated sample of the essential oil's chemical constituent. Additionally, a polarimeter can reveal adulterations. For example, since synthetic molecules result in the production of an equal mixture of both enantiomers, the optical rotation of a synthetic substance would differ from a natural, pure substance. As you can see in Figure 7, the optical rotation of an equal mixture of both

enantiomers results in no light rotation. This is because both molecules rotate the light in an equal but opposite way, and thus cancel out any optical rotation. Therefore, a lack of optical rotation can indicate that the sample of molecule was created synthetically.

Up until now, the discussion has focused on the optical rotation of a single molecule or pair of enantiomers. However, scientists can also discern the quality of an essential oil by measuring the optical rotation of the entire oil, without separating the oil into its chemical constituents. For example, lime oil adulterated with terpenes can be detected by an increase in optical rotation from normal values (Board, 2003). Furthermore, the optical rotation of an oil can also be affected by unripe fruit or high wax content, both signs of poor quality oils (Board, 2003).

—Modern Chemical Analysis

In 1833, the French chemist M. J. Dumas published the first analysis of an essential oil's chemical constituents (Baser et al., 2009). Since Dumas, many chemists have also focused their efforts on identifying the countless chemicals found in

EO Science in Depth

essential oils. In the late 19th century, chemical reactions and optical rotation measurements were the only methods available for identifying chemical constituents in essential oils (Baser et al., 2009). However, with the recent introduction of modern chemical analysis methods, including Gas Chromatography Mass Spectrometry (GCMS) and Fourier Transform Infrared Spectroscopy (FTIS), the structural identification and analysis of chemical constituents is now possible. Modern chemical analysis goes beyond physical analysis by identifying the structure and quantity of chemical constituents in an essential oil. The use of modern chemical analysis provides the clearest information on the quality and purity of an essential oil. To ensure quality, essential oils should only be obtained from suppliers who require modern chemical testing on all their oils.

Gas Chromatography Mass Spectrometry (GCMS) is the most common technique used for analyzing essential oils (Baser et al., 2009). GCMS involves two main procedures. First, an essential oil is separated into its individual constituents by a process called gas chromatography. Next, an instrument called a mass spectrometer is used to identify the mass and quantity of the individual constituents.

The basic process of gas chromatography begins by injecting a sample substance into a heated column that then vaporizes the substance (see Figure 8). The components of a substance are separated based on their volatility, with the most volatile components reaching the end of the column first. Since essential oils are highly volatile substances, this technique is ideal for analyzing essential oils.

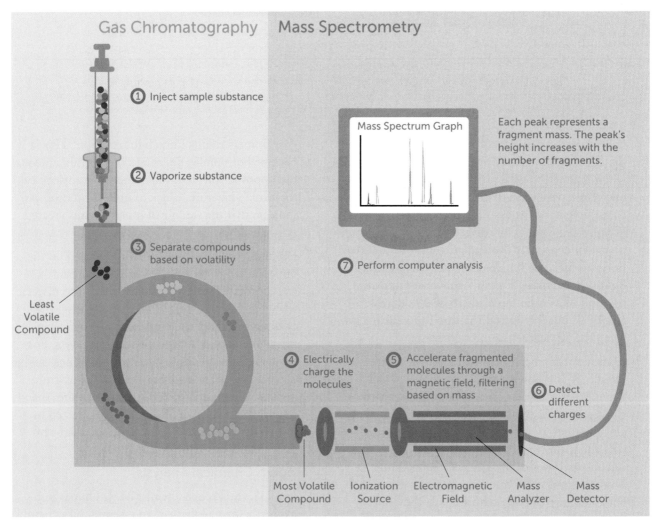

Figure 8: This diagram displays an overview of the Gas Chromatography Mass Spectrometry process. First, the gas chromatography process (highlighted in blue) separates the chemical constituents of an essential oil. Second, the mass spectrometry (highlighted in yellow) calculates the mass of the original whole substance, the mass of the fragments, and the quantity of each fragment.

To clarify, gas chromatography can be compared to an uphill race. All the contestants begin together at the start line. As the race begins, the competitive athletes quickly separate from the crowd as the slower contenders struggle to move up the inclined track. The hill creates a gradient of runners based on their training and ability. Similarly, gas chromatography separates chemicals based on their physical and chemical characteristics.

Once an essential oil is separated by gas chromatography, it is then analyzed by mass spectrometry. A molecule that enters the mass spectrometer is first blasted with electrons. This causes the molecule to separate into positively charged fragments called ions. The ions then travel through an electromagnetic field that filters the ions based on mass. At the end of the filter, a mass detector counts the number of ions associated with each mass. Lastly, a computer generates a mass spectrum graph that shows the number of fragments that fall into each mass group.

To simplify mass spectrometry, the process can be thought of as a money coin counter. For example, a handful of various coins can be inserted into the coin counter machine and the machine is able to sort the coins based on their size. Furthermore, the machine is able to calculate the quantity of each coin and the grand total value of all the coins

together. Similarly, the mass spectrometer is able to sort molecule fragments by their mass to generate a graph that reveals the mass of the original whole substance, the mass of the fragments, and the quantity of each fragment.

GCMS is an extremely useful method for testing essential oils because the chemical constituents can be identified, and the percentage of each constituent can be calculated. Chemical constituent percentages fluctuate due to the inherent variability of plant growth and the distillation processes. Identifying the chemical constituent percentages of an essential oil can elucidate the quality of an essential oil. Even pure essential oils will be rejected for therapeutic use if the chemical constituent percentages measured during GCMS are found to be abnormal.

Furthermore, GCMS can also reveal adulterants that have been added to an essential oil. Specifically, GCMS is useful for detecting nonvolatile adulterants like heavy metals. However, no one test is completely reliable; so essential oils are often additionally tested using other modern methods.

Fourier Transform Infrared Spectroscopy (FTIS) is another common technique used to analyze essential oils. Specifically, FTIS is used to identify the characteristics of bonds between different atoms.

Electromagnetic Spectrum

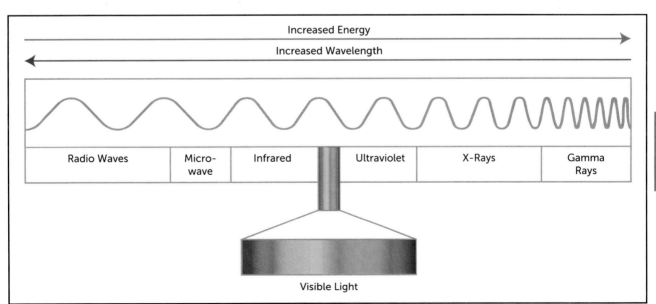

Figure 9: Infrared radiation is a type of electromagnetic radiation with a wavelength greater than red visible light. Infrared radiation is emitted by heated objects.

Therefore, FTIS, like GCMS, can be used for the identification of chemical constituents. Since FTIS uses a different technology but obtains the same information as GCMS, it is often used to substantiate results obtained from GCMS. Unlike GCMS, FTIS has the ability to discriminate between different chiral molecules (Baser et al., 2009).

FTIS consists of a process called infrared spectroscopy in which infrared radiation (see Figures 9 and 10) is passed through a sample substance. Some of the infrared radiation is absorbed by the sample, and some is allowed to pass through the sample. A detector measures the pattern of absorption created by the sample. The pattern of absorption is unique, like a fingerprint, for each sample.

After the detector obtains a pattern of absorption, a computer performs a mathematical calculation called a Fourier transform. The Fourier transform converts the raw data into a readable spectrum. The absorption spectrum of the sample can determine the quality or consistency of a sample and determine the amount of components in a mixture (Thermo Nicolet Corporation, 2001).

Since the absorption peaks produced by infrared spectroscopy are unique for each compound, the results can be used to identify substances. Furthermore, the size of each peak is a direct indication of the amount of material present in the sample.

Understanding these methods of testing essential oils will help you to make educated essential oil purchases. Although there are many more testing methods, the methods presented in this section are the most widely used. To ensure the quality and purity of an essential oil, multiple tests should be used. You can contact an essential oil provider to obtain information on the testing performed on their essential oils.

Fourier Transform Infrared Spectroscopy

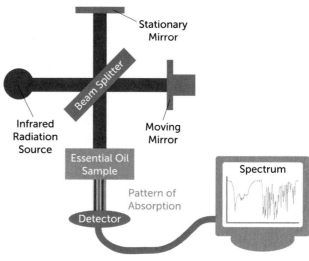

Figure 10: This simplified diagram illustrates the process of FTIS. First, an infrared beam is split and reflected off two mirrors. The beam reunites and passes through a sample substance. The absorption pattern created by the substance is recorded by a detector and then processed by a computer. Fourier transform calculations performed by the computer produce a spectrum that can be used to identify the substance.

Essential Oil Constituents

In general, pure essential oil constituents can be subdivided into two distinct groups: the hydrocarbons, which are made up almost exclusively of terpenes (monoterpenes, sesquiterpenes, and diterpenes), and the oxygenated compounds, which are mainly esters, aldehydes, ketones, alcohols, phenols, and oxides.

Terpenes

Terpenes are the largest family of natural products and are found throughout nature. High concentrations of terpenes are found directly after flowering (Paduch et al., 2007). The basic molecular structure of a terpene is an isoprene unit (which has a C_5H_8 molecular formula):

Isoprene Unit (C_5H_8)

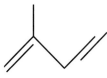

Figures such as the one shown at left represent the bonds between carbon (C) atoms in a molecule. Single lines represent a single bond, while double lines represent a double bond. Each intersecting point and the end of each line represents a carbon molecule along with any hydrogen molecules it is bonded to. Since each carbon molecule can have up to four bonds with other atoms, the number of hydrogen atoms can be determined by subtracting the number of bonds (lines) coming to each carbon atom from four. Thus the shorthand figure at top represents the same molecule shown below it.

Isoprene Unit (C_5H_8)

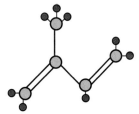

⬤ = carbon
● = hydrogen

Classes of terpenes are named according to how many isoprene units are present.

- Monoterpenes (C10)   = two isoprene units
- Sesquiterpenes (C15) = three isoprene units
- Triterpenes (C30)   = six isoprene units
- Tetraterpenes (C40) = eight isoprene units

Terpenes may also have oxygen-containing functional groups. Terpenes with these oxygen-containing functional groups are referred to as terpenoids (McGarvey et al., 1995).

—Monoterpenes

Monoterpenes occur in practically all essential oils and have many different activities. Most tend to inhibit the accumulation of toxins and help discharge existing toxins from the liver and kidneys. Some are antiseptic, antibacterial, stimulating, analgesic (weak), and expectorant; while other specific terpenes have antifungal, antiviral, antihistaminic, antirheumatic, antitumor (antiblastic, anticarcinogenic), hypotensive, insecticidal, purgative, and pheromonal properties. Monoterpenes, in general, have a stimulating effect and can be very soothing to irritated tissues as well. Most citrus oils (not bergamot) and conifer oils contain a high proportion of monoterpenes.

Found as a Significant Constituent in ALL Essential Oils Except: Basil, birch, cassia, cinnamon, clary sage, clove, geranium, sandalwood, vetiver, wintergreen, and ylang ylang.

Examples of Monoterpenes:

– Pinenes (α- & β-)

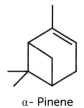
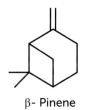

α- Pinene   β- Pinene

α- and β- pinene are isomers (meaning they have the same chemical formula but differing structures). They get their name because they are major constituents in pine resin or pine oil. They give off a resiny, piney smell. Pinenes have strong antiseptic, antibacterial, antifungal, and expectorant properties.

Bone Resorption Inhibition: α- and β-pinene (found in pine oil) were found in animal studies to inhibit bone resorption. Bone resorption is the process by which osteoclasts—macrophage cells that reside in the bones—break down bone and release the minerals, which can lead to the loss of bone, such as in osteoporosis. Further studies have indicated that while α- and β-pinene may not directly influence osteoclast activity and bone resorption rates, a metabolite (a product created by the body from the original molecule when taken internally) of the pinenes, cis-verbenol, did directly inhibit bone

EO Science in Depth

resorption and the formation of osteoclasts (Eriksson et al., 1996; Muhlbauer et al., 2003).

Mosquito Larvicide: α-pinenes found in *Alpinia speciosa* and *Rosmarinus officinalis* (ginger and rosemary) demonstrated effective larvicidal activity against the mosquito *Aedes aegypti L.* The *A. aegypti* is a carrier of the dengue virus that causes dengue fever in tropical areas of the world (Freitas et al., 2010).

Antibacterial: It has been observed that the larvae of the Douglas fir tussock moth have digestive systems that are relatively clear of bacterial flora. These larvae feed on terpenes found in the bark of Douglas fir trees, of which α-pinene is a major constituent. α-pinene inhibits the growth of *Bacillus* species (gram-positive bacteria). The concentration needed for maximum inhibition is well below the concentrations of α-pinene found in Douglas fir pine trees. Bacterial inhibition occurs because α-pinene disrupts the cytoplasmic membranes of the bacterial species. α-pinene seems to perform more effectively against gram-positive bacteria than gram-negative bacteria due to the extra outer membrane found in the cell walls of gram-negative bacteria (Andrews et al., 1980; Uribe et al., 1985).

Anti-inflammatory: NF_KB is an important transcription factor in the body that regulates proinflammatory responses (signals proteins, specifically cytokines, to cause inflammation). When NF_KB is activated, it goes to the nucleus of the cells, binds to DNA, and activates transcription needed to produce cytokines, chemokines, and cell adhesion molecules. These molecules all help in producing inflammation in the body.

α-pinene has been shown to inhibit/block NF_KB from going to the nucleus. LPS (lipopolysaccharide, an endotoxin produced by gram-negative bacteria that causes inflammation in the body) was introduced to the cell culture of THP-1 cells to induce the activation of NF_KB. However, when α-pinene was present, activation was markedly reduced.

α-pinene inhibits NF_KB by blocking the degradation of $I_KB\alpha$. $I_KB\alpha$ is a protein that binds to NF_KB to prevent it from constantly transcribing proinflammatory genes. If LPS, a virus, or some stimulant of the immune system is recognized, $I_KB\alpha$ will degrade and release/activate NF_KB. NF_KB will then transcribe genes to make proteins that cause inflammation at the site of "invasion," such as a cut, scrape, or burn.

Even in the presence of an immune system stimulant (LPS), α-pinene blocks $I_KB\alpha$. During experimentation, it was also noted that the THP-1 cells received no cytotoxicity from the addition of α-pinene (Zhou et al., 2004; Weaver, 2008).

–Camphene

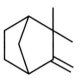

Camphene

Camphene is found in many oils, such as cypress, citronella, neroli, ginger, and others. It is an insect repellent. According to the *Phytochemical Dictionary*, it is "used to reduce cholesterol saturation index in the treatment of gallstones."

– β-Myrcene

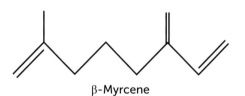

β-Myrcene

β-Myrcene is found in oils such as lemongrass, verbena, and bay. It has cancer-preventative properties.

Antioxidant: Studies have elucidated that β-myrcene can reverse and prevent the damaging effects of TCDD (2,3,7,8-Tetrachloro-p-dibenzodioxin) to the liver of rats by increasing GSH (glutathione), SOD (superoxide dismutase), and catalase activation (Ciftci et al., 2011; Gaetani et al., 1996).

– d-Limonene

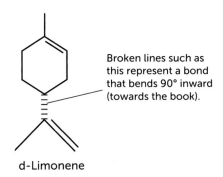

Broken lines such as this represent a bond that bends 90° inward (towards the book).

d-Limonene

d-Limonene is found in 90% of the citrus peel oils and in caraway seeds and dill. It is anti-cancer, antibacterial, antifungal, antiseptic (5x phenol), and highly antiviral.

Cancer Cell Inhibition: d-limonene has been found to be cancer-preventive in vitro and in human mammary cells. It acts as a selective isoprenylation inhibitor. d-Limonene specifically inhibits small g-proteins known as Ras p21 (or p21ras). p21ras is a critical protein for oncogenesis (formation of cancer cells) in the body. In order for oncogenesis to commence, the p21ras protein must be transferred within the cell to the plasma membrane. Once p21ras is able to interact with the plasma membrane of the cell, it causes abnormal cell growth, intracellular localization, and transformations.

d-limonene inhibits the transferral of p21ras within the cell, blocking its access to the plasma membrane.

Researchers also found that d-limonene is selectively inhibitive. It targets only the transferral of Ras proteins and leaves all other ordinary cell functions alone. This makes d-Limonene a potentially effective chemopreventive agent because it targets areas of high oncogenic susceptibility and has no harmful side effects against critical cell components (low toxicity) (Kato et al., 1992; Crowell et al., 1991; and Morse et al., 1993).

Researchers have also observed that a continuous dose of limonene in the diets of rats with chemical-induced cancer helps inhibit the formation of secondary tumors and reduces the size of primary tumors. However, when limonene was removed from the rats' daily diet, tumors were more likely to return. This gives evidence that limonene works as a cytostatic agent (an agent that stops the tumor cells from creating new tumor cells) rather than a cytotoxic agent (an agent that kills the tumor cells). These researchers also observed that little toxicity occurred to the rats from the high doses of d-limonene (Haag et al., 1992).

Cholesterol Suppression: Researchers have discovered that when d-limonene is included in the daily diet of rats treated with a chemical (7,12-dimetylbenzantracene) that induced high cholesterol, there was a 45% decrease in hepatic HMG-CoA reductase activity. HMG-CoA reductase is an enzyme that converts HMG-CoA (93-hydroxy-3-methylglutaryl coenzyme A) to mevalonic acid, which acts as a precursor to the production of cholesterol. Inhibiting HMG-CoA reductase halts this process and, in effect, lowers cholesterol rates (Sorentino et al., 2005; Qureshi et al., 1988).

—Sesquiterpenes

Sesquiterpenes are found in great abundance in essential oils. They are antibacterial, strongly anti-inflammatory, slightly antiseptic and hypotensive, and sedative. Some have analgesic properties, while others are highly antispasmodic. They are soothing to irritated skin and tissue and are calming. They also work as liver and gland stimulants. Research from the universities of Berlin and Vienna shows that sesquiterpenes increase oxygenation around the pineal and pituitary glands. Further research has shown that sesquiterpenes have the ability to surpass the blood-brain barrier and enter the brain tissue. They are larger molecules than monoterpenes and have a strong aroma.

Found as a Major Constituent In: Ginger, myrrh, sandalwood, vetiver, and ylang ylang.

Found as a Minor Constituent In: Bergamot, cinnamon, clary sage, clove, cypress, white fir, frankincense, geranium, helichrysum, lavender, lemongrass, melaleuca, and peppermint.

Examples of Sesquiterpenes:

–β-Caryophyllene

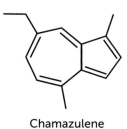

β-Caryophyllene

β-caryophyllene is found in clove and cinnamon essential oils and is found in high proportions in plants from the Labiatae family. It is antiedema, anti-inflammatory, antispasmodic, and an insect and termite repellent.

Anesthetic: β-caryophyllene has been shown to act as a local anesthetic in vitro and in vivo. In an in vitro experiment, β-caryophyllene reduced the number of contractions electrically invoked in rat phrenic nerve-hemidiaphragms. Phrenic nerves are found in the spine, specifically at the 3rd, 4th, and 5th cervical vertebrae. These nerves provide sole motor control to the diaphragm. In this experiment, electrical impulses through the phrenic nerves induced diaphragm contractions, but the addition of β-caryophyllene reduced the number of contractions (Bulbring, 1946).

In an in vivo (real life) experiment, researchers performed a conjunctival reflex test on rabbits in which the conjunctival sac, found in the eye, was stimulated with a cat whisker to promote palpebral closure (or blinking). β-caryophyllene acted as a local anesthetic: when it was applied to the eye, more stimulation with the cat whisker was required in order to promote blinking in the rabbit (Ghelardini et al., 2001).

–Chamazulene

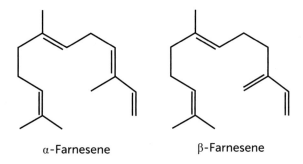

Chamazulene

Chamazulene is found in chamomile oil and is very high in anti-inflammatory and antibacterial activity.

–Farnesene

α-Farnesene   β-Farnesene

Farnesene refers to several isomers with the chemical formula $C_{15}H_{24}$. Farnesene is found in ylang ylang, valerian, and German chamomile oil and is antiviral in action.

Alcohols

Alcohols are any organic molecule with a carbon atom bound to a hydroxyl group. A hydroxyl group is an oxygen and hydrogen molecule (-OH). Alcohols are commonly recognized for their antibacterial, anti-infectious, and antiviral activities. They are somewhat stimulating and help to increase blood circulation. Because of their high resistance to oxidation and their low toxicity levels, they have been shown in animal studies to revert cells to normal function and activity. They create an uplifting quality and are regarded as safe and effective for young and old alike.

Found as a Significant Constituent in ALL Essential Oils Except: Birch, cassia, clove, white fir, grapefruit, myrrh, oregano, and wintergreen.

–Monoterpene Alcohols (or Monoterpenols)

Like monoterpenes, monoterpene alcohols are comprised of two isoprene units but have a hydroxyl group bound to one of the carbons instead of a hydrogen. Monoterpene alcohols are known for their ability to stimulate the immune system and to work as a diuretic and a general tonic. They are antibacterial and mildly antiseptic as well.

Examples of Monoterpene Alcohols:

Methanol (CH₃OH)

—OH

Methanol (CH₃OH)

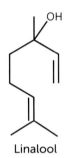

Shorthand model of methanol, the simplest alcohol, and the molecular model it represents, below.

◯ = carbon
● = hydrogen
◯ = oxygen

–Linalool

OH

Linalool

Linalool is found in rosewood, bergamot, coriander, rose, jasmine, and lavender essential oils. It has a flowery aroma and is used to scent soaps, shampoos, and perfumes. Linalool can help relieve discomfort. It has antibacterial, antifungal, antiseptic (5x phenol), antispasmodic, antiviral, and sedative properties.

Anti-inflammatory: Linalool has been used to reduce paw swelling induced by carrageenan in mice. The effects of linalool work against swelling in a dose-dependent manner (Peana et al., 2002; Skold et al., 2002). Linalool also mediates pain caused by inflammation. In a particular study, acetic acid was administered to mice via intraperitoneal (gut) injections. Mice that received a dose of linalool following administration of acetic acid exhibited less writhing (due to pain) than mice that acted as controls (Peana et al., 2003).

Antifungal: *Candida albicans* is the primary fungus responsible for yeast infections. Yeast infections are commonly exhibited as vulvovaginal candidiasis and thrush (oropharyngeal candidiasis, in the mouth). Thrush is commonly expressed in newborns and AIDS patients.

Candida albicans is also becoming a concern due to its emergence as a nosocomial infection (an infection contracted in a hospital) and its increasing resistance to fluconazole—an antifungal drug. *C. albicans* can form biofilms (aggregated colonies) on medical devices such as catheters and dentures (Mukherjee et al., 2003; *Microbiology* 9th ed., 2007).

Topical application of linalool to colonies of the polymorphic fungus *Candida albicans* results in growth inhibition and fungal death. Linalool affects growth by blocking passage beyond the G1 (cell growth) phase of the cell cycle (Zore et al., 2011).

Sedative: Linalool is a common sedative used in Brazilian folk medicine. According to studies using mice, inhaled linalool induces sleep or sedation (Linck et al., 2009; de Almeida et al., 2009).

Nerve Cells

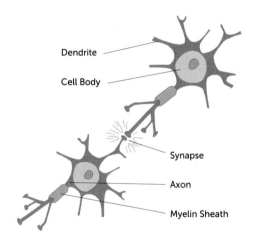

Dendrite

Cell Body

Synapse

Axon

Myelin Sheath

Synapse

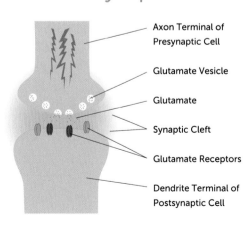

Axon Terminal of Presynaptic Cell

Glutamate Vesicle

Glutamate

Synaptic Cleft

Glutamate Receptors

Dendrite Terminal of Postsynaptic Cell

EO Science in Depth

Antiepileptic/Anticonvulsant: Epilepsy is characterized by seemingly spontaneous spasms of electrical activity in the brain. These spasms can cause seizures and convulsions. One hypothesis for the cause of epilepsy is excessive glutamate levels in neurons (nerve cells)(Chapman et al., 2000; Meldrum et al., 1999; Meldrum, 1994; and Chapman, 1998). Glutamates are a common form of neurotransmitter that are stored in special vesicles (storage containers) near nerve synapses (locations where nerve cells come close to each other in order to pass along electrical impulses and signals). Impulses along the nerve cause one nerve cell to release glutamate across the synapse where it is received by receptors on the second nerve cell, opening channels in that cell to allow it to pass ions through the cell membrane, changing the electrical potential of that cell (*Medical Physiology* 10th ed., 2000).

Studies have shown that the release of large concentrations of glutamate will lead to too many open channels, which will cause high, intense depolarization sequences of the action potential. Disproportionate depolarizations are the basis for seizures and convulsions in epilepsy (Chapman et al., 2000; Meldrum et al., 1994; and Paolette et al., 2007).

Using mouse models, researchers have found that applications of linalool on cortical synaptosomes (isolated nerve terminals, or synapses) significantly inhibited glutamate uptake. Inhibition of glutamate is a method to reduce occurrences of epileptic seizures. These observations provide significant evidence for linalool acting as a possible antiepileptic agent (Silva Brum et al., 2001a and Silva Brum et al., 2001b).

–Citronellol

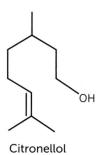

Citronellol

Citronellol is found in citronella, rose, melissa, and eucalyptus essential oils. It has antibacterial, antifungal, antiseptic (3.8x phenol), and sedative properties.

Anticonvulsant Activity: Administered doses of citronellol given via the intraperitoneal cavity (gut) to rodents have been observed to reduce the convulsive effects in induced epileptic attacks. Epilepsy is studied in animal models by inducing convulsions with compounds such as pentylenetetrazol (PTZ) and picrotoxin. Citronellol, over time, reduces the amplitude of the compound action potential (CAP) in neurons. This decreases the effect and intensity of convulsions (de Sousa et al., 2006).

Blood Pressure: Injections of citronellol into the blood were found by researchers to reduce blood pressure in animal models. Citronellol is theorized to decrease the flux of Ca^{2+} ions into smooth vascular muscle cells by deactivating VOCCs (voltage-operated calcium channels). Calcium is the principal regulator of tension in vascular smooth muscle (blood vessels). When the transport of Ca^{2+} into the cell is blocked, smooth muscle relaxation occurs. This leads to increased vasodilation (an increase in the diameter of the blood vessels, allowing a higher volume of blood flow) and, thus, lowered blood pressure (Bastos et al., 2009; Gurney, 1994; and Munzel et al., 2003).

–Geraniol

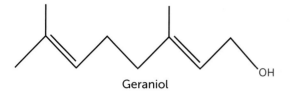

Geraniol

Geraniol is found in rose, citronella, and lemon essential oils. It has antifungal, antiseptic (7x phenol), cancer-preventative, and sedative properties.

–Other Monoterpene Alcohols:

Borneol, menthol, nerol, terpineol (which Dr. Gattefossé considered to be a decongestant), vetiverol, and cedrol.

–Sesquiterpene Alcohols (Sesquiterpenols)

Like sesquiterpenes, sesquiterpene alcohols are comprised of three isoprene units but have a hydroxyl group bound to one of the carbons instead of a hydrogen. Sesquiterpene alcohols are known to be antiallergic, antibacterial, anti-inflammatory, ulcer-protective (preventative), and liver and glandular stimulant.

Examples of Sesquiterpene Alcohols:

–Farnesol

Farnesol

Farnesol is found in rose, neroli, ylang ylang, and Roman chamomile essential oils. It is known to be good for the mucous membranes and to help prevent bacterial growth from perspiration.

–Bisabolol

Bisabolol

Bisabolol is found in German chamomile essential oil. It is one of the strongest sesquiterpene alcohols.

–Other Sesquiterpene Alcohols:

Others include nerolidol and zingiberol.

Esters

Methyl Acetate
(CH_3COOCH_3)

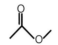

Methyl acetate (shown here) is a simple organic ester molecule.

Methyl Acetate
(CH_3COOCH_3)

○ = carbon
● = hydrogen
● = oxygen

Esters are the compounds resulting from the reaction of an alcohol with an acid (known as esterification). Esters consist of a carboxyl group (a carbon atom double bonded to an oxygen atom) bound to a hydrocarbon group on one side and bound to an oxygen and a hydrocarbon group on the opposite side.

Esters are very common and are found in the mildest essential oils. Mostly free of toxicity and irritants, they tend to be the most calming, relaxing, and balancing of all the essential oil constituents. They are also antifungal and antispasmodic. They have a balancing or regulatory effect, especially on the nervous system. Some examples are linalyl acetate, geranyl acetate (with strong antifungal properties), and bornyl acetate (effective on bronchial candida). Other esters include eugenyl acetate, lavendulyl acetate, and methyl salicylate.

Found as a Major Constituent In: Birch, bergamot, clary sage, Douglas fir, geranium, helichrysum, lavender, wintergreen, and ylang ylang.

Found as a Minor Constituent In: Cassia, clove, cypress, white fir, lemon, lemongrass, marjoram, and orange.

EO Science in Depth

Aldehydes

Acetaldehyde
(CH₃CHO)

Acetaldehyde (shown here) is a simple organic aldehyde molecule.

Acetaldehyde
(CH₃CHO)

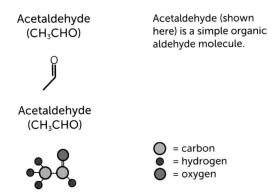

○ = carbon
● = hydrogen
⬤ = oxygen

Aldehydes are often responsible for the fragrance of an oil. They exert powerful aromas and are often calming to the emotions. They are highly reactive and are characterized by a carboxyl group (a carbon atom double bonded to an oxygen atom) with a hydrogen atom on one side and a hydrocarbon group on the opposite side.

In general, they are anti-infectious, anti-inflammatory, calming to the central nervous system, fever-reducing, hypotensive, and tonic. Some are antiseptic, antimicrobial, and antifungal, while others act as vasodilators. They can be quite irritating when applied topically (citrals being an example). However, it has been shown that adding an essential oil with an equal amount of d-Limonene can negate the irritant properties of a high citral oil.

Found as a Major Constituent In: Cassia, cinnamon, and lemongrass.

Found as a Minor Constituent In: Douglas fir, *Eucalyptus radiata*, grapefruit, lemon, myrrh, and orange.

Examples of Aldehydes:

—Citrals

Geranial

Citrals (like neral, geranial, and citronellal) are very common and have a distinct antiseptic action. They also show antiviral properties (as is the case with melissa oil) when applied topically on herpes simplex.

—Other Aldehydes

Benzaldehyde, cinnamic aldehyde, cuminic aldehyde, and perillaldehyde.

Ketones

Acetone
(CH₃COCH₃)

Acetone (shown here) is a simple ketone molecule.

Acetone
(CH₃COCH₃)

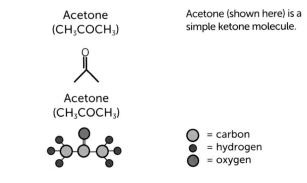

○ = carbon
● = hydrogen
⬤ = oxygen

Ketones are organic compounds characterized by a carboxyl group (a carbon atom double bonded to an oxygen atom) with a hydrocarbon on both sides. Ketones are sometimes mucolytic and neurotoxic when isolated from other constituents. However, all recorded toxic effects come from laboratory testing on guinea pigs and rats. No documented cases exist where oils with a high concentration of ketones (such as mugwort, tansy, sage, and wormwood) have ever caused a toxic effect on a human being. Also, large amounts of these oils would have to be consumed for them to result in a toxic neurological effect. Ketones stimulate cell regeneration, promote the formation of tissue, and liquefy mucus. They are helpful with conditions such as dry asthma, colds, flu, and dry cough and are largely found in oils used for the upper respiratory system, such as hyssop, rosemary, and sage.

Found as a Major Constituent In: rosemary (CT verbenon).

Found as a Minor (but significant) Constituent In: Dougas fir, fennel, geranium, helichrysum, lemongrass, myrrh, peppermint, and vetiver.

Examples of Ketones:

—Thujone

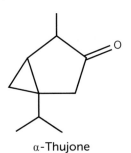

α-Thujone

Thujone is one of the most toxic members of the ketone family. It can be an irritant and upsetting to the central nervous system and may be neurotoxic when taken internally, such as in the banned drink absinthe. Although oils containing thujone may be inhaled to relieve respiratory distress and may stimulate the immune system, they should usually be used in dilution (1–2%) and/or for only short periods of time.

—Jasmone

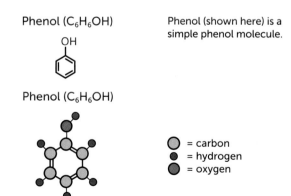

Jasmone

Jasmone is found in jasmine essential oil and is nontoxic.

—Fenchone

Fenchone

Fenchone is found in fennel essential oil and is nontoxic.

—Other Ketones:

Camphor, carvone, menthone, methyl nonyl ketone, and pinocamphone.

Phenols

Phenol (C_6H_6OH)

OH

Phenol (C_6H_6OH)

Phenol (shown here) is a simple phenol molecule.

○ = carbon
● = hydrogen
● = oxygen

Phenols are a diverse group of compounds derived from a phenol group, which is comprised of a benzene ring (six carbon atoms bound in a circle) and a hydroxyl group (oxygen and hydrogen).

Phenols comprise some of the most powerful antibacterial, anti-infectious, and antiseptic constituents in the plant world. They are also very stimulating to both the nervous and immune systems. They contain high levels of oxygenating molecules and have antioxidant properties. However, they can be quite caustic to the skin, and they present some concerns regarding liver toxicity. Essential oils that contain a high proportion of phenols should be diluted and/or used only for short periods of time.

Found as a Major Constituent In: Basil, birch, cinnamon, clove, fennel, melaleuca, oregano, peppermint, thyme, and wintergreen.

Found as a Minor Constituent In: Cassia, marjoram, and ylang ylang.

Examples of Phenols:

—Eugenol

Eugenol

Eugenol is found in clove, nutmeg, cinnamon, bay, and basil essential oils. It has analgesic, anesthetic (in dentistry), anticonvulsant, antifungal, anti-inflammatory, antioxidant, antiseptic, cancer-preventative, and sedative properties.

Vasodilator: Eugenol was found to increase vasodilation (increase the diameter of the opening through the blood vessels) in animal models. When blood vessels expand, the result is larger amounts of blood flow and, thus, a decrease in heart rate. In these particular studies, it was observed that heart rate decreased in conjunction with increased vasodilation, as compared to controls (Lahlou et al., 2004; Damiani et al., 2003).

Eugenol is thought to increase vasodilation by inhibiting the action of calcium (Ca^{2+}) in voltage-operated calcium channels (VOCCs). Ca^{2+} is the main regulator of vascular smooth muscle (blood vessel) tension. When Ca^{2+} is blocked, blood vessels relax and widen, allowing for an increase in blood flow (Gurney, 1994; Munzel et al., 2003).

EO Science in Depth

—Thymol

Thymol

Thymol is found in thyme and oregano essential oils. It may not be as caustic as other phenols. It has antibacterial, antifungal, anti-inflammatory, antioxidant, antiplaque, antirheumatic, antiseptic (20x phenol), antispasmodic, deodorizing, and expectorant properties.

Antibacterial: Thymol has been shown to inhibit the growth of microorganisms such as *Escherichia coli, Campylobacter jejuni, Porphyromonas gingivalis, Staphylococcus aureus,* and *Pseudomonas aeruginosa.* Thymol is thought to disrupt (or impair) the cytoplasmic membranes of microbes, causing cell leakage. Without the protective barrier of the cytoplasmic membrane, viability of these microorganisms significantly decreases (Shapiro et al., 1995; Xu et al., 2008; Lambert et al., 2001; and Evans et al., 2000).

—Carvacrol

Carvacrol

Carvacrol is a product of auto-oxidation of d-Limonene. It is antibacterial, antifungal, anti-inflammatory, antiseptic (1.5x phenol), antispasmodic, and expectorant. Researchers believe it may possibly have some anticancer properties as well.

—Other Phenols

Methyl eugenol, methyl chavicol, anethole, and safrole.

Oxides

An organic oxide typically refers to an organic molecule (one that contains carbon and hydrogen) that has been oxidized, meaning an oxygen atom has become bound between two carbon atoms. According to the American Heritage® Dictionary of the English Language, an oxide is "a binary compound of an element or a radical with oxygen." Oxides often act as expectorants and are mildly stimulating.

Found as a Major Constituent In: *Eucalyptus radiata* and rosemary.

Found as a Minor Constituent In: Douglas fir, basil, lemongrass, melaleuca, thyme, and ylang ylang.

Examples of Oxides:

—1,8-Cineol (Eucalyptol)

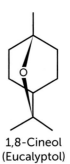

1,8-Cineol
(Eucalyptol)

1,8-cineol is, by far, the most prevalent member of the oxide family and virtually exists in a class of its own. It is anesthetic, antiseptic, and works as a strong mucolytic as it thins mucus in respiratory tract infections.

Anti-Inflammatory: Researchers found in an animal experiment that rats that were given oral doses of 1,8-cineole before injection with lambda carrageenan (a sweetener that causes inflammation) had markedly decreased swelling when compared to rats that were given the injection without a dosage of 1,8-cineole.

It has been suggested by scientists that 1,8-cineole inhibits cytokine production. Inhibiting cytokine production would decrease inflammation despite having a stimulant present (such as carrageenan) (Santos et al., 2000; Juergens et al., 2003).

Asthma: Asthma is a chronic inflammatory disease that restricts air flow to the lungs (specifically in the bronchial tubes). A double-blind, placebo-controlled study was performed to test the ability of 1,8-cineole to alleviate asthmatic symptoms. All subjects in the study suffered from bronchial asthma and required daily administration of oral glucocorticosteroids in order to maintain stable conditions.

At the conclusion of the study, which lasted over a course of 12 weeks, patients who received daily doses of 1,8-cineole were able to maintain stable conditions despite significantly reduced oral doses of glucocorticosteroids, as compared to the placebo group. Proper lung function was also maintained four times longer in the test group than in the placebo group (Juergens et al., 2003; Goodwin et al., 1986).

Pain: In one study, mice were injected in the hind paw with a dose of 1% formalin (a common substance used to model pain in experimental studies)/99% saline solution. A portion of mice were given 1,8-cineole. It was observed that these mice who received 1,8-cineole licked their paw substantially less (meaning they did not feel as much pain) than mice that did not receive the 1,8-cineole treatment. In this study, researchers found that 1,8-cineole treatment produced antinociceptive (pain-blocking) effects comparable to those observed for morphine (Santos et al., 2000 and Shibata et al., 1989).

—Other oxides

Linalool oxide, ascaridol, bisabolol oxide, 1,4-cineol, and bisabolone oxide.

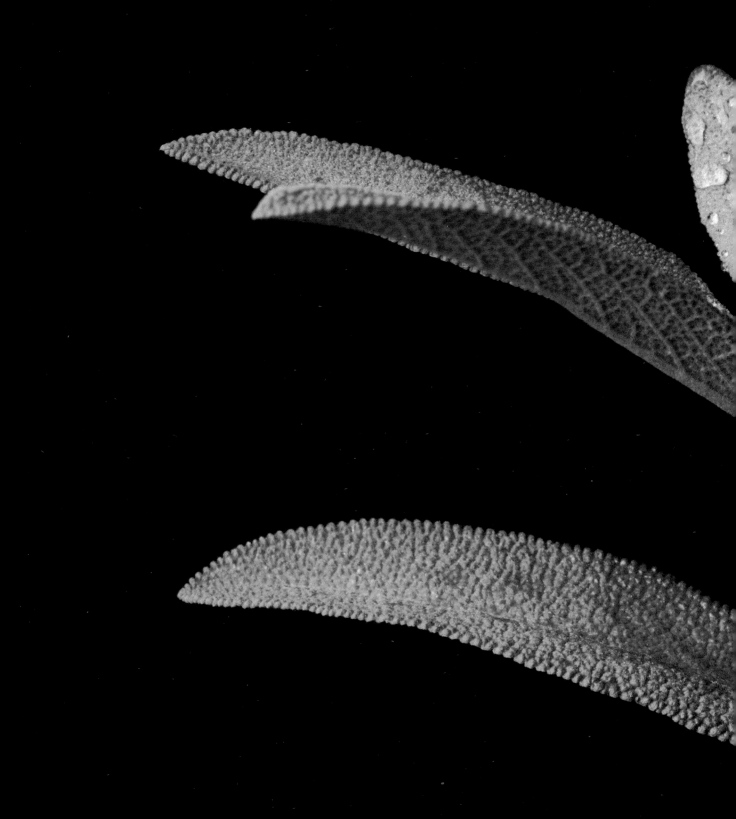

Appendix and References

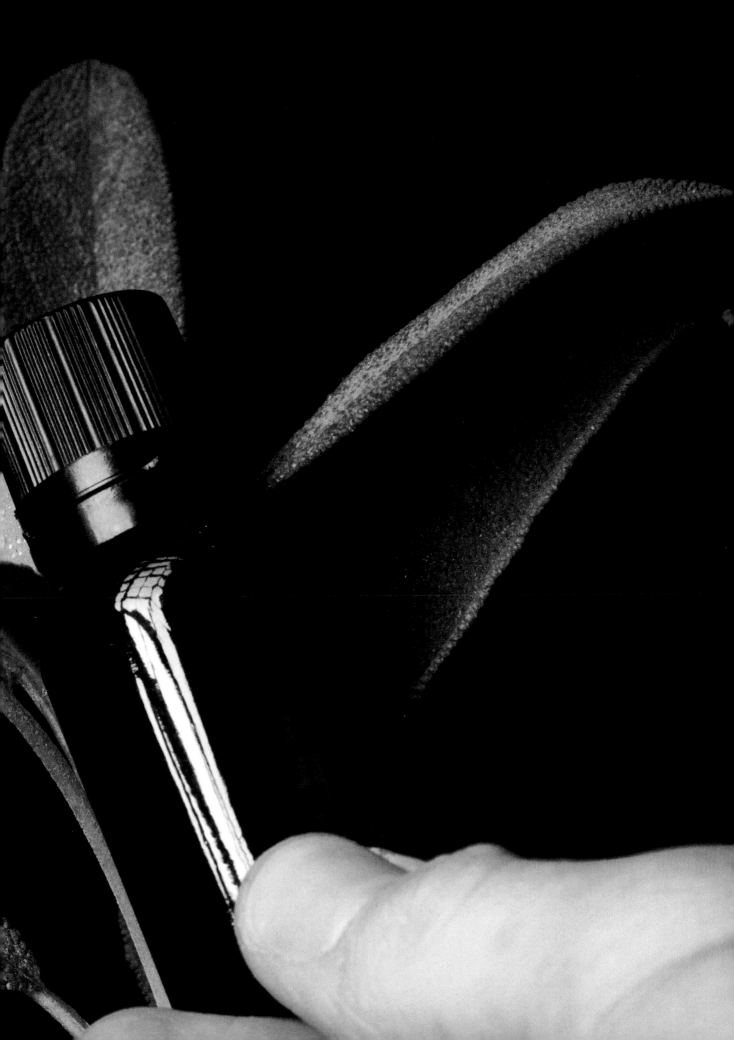

Appendix A: Body Systems Chart

The following chart lists the oils and products discussed within this book and indicates which body systems they primarily affect. While this chart does not include every system that could possibly be affected by each formulation, it attempts to list the primary systems that are most often affected. It is provided to give the beginning aromatherapy student a starting point for personal use and analysis.

Product Name	Cardiovascular System	Digestive System	Emotional Balance	Hormonal System	Immune System	Muscles and Skeletal System	Nervous System	Respiratory System	Skin and Hair
A2z Chewable	●	●		●	●	●	●	●	●
Alpha CRS+	●				●	●	●	●	●
Arborvitae			●					●	●
AromaTouch			●	●	●	●	●		
Balance			●			●	●		●
Basil	●					●			
Bergamot		●	●						●
Birch						●			
Black Pepper		●					●		
Blue Tansy							●		
Bone Nutrient Lifetime Complex			●			●	●		●
Brave			●				●		
Breathe								●	
Calmer			●				●		
Cardamom		●						●	
Cassia					●				
Cedarwood							●	●	
Cheer			●						
Cilantro		●	●						
Cinnamon Bark					●				
Citrus Bliss			●		●		●		
ClaryCalm			●	●					●
Clary Sage				●					
Clove	●	●			●			●	
Console			●						
Copaiba	●	●	●		●	●			●
Coriander		●		●					
Cypress	●					●			
DDR Prime	●				●	●		●	
Deep Blue						●	●		
DigestZen		●							
Dill	●	●							
Douglas Fir						●		●	

Product Name	Cardiovascular System	Digestive System	Emotional Balance	Hormonal System	Immune System	Muscles and Skeletal System	Nervous System	Respiratory System	Skin and Hair
Elevation			•	•					
Eucalyptus								•	•
Fennel		•		•					
Forgive			•						
Frankincense			•		•		•		•
Geranium			•						•
Ginger		•					•		
Grapefruit	•								
Green Mandarin		•	•		•				•
GX Assist		•			•				
HD Clear					•				•
Helichrysum	•					•			
Hinoki			•		•			•	•
InTune			•	•	•		•		
IQ Mega	•	•			•		•		•
Jasmine			•	•					
Juniper Berry		•	•				•		•
Lavender	•		•				•		•
Lemon		•			•			•	
Lemon Myrtle					•	•		•	
Lemongrass					•	•			
Lime		•			•			•	
Litsea		•			•			•	
Magnolia				•	•				•
Manuka						•		•	•
Marjoram	•					•			
Melaleuca					•	•		•	•
Melissa			•						•
Microplex MVp	•	•	•	•	•	•	•	•	•
Mito2Max	•				•	•	•		
Motivate			•						
Myrrh				•	•		•		•
Neroli		•	•						•
On Guard					•				•
Orange		•	•		•				•
Oregano					•	•		•	
Passion			•						
PastTense						•	•		
Patchouli									•

Appendix

Product Name	Cardiovascular System	Digestive System	Emotional Balance	Hormonal System	Immune System	Muscles and Skeletal System	Nervous System	Respiratory System	Skin and Hair
Peace			●						
Peppermint		●				●	●	●	●
Petitgrain			●		●				
Phytoestrogen Lifetime Complex			●	●		●			●
Pink Pepper					●			●	●
Purify		●	●		●				●
Rescuer						●	●		
Roman Chamomile			●				●		●
Rose			●						●
Rosemary					●		●	●	
Sandalwood			●			●	●		●
Serenity			●				●		
Siberian Fir						●		●	
Slim & Sassy		●	●						
Slim & Sassy TrimShake and V Shake		●		●		●			
Spearmint		●	●						
Spikenard			●						●
Star Anise	●	●		●				●	
Steady			●				●		
Stronger					●				●
TerraShield									●
Terrazyme		●							
Thinker			●				●		
Thyme					●	●			
Turmeric		●			●				●
Vetiver			●	●			●		●
Whisper			●	●			●		
White Fir								●	
Wintergreen						●			
xEO Mega	●	●			●		●		●
Yarrow				●	●				●
Yarrow Pom	●		●	●	●		●		●
Ylang Ylang	●		●	●					
Yoga Blends			●	●			●		
Yuzu		●			●				●
Zendocrine		●		●	●			●	●

459

Appendix B: Single Essential Oils Property Chart

The following chart presents some of the properties of each of the single oils. An attempt has been made to indicate the effectiveness of the oils for each property, where supporting information existed. However, this information should not be considered conclusive. It is provided to give the beginning aromatherapy student a starting point for personal use and analysis. Also, keep in mind the applicable safety data when applying an oil for its property. For example, cinnamon bark is one of the best known antiseptics, but it is also extremely irritating to the skin. It may work well to sanitize the bathroom with, but it should be used with extreme caution on the skin.

Properties of Essential Oils

Antibacterial: an agent that prevents the growth of (or destroys) bacteria.

Anticatarrhal: an agent that helps remove excess catarrh from the body. Expectorants help promote the removal of mucus from the respiratory system.

Antidepressant: an agent that helps alleviate depression.

Antifungal: an agent that prevents and combats fungal infection.

Anti-infectious: an agent that prevents and combats the spread of germs.

Anti-inflammatory: an agent that alleviates inflammation.

Antimicrobial: an agent that resists or destroys pathogenic microorganisms.

Antiparasitic: an agent that prevents and destroys parasites.

Antirheumatic: an agent that helps prevent and relieve rheumatism.

Antiseptic: an agent that destroys and prevents the development of microbes.

Antispasmodic: an agent that prevents and eases spasms or convulsions.

Antiviral: a substance that inhibits the growth of a virus.

Analgesic: a substance that relieves pain.

Immune-stimulant: an agent that stimulates the natural defense mechanism of the body.

Single Oil Name	Antibacterial	Anticatarrhal	Antidepressant	Antifungal	Anti-infectious	Anti-inflammatory	Antimicrobial	Antiparasitic	Antirheumatic	Antiseptic	Antispasmodic	Antiviral	Analgesic	Immune-stimulant
Arborvitae	++		+++	+		++	++		++					
Basil	++	+	+		+	+++				+	+	+		
Bergamot			+		+++		+			+	+		+	
Birch					+			+	+++	+				
Black Pepper	+					+			+	+	+	++		
Blue Tansy	+		++		+	++			+			+		
Cardamom	++			+	++	+			+	+				
Cassia	+		+	+	+	+	++	+		++++	+	+		
Cedarwood			+	+					++					
Cilantro	+		+											
Cinnamon	+		+	+	+	+	++	+		++++	+	+		
Clary Sage	+		+		+					+	+			
Clove	+++	+		++	+			++	+	+		+++		
Copaiba	++				++++					++			++	
Coriander	++		++		++		+			+		+		
Cypress	+			+			+	+	+	+				
Dill	+			+		+					++			
Douglas Fir		+++			+	+			+					
Eucalyptus	++	++		+	+						+++	++	+	

Single Oil Name	Antibacterial	Anticatarrhal	Antidepressant	Antifungal	Anti-infectious	Anti-inflammatory	Antimicrobial	Antiparasitic	Antirheumatic	Antiseptic	Antispasmodic	Antiviral	Analgesic	Immune-stimulant
Fennel	+	++			+	+	+			+	+			
Frankincense		++	++			+++	+				+			+++
Geranium	+++		++	++	+	+				+				
Ginger		++								++			++	
Grapefruit	++									++				
Green Mandarin						++	+				+	+		
Helichrysum	++	+++		+		++	++			+	+++			
Hinoki	++			+	+	++				+		+		
Jasmine		+	++				++				+	+	+	
Juniper Berry										++	+		+	
Lavender			++		+	++	+	+	+	+	++		++	
Lemon	++			+			++		+	+++	+			++
Lemon Myrtle	++			+++		+	++						+	
Lemongrass	+		+	+		++	+			+			++	
Lime	++									++		+		
Litsea	++			+			+			+		+		
Magnolia	+					+	+						++	
Manuka	+++	+		++	+		+			+++		+	+	
Marjoram	+	+		+	+					++	++	+	++	
Melissa	+		++				+				++	++		
Melaleuca	+++			++++	+	+		+		+		+++		++
Myrrh		+		+	+	+++	++	+		+		+++		
Neroli	+		++		+			+		++	++	+		
Orange	++		++	+		+				++				
Oregano	+++	+		+++	+++			+++	++	+	+	++	++	++
Patchouli	+		+	+	+	+	+			+	+			
Peppermint	+	+		+	+	++	+			+	+	+	++	
Petitgrain	++				+	+	+			++				
Pink Pepper	++			+		+					+			
Roman Chamomile	+		+		+	+++				+	+		++	
Rose					+									
Rosemary	+++	+		+++	+	+++							+++	
Sandalwood	+	+++	++	+						++	+			
Siberian Fir		+								++		+		
Spearmint	++			+	+					+	+			+
Spikenard	+		++	+	+			+						+
Star Anise				++						+	+			
Thyme	+	+		+++			++	+	++	+	+			++
Turmeric						++	+						+	
Vetiver					+					+	+			+
White Fir		+								++			+	
Wintergreen						+++			+	+	+		+	
Yarrow						+				++				
Ylang Ylang			+		+					+	+			
Yuzu	+													+

Appendix

Appendix C: Single Oil & Blend Quick Usage Chart

ESSENTIAL OILS	COMMON USES
ARBORVITAE	🌿: Protects against environmental and seasonal threats. 🌿: Promotes healthy cell function. 🌿🌿: Powerful cleansing and purifying agent. 🌿: Natural insect repellent. ✚: Body System(s) Affected: Emotional Balance, Respiratory System, Skin, and Hair.
BASIL	🌿: Soothes sore muscles and joints. 🌿: Assists with clear breathing. 🌿: Acts as a cooling agent for the skin. ✚: Body System(s) Affected: Cardiovascular System, Muscles, and Bones.
BERGAMOT	🌿: Reduces tension and stress. 🌿: Promotes healthy, clear skin. 🌿: Soothes and rejuvenates skin. ✚: Body System(s) Affected: Digestive System, Emotional Balance, Skin, and Hair.
BIRCH	🌿: Soothes muscles and joints. 🌿: Supports healthy circulation. 🌿🌿: Promotes clear breathing and healthy respiratory function. 🌿: Beneficial for oily skin conditions. ✚: Body System(s) Affected: Muscles and Bones.
BLACK PEPPER	🌿🌿: Rich source of antioxidants. 🌿: Supports healthy circulation. 🌿: Aids digestion. 🌿: Enhances food flavor. ✚: Body System(s) Affected: Digestive System and Nervous System.
BLUE TANSY	🌿🌿: Helps calm and support the nervous system. 🌿: Helps soothe minor skin irritations. 🌿: Helps promote a feeling of calming and relaxation. ✚: Body System(s) Affected: Nervous System
CARDAMOM	🌿: Eases occasional indigestion. 🌿🌿: Promotes clear breathing and respiratory health. 🌿: Flavorful spice for cooking and baking. 🌿🌿: Calms occasional stomach upset. ✚: Body System(s) Affected: Digestive System and Respiratory System.
CASSIA	🌿: Promotes healthy digestion. 🌿: Supports healthy immune function. 🌿: Warming, uplifting aroma. 🌿: Helps soothe sore, achy joints. ✚: Body System(s) Affected: Immune System.
CEDARWOOD	🌿: Supports and maintains healthy respiratory function. 🌿: Promotes clear, healthy skin. 🌿🌿: Evokes feelings of wellness and vitality. 🌿: Relaxing, soothing aroma. ✚: Body System(s) Affected: Nervous System and Respiratory System.
CILANTRO	🌿: Aids digestion. 🌿🌿: Rich in antioxidants. 🌿: Gives food a fresh and tasty flavor. 🌿: Soothing to the skin. ✚: Body System(s) Affected: Digestive System and Skin.
CINNAMON	🌿: Promotes circulation. 🌿: Helps alleviate sore muscles and joints. 🌿: Maintains a healthy immune system. 🌿: Long used as a natural flavoring and for its internal health benefits. ✚: Body System(s) Affected: Immune System.
CLARY SAGE	🌿🌿: Soothes monthly discomfort associated with menstrual cycles. 🌿🌿: Helps balance hormones. 🌿: Soothes nervous tension and lightens mood. 🌿: Calming and soothing to the skin. ✚: Body System(s) Affected: Hormonal System.
CLOVE	🌿: Powerful antioxidant properties. 🌿🌿: Supports cardiovascular health. 🌿: Promotes oral health and helps soothe teeth and gums. ✚: Body System(s) Affected: Cardiovascular System, Digestive System, Immune System, and Respiratory System.

ESSENTIAL OILS	COMMON USES
COPAIBA	◐: Powerful antioxidant. ◐: Helps calm and support the nervous system. ◑: Promotes clear, smooth skin. ✚: Body System(s) Affected: Cardiovascular System, Digestive System, Nervous System, Immune System, and Respiratory System
CORIANDER	◐: Promotes digestion and eases occasional stomach upset. ◐: Helps maintain an already healthy insulin response. ◑: Soothes joint and muscle discomfort. ◑: Helps oily skin areas to reduce breakouts. ✚: Body System(s) Affected: Digestive System and Hormonal System.
CYPRESS	◎: Assists with clear breathing. ◎: Promotes healthy respiratory function. ◑: Soothes tight, tense muscles. ◑: Supports localized blood flow. ✚: Body System(s) Affected: Cardiovascular System, Muscles, and Bones.
DOUGLAS FIR	◎: Promotes feelings of clear airways and easy breathing. ◑: Cleansing and purifying to the skin. ◎◑: Promotes a positive mood and sense of focus. ✚: Body System(s) Affected: Respiratory System, Muscles, and Bones.
EUCALYPTUS	◎: Assists with clear breathing. ◎◑: Supports overall respiratory health. ◑: Soothes tired, sore muscles. ◎: Helps to lessen stress. ✚: Body System(s) Affected: Respiratory System and Skin.
FENNEL (SWEET)	◐◑◑: Relieves occasional indigestion and digestive troubles. ◑◑: Eases monthly menstrual cycles. ◑: Supports a healthy lymphatic system. ◑: Calms minor skin irritation. ✚: Body System(s) Affected: Digestive System and Hormonal System.
FRANKINCENSE	◑◑: Helps build and maintain a healthy immune system. ◑◑◐: Promotes cellular health. ◑: Reduces the appearance of blemishes and rejuvenates skin. ✚: Body System(s) Affected: Emotional Balance, Immune System, Nervous System, and Skin.
GERANIUM	◑: Promotes clear, healthy skin. ◎◑: Helps calm nerves and lessen stress. ◑◎: Supports liver health. ✚: Body System(s) Affected: Emotional Balance and Skin.
GINGER	◐◑: Helps ease occasional indigestion and nausea. ◐◎: Promotes digestion. ◐◑: Supports overall digestive health. ✚: Body System(s) Affected: Digestive System and Nervous System.
GRAPEFRUIT	◑◎◐: Cleanses and purifies. ◑: Beneficial for oily skin issues. ◎◐: Supports healthy metabolism. ◎◑: Helps reduce mental and physical fatigue. ✚: Body System(s) Affected: Cardiovascular System.
GREEN MANDARIN	◎◑: Calming. ◑◎◐: Relieves occasional stomach upset. ◑◎◐: Soothing and uplifting. ◑: Tones skin. ✚: Body System(s) Affected: Emotional Balance, Digestive System, Immune System, Skin.
HAWAIIAN SANDALWOOD	◑: Promotes healthy, smooth skin. ◑: Reduces the appearance of scars and blemishes. ◎: Frequently used in meditation for its grounding and uplifting properties. ✚: Body System(s) Affected: Emotional Balance, Muscles, Bones, Nervous System, and Skin.
HELICHRYSUM	◑: Helps skin recover quickly. ◑◎: Promotes healthy liver function. ◑: Supports localized blood flow. ◑: Helps reduce the appearance of wrinkles and other blemishes. ✚: Body System(s) Affected: Cardiovascular System, Muscles, and Bones.
HINOKI	◎◑: Calming. ◑: Cleansing. ◎◑: Supports healthy respiratory system. ◑: Soothes occasional skin irritations. ✚: Body System(s) Affected: Emotional Balance, Immune System, Respiratory System, and Skin.

ESSENTIAL OILS	COMMON USES
JASMINE	⬡: Helps balance hormones and manage the symptoms of PMS. ⬡: Promotes a healthy, glowing complexion. ⬡: Nourishes and protects the skin and scalp. ✛: Body System(s) Affected: Emotional Balance and Hormonal System.
JUNIPER BERRY	⬡: Supports healthy kidney and urinary function. ⬡: May benefit problematic skin areas. ⬡: Acts as a natural cleansing and detoxifying agent. ⬡: Helps relieve tension and stress. ✛: Body System(s) Affected: Digestive System, Emotional Balance, Nervous System, and Skin.
LAVENDER	⬡: Widely used for its calming and relaxing qualities. ⬡: Soothes occasional skin irritations. ⬡: Helps skin recover quickly. ⬡: Eases muscle tension in the head and neck. ✛: Body System(s) Affected: Cardiovascular System, Emotional Balance, Nervous System, and Skin.
LEMON	⬡: Cleanses and purifies the air and surfaces. ⬡: Aids in digestion. ⬡: Supports healthy respiratory function. ⬡: Promotes a positive mood and cognitive ability. ✛: Body System(s) Affected: Digestive System, Immune System, and Respiratory System.
LEMON MYRTLE	⬡: Supports healthy respiratory system. ⬡: Refreshing. ⬡: Calming and Relaxing. ⬡: Uplifting. ✛: Body System(s) Affected: Immune System, Respiratory System, and Muscles and Bones.
LEMONGRASS	⬡: Promotes healthy, smooth skin. ⬡: Reduces the appearance of scars and blemishes. ⬡: Frequently used in meditation for its grounding and uplifting properties. ✛: Body System(s) Affected: Emotional Balance, Muscles, Bones, Nervous System, and Skin.
LIME	⬡: Supports healthy immune function. ⬡: Positively affects mood. ⬡: Used as an aromatic, topical, and internal cleanser. ⬡: Promotes emotional balance and well-being. ✛: Body System(s) Affected: Digestive System, Immune System, and Respiratory System.
LITSEA	⬡: Supports healthy immune function. ⬡: Helps clean and purify surfaces. ⬡: Use to support meditation and yoga. ⬡: Used as a flavoring in food. ✛: Body System(s) Affected: Digestive System, Immune System, and Respiratory System.
MAGNOLIA	⬡: Calming and relaxing. ⬡: Helps keep skin clean and healthy. ⬡: Soothing to the skin. ⬡: May help reduce feelings of anxiousness. ✛: Body System(s) Affected: Hormonal System, Immune System, and Skin.
MANUKA	⬡: Supports healthy respiratory function. ⬡: Helps support the appearance of youthful, clear skin. ⬡: Provides soothing support to sore muscles and joints. ✛: Body System(s) Affected: Muscles and Bones, Respiratory System, Skin.
MARJORAM	⬡: Valued for its calming properties and positive effect on the nervous system. ⬡: Soothes tired, stressed muscles. ⬡: Supports a healthy respiratory system. ⬡: Benefits the cardiovascular system. ✛: Body System(s) Affected: Cardiovascular System and Muscles.
MELALEUCA	⬡: Renowned for its cleansing and rejuvenating effects on the skin. ⬡: Promotes healthy immune function. ⬡: Protects against environmental and seasonal threats. ✛: Body System(s) Affected: Immune System, Respiratory System, Muscles, Bones, and Skin.

ESSENTIAL OILS	COMMON USES
MELISSA	: Supports and helps boost a healthy immune system. : Calms tension and nerves. : Addresses occasional stomach discomfort. : Body System(s) Affected: Emotional Balance and Skin.
MYRRH	: Powerful cleansing properties. : Soothing to the skin; promotes a smooth, youthful-looking complexion. : Promotes emotional balance and well-being. : Body System(s) Affected: Hormonal System, Immune System, Nervous System, and Skin.
NEROLI	: Promotes a positive mood. : May help reduce feelings of anxiousness. : Soothes skin. : Encourages relaxation. : Body System(s) Affected: Digestive System, Emotional Balance, and Skin
ORANGE	: Powerful cleanser and purifying agent. : Protects against environmental and seasonal threats. : High in antioxidants. : Uplifting to the mind and body. : Body System(s) Affected: Digestive System, Immune System, Emotional Balance, and Skin.
OREGANO	: Used as a powerful cleansing and purifying agent. : Supports healthy digestion and respiratory function. : Excellent source of antioxidants. : Body System(s) Affected: Immune System, Respiratory System, Muscles, and Bones.
PATCHOULI	: Grounding, balancing effect on emotions. : Helps skin recover quickly. : Soothes minor skin irritations. : Helps with head and neck tension. : Body System(s) Affected: Skin.
PEPPERMINT	: Promotes healthy respiratory function. : Alleviates occasional stomach upset. : Frequently used in toothpaste and chewing gum for oral health. : Body System(s) Affected: Digestive System, Muscles, Bones, Nervous System, Respiratory System, and Skin.
PETITGRAIN	: Supports healthy cardiovascular function. : Provides antioxidant support. : Supports healthy immune function. : Grounding, balancing effect on emotions. Promote Restful Sleep. : Body System(s) Affected: Emotional Balance
PINK PEPPER	: Promotes alertness and awareness. :Cleansing. : Body System(s) Affected: Immune System, Respiratory System, and Skin.
ROMAN CHAMOMILE	: Has a therapeutic, calming effect on the skin, mind, and body. : Soothes the systems of the body. : Supports healthy immune system function. : Body System(s) Affected: Emotional Balance, Nervous System, and Skin.
ROSE	: Helps balance moisture levels in the skin. : Reduces the appearance of skin imperfections. : Promotes an even skin tone and healthy complexion. : Emotionally uplifting. : Body System(s) Affected: Emotional Balance and Skin.
ROSEMARY	: Supports healthy digestion. : Soothes sore muscles and joints. : Helps reduce nervous tension and fatigue. : Body System(s) Affected: Immune System, Respiratory System, and Nervous System.

ESSENTIAL OILS	COMMON USES
SANDALWOOD	🝆: Promotes healthy, smooth skin. 🝆: Reduces the appearance of blemishes. 🝆: Enhances mood. 🝆: Frequently used in meditation for its grounding properties. ✚: Body System(s) Affected: Emotional Balance, Muscles, Bones, Nervous System, Skin.
SIBERIAN FIR	🝆: Provides soothing support to sore muscles and joints in massage. 🝆🝆: Supports clear breathing and respiratory function. 🝆: Promotes a feeling of relaxation. ✚: Body System(s) Affected: Muscles, Bones, Respiratory System.
SPEARMINT	🝆: Promotes digestion and helps reduce occasional stomach upset. 🝆: Promotes a sense of focus and uplifts mood. 🝆🝆: Cleanses the mouth and promotes fresh breath. ✚: Body System(s) Affected: Digestive System and Emotional Balance.
SPIKENARD	🝆🝆: Promotes feelings of calmness and relaxation. 🝆: Purifying to the skin. 🝆: Uplifting aroma. ✚: Body System(s) Affected: Emotional Balance, Skin.
STAR ANISE	🝆🝆🝆: Helps with occasional indigestion. 🝆🝆🝆: Relaxing. ✚: Body System(s) Affected: Cardiovascular System, Digestive System, Hormonal System, and Respiratory System.
THYME	🝆: Provides cleansing and purifying effects for the skin. 🝆🝆: Broad-spectrum activity in promoting wintertime health. ✚: Body System(s) Affected: Immune System, Muscles, and Bones.
TURMERIC	🝆🝆🝆: Powerful antioxidant. 🝆🝆🝆: Promotes healthy digestion. 🝆: May reduce appearance of blemishes. 🝆: Supports clean, healthy skin. ✚: Body System(s) Affected: Digestive System, Immune System, Skin.
VETIVER	🝆: Supports healthy circulation. 🝆: Calming, grounding effect on emotions. 🝆: Immune-enhancing properties. ✚: Body System(s) Affected: Emotional Balance, Hormonal System, Nervous System, and Skin.
WHITE FIR	🝆: Provides soothing support to sore muscles and joints. 🝆🝆: Supports clear breathing and respiratory function. 🝆🝆: Energizes the body and the mind. 🝆: Evokes feelings of stability, energy, and empowerment. ✚: Body System(s) Affected: Respiratory System.
WINTERGREEN	🝆: Soothes achy muscles and joints. 🝆: Promotes healthy respiratory function. ✚: Body System(s) Affected: Muscles and Bones.
YARROW	🝆🝆🝆: Powerful antioxidant. 🝆: Calming effect. 🝆: Uplifts mood. 🝆: Helps skin recover quickly. 🝆: Promotes clean, clear skin. ✚: Body System(s) Affected: Hormonal System, Immune System, and Skin.
YLANG YLANG	🝆🝆: Helps balance hormones. 🝆: Promotes healthy skin and hair. 🝆: Lifts mood while having a calming effect. 🝆🝆: Helps to lessen tension and stress. ✚: Body System(s) Affected: Emotional Balance, Cardiovascular System, and Hormonal System.
YUZU	🝆🝆: Calming. 🝆: Warming. ✚: Body System(s) Affected: Digestive System, Immune System, and Skin.

ESSENTIAL OILS	COMMON USES
AROMATOUCH	⊘⊜: Relaxes muscles and soothes joints. ⊜: Promotes circulation. ⊜: Helps to calm and soothe target areas. ✛: Body System(s) Affected: Respiratory System, Cardiovascular System, Muscles, and Bones.
BALANCE	⊘⊜: Creates a sense of calm and well-being. ⊜: Soothes sore muscles and joints. ⊜: Promotes circulation. ⊜: Supports cellular health and overall well-being. ✛: Body System(s) Affected: Muscles, Bones, Skin, Nervous System, and Emotional Balance.
BREATHE	⊜⊘: Maintains clear airways and breathing. ⊜⊘: Supports overall respiratory health. ⊜⊘: Helps minimize the effects of seasonal threats. ✛: Body System(s) Affected: Respiratory System and Skin.
CHEER	⊘⊜: Promotes feelings of optimism, cheerfulness, and happiness. ⊘⊜: Counteracts negative emotions of feeling down, blue, or low. ✛: Body System(s) Affected: Hormonal System and Emotional Balance.
CITRUS BLISS	⊘⊜: Cleanses and purifies the air and surfaces. ⊘⊜: Helps reduce stress and uplift mood. ⊘⊜: Positively affects mood with energizing and refreshing properties. ✛: Body System(s) Affected: Immune System and Emotional Balance.
CONSOLE	⊘⊜: Promotes feelings of comfort and hope. ⊘⊜: Counteracts negative emotions of grief, sadness, and hopelessness. ✛: Body System(s) Affected: Hormonal System and Emotional Balance.
DDR PRIME	◐: Supports healthy cellular integrity. ◐: Supports healthy cellular function and metabolism. ◐: Protects the body and cells from oxidative stress. ✛: Body System(s) Affected: Cardiovascular System, Immune System, Nervous System, Muscles, Bones, Skin, and Hair.
DEEP BLUE	⊜: Soothes sore muscles and achy joints. ⊜: Supports healthy circulation. ✛: Body System(s) Affected: Nervous System, Muscles, and Bones.
DIGESTZEN	◐⊜: Aids in the digestion of foods. ◐⊜: Soothes occasional stomach upset. ◐⊜: Maintains a healthy gastrointestinal tract. ✛: Body System(s) Affected: Digestive System.
ELEVATION	⊘⊜: Elevates mood and increases vitality. ⊘: Energizing, refreshing aroma. ⊘⊜: Helps to lessen sad and anxious feelings. ⊘⊜: Promotes a positive mood and energized mind and body. ✛: Body System(s) Affected: Emotional Balance.
FORGIVE	⊘⊜: Promotes feelings of contentment, relief, and patience. ⊘⊜: Counteracts negative emotions of anger and guilt. ✛: Body System(s) Affected: Hormonal System and Emotional Balance.
HD CLEAR	⊜: Helps keep skin clean, clear, and hydrated. ⊜: Promotes clear, smooth skin. ⊜: Soothes skin irritations. ⊜: Assists in cell renewal. ✛: Body System(s) Affected: Immune System.
IMMORTELLE	⊜: Reduces the appearance of fine lines and wrinkles. ⊜: Helps reduce contributing factors to aging skin. ⊜: Supports skin at a cellular level. ⊜: Helps sustain smoother, more radiant, and youthful skin. ✛: Body System(s) Affected: Skin.

ESSENTIAL OILS	COMMON USES
INTUNE	👁️👃: Enhances and sustains focus. 👁️👃: Supports efforts of those who have difficulty paying attention and staying on task. 👃: Promotes healthy thought processes. ✚: Body System(s) Affected: Emotional Balance, Hormonal System, and Nervous System.
KIDS: BRAVE	👁️👃: Helps reduce anxious feelings. 👁️👃: Uplifting to the mood. 👁️👃: Promotes courage. ✚: Body System(s) Affected: Nervous System and Emotional Balance.
KIDS: CALMER	👁️👃: Helps reduce stress and anxious feelings. 👁️👃: Calming. 👁️👃: Promotes restful sleep. 👁️👃: Lessens feelings of tension. ✚: Body System(s) Affected: Nercous System and Emotional Balance.
KIDS: RESCUER	👃: Soothes sore muscles and achy joints. 👁️👃: Helps reduce stress. 👁️👃: Eases muscle tension in the head and neck. ✚: Body System(s) Affected: Nervous System and Muscles and Bones.
KIDS: STEADY	👃: Enhances and sustains focus. 👁️👃: Helps reduce anxious feelings. 👁️👃: Creates a sense of calm and well-being. 👁️👃: Uplifts mood. 👁️👃: Energizes. ✚: Body System(s) Affected: Nervous System and Emotional Balance.
KIDS: STRONGER	👃: Promotes healthy skin. 👁️👃: Cleansing. 👃: Promotes skin healing. 👁️👃: Supports immune system. ✚: Body System(s) Affected: Immune System and Skin.
KIDS: THINKER	👁️👃: Enhances and sustains focus. 👁️👃: Promotes alertness. 👁️👃: Helps reduce stress and anxious feelings. 👁️👃: Calming. ✚: Body System(s) Affected: Nervous System and Emotional Balance.
MOTIVATE	👁️👃: Promotes feelings of confidence, courage, and belief. 👁️👃: Counteracts negative emotions of doubt, pessimism, and cynicism. ✚: Body System(s) Affected: Hormonal System and Emotional Balance.
ON GUARD	👁️👃💧: Supports healthy immune function. 👁️👃💧: Protects against environmental threats. 👃: Cleans surfaces. 👃: Purifies the skin while promoting healthy circulation. ✚: Body System(s) Affected: Immune System.
PASSION	👁️👃: Ignites feelings of excitement, passion, and joy. 👁️👃: Counteracts negative feelings of boredom and disinterest. ✚: Body System(s) Affected: Hormonal System and Emotional Balance.
PASTTENSE	👁️👃: Eases muscle tension in the head and neck. 👁️👃: Helps reduce tension, stress, and worry. 👃: Soothes the mind and body. 👃: Calms emotions. ✚: Body System(s) Affected: Nervous System, Muscles, and Bones.
PEACE	👁️👃: Promotes feelings of peace, reassurance, and contentment. 👁️👃: Counteracts anxious and fearful emotions. ✚: Body System(s) Affected: Hormonal System and Emotional Balance.
PURIFY	👃: Refreshing aroma. 👃: Eradicates unpleasant odors and clears the air. 👁️👃: Protects against environmental threats. ✚: Body System(s) Affected: Digestive System, Emotional Balance, and Skin.

ESSENTIAL OILS	COMMON USES
SERENITY	*⊘*: Calming, renewing fragrance. *⊘◒*: Promotes relaxation and restful sleep. *⊘*: Diffuses into a subtle aroma; ideal for aromatic benefits. *⊘◒*: Lessens tension and calms emotions. ✛: Body System(s) Affected: Nervous System and Emotional Balance.
SLIM & SASSY	*⊘◯*: Promotes healthy metabolism. *⊘◯*: Stimulates the endocrine system. *⊘◯*: Helps manage hunger cravings. *⊘◯*: Calms the stomach and lifts mood. *⊘*: Promotes a positive mood. ✛: Body System(s) Affected: Digestive System and Emotional Balance.
TERRASHIELD	*◒⊘*: Acts as an effective, natural repellent. *◒⊘*: Helps ward off insects. ✛: Body System(s) Affected: Skin.
WHISPER	*⊘*: Combines with each individual's chemistry to create a beautiful, unique, and personal fragrance. *⊘*: Provides a warming aroma that entices the senses and intrigues the mind. *◒⊘*: Calms the skin and emotions. ✛: Body System(s) Affected: Emotional Balance and Skin.
WOMEN'S MONTHLY BLEND	*◒⊘*: Helps balance hormones. *◒⊘*: Provides temporary respite from cramps, hot flashes, and emotional swings. ✛: Body System(s) Affected: Hormonal System, Emotional Balance, and Skin.
YARROW POM	*◯*: Promotes youthful looking skin. *◯*: Promotes healthy skin. *◯*: Antioxidant. *◯*: Supports cellular health. ✛: Body System(s) Affected: Cardiovascular System, Immune System, Nervous System, Emotional Balance, and Skin.
ZENDOCRINE	*◯◒*: Supports the body's natural ability to rid itself of unwanted substances. *◯◒*: Supports healthy liver function. *◯◒*: Purifying and detoxifying to the body's systems. ✛: Body System(s) Affected: Hormonal System, Emotional Balance, Skin, and Hair.

Appendix D: Taxonomical Information

The following chart is the taxonomical breakdown of the plant families for each of the essential oils found in this book. Following this division chart, there is further information for each family—including the plants within that family that essential oils are derived from, the body systems affected by these essential oils, the properties of these oils, and general uses for these oils.

Division: Embryophyte Siphonogama (plants with seeds)

Subdivision: Gymnosperm (plants with concentric rings, exposed seeds, and resinous wood)

Class: Coniferae (cone-bearing plants) and Taxaceae (yew-like plants)

Family: Pinaceae (trees or shrubs with cones and numerous "scales")

Genus: Abies (firs, balsam trees), Cedrus (cedars), Pinus (pines), Picea (spruces), Pseudotsuga (false hemlock), Tsuga (hemlocks)

Family: Cupressaceae

Genus: Callitris (blue cypress), Cupressus (cypresses), Juniperus (junipers), Thuja (arborvitae or cedars)

Subdivision: Angiosperm (highly evolved plants with seeds enclosed by fruits)

Class: Monocotyledons (plants with one-leaf embryos)

Family: Gramineae, Zingiberaceae

Class: Dicotyledons (plants with multiple-leaf embryos)

Family: Annonaceae, Betulaceae, Burseraceae, Cistaceae, Compositae, Ericaceae, Geraniaceae, Guttiferae, Labiatae, Lauraceae, Myrtaceae, Oleaceae, Piperaceae, Rosaceae, Rutaceae, Santalaceae, Styracaceae, Umbelliferae

Annonaceae
Shrubs, trees, climbers; fragrant flowers; 128 genera, 2000 species; mostly tropical, found in Old World and rain forest.

Body Systems: Cardiovascular System, Nervous System (calming), Hormonal System (aphrodesiac)

Properties: extreme fire and water; nervous sedative, balancing

General Uses: depression, frigidity, impotence, palpitations, skin care

Cananga odorata: two forms exist: var. odorata (var. genuina., *Unona odorantissimum*): ylang-ylang; var. macrophylla: cananga

Betulaceae
Shrubs, trees; fruit is one-seeded nut, often winged; includes birches, alders, hornbeams, and hazels; 6 genera, 150 species; from northern hemisphere to tropical mountains.

Body Systems: Digestive and Respiratory Systems, Muscles and Bones

Properties: analgesic, draining (lymph), purifying

General Uses: auto intoxication, muscle pain

Betula lenta: sweet birch

Burseraceae
Means "dry fire"; resinous tropical timber trees; drupe or capsule fruit; 21 genera, 540 species.

Body Systems: Respiratory System (secretions), Emotional Balance (psychic centers)

Skin Properties: cooling, drying, fortifying

General Uses: anti-inflammatory, expectorant, scar tissue (reducing), ulcers, wounds (healing)

Boswellia frereana: frankincense

Commiphora myrrha: myrrh

Compositae (Asteraceae)
Largest family of flowering plants; inflorescent, small flowers; 1317 genera, 21,000 species; found everywhere, especially around Mediterranean.

Body Systems: Digestive System, Skin

Properties: "perfect balance of etheric and astral forces, promoting realization, reorganization, structure" [Lavabre, *Aromatherapy Workbook*]; adaptive, calming, regeneration (note: because of the large variety of plants within this family, the therapeutic activity is very diversified; some plants are neurotoxic)

General Uses: infections, inflammation, regeneration

Chamaemelum nobile: Roman chamomile

Helichrysum angustifolium (var. Italicum): helichrysum

Cupressaceae

Conifer cypress family, needle-like leaves and cones; 17 genera, 113 species, most in northern temperate zones.

Body Systems: Hormonal, Respiratory, and Nervous Systems

Properties: appeasing, reviving, tonic, warming

General Uses: antirheumatic, astringent, cellulite (reduces), insomnia, nervous tension (reduces), respiration (when taken through inhalation), stress-related conditions

Cupressus sempervirens: cypress

Juniperus virginiana: red cedarwood

Juniperus communis: juniper

Ericaceae

Shrubs and small trees with leathery evergreen leaves, fruit berry, drupe, or capsule; 103 genera, 3350 species; cosmopolitan centered in northern hemisphere.

Body Systems: Cardiovascular and Digestive Systems

Properties: detoxifying

General Uses: hypertension, kidney and liver stimulant

Gaultheria procumbens: wintergreen

Geraniaceae

Herbs or low shrubs, 14 genera, 730 species; temperate and tropical zones.

Body Systems: Hormonal System, Digestive System (kidneys (excretion), liver and pancreas (metabolism)), Nervous System, Emotional Balance

Properties: balancing (nervous system)

General Uses: burns, depression, diabetes, hemorrhaging, nervous tension, skin, sore throat, ulcers, wounds

Pelargonium graveolens: geranium

Gramineae (or Poaceae)

Nutritious grass family; used for ground covering and food (wheat, rice, corn, barley); large root systems; 737 genera, 7950 species; distributed throughout the world.

Body Systems: Cardiovascular System, Digestive System (stimulant), Respiratory System, Skin

Properties: air purifier, calming, refreshing, sedative

General Uses: air deodorizer, calm digestion, cleanse and balance skin (acne)

Cymbopogon flexuosus: lemongrass

Vetiveria zizanoides: vetiver

Labiatae (Lamiaceae)

Herbs or low shrubs with quadrangular stems; largest of all essential oil–producing plant families; oils are mostly nontoxic and non-hazardous; some antiseptic oils; some oils used for flavoring; most oils helpful for headaches, congestion, muscular problems (analgesic, anti-inflammatory); oils stimulate one or more body systems; 224 genera, about 5600 species; main distribution in tropical and warmer temperate regions.

Body Systems: Digestive and Respiratory Systems

Properties: appeases overactive astral body [Lavabre, *Aromatherapy Workbook*], curative, stimulates, warms

General Uses: anemia, diabetes, digestion (poor), headaches, respiratory problems; "good for people with intense psychic activity to prevent exhaustion and loss of self" [Lavabre, Aromatherapy Workbook]

Lavandula angustifolia: lavender

Mentha piperita: peppermint

Origanum majorana: marjoram

Origanum vulgare: oregano

Rosmarinus officinalis: rosemary; several varieties—var. officinalis: common rosemary; numerous cultivars and forms; chemotypes: CT I: camphor; CT II: cineole; CT III: verbenone

Salvia sclarea: clary sage

Thymus vulgaris: thyme; chemotypes: linalool; thymol (or geraniol)

Appendix

Lauraceae

Trees and shrubs with evergreen leaves and aromatic oils; some valued for timber, as ornamentals, or for oils or spices; 45 genera, 2500-3000 species; found in tropics and subtropics in Amazona and Southeast Asia.

Body Systems: Cardiovascular System (cardiac stimulant, pulmonary stimulant), Nervous System (regulator), Hormonal System (aphrodisiac), Skin (cellular regenerator)

Properties: antifungal, antiviral, antibacterial, stimulant, tonic (some oils in this family are irritant)

General Uses: depression, headache, hypotension, scars, sexual debility

Cinnamomum cassia: cassia

Cinnamomum zeylanicum: cinnamon bark

Laurus nobilis: laurel (bay)

Ravensara aromatica: ravensara

Myrtaceae

Mainly tropical and subtropical plants with dotted leaves and oil glands; fruit is woody capsule or berry with one or many seeds; some have ornamental or showy flowers; many produce valuable timber; 121 genera, 3850 species; found in tropical and warm regions, especially Australia.

Body Systems: Respiratory and Immune Systems

Properties: "balances interaction of four elements (earth, air, fire, water)" [Lavabre, Aromatherapy Workbook], antiseptic, stimulant, tonic

General Uses: antiseptic, energy (balances), respiratory (infections), stimulant, tonic

Backhousia citriodora: lemon myrtle

Eucalyptus globulus: eucalyptus

Eucalyptus radiata: eucalyptus radiata

Eugenia caryophyllata: clove bud

Melaleuca alternifolia: melaleuca (tea tree)

Oleaceae

Trees or shrubs, including olive and ash; used for timber; 24 genera, 900 species; widely distributed, centered on Asia.

Body Systems: Emotional Balance, Hormonal System (aphrodisiac)

Properties: calming, soothing, uplifting

General Uses: anxiety, depression, frigidity, impotence, stress

Jasminum officinale: jasmine

Pinaceae (Abietaceae)

Conifers with male and female cones; 9 genera, 194 species; found in northern hemisphere, temperate climates.

Body Systems: Hormonal, Nervous, and Respiratory Systems; signifies air element

Properties: antiseptic, appeasing, reviving, tonic, warming

General Uses: arthritis, congestion (inhaled), oxygen deficiency, respiratory disorders, rheumatism, stress

Abies alba: white fir, silver fir

Picea mariana: spruce, black spruce

Pinus sylvestris: pine, Scotch pine

Rosaceae

Trees, shrubs, and herbs; some edible fruits; many cultivated for fruits (almond) or flowers (rose); 107 genera, 3100 species; found in temperate climates throughout the world.

Body Systems: Hormonal System (female reproductive); heart chakra

Properties: aphrodisiac, harmonizing, tonic, uplifting

General Uses: emotional shock, frigidity, grief, impotence

Rosa damascena: Bulgarian rose

Rutaceae

Aromatic trees and shrubs; sometimes thorny; dotted, compound leaves with aromatic glands; includes citrus fruits; 161 genera, about 1650 species; found in tropical and warm temperate regions, especially Australia and South Africa.

Body Systems: Digestive (kidneys, liver) and Nervous Systems, Skin

Properties: cooling, refreshing, secretion (fruits), sedative (flowers)

General Uses: inflammation, oversensitivity, water balance

Citrus aurantifolia: lime

Citrus bergamia: bergamot

Citrus limon: lemon

Citrus nobilis: tangerine

Citrus x paradisi: grapefruit

Citrus reticulate: mandarin

Citrus sinensis: orange

Santalaceae

Herbs, shrubs, and trees which are semiparasitic on roots and stems of other plants; 36 genera, about 500 species; found in tropical and temperate regions.

Body Systems: Digestive System (excretory balance, genitourinary disinfectant), Nervous System (balances), and Respiratory System (balances)

Properties: balancing, calming, constriction, grounding

General Uses: genitourinary tract infections, impotence, lung congestion, stress-related disorders

Santalum album: East Indian sandalwood, Mysore sandalwood, sandalwood

Umbelliferae (Apiaceae)

Herbs and a few shrubs, flowers borne in umbels (flowers radiating from a central point, like an umbrella); some important as food (carrot, celery), while others are very poisonous; some have medicinal actions; 420 genera, 3100 species; found throughout the world, mainly in northern temperate regions.

Body Systems: Digestive System (balances), Hormonal System (stimulates uterus), Respiratory System, Skin (regenerates)

Properties: air element; accumulation (elimination, excretion), secretion

General Uses: gas, glandular problems, spasms

Carum carvi: caraway

Coriandrum sativum: coriander (from seeds), cilantro (from leaves)

Cuminum cyminum: cumin

Foeniculum vulgare: fennel

Pimpinella anisum: anise

Zingiberaceae

Ginger family comprising rhizomatous herbs; 53 genera, 1200 species; found mostly in rain forests throughout the tropics, but mainly in Indo-Malaysia.

Body Systems: Digestive and Hormonal Systems, Muscles and Bones

Properties: analgesic, fever reducing, scurvy (prevents), stimulant, tonic, warming

General Uses: digestive (stimulant), rheumatism, sexual tonic

Zingiber officinale: ginger

Research References

Aalinkeel R et al. (2008 Aug 25). "The dietary bioflavonoid, quercetin, selectively Aalinkeel R et al. (2008 Aug 25). "The dietary bioflavonoid, quercetin, selectively induces apoptosis of prostate cancer cells by down-regulating the expression of heat shock protein 90," Prostate.

Abbasi M N, Abbasi M S, Bekhradi R (2013). "Suppressive effects of rosa damascena essential oil on naloxone-precipitated morphine withdrawal signs in male mice," Iran J Pharm Res. 12(3):357-61.

Abdel-Aal el, S. M., Akhtar, H., Zaheer, K., & Ali, R. (2013 Apr). Dietary sources of lutein and zeaxanthin carotenoids and their role in eye health. Nutrients, 5(4), 1169-1185.

Abdel-Sattar E, Zaitoun AA, Farag MA, El Gayed SH, Harraz FM (2009 Feb 25). "Chemical composition, insecticidal and insect repellent activity of Schinus molle L. leaf and fruit essential oils against Trogoderma granarium and Tribolium castaneum," Nat Prod Res. Epub ahead of print: 1-10.

Abdullah, D., Ping, Q. N., & Liu, G. J. (1996 Jan). Enhancing effect of essential oils on the penetration of 5-fluorouracil through rat skin. Yao Xue Xue Bao, 31(3), 214-221.

Abebe, W. (2002). Herbal medication: potential for adverse interactions with analgesic drugs. Journal of Clinical Pharmacy and Therapeutics, 27(6), 391-401.

Abedon, B (2008). "Essentra - a patented extract that reduces stress and enhances sleep," (http://www.nutragenesisnutrition.com/images/stories/pdf/ess_stress_wp.pdf):1-4.

Abenavoli L, Capasso R, Milic N, Capasso F (2010 Jun 7). "Milk thistle in liver diseases: past, present, future," Phytother Res. Epub ahead of print.

Adam B, Liebregts T, Best J, Bechmann L, Lackner C, Neumann J, Koehler S, Holtmann G (2006 Feb). "A combination of peppermint oil and caraway oil attenuates the post-inflammatory visceral hyperalgesia in a rat model," Scand J Gastroenterol. 41(2):155-60.

Adib-Hajbaghery M, Mousavi SN (2017 Dec). "The effects of chamomile extract on sleep quality among elderly people: A clinical trial," Complement Ther Med. 35:109-114.

Agero A.L.C., Verallo-Rowell V.M (2004 Sep). "A randomized double-blind controlled trial comparing extra virgin coconut oil with mineral oil as a moisturizer for mild to moderate xerosis," Dermatitis. 15(3):109-116.

Agrawal, P., Rai, V., & Singh, R. B. (1996 Sep). Randomized placebo-controlled, single blind trial of holy basil leaves in patients with noninsulin-dependent diabetes mellitus. Int J Clin Pharmacol Ther, 34(9), 406-409.

Ahmad A, Khan A, Kah L.A., Manzoor N (2012 Oct). "In vitro synergy of eugenol and methyleugenol with fluconazole against clinical Candida isolates," J. Med. Microbiol. 59(10):1178-1184.

Ahmad S, Beg Z.H. (2013 Jun). "Hypolipidemic and antioxidant activities of thymoquinone and limonene in atherogenic suspension fed rats," Food Chem. 138(2-3):1116-1124.

Ahmed H.H., Abd-Rabou A.A., Hassan A.Z., "Phytochemical Analysis and Anticancer Investigation of Bswellia serrata Bioactive Constituents In Vitro," Asian Pac. J. Cancer Prev. 16(16):7179-7188.

Akha, O., Rabiei, K., Kashi, Z., Bahar, A., Zaeif-Khorasani, E., Kosaryan, M., . . . Emadian, O. (2014). The effect of fennel (Foeniculum vulgare) gel 3% in decreasing hair thickness in idiopathic mild to moderate hirsutism, A randomized placebo controlled clinical trial. Caspian J Intern Med, 5(1), 26-29.

Akhondzadeh S, Naghavi HR, Vazirian M, Shayeganpour A, Rashidi H, Khani M (2001 Oct). "Passionflower in the treatment of generalized anxiety: a pilot double-blind randomized controlled trial with oxazepam," J Clin Pharm Ther. 26(5):363-7.

Akhtar, S., Ismail, T., & Riaz, M. (2013). Flaxseed - a miraculous defense against some critical maladies. Pak J Pharm Sci, 26(1), 199-208.

Al-Ali, K. H., El-Beshbishy, H. A., El-Badry, A. A., & Alkhalaf, M. (2013 Dec). Cytotoxic activity of methanolic extract of Mentha longifolia and Ocimum basilicum against human breast cancer. Pak J Biol Sci, 16(23), 1744-1750.

Alam, P., Ansari, M.J., Anwer, M.K., Raish, M. Kamal, Y.K., & Shakeel, F. (2017 May). "Wound healing effects of nanoemulsion containing clove essential oil," Artif Cells Nanomed Biotechnol. 45(3):591-597.

Al-Anati L, Essid E, Reinehr R, Petzinger E (2009 Apr). "Silibinin protects OTA-mediated TNF-alpha release from perfused rat livers and isolated rat Kupffer cells," Mol Nutr Food Res. 53(4):460-6.

al-Bagieh N.H., Idowu A, Salako N.O. (1994). "Effect of aqueous extract of miswak on the in vitro growth of Candida albicans," Microbios. 80(323):107-113.

Alberti, T.B., Barbosa, W. L.R., Vieira, J.L.F., Raposo, N.R.B., & Dutra, R.C. (2017). "(-)-β-Caryophyllene, a CB2 Receptor-Selective Phytocannabinoid, Suppresses Motor Paralysis and Neuroinflammation in a Murine Model of Multiple Sclerosis," Int J Mol Sci. 18(4):691.

Alberts, B., Bray, D., Hopkin, K., Johnson, A., Lewis, J., Raff, M., . . . Walter, P. (2013). Essential cell biology. New York, NY: Garland Science.

Albertsson, P. A., Kohnke, R., Emek, S. C., Mei, J., Rehfeld, J. F., Akerlund, H. E., & Erlanson-Albertsson, C. (2007 Feb 1). Chloroplast membranes retard fat digestion and induce satiety: effect of biological membranes on pancreatic lipase/co-lipase. Biochem J, 401(3), 727-733.

Alexandrovich I, Rakovitskaya O, Kolmo E, Sidorova T, Shushunov S (2003 Jul-Aug). "The effect of fennel (Foeniculum Vulgare) seed oil emulsion in infantile colic: a randomized, placebo-controlled study," Altern Ther Health Med. 9(4):58-61.

Alfthan G, Tapani K, Nissinen A, et al. (2004). "The effect of low doses of betaine on plasma homocysteine in healthy volunteers," Br J Nutr. 92:665-669.

al-Hader AA, Hasan ZA, Aqel MB (1994 Jul 22). "Hyperglycemic and insulin release inhibitory effects of Rosmarinus officinalis," J Ethnopharmacol. 43(3):217-21.

Al-Harrasi A. et al (2014 Sep). "Analgesic effects of crude extracts and fractions of Omani frankincense obtained from traditional medicinal plant Boswellia sacra on animal models," Asian Pac J Trop Med. 7S1:S485-49

Al-Howiriny, T., Alsheikh, A., Alqasoumi, S., Al-Yahya, M., ElTahir, K., & Rafatullah, S. (2009 Aug). Protective Effect of Origanum majorana L. 'Marjoram' on various models of gastric mucosal injury in rats. Am J Chin Med, 37(3), 531-545.

Ali, S. A., Rizk, M. Z., Ibrahim, N. A., Abdallah, M. S., Sharara, H. M., & Moustafa, M. M. (2010 Dec). Protective role of Juniperus phoenicea and Cupressus sempervirens against CCl(4). World J Gastrointest Pharmacol Ther, 1(6), 123-131.

Allman-Farinelli, M. A., Gomes, K., Favaloro, E. J., & Petocz, P. (2005 Jul 29). A diet rich in high-oleic-acid sunflower oil favorably alters low-density lipoprotein cholesterol, triglycerides, and factor VII coagulant activity. J Am Diet Assoc, 105(7), 1071-1079.

Almas K., Al-Zeid Z (2004 Feb). "The immediate antimicrobial effect of a toothbrush and miswak on cariogenic bacteria: a clinical study," J. Contemp. Dent. Pract. 5(1):105-114.

Almela L, Sánchez-Muñoz B, Fernández-López JA, Roca MJ, Rabe V (2006 Jul). "Liquid chromatograpic-mass spectrometric analysis of phenolics and free radical scavenging activity of rosemary extract from different raw material," J Chromatogr A. 1120(1-2):221-9.

Aloisi AM, Ceccarelli I, Masi F, Scaramuzzino A (2002 Oct 17). "Effects of the essential oil from citrus lemon in male and female rats exposed to a persistent painful stimulation," Behav Brain Res. 136(1):127-35.

Alqareer A, Alyahya A, Andersson L (2006 Nov). "The effect of clove and benzocaine versus placebo as topical anesthetics," J Dent. 34(10):747-50.

Al-Saidi S, Rameshkumar K.B., Hisham A, Sivakumar N, Al-Kind (2012 Mar). "Composition and antibacterial activity of the essential oils of four commercial grades of Omani luban, the oleo-gum resin of Boswellia sacra FLUECK," Chem. Biodivers. 9(3):615-624.

Al-Snafi, A.E. (2015). "The Pharmacological importance of Bellis perennis - A review," Int J Phytotherapy. 5(2):63-69.

al-Zuhair H, el-Sayeh B, Ameen HA, al-Shoora H (1996 Jul-Aug). "Pharmacological studies of cardamom oil in animals," Pharmacol Res. 34(1-2):79-82.

Amano S, Akutsu N, Ogura Y, Nishiyama T (2004 Nov). "Increase of laminin 5 synthesis in human keratinocytes by acute wound fluid, inflammatory cytokines and growth factors, and lysophospholipids," Br J Dermatol. 151(5):961-70.

Amantea D, Fratto V, Maida S, Rotiroti D, Ragusa S, Nappi G, Bagetta G, Corasaniti MT (2009). "Prevention of Glutamate Accumulation and Upregulation of Phospho-Akt may Account for Neuroprotection Afforded by Bergamot Essential Oil against Brain Injury Induced by Focal Cerebral Ischemia in Rat," Int Rev Neurobiol. 85:389-405.

Ambrosone CB, McCann SE, Freudenheim JL, Marshall JR, Zhang Y, Shields PG (2004 May). "Breast cancer risk in premenopausal women is inversely associated with consumption of broccoli, a source of isothiocyanates, but is not modified by GST genotype," J Nutr. 134(5):1134-8.

American Cancer Society (2008). "Cancer Facts and Figures." Downloaded at http://www.cancer.org/downloads/STT/2008CAFFfinalsecured.pdf.

Amine, E., Baba, N., Belhadj, M., Deurenberg-Yap, M., Djazayery, A., Forrester, T., ... & Yoshiike, N. (2002). Diet, nutrition and the prevention of chronic diseases: Report of a Joint WHO/FAO Expert Consultation. World Health Organization.

Ammar, A.H., Bouajila, J., Lebrihi, A., Mathieu, F., Romdhane, M., Zagrouba, F. (2012). "Chemical composition and in vitro antimicrobial and antioxidant activities of Citrus aurantium l. flowers essential oil (Neroli oil)," Pak J Biol Sci. 15(21):1034-40.

Ammon HP (2002). "Boswellic acids (components of frankincense) as the active principle in treatment of chronic inflammatory diseases," Wien Med Wochenschr. 152(15-16):373-8.

Amoian B, Moghadamnia A.A., Barzi S, Sheykholeslami S, Rangiani A (2010 Aug). "Salvadora Persica extract chewing gum and gingival health: Improvement of gingival and probebleeding index," Complement. Ther. Clin. Pract. 16(3):121-123.

An, R., Chiu, C. Y., Zhang, Z., & Burd, N. A. (2014). Nutrient intake among US adults with disabilities. Journal of Human Nutrition and Dietetics.

Anderson, J. W., Weiter, K. M., Christian, A. L., Ritchey, M. B., & Bays, H. E. (2014 Jan 1). Raisins compared with other snack effects on glycemia and blood pressure: a randomized, controlled trial. Postgrad Med, 126(1), 37-43.

Anderson KJ, Teuber SS, Gobeille A, Cremin P, Waterhouse AL, Steinberg FM (2001 Nov). "Walnut polyphenolics inhibit in vitro human plasma and LDL oxidation," J Nutr. 131(11):2837-42.

Ando Y (1994 Aug). "[Breeding control and immobilizing effects of wood microingredients on house dust mites]," Nihon Koshu Eisei Zasshi. 41(8):741-50.

Andradea, E. H. A., Alves, C. N., Guimarães, E. F., Carreira, L. M. M., & Maia, J. G. S. (2011 Sep). Variability in essential oil composition of Piper dilatatum L.C. Rich. Biochemical Systematics and Ecology, 39, 669-675.

Andrews R.E., Parks L.W., Spence K.D. (1980) Some Effects of Douglas Fir Terpenes on Certain Microorganisms. Applied and Environmental Microbiology. 40: 301-304.

Andrian E., Grenier D., Rouabhia M. (2006) Porphyromonas gingivalis-Epithelial Cell Interactions in Periodontitis. Journal of Dental Research. 85: 392-403.

Antimutagenic effects of extracts from sage (Salvia officinalis) in mammalian system in vivo. (2006 Jul 19). "Relaxant effects of Rosa damascena on guinea pig tracheal chains and its possible mechanism(s)," J Ethnopharmacol. 106(3):377-82.

Apay S.E., Arslan S, Akpinar R.B., Celebioglu A (2012 Dec). "Effect of aromatherapy massage on dysmenorrhea in Turkish students," Pain Manag. Nurs. Off. J. Am. Soc. Pain Manag. Nurses. 13(4): 236-240.

Appendino G, Ottino M, Marquez N, Bianchi F, Giana A, Ballero M, Sterner O, Fiebich BL, Munoz E (2007 Apr). "Arzanol, an anti-inflammatory and anti-HIV-1 phloroglucinol alpha-Pyrone from Helichrysum italicum ssp. microphyllum," J Nat Prod. 70(4):608-12.

Aqel MB (1991 May-Jun). "Relaxant effect of the volatile oil of Rosmarinus officinalis on tracheal smooth muscle," J Ethnopharmacol. 33(1-2):57-62.

Arasada BL, Bommareddy A, Zhang X, Bremmon K, Dwivedi C. (2008 Jan-Feb). "Effects of alpha-santalol on proapoptotic caspases and p53 expression in UVB irradiated mouse skin," Anticancer Res. 28(1A):129-32.

Arash, A., Mohammad, M. Z., Jamal, M. S., Mohammad, T. A., & Azam, A. (2013 Oct). Effects of the Aqueous Extract of Anethum graveolens Leaves on Seizure Induced by Pentylenetetrazole in Mice. Malays J Med Sci, 20(5), 23-30.

Archana R, Namasivayam A (1999 Jan). "Antistressor effect of Withania somnifera," J Ethnopharmacol. 64(1):91-3.

Arima, Y., Nakai, Y., Hayakawa, R., & Nishino, T. (2003 Jan). Antibacterial effect of beta-thujaplicin on staphylococci isolated from atopic dermatitis: relationship between changes in the number of viable bacterial cells and clinical improvement in an eczematous lesion of atopic dermatitis. J Antimicrob Chemother, 51(1), 113-122.

Arunakul M, Thaweboon B, Thaweboon S, Asvanund Y, Charoenchaikorn K (2011 Dec). "Efficacy of xylitol and fluoride mouthrinses on salivary Mutans streptococci," Asian Pac. J. Trop. Biomed. 1(6):488-490.

Arzi A, Sela L, Green A, Givaty G, Dagan Y, Sobel N (2010 Jan). "The influence of odorants on respiratory patterns in sleep," Chem. Senses. 35(1):31-40.

Asakura, K., Matsuo, Y., Oshima, T., Kihara, T., Minagawa, K., Araki, Y., . . . Ninomiya, M. (2000 Apr). omega-agatoxin IVA-sensitive Ca(2+) channel blocker, alpha-eudesmol, protects against brain injury after focal ischemia in rats. Eur J Pharmacol, 394(1), 57-65.

Asao T, Kuwano H, Ide M, Hirayama I, Nakamura JI, Fujita KI, Horiuti R (2003 Apr). "Spasmolytic effect of peppermint oil in barium during double-contrast barium enema compared with Buscopan," Clin Radiol. 58(4):301-5.

Asensio, C. M., Nepote, V., & Grosso, N. R. (2011 Sep). Chemical stability of extra-virgin olive oil added with oregano essential oil. J Food Sci, 76(7), S445-450.

Asnaashari, S., Delazar, A., Habibi, B., Vasfi, R., Nahar, L., Hamedeyazdan, S., & Sarker, S. D. (2010 Dec). Essential oil from Citrus aurantifolia prevents ketotifen-induced weight-gain in mice. Phytother Res, 24(12), 1893-1897.

Astani A, Reichling J, Schnitzler P (2011). "Screening for antiviral activities of isolated compounds from essential oils," Evid.-Based Complement. Altern. Med. ECAM. 2011:253643.

Atsumi T, Tonosaki K (2007 Feb). "Smelling lavender and rosemary increases free radical scavenging activity and decreases cortisol level in saliva," Psychiatry Res. 150(1):89-96.

Auffray, B. (2007 Feb). Protection against singlet oxygen, the main actor of sebum squalene peroxidation during sun exposure, using Commiphora myrrha essential oil. Int J Cosmet Sci, 29(1), 23-29.

Australia Rural Industries Research and Development Corporation. (n.d.). Essential Oils and Plant Extracts. Retrieved Sept. 29, 2014 from http://www.rirdc.gov.au/research-programs/plant-industries/essential-oils-and-plant-extracts.

Awale, S., Tohda, C., Tezuka, Y., Miyazaki, M., & Kadota, S. (2011). Protective Effects of Rosa damascena and Its Active Constituent on Abeta(25-35)-Induced Neuritic Atrophy. Evid Based Complement Alternat Med, 2011, 1-8.

Azanchi, T., Shafaroodi, H., and Asgarpanah, J. (2014). "Anticonvulsant activity of Citrus aurantium blossom essential oil (neroli): involvment of the GABAergic system," Nat Prod Commun. 9(11):1615-8.

Baba, T., Nakano, H., Tamai, K., Sawamura, D., Hanada, K., Hashimoto, I., & Arima, Y. (1998 Jan). Inhibitory effect of beta-thujaplicin on ultraviolet B-induced apoptosis in mouse keratinocytes. J Invest Dermatol, 110(1), 24-28.

Babu, K. G., Singh, B., Joshi, V. P., & Singh, V. (2002). Essential oil composition of Damask rose (Rosa damascena Mill.) distilled under different pressures and temperatures. Flavour and Fragrance Journal, 17(2), 136-140.

Badia P, Wesensten N, Lammers W, Culpepper J, Harsh J (1990 Jul). "Responsiveness to olfactory stimuli presented in sleep," Physiol Behav. 48(1):87-90.

Bae GS et al (2012 Oct). "Protective effects of alpha-pinene in mice with cerulein-induced acute pancreatitis," Life Sciences. 91(17-18):866-871.

Bagchi D, Hassoun EA, Bagchi M, Stohs SJ (1993 Aug). "Protective effects of antioxidants against endrin-induced hepatic lipid peroxidation, DNA damage, and excretion of urinary lipid metabolites," Free Radic Biol Med. 15(2):217-22.

Bagchi D, Sen CK, Ray SD, Das DK, Bagchi M, Preuss HG, Vinson JA (2003 Feb-Mar). "Molecular mechanisms of cardioprotection by a novel grape seed proanthocyanidin extract," Mutat Res. 523-24:87-97.

Bagg J, Jackson MS, Petrina Sweeney M, Ramage G, Davies AN (2006 May). "Susceptibility to Melaleuca alternifolia (tea tree) oil of yeasts isolated from the mouths of patients with advanced cancer," Oral Oncol. 42(5):487-92.

Bagheri-Nesami M, Espahbodi F, Nikkhah A, Shorofi S.A., Charati J.Y. (2014 Feb). "The effects of lavender aromatherapy on pain following needle insertion into a fistula in hemodialysis patients," Complement. Ther. Clin. Pract. 20(1):1-4.

Bahramikia, S., & Yazdanparast, R. (2009 Aug). Efficacy of different fractions of Anethum graveolens leaves on serum lipoproteins and serum and liver oxidative status in experimentally induced hypercholesterolaemic rat models. Am J Chin Med, 37(4), 685-699.

Bakirel T, Bakirel U, Keleş OU, Ulgen SG, Yardibi H (2008 Feb 28). "In vivo assessment of antidiabetic and antioxidant activities of rosemary (Rosmarinus officinalis) in alloxan-diabetic rabbits," J Ethnopharmacol. 116(1):64-73.

Balazs L, Okolicany J, Ferrebee M, Tolley B, Tigyi G (2001 Feb). "Topical application of the phospholipid growth factor lysophosphatidic acid promotes wound healing in vivo," Am J Physiol Regul Integr Comp Physiol. 280(2):R466-72.

Balestrieri, E., Pizzimenti, F., Ferlazzo, A., Giofre, S. V., Iannazzo, D., Piperno, A., . . . Macchi, B. (2011 Mar). Antiviral activity of seed extract from Citrus bergamia towards human retroviruses. Bioorg Med Chem, 19(6), 2084-2089.

Balick, MJ, Cox PA. (1996). Plants, People and Culture: The Science of Ethnobotany. Scientific American Library, New York.

Ballard CG, O'Brien JT, Reichelt K, Perry EK (2002 Jul). "Aromatherapy as a safe and effective treatment for the management of agitation in severe dementia: the results of a double-blind, placebo-controlled trial with Melissa," J Clin Psychiatry. 63(7):553-8.

Baldissera MD, Da Silva AS, Oliveira CB, Zimmermann CE, Vaucher RA, Santos RC, Rech VC, Tonin AA, Giongo JL, Mattos CB, Koester L, Santurio JM, Monteiro SG (2013 Apr). "Trypanocidal activity of the essential oils in their conventional and nanoemulsion forms: in vitro tests," Exp Parasitol. 134(3):356-61.

Ballabeni V, Tognolini M, Bertoni S, Bruni R, Guerrini A, Rueda GM, Barocelli E (2007 Jan). "Antiplatelet and antithrombotic activities of essential oil from wild Ocotea quixos (Lam.) Kosterm. (Lauraceae) calices from Amazonian Ecuador," Pharmacol Res. 55(1):23-30.

Ballabeni V, Tognolini M, Giorgio C, Bertoni S, Bruni R, Barocelli E (2009 Oct 13). "Ocotea quixos Lam. essential oil: In vitro and in vivo investigation on its anti-inflammatory properties," Fitoterapia. Epub ahead of print.

Banerjee S, Ecavade A, Rao AR (1993 Feb). "Modulatory influence of sandalwood oil on mouse hepatic glutathione S-transferase activity and acid soluble sulphydryl level," Cancer Lett. 68(2-3):105-9.

Banes-Marshall L, Cawley P, Phillips CA (2001). "In vitro activity of Melaleuca alternifolia (tea tree) oil against bacterial and Candida spp. isolates from clinical specimens," Br J Biomed Sci. 58(3):139-45.

Bani, S., Hasanpour, S., Mousavi, Z., Mostafa Garehbaghi, P., & Gojazadeh, M. (2014 Jan). The Effect of Rosa Damascena Extract on Primary Dysmenorrhea: A Double-blind Cross-over Clinical Trial. Iran Red Crescent Med J, 16(1), 1-6.

Banno N, Akihisa T, Yasukawa K, Tokuda H, Tabata K, Nakamura Y, Nishimura R, Kimura Y, Suzuki T (2006 Sep 19). "Anti-inflammatory activities of the triterpene acids from the resin of Boswellia carteri," J Ethnopharmacol. 107(2):249-53.

Bao L, Yao XS, Tsi D, Yau CC, Chia CS, Nagai H, Kurihara H (2008 Jan 23). "Protective effects of bilberry (Vaccinium myrtillus L.) extract on KbrO3-induced kidney damage in mice," J Agric Food Chem. 56(2):420-5.

Baqui, A. A., Kelley, J. I., Jabra-Rizk, M. A., Depaola, L. G., Falkler, W. A., & Meiller, T. F. (2001 Jul). In vitro effect of oral antiseptics on human immunodeficiency virus-1 and herpes simplex virus type 1. J Clin Periodontol, 28(7), 610-616.

Barak AJ, Beckenhauer HC, Badkhsh S, Tuma DJ (1997). "The effect of betaine in reversing alcoholic steatosis", Alcohol Clin Exp Res. 21(6):1100-1102.

Barceloux D.G. (2009 Jun). "Cinnamon (Cinnamomum Species)," Disease-a-Month. 55(6):327-335.

Barchiesi, F., Silvestri, C., Arzeni, D., Ganzetti, G., Castelletti, S., Simonetti, O., Cirioni, O., Kamysz, W., Kamysz, E., Spreghini, E., Abruzzetti, A., Riva, A., Offidani, A.M., Giacometti, A., and Scalise, G. "In vitro susceptibility of dermatophytes to conventional and alternative antifungal agents," Med. Mycol. 2009;47(3):321–326.

Barker S, Grayhem P, Koon J, Perkins J, Whalen A, Raudenbush S (2003 Dec). "Improved performance on clerical tasks associated with administration of peppermint odor," Percept. Mot. Skills. 97(3):1007-1010.

Barocelli E et al (2004 Nov). "Antinociceptive and gastroprotective effects of inhaled and orally administered Lavandula hybrida Reverchon 'Grosso' essential oil," Life Sci. 76(2):213-23.

Barthelman M., Chen W., Gensler H.L., Huang C., Dong Z., Bowden G.T. (1998) Inhibitory Effects of Perillyl Alcohol on UVB-induced Murine Skin Cancer and AP-1 Transactivation. Cancer Research. 58: 711-716.

Basholli-Salihu, M., Schuster, R., Hajardi, A., Mulla, D., Viernstein, H., Mustafa, B., & Mueller, M. (2017 Dec). "Phytochemical composition, anti-inflammatory activity and cytotoxic effects of essential oils from three Pinus spp," Pharm Biol. 55(1):1553-1560.

Bassett IB, Pannowitz DL, Barnetson RS (1990 Oct 15). "A comparative study of tea-tree oil versus benzoylperoxide in the treatment of acne," Med J Aust. 153(8):455-8.

Appendix

Bastiaens M, Hoefnagel J, Westendorp R, Vermeer BJ, Bouwes Bavinck JN (2004 Jun). "Solar lentigines are strongly related to sun exposure in contrast to ephelides," Pigment Cell Res. 17(3).

Bastos J.F.A., Moreira I.J.A., Ribeiro T.P., Medeiros I.A., Antoniolli A.R., De Sousa D.P., Santos M.R.V. (2009) Hypotensive and Vasorelaxant Effects of Citronellol, a Monoterpene Alcohol, in Rats. Basic & Clinical Pharmacology & Toxicology. 106: 331-337.

Basu A, Lucas EA (2007 Aug). "Mechanisms and effects of green tea on cardiovascular health," Nutr Rev. 65(8 Pt 1):361-75.

Batista LC, Cid YP, De Almeida AP, Prudêncio ER, Riger CJ, De Souza MA, Coumendouros K, Chaves DS (2016 Feb). "In vitro efficacy of essential oils and extracts of Schinus molle L. against Ctenocephalides felis felis," Parasitology. 143(5):627-38.

Bayala B. et al (2014 Mar). "Chemical Composition, Antioxidant, Anti-Inflammatory and Anti-Proliferative Activities of Essential Oils of Plants from Burkina Faso," PLoS ONE. 9(3):92122.

Baylac S (2003). "Inhibition of 5-lipoxygenase by essential oils and other natural fragrant extracts," Int. J. Aromather. 13(2-3):138-142.

Behnam S, Farzaneh M, Ahmadzadeh M, Tehrani AS (2006). "Composition and antifungal activity of essential oils of Mentha piperita and Lavendula angustifolia on post-harvest phytopathogens," Commun Agric Appl Biol Sci. 71(3 Pt B):1321-6.

Belardinelli R, Mucaj A, Lacalaprice F, Solenghi M, Principi F, Tiano L, Littarru GP (2005). "Coenzyme Q10 improves contractility of dysfunctional myocardium in chronic heart failure," Biofactors. 25(1-4):137-45.

Belhamel K, Abderrahim A, Ludwig R (2008). "Chemical composition and antibacterial activity of the essential oil of Schinus molle L. grown in Algeria," Int. J. Essent. Oil Ther. 2(4):175-177.

Benencia F, Courrèges MC (2000 Nov). "In vitro and in vivo activity of eugenol on human herpes virus," Phytother Res. 14(7):495-500.

Benencia, F., & Courreges, M. C. (1999 May). Antiviral activity of sandalwood oil against herpes simplex viruses-1 and -2. Phytomedicine, 6(2), 119-123.

Ben Othman, S., Katsuno, N., Kanamaru, Y., & Yabe, T. (2015). Water-soluble extracts from defatted sesame seed flour show antioxidant activity in vitro. Food Chemistry, 175(0), 306-314

Bemben, Michael G, Massey Benjamin H, Bemben, Debra A, Boileau Richard A, Misner James E (1995 Feb). "Age-related patterns in body composition for men aged 20-79 yr," Med Sci Sports Exerc, 27(2):264-9.

Bendaoud H, Romdhane M, Souchard J.P., Cazaux S, Bouajila J (2010 Aug). "Chemical composition and anticancer and antioxidant activities of Schinus molle L. and Schinus terebinthifolius Raddi berries essential oils," J. Food Sci. 75(6):C466-472.

Benedek B. et al (2008 Jan). "Yarrow (Achillea millefolium L. s.l.): pharmaceutical quality of commercial samples," Pharm. 63(1):23-26.

Benzi VS, Murrayb AP, Ferrero AA (2009 Sep). "Insecticidal and insect-repellent activities of essential oils from Verbenaceae and Anacardiaceae against Rhizopertha dominica," Nat Prod Commun. 4(9):1287-90.

Berić T, Nikolić B, Stanojević J, Vuković-Gacić B, Knezević-Vukcević J (2008 Feb). "Protective effect of basil (Ocimum basilicum L.) against oxidative DNA damage and mutagenesis," Food Chem Toxicol. 46(2):724-32.

Bezanilla F. (2006) The action potential: From voltage-gated conductances to molecular structures. Biological Research. 39: 425-435.

Bhalla Y, Gupta V.K., Jaitak V (2013 Dec). "Anticancer activity of essential oils: a review: Anticancer activity of essential oils," Journal of the Science of Food and Agriculture. 93(15):3643-3

Bhatia S.P., McGinty D, Letizia C.S., Api A.M. (2008 Nov). "Fragrance material review on cedrol," Food and Chemical Toxicology. 46(11):S100-S102.

Bhattacharya SK, Goel RK (1987 Mar). "Anti-stress activity of sitoindosides VII and VIII, new acylsterylglucosides from Withania somnifera," Phytother Res. 1(1):32-7.

Bhattacharya SK, Kumar A, Ghosal S (1995). "Effects of glycowithanolides from Withania somnifera on animal model of Alzheimer's disease and perturbed central cholinergic markers of cognition in rats," Phytother. Res. 9:110-3.

Bhuinya T, Singh P, Mukherjee S et al (2010). "Litsea cubeba—Medicinal values—Brief summary," J. Trop. Med. Plants. 11(2):179-183.

Bhushan S, Kumar A, Malik F, Andotra SS, Sethi VK, Kaur IP, Taneja SC, Qazi GN, Singh J (2007 Oct). "A triterpenediol from Boswellia serrata induces apoptosis through both the intrinsic and extrinsic apoptotic pathways in human leukemia HL-60 cells," Apoptosis. 12(10):1911-26.

Bixby WR, Spalding TW, Haufler AJ, Deeny SP, Mahlow PT, Zimmerman JB, Hatfield BD (2007 Aug). "The unique relation of physical activity to executive function in older men and women," Med Sci Sports Exerc, 39(8):1408-16.

Bixquert JM (2009). "Treatment of irritable bowel syndrome with probiotics: An etiopathogenic approach at last?," Revista Espanola de Enfermadaded Digestivas. 101(8):553-64.

Blain EJ, Ali AY, Duance VC (2010 Jun). "Boswellia frereana (frankincense) supresses cytokine-induced matrix metalloproteinase expression and production of pro-inflammatory molecules in articular cartilage," Phytother Res. 24(6):905-12.

Blanes-Mira C, Clemente J, Jodas G, Gil A, Fernandez-Ballester G, Ponsati B, Gutierrez L, Perez-Paya E, Ferrer-Montiel A (2002 Oct). "A synthetic hexapeptide (Argireline) with antiwrinkle activity," Int J Cosmet Sci. 24(5):303-10.

Blumenthal JA, Sherwood A, Babyak MA, Watkins LL, Smith PJ, Hoffman BM, O'Hayer CV, Mabe S, Johnson J, DOraiswamy PM, Jiang W, Schocken DD, Hinderliter AL (2012 Sep). "Exercise and pharmacological treatment of depressive symptoms in patients with coronary heart disease: results from the UPBEAT (Understanding the Prognostic Benefits of Exercise and Antidepressant Therapy study)," J Am Coll Cardiol, 60(12):1053-63.

Bobe G et al. (2008 Mar). "Flavonoid intake and risk of pancreatic cancer in male smokers (Finland)," Cancer Epidemiol Biomarkers Prev. 17(3):553-62.

Bonan, R.F., Bonan, P.R., Batista, A.U., Sampaio, F.C., Albuquerque, A.J., Moraes, M.C., Mattoso, L.H., Glenn, G.M., Medeiros, E.S., and Oliveira J.E. (2015). "In vitro antimicrobial activity of solution blow spun poly(lactic acid)/polyvinylpyrrolidone nanofibers loaded with Copaiba (Copaifera sp.) oil," Mater Sci Eng C Mater Biol Appl. 48:372-7.

Bone ME, Wilkinson DJ, Young JR, McNeil J, Charlton S (1990 Aug). "Ginger root--a new antiemetic. The effect of ginger root on postoperative nausea and vomiting after major gynaecological surgery," Anaesthesia. 45(8):669-71.

Boots AW, Wilms LC, Swennen EL, Kleinjans JC, Bast A, Haenen GR (2008 Jul-Aug). "In vitro and ex vivo anti-inflammatory activity of quercetin in healthy volunteers," Nutrition. 24(7-8):703-10.

Boque, N., Campion, J., de la Iglesia, R., de la Garza, A. L., Milagro, F. I., San Roman, B., . . . Martinez, J. A. (2013 Mar). Screening of polyphenolic plant extracts for anti-obesity properties in Wistar rats. J Sci Food Agric, 93(5), 1226-1232.

Bora, K. S., Arora, S., & Shri, R. (2011 Oct). Role of Ocimum basilicum L. in prevention of ischemia and reperfusion-induced cerebral damage, and motor dysfunctions in mice brain. J Ethnopharmacol, 137(3), 1360-1365.

Borgatti, M., Mancini, I., Bianchi, N., Guerrini, A., Lampronti, I., Rossi, D., . . . Gambari, R. (2011 Apr). Bergamot (Citrus bergamia Risso) fruit extracts and identified components alter expression of interleukin 8 gene in cystic fibrosis bronchial epithelial cell lines. BMC Biochem, 12, 15.

Borkow G (2014). "Using copper to improve the well-being of the skin," Current Chemical Biology. 8:89-102.

Bose M, Lambert JD, Ju J, Reuhl KR, Shapses SA, Yang CS (2008 Sep). "The major green tea polyphenol, (-)-epigallocatechin-3-gallate, inhibits obesity, metabolic syndrome, and fatty liver disease in high-fat-fed mice," J Nutr. 138(9):1677-83.

Boudier D, Breugnot J, Vignau E, Loumonier J, Li L, Closs B (2010 Jun). "Skin care—The refinement of pores," Cosmeticbusiness.com.

Boudier D, Perez E, Rondeau D, Bordes S, Closs B (2008 Mar). "Innovatory approach fights pigment disturbances," Personal Care.

Bounihi A, Hajjaj G, Alnamer R, Cherrah Y, Zellou A (2013). "In vivo potential anti-inflammatory activity of melissa officinalis l. essential oil," Adv Pharmacol Sci.

Bourgou, S., Rahali, F.Z., Ourghemmi, I., and Saïdani Tounsi, M. (2012.) "Changes of peel essential oil composition of four Tunisian citrus during fruit maturation," Scientific World J. 2012:528593.

Boussetta T, Raad H, Lettéron P, Gougerot-Pocidalo MA, Marie JC, Driss F, El-Benna J (2009 Jul 31). "Punicic acid a conjugated linoleic acid inhibits TNFalpha-induced neutrophil hyperactivation and protects from experimental colon inflammation in rats," PLoS One. 4(7):e6458.

Bouwstra J.A., Gooris G.S., Dubbelaar F.E.R., Weeheim A.M., Ijzerman A.P., Ponec M. (1998) Role of ceramide 1 in the molecular organization of the stratum corneum lipids. Journal of Lipid Research. 39: 186-196.

Bouzenna, H., Hfaiedh, N., Giroux-Metges, M.A., Elfeki, A., & Talarmin, H. (2017 May). "Protective effects of essential oil of Citrus limon against aspirin-induced toxicity in IEC-6 cells," Appl Physiol Nutr Metab. 42(5):479-486.

Bowen, R. (2006). The gastrointestinal barrier. In W.E. Wingfield & M.R. Raffe (Eds.), The veterinary ICU book (40-46). Alpine, WY: Teton NewMedia.

Bowles, E. J. (2003). The chemistry of aromatherapeutic oils (3rd ed.). Australia: Allen & Unwin.

Bradley BF, Brown SL, Chu S, Lea RW (2009 Jun). "Effects of orally administered lavender essential oil on responses to anxiety-provoking film clips," Hum Psychopharmacol. 24(4):319-30.

Bradley BF, Starkey NJ, Brown SL, Lea RW (2007 May 22). "Anxiolytic effects of Lavandula angustifolia odour on the Mongolian gerbil elevated plus maze," J Ethnopharmacol. 111(3):517-25.

Brady A, Loughlin R, Gilpin D, Kearney P, Tunney M (2006 Oct). "In vitro activity of tea-tree oil against clinical skin isolates of methicillin-resistant and -sensitive Staphylococcus aureus and coagulase-negative staphylococci growing planktonically and as biofilms," J Med Microbiol. 55(Pt 10):1375-80.

Brand C, Ferrante A, Prager RH, Riley TV, Carson CF, Finlay-Jones JJ, Hart PH. (2001 Apr). "The water-soluble components of the essential oil of Melaleuca alternifolia (tea tree oil) suppress the production of superoxide by human monocytes, but not neutrophils, activated in vitro.," Inflamm Res. 50(4):213-9.

Brand C, Grimbaldeston MA, Gamble JR, Drew J, Finlay-Jones JJ, Hart PH (2002 May). "Tea tree oil reduces the swelling associated with the efferent phase of a contact hypersensitivity response," Inflamm Res. 51(5):236-44.

Brand C, Townley SL, Finlay-Jones JJ, Hart PH (2002 Jun). "Tea tree oil reduces histamine-induced oedema in murine ears," Inflamm Res. 51(6):283-9.

Bras C, Gumilar F, Gandini N, Minetti A, Ferrero A (2011 Oct). "Evaluation of the acute dermal exposure of the ethanolic and hexanic extracts from leaves of Schinus molle var. areira L. in rats," J.Ethnopharmacol. 137 (3):1450-56.

Brass EP, Adler S, Sietsema KE, Hiatt WR, Orlando AM, Amato A; CHIEF Investigators (2001 May). "Intravenous L-carnitine increases plasma carnitine, reduces fatigue, and may preserve exercise capacity in hemodialysis patients," Am J Kidney Dis. 37(5):1018-28.

Brenner, G. M., & Stevens, C. (2009). Pharmacology (3rd ed.). Philadelphia, PA: Saunders Elsevier.

Brien S, Lewith G, Walker A, Hicks SM, Middleton D (2004 Dec). "Bromelain as a Treatment for Osteoarthritis: a Review of Clinical Studies," Evid Based Complement Alternat Med. 1(3):251-257.

Brown AL et al. (2008 Aug). "Effects of dietary supplementation with the green tea polyphenol epigallocatechin-3-gallate on insulin resistance and associated metabolic risk factors: randomized controlled trial," Br J Nutr. 19:1-9.

Brown T.L., LeMay H.E., Bursten B.E. Chemistry: The Central Science. 10th ed. Upper Saddle River: Pearson Prentice Hall, 2006.

Brum LF, Elisabetsky E, Souza D (2001 Aug). "Effects of linalool on [(3)H]MK801 and [(3)H] muscimol binding in mouse cortical membranes," Phytother Res. 15(5):422-5.

Brussow, H. (2013). Microbiota and healthy ageing: observational and nutritional intervention studies. Microb Biotechnol, 6(4), 326-334.

Buchbauer G, Jirovetz L, Jäger W, Dietrich H, Plank C (1991 Nov-Dec). "Aroma-therapy: evidence for sedative effects of the essential oil of lavender after inhalation," Z Naturforsch C. 46(11-12):1067-72.

Bucheli, P., Vidal, K., Shen, L., Gu, Z., Zhang, C., Miller, L. E., & Wang, J. (2011 Feb). Goji berry effects on macular characteristics and plasma antioxidant levels. Optom Vis Sci, 88(2), 257-262.

Bucher HC, Hengstler P, Schindler C, Meier G (2002 Mar). "N-3 polyunsaturated fatty acids in coronary heart disease: a meta-analysis of randomized controlled trials," Am J Med. 112(4):298-304.

Budiyanto, A., Ahmed, N.U., Wu, A., Bito, T., Nikaido, O., Osawa, T., Ueda, M., Ichihashi, M. (200 Nov). "Protective effect of topically applied olive oil against photocarcinogenesis following UVB exposure of mice," Carcinogenesis, 21(11): 2085-2090.

Buck DS, Nidorf DM, Addino JG (1994 Jun). "Comparison of two topical prepara-tions for the treatment of onychomycosis: Melaleuca alternifolia (tea tree) oil and clotrimazole," J Fam Pract. 38(6):601-5.

Bukovska, A., Cikos, S., Juhas, S., Il'kova, G., Rehak, P., & Koppel, J. (2007 Feb). Ef-fects of a combination of thyme and oregano essential oils on TNBS-induced colitis in mice. Mediators Inflamm, 2007, 23296.

Bulbring E. (1946) Observations on the Isolated Phrenic Nerve Diaphragm Preparation of the Rat. British Journal of Pharmacology. 1: 38-61.

Burke BE, Baillie JE, Olson RD (2004 May). "Essential oil of Australian lemon myrtle (Backhousia citriodora) in the treatment of molluscum contagiosum in children," Biomed Pharmacother. 58(4):245-7.

Bushra, R., Aslam, N., & Khan, A. Y. (2011 Mar). Food-drug interactions. Oman Med J, 26(2), 77-83.

Butte NF, Puyau MR, Adoph AL, Vohra FA, Zakeri I (2007 Aug). "Physical activity in nonoverweight and overweight Hispanic children and adolescents," Med Sci Sports Exerc, 39(8):1257-66.

Cabrera, C., Artacho, R., & Giménez, R. (2006 Apr). Beneficial Effects of Green Tea—A Review. J Am Coll Nutr, 25(2), 79-99.

Cabrera-Vique C, Marfil R, Gimenez R, Martinez-Augustin O (2012 May). "Bioactive compounds and nutritional significance of virgin argan oil—an edible oil with poten-tial as a functional food,' Nutr Rev. 70(5):266-79.

Caccioni DR, Guizzardi M, Biondi DM, Renda A, Ruberto G (1998 Aug 18). "Rela-tionship between volatile components of citrus fruit essential oils and antimicrobial action on Penicillium digitatum and penicillium italicum," Int J Food Microbiol. 43(1-2):73-9.

Caceres, A.I., Liu, B., Jabba S.V., Achanta, S., Morris, J.B., & Jordt, S.E. (2017 May). "Transient Receptor Potential Cation Channel Subfamily M Member 8 channels mediate the anti-inflammatory effects of eucalyptol," Br J Pharmacol. 174(9):867-879.

Cai, X., Zhou, Y. F., & Hu, Z. H. (2008 Apr). Ultrastructure and secretion of secretory canals in vegetative organs of Bupleurum chinense DC. Journal of Molecular Cell Biology, 41(2), 96-106.

Cal K, Janicki S, Sznitowska M (2001 Aug). "In vitro studies on penetration of terpenes from matrix-type transdermal systems through human skin," Int. J. Pharm. 224(1-2):81-88.

Caldefie-Chézet F, Fusillier C, Jarde T, Laroye H, Damez M, Vasson MP, Guillot J (2006 May). "Potential anti-inflammatory effects of Melaleuca alternifolia essential oil on human peripheral blood leukocytes," Phytother Res. 20(5):364-70.

Caldefie-Chézet F, Guerry M, Chalchat JC, Fusillier C, Vasson MP, Guillot J (2004 Aug). "Anti-inflammatory effects of Melaleuca alternifolia essential oil on human polymorphonuclear neutrophils and monocytes," Free Radic Res. 38(8):805-11.

Camarda L, Dayton T, Di Stefano V, Pitonzo R, Schillaci D (2007 Sep). "Chemical composition and antimicrobial activity of some oleogum resin essential oils from Boswellia spp. (Burseraceae)," Ann Chim. 97(9):837-844.

Campelo, L. M., Goncalves, F. C., Feitosa, C. M., & de Freitas, R. M. (2011 Jul). Antioxidant activity of Citrus limon essential oil in mouse hippocampus. Pharm Biol, 49(7), 709-715.

Candan F, Unlu M, Tepe B, Daferera D, Polissiou M, Sökmen A, Akpulat HA (2003 Aug). "Antioxidant and antimicrobial activity of the essential oil and methanol ex-tracts of Achillea millefolium subsp. millefolium Afan. (Asteraceae)," J Ethnophar-macol. 87(2-3):215-20.

Cannas S. et al (2015 Jun). "Essential oils in ocular pathology: an experimental study," J. Infect. Dev. Ctries. 9(6):650-654.

Canyon DV, Speare R (2007 Apr). "A comparison of botanical and synthetic substances commonly used to prevent head lice (Pediculus humanus var. capitis) infestation," Int J Dermatol. 46(4):422-6.

Capasso R, Savino F, Capasso F (2007 Oct). "Effects of the herbal formulation ColiMil on upper gastrointestinal transit in mice in vivo," Phytother Res. 21(10):999-1101.

Cappello G, Spezzaferro M, Grossi L, Manzoli L, Marzio L (2007 Jun). "Peppermint oil (Mintoil) in the treatment of irritable bowel syndrome: a prospective double blind placebo-controlled randomized trial," Dig Liver Dis. 39(6):530-6.

Capuzzo A, Occhipinti A, Maffei M.E. (2014 Dec). "Antioxidant and radical scaveng-ing activities of chamazulene," Nat. Prod. Res. 28(24):2321-2323.

Carnesecchi S., Bradaia A., Fischer B., Coelho D., Scholler-Guinard M., Gosse F., Raul F. (2002) Perturbation by Geraniol of Cell Membrane Permeability and Signal Transduction Pathways in Human Colon Cancer Cells. The Journal of Pharmacol-ogy and Experimental Therapeutics. 303: 711-715.

Carnesecchi S., Bras-Goncalves R., Bradaia A., Zeisel M., Gosse F., Poupon M-F., Raul F. (2004) Geraniol, a component of plant essential oils, modulates DNA synthesis and potentiates 5-fluorouracil efficacy on human colon tumor xenografts. Cancer Letters. 215: 53-59.

Carnesecchi S., Langley K., Exinger F., Gosse F., Raul F. (2002) Geraniol, a Compo-nent of Plant Essential Oils, Sensitizes Human Colonic Cancer Cells to 5-Fluroura-cil Treatment. The Journal of Pharmacology and Experimental Therapeutics. 301: 625-630.

Carnesecchi S, Schneider Y, Ceraline J, Duranton B, Gosse F, Seiler N, Raul F (2001 Jul). "Geraniol, a component of plant essential oils, inhibits growth and polyamine biosynthesis in human colon cancer cells," J Pharmacol Exp Ther. 298(1):197-200.

Carson CF, Cookson BD, Farrelly HD, Riley TV (1995 Mar). "Susceptibility of methicillin-resistant Staphylococcus aureus to the essential oil of Melaleuca alterni-folia," J Antimicrob Chemother. 35(3):421-4.

Carvalho-Freitas MI, Costa M (2002 Dec). "Anxiolytic and sedative effects of extracts and essential oil from Citrus aurantium L," Biol Pharm Bull. 25(12):1629-33.

Catalán A, Pacheco JG, Martínez A, Mondaca MA (2008 Mar). "In vitro and in vivo activity of Melaleuca alternifolia mixed with tissue conditioner on Candida albicans," Oral Surg Oral Med Oral Pathol Oral Radiol Endod. 105(3):327-32.

Cavaleiro C, Salgueiro L, Goncalves MJ, Hrimpeng K, Pinto J, Pinto E (2015 Apr). "Antifungal activity of the essential oil of Angelica major against Candida, Crypto-coccus, Aspergillus and dermatophyte species," J Nat Med. 69(2):241-248.

Ceccarelli I, Lariviere WR, Fiorenzani P, Sacerdote P, Aloisi AM (2004 Mar 19). "Ef-fects of long-term exposure to lemon essential oil odor on behavioral, hormonal and neuronal parameters in male and female rats," Brain Res. 1001(1-2):78-86.

Cencic A, Chingwaru W (2010). The Role of Functional Foods, Nutraceuticals, and Food Supplements in Intestinal Health. Nutrients, 2(6):611-625.

Cenizo, V., Andre, V., Reymermier, C., Sommer, P., Damour, O., & Perrier, E. (2006 Aug). LOXL as a target to increase the elastin content in adult skin: a dill extract induces the LOXL gene expression. Exp Dermatol, 15(8), 574-581.

Centers for Disease Control and Prevention (CDC) (2004 May 7). "Spina bifida and anencephaly before and after folic acid mandate--United States, 1995-1996 and 1999-2000," MMWR Morb Mortal Wkly Rep. 53(17):362-5.

Ceriotti G, Spandrio L, Gazzaniga A (1967 Jul-Aug). "[Demonstration, isolation and physical and chemical characteristics of narciclasine, a new antimitotic of plant origin]," Tumori. 53(4):359-71.

Cermelli C, Fabio A, Fabio G, Quaglio P (2008 Jan). "Effect of eucalyptus essential oil on respiratory bacteria and viruses," Curr Microbiol. 56(1):89-92.

Cetinkaya B, Basbakkal Z (2012 Apr). "The effectiveness of aromatherapy massage us-ing lavender oil as a treatment for infantile colic," Int. J. Nurs. Pract. 18(2):164-169.

Chaiyana W, Okonogi S (2012 Jun). "Inhibition of cholinesterase by essential oil from food plant," Phytomedicine Int. J. Phytother. Phytopharm. 19(8-9):836-839.

Chaudhuri, R.K., and Bojanowski, K. (2014). "Bakuchiol: a retinol-like functional com-pound revealed by gene expression profiling and clinically proven to have anti-aging effects," Int J Cosmet Sci. 36(3):221-30.

Cháfer, M., Sanchez-Gonzalez, L., Gonzalez-Martinez, C., & Chiralt, A. (2012 Aug). Fungal decay and shelf life of oranges coated with chitosan and bergamot, thyme, and tea tree essential oils. J Food Sci, 77(8), E182-187.

Chaieb K, Zmantar T, Ksouri R, Hajlaoui H, Mahdouani K, Abdelly C, Bakhrouf A (2007 Sep). "Antioxidant properties of the essential oil of Eugenia caryophyllata and its antifungal activity against a large number of clinical Candida species," Mycoses. 50(5):403-6.

Chaiyakunapruk N, Kitikannakorn N, Nathisuwan S, Leeprakobboon K, Leelasettagool C (2006 Jan). "The efficacy of ginger for the prevention of postoperative nausea and vomiting: a meta-analysis," Am J Obstet Gynecol. 194(1):95-9.

Chakraborty PK, Mustafi SB, Raha S (2008 Sep). "Pro-survival effects of repetitive low-grade oxidative stress are inhibited by simultaneous exposure to resveratrol," Phamacol Res. 2.

Chambers H.F. (2001) The Changing Epidemiology of Staphylococcus aureus?. Emerging Infectious Diseases. 7: 178-182.

Chan YS, Cheng LN, Wu JH, Chan E, Kwan YW, Lee SM, Leung GP, Yu PH, Chan SW (2011 Oct). "A review of the pharmacological effects of Arctium lappa (burdock)," Inflammopharmacology. 19(5):245-54.

Chang, K. S., Tak, J. H., Kim, S. I., Lee, W. J., & Ahn, Y. J. (2006 Nov). Repellency of Cinnamomum cassia bark compounds and cream containing cassia oil to Aedes aegypti (Diptera: Culicidae) under laboratory and indoor conditions. Pest Manag Sci, 62(11), 1032-1038.

Chang SM, Chen CH (2016 Feb). "Effects of an intervention with drinking chamomile tea on sleep quality and depression in sleep disturbed postnatal women: a random-ized controlled trial," J Adv Nurs. 72(2):306-15.

Chang WC, Yu YM, Chiang SY, Tseng CY (2008 Apr). "Ellagic acid supresses oxidised low-density lipoprotein-induced aortic smooth muscle cell proliferation: studies on the activation of extracellular signal-regulated kinase ½ and proliferating cell nuclear antigen expression," Br J Nutr. 99(4):709-14.

Appendix

Chang WL, Cheng FC, Wang SP, Chou ST, Shih Y (2016 Feb). "Cinnamomum cassia essential oil and its major constituent cinnamaldehyde induced cell cycle arrest and apoptosis in human oral squamous cell carcinoma HSC-3 cells," Environ. Toxicol.

Chang YT, Chu FH (2011 Mar). "Molecular cloning and characterization of monoterpene synthases from Litsea cubeba (Lour.) Persoon," Tree Genetics & Genomes. 7(4):835-844.

Chapman A.G. (1998) Glutamate receptors in epilepsy. Progress in Brain Research. 116: 371-383.

Chapman A.G. (2000) Glutamate and Epilepsy. The Journal of Nutrition. 130: 1043S-1045S.

Charles C.A. et al (2014). "Early benefits with daily rinsing on gingival health improvements with an essential oil mouthrinse--post-hoc analysis of 5 clinical trials," J. Dent. Hyg. JDH Am. Dent. Hyg. Assoc. 88L40-50.

Charles CH, Vincent JW, Borycheski L, Amatnieks Y, Sarina M, Qaqish J, Proskin HM (2000 Sep). "Effect of an essential oil-containing dentifrice on dental plaque microbial composition," Am J Dent. 13():26C-30C.

Charrouf Z, Guillaume D (2010 May). "Should the amazigh diet (regular and moderate argan-oil consumption) have a beneficial impact on human health?," Crit Rev Food Sci Nutr. 50(5):473-7.

Chaturvedi AP, Kumar M, Tripathi YB (2013 Dec). "Efficacy of Jasminum grandiflorum L. leaf extract on dermal wound healing in rats," Int Wound J. 10(6):675-82.

Chaudhary S.C., Siddiqui M.S., Athar M, Alam M.S. (2012 Aug). "D-Limonene modulates inflammation, oxidative stress and Ras-ERK pathway to inhibit murine skin tumorigenesis," Hum. Exp. Toxicol. 31(8):798-811.

Chaudhuri RK, Bojanowski K (2014 Jun). "Bakuchiol: a retinol-like functional compound revealed by gene expression profiling and clinically proven to have anti-aging effects," Int J Cosmet Sci. 36(3):221-30.

Checker R, Chatterjee S, Sharma D, Gupta S, Variyar P, Sharma A, Poduval TB (2008 May). "Immunomodulatory and radioprotective effects of lignans derived from fresh nutmeg mace (Myristica fragrans) in mammalian splenocytes," Int Immunopharmacol. 8(5):661-9.

Chee H.Y., Lee M.H. (2007 Dec). "Antifungal activity of clove essential oil and its volatile vapour against dermatophytic fungi," Mycobiology. 35(4):241-243.

Cheeke PR, Piacente S, Oleszek W (2006). "Anti-inflammatory and anti-arthritic effects of yucca schidigera: A review", J Inflamm (Lond). 3:6.

Chen CJ. et al (2012 Dec). "Neuropharmacological activities of fruit essential oil from Litsea cubeba Persoon," Journal of Wood Science. 58(6):538-543.

Chen CJ, Kumar KJ, Chen YT, Tsao NW, Chien SC, Chang ST, Chu FH, Wang SY (2015). "Effect of Hinoki and Meniki Essential Oils on Human Autonomic Nervous System Activity and Mood States," Nat Prod Commun. 10(7):1305-8.

Chen HC et al (2016 Aug). "Immunosuppressive Effect of Litsea cubeba L. Essential Oil on Dendritic Cell and Contact Hypersensitivity Responses," International Journal of Molecular Sciences. 17(8):1319.

Chen M, Zhang J, Yu S, Wang S, Zhang Z, Chen J, Xiao J, Wang Y (2012). "Anti-lung-cancer activity and liposome -based delivery systems of beta-elemene," Evid Based Complement Alternat Med. 2012:259523.

Chen MC, Fang SH, Fang L (2015 Feb). "The effects of aromatherapy in relieving symptoms related to job stress among nurses: Aromatherapy," Int. J. Nurs. Pract. 21(1):87-93.

Chen YC, Chiu WT, Wu MS (2006 Jul). "Therapeutic effect of topical gamma-linolenic acid on refractory uremic pruritus," Am J Kidney Dis. 48(1):69-76.

Chen Y. et al (2013 Oct "Composition and potential anticancer activities of essential oils obtained from myrrh and frankincense," Oncol Lett. 6(4):1140-1146.

Chen, Y., Zeng, H., Tian, J., Ban, X., Ma, B., & Wang, Y. (2014 Apr). Dill (Anethum graveolens L.) seed essential oil induces Candida albicans apoptosis in a metacaspase-dependent manner. Fungal Biol, 118(4), 394-401.

Cheung S, Tai J (2007 Jun). "Anti-proliferative and antioxidant properties of rosemary Rosmarinus officinalis," Oncol Rep. 17(6):1525-31.

Chevrier MR, Ryan AE, Lee DY, Zhongze M, Wu-Yan Z, Via CS (2005 May). "Boswellia carterii extract inhibits TH1 cytokines and promotes TH2 cytokines in vitro," Clin Diagn Lab Immunol. 12(5):575-80.

Chidambara Murthy K.N., Jayaprakasha G.K., Patil B.S. (2012 Oct). "D-limonene rich volatile oil from blood oranges inhibits angiogenesis, metastasis and cell death in human colon cancercells," Life Sci. 91(11-12):429-439.

Chien, L. W., Cheng, S. L., & Liu, C. F. (2012 Aug). The effect of lavender aromatherapy on autonomic nervous system in midlife women with insomnia. Evid Based Complement Alternat Med, 2012.

Chinou IB, Roussis V, Perdetzoglou D, Loukis A (1996 Aug). "Chemical and biological studies on two Helichrysum species of Greek origin," Planta Med. 62(4):377-9.

Chioca L.R., Antunes V.D.C., Ferro M.M., Losso E.M., Andreatini R (2013 May). "Anosmia does not impair the anxiolytic-like effect of lavender essential oil inhalation in mice," Life Sci. 92(20-21):971-975.

Chioca L.R. et al (2013 May). "Anxiolytic-like effect of lavender essential oil inhalation in mice: participation of serotonergic but not GABAA/benzodiazepine neurotransmission," J. Ethnopharmacol. 147(2):412-418.

Cho, M. Y., Min, E. S., Hur, M. H., & Lee, M. S. (2013 Feb). Effects of aromatherapy on the anxiety, vital signs, and sleep quality of percutaneous coronary intervention patients in intensive care units. Evid Based Complement Alternat Med, 2013, 1-6.

Cho, S., Choi, Y., Park, S., & Park, C. (2012 Feb). Carvacrol prevents diet-induced obesity by modulating gene expressions involved in adipogenesis and inflammation in mice fed with high-fat diet. J Nutr Biochem, 23(2), 192-201.

Choi, H. Y., Yang, Y. C., Lee, S. H., Clark, J. M., & Ahn, Y. J. (2010 May). Efficacy of spray formulations containing binary mixtures of clove and eucalyptus oils against susceptible and pyrethroid/ malathion-resistant head lice (Anoplura: Pediculidae). J Med Entomol, 47(3), 387-391.

Choi, S. Y., Kang, P., Lee, H. S., and Seol, G. H. (2014). "Effects of Inhalation of Essential Oil of Citrus aurantium L. var. amara on Menopausal Symptoms, Stress, and Estrogen in Postmenopausal Women: A Randomized Controlled Trial," Evid Based Complement Alternat Med. 2014:796518.

Choi, U. K., Lee, O. H., Yim, J. H., Cho, C. W., Rhee, Y. K., Lim, S. I., & Kim, Y. C. (2010 Feb). Hypolipidemic and antioxidant effects of dandelion (Taraxacum officinale) root and leaf on cholesterol-fed rabbits. Int J Mol Sci, 11(1), 67-78.

Choi, Y. Y., Kim, M. H., Han, J. M., Hong, J., Lee, T. H., Kim, S. H., & Yang, W. M. (2014 Feb 8). "The anti-inflammatory potential of Cortex Phellodendron in vivo and in vitro: down-regulation of NO and iNOS through suppression of NF-kappaB and MAPK activation," Int Immunopharmacol, 19(2): 214-220.

Chou ST, Peng HY, Hsu JC, Lin CC, Shih Y (2013 Jun). "Achillea millefolium L. Essential Oil Inhibits LPS-Induced Oxidative Stress and Nitric Oxide Production in RAW 264.7 Macrophages," Int. J. Mol. Sci. 14(7):12978-12993.

Chow H.S., Salazar D, Hakin I.A. (2002 Nov). "Pharmacokinetics of perillic acid in humans after a single dose administration of a citrus preparation rich in d-limonene content," Cancer Epidemiol. Biomark. Prev. Publ. Am. Assoc. Cancer Res. Cosponsored Am. Soc. Prev. Oncol 11(11):1472-1476.

Chung, H. S., Harris, A., Kristinsson, J. K., Ciulla, T. A., Kagemann, C., & Ritch, R. (1999 Jun). Ginkgo biloba extract increases ocular blood flow velocity. J Ocul Pharmacol Ther, 15(3), 233-240.

Chung, M. J., Cho, S. Y., Bhuiyan, M. J., Kim, K. H., & Lee, S. J. (2010 Jul). Anti-diabetic effects of lemon balm (Melissa officinalis) essential oil on glucose- and lipid-regulating enzymes in type 2 diabetic mice. Br J Nutr, 104(2), 180-188.

Chungchunlam, S. M., Henare, S. J., Ganesh, S., & Moughan, P. J. (2014 Apr 5). Effect of whey protein and glycomacropeptide on measures of satiety in normal-weight adult women. Appetite, 78, 172-178.

Chunmuang S, Jitpukdeebodintra S, Chuenarrom C, Benjakul P (2007). "Effect of xylitol and fluoride on enamel erosion in vitro," J. Oral Sci. 49(4):293-297.

Ciacci G, Peluso G, Iannoni E, Siniscalchi M, Iovino P, Rispo A, Tortora R, Bucci C, Zingone F, Margarucci S, Calvani M (2007 Oct). "L-Carnitine in the treatment of fatigue in adult celiac disease patients: a pilot study," Dig Liver Dis. 39(10):922-8.

Cibulka MT, Sinacore DR, Cromer GS, Delitto A (1998). "Unilateral hip rotation range of motion asymmetry in patients with sacroiliac joint regional pain," Spine, 23(9):1009-15.

Ciftci O., Ozdemir I., Tanyildizl S., Yildiz S., Oguzturk H. (2011) Antioxidative effects of curcumin, β-myrcene and 1,8-cineole against 2,3,7,8-tetracholorodibenzo-p-dioxin - induced oxidative stress in rats liver. Toxicology and Industrial Health. 27: 447-453.

Cioanca, O., Hritcu, L., Mihasan, M., Trifan, A., & Hancianu, M. (2014 May). Inhalation of coriander volatile oil increased anxiolytic-antidepressant-like behaviors and decreased oxidative status in beta-amyloid (1-42) rat model of Alzheimer's disease. Physiol Behav, 131, 68-74.

Cioanca, O., Hritcu, L., Mihasan, M., & Hancianu, M. (2013 Aug). Cognitive-enhancing and antioxidant activities of inhaled coriander volatile oil in amyloid beta(1-42) rat model of Alzheimer's disease. Physiol Behav, 120, 193-202.

Cline M, Taylor J.E., Flores J, Bracken S, McCall S, Ceremuga T.E. (2008 Feb). "Investigation of the anxiolytic effects of linalool, a lavender extract, in the male Sprague-Dawley rat," AANA J. 76(1):47-52.

Coderch L, Lopez O., de la Maza A., Parra J.L. (2003) Ceramides and Skin Function. American Journal of Clinical Dermatology. 4: 107-129.

Conrad P, Adams C (2012 Aug). "The effects of clinical aromatherapy for anxiety and depression in the high risk postpartum woman - a pilot study," Complement. Ther. Clin. Pract. 18(3):164-168.

Cooley K, Szczurko O, Perri D, Mills EJ, Bernhardt B, Zhou Q, Seely D (2009 Aug 31). "Naturopathic care for anxiety: a randomized controlled trial IS-RCTN78958974," PLoS One. 4(8):e6628.

Corasaniti, M. T., Maiuolo, J., Maida, S., Fratto, V., Navarra, M., Russo, R., . . . Bagetta, G. (2007 Jun). Cell signaling pathways in the mechanisms of neuroprotection afforded by bergamot essential oil against NMDA-induced cell death in vitro. Br J Pharmacol, 151(4), 518-529.

Costalonga M., Herzberg M.C. (2014 Dec). "The oral microbiome and the immunobiology of periodontal disease and caries," Immunol. Lett. 162(200):22-38.

Couse JF, Lindzey J, Grandien K, Gustafsson JA, Korach KS (1997 Nov). "Tissue distribution and quantitative analysis of estrogen reseptor-alpha (ERalpha) and estrogen receptor-beta (ERbeta) messenger ribonucleic acid in the wild-type and ERalpha-knockout mouse," Endocrinology. 138*11):4613-21.

Cowan M.K., Talaro K.P. Microbiology: A Systems Approach. 2nd ed. New York: McGraw Hill, 2009.

Cox SD, Mann CM, Markham JL, Bell HC, Gustafson JE, Warmington JR, Wyllie SG (2000 Jan). "The mode of antimicrobial action of the essential oil of Melaleuca alternifolia (tea tree oil)," J Appl Microbiol. 88(1):170-5.

Cronin H, Draelos Z.D. (2010 Sep). "Top 10 botanical ingredients in 2010 anti-aging creams," J Cosmet Dermatol. 9(3):218-225.

Cross SE, Russell M, Southwell I, Roberts MS (2008 May). "Human skin penetration of the major components of Australian tea tree oil applied in its pure form and as a 20% solution in vitro," Eur J Pharm Biopharm. 69(1):214-22.

Crowell P.L., Chang R.R., Ren Z., Elson C.E., Gould M.N. (1991) Selective Inhibition of Isoprenylation of 21-26kDa Proteins by the Anticarcinogen d-Limonene and Its Metabolites. J. Biol. Chem. 266: 17679-17685.

Crowell P.L., Elson C.E., Bailey H.H., Elegbede A, Haag J.D., Gould M.N. (1994). "Human metabolism of the experimental cancer therapeutic agent d-limonene," Cancer Chemother. Pharmacol. 35 (1):31-37.

Crowell, P.L., & Gould M.N. (1994). "Chemoprevention and therapy of cancer by d-limonene," Crit Rev Oncog. 5(1):1-22.

Crowell P.L., Lin S, Vedejs E, Gould M.N. (1992). "Identification of metabolites of the antitumor agent d-limonene capable of inhibiting protein isoprenylation and cell growth," Cancer Chemother. 13(3):205-212.

Cuellar, M. J., Giner, R. M., Recio, M. C., Manez, S., & Rios, J. L. (2001 Mar). Topical anti-inflammatory activity of some Asian medicinal plants used in dermatological disorders. Fitoterapia, 72(3), 221-229.

Cui Y et al. (2008 May 15). "Dietary flavonoid intake and lung cancer—a population-based case-control study," Cancer. 112(10):2241-8.

Curi R, Alvarez M, Bazotte RB, Botion LM, Godoy JL, Bracht A (1986). "Effect of Stevia rebaudiana on glucose tolerance in normal adult humans," Braz J Med Biol Res. 19(6):771-4.

Curio M, Jacone H, Perrut J, Pinto AC, Filho VF, Silva RC (2009 Aug). "Acute effect of Copaifera reticulata Ducke copaiba oil in rats tested in the elevated plus-maze: an ethological analysis," J Pharm Pharmacol. 61(8):1105-10.

Dahham S.S. et al (2015). "The Anticancer, Antioxidant and Antimicrobial Properties of the Sesquiterpene β-Caryophyllene from the Essential Oil of Aquilaria crassna," Mol. Basel Switz. 20(7):11808-11829.

Dai ZJ, Tang W, Lu WF, Gao J, Kang HF, Ma XB, Min WL, Wang XJ, Wu WY (2013 Mar 14). "Antiproliferative and apoptotic effects of beta-elemne on human hepatoma HepG2 cells," Cancer Cell Int. 13(1):27.

Dagli N, Dagli R, Mahmoud R.S., Baroudi K (2015). "Essential oils, their therapeutic properties, and implication in dentistry: A review," J. Int. Soc. Prev. Community Dent. 5(5):335-340.

d'Alessio P.A., Mirshani M, Bisson JF, Bene M.C. (2014 Mar). "Skin repair properties of d-Limonene and perillyl alcohol in murine models," Anti-Inflamm. Anti-Allergy Agents Med. Chem. 13(1):29-35.

d'Alessio P.A., Ostan R, Bisson JF, Schulzke J.D., Ursini M.V., Béné M.C (2013 Jul). "Oral administration of d-limonene controls inflammation in rat colitis and displays anti-inflammatory properties as diet supplementation in humans," Life Sci. 92(24-26):1151-1156.

Danner G.R., Muto K.W., Zieba A.M., Stillman C.M., Seggio J.A., Ahmad S.T. (2011 Dec). "Spearmint (1 -Carvone) Oil and Wintergreen (Methyl Salicylate) Oil Emulsion Is an Effective Immersion Anesthetic of Fishes," J. Fish Wildl. Manag. 2(2):146-155.

Darmstadt GL, Mao-Qiang M, Chi E, Saha SK, Ziboh VA, Black RE, Santosham M, Elias PM (2002). "Impact of topical oils on the skin barrier: possible implications for neonatal health in developing countries," Acta Paediatr. 91(5):546-54.

Darmstadt GL, Saha SK, Ahmed AS, Chowdhury MA, Law PA, Ahmed S, Alam MA, Black RE, Santosham M (2005 Mar 19-25). "Effect of topical treatment with skin barrier-enhancing emollients on nosocomial infections in preterm infants in Bangladesh: a randomised controlled trial," Lancet. 365(9464):1039-45.

Damiani C.E.N., Rossoni L.V., Vassallo D.V. (2003) Vasorelaxant effects of eugenol on rat thoracic aorta. Vascular Pharmacology. 40: 59-66.

Das, I., Acharya, A., Berry, D. L., Sen, S., Williams, E., Permaul, E., . . . Saha, T. (2012 Sep). Antioxidative effects of the spice cardamom against non-melanoma skin cancer by modulating nuclear factor crythroid-2-related factor 2 and NF-kappaB signalling pathways. Br J Nutr, 108(6), 984-997.

da Silva, A.G., Puziol Pde, F., Leitao, R.N., Gomes, T.R., Scherer, R., Martins, M.L., Cavalcanti, A.S., and Cavalcanti, L.C. (2012). "Application of the essential oil from copaiba (Copaifera langsdori Desf.) for acne vulgaris: a double-blind, placebo-controlled clinical trial," Altern Med Rev. 17(1):69-75.

da Silva E.B.P., Matsuo A.L., Figueiredo C.R., Chaves M.H., Sartorelli P., Lago J.H.G. (2013 Feb). "Chemical constituents and cytotoxic evaluation of essential oils from leaves of Porcelia macrocarpa (Annonaceae)," Nat. Prod. Commun. 8(2):277-279.

D'Auria FD, Laino L, Strippoli V, Tecca M, Salvatore G, Battinelli L, Mazzanti G (2001 Aug). "In vitro activity of tea tree oil against Candida albicans mycelial conversion and other pathogenic fungi," J Chemother. 13(4):377-83.

D'Auria FD, Tecca M, Strippoli V, Salvatore G, Battinelli L, Mazzanti G (2005 Aug). "Antifungal activity of Lavandula angustifolia essential oil against Candida albicans yeast and mycelial form," Med Mycol. 43(5):391-6.

Darvesh S, Hopkins A, Guela C (2003 Feb). "Neurobiology of butyrylcholinesterase," Nat. Rev. Neurosci. 4(2):131-138.

Davaatseren, M., Hur, H. J., Yang, H. J., Hwang, J. T., Park, J. H., Kim, H. J., . . . Sung, M. J. (2013 Aug). Taraxacum official (dandelion) leaf extract alleviates high-fat diet-induced nonalcoholic fatty liver. Food Chem Toxicol, 58, 30-36.

Davenport MH, Hogan DB, Exkes GA, Longman RS, Poulin MJ (2012). "Cerebrovascular Reserve: The LInk Between Fitness and Cognitive Function?," Sport Sci Rev, 40(3):153-8.

Davies K (1995). "Oxidative stress: the paradox of aerobic life," Biochem Soc Symp. 61:1-31.

d'Avila Farias M et al (2014 May). "Eugenol derivatives as potential anti-oxidants: is phenolic hydroxyl necessary to obtain an effect?," J. Pharm. Pharmacol. 66(5):733-746.

Dayan N., Sivalenka R, Chase J (2009 Feb). "Skin Moisturization by hydrogenated polyisobutene - Quantitative and visual evaluation," Journal of Cosmetic Science. 60.

de Almeida R.N., Araujo D.A.M., Goncalvevs J.C.R., Montenegro F.C., de Sousa D.P., Leite J.R., Mattei R., Benedito M.A.C., de Carvalho J.G.B., Cruz J.S., Maia J.G.S. (2009) Rosewood oil induces sedation and inhibits compound action petential in rodents. Journal of Ethnopharmacology. 124: 440-443.

de Almeida R.N., de Sousa D.P., Nobrega F.F.F., Claudino F.S., Araujo D.A.M., Leite J.R., Mattei R. (2008) Anticonvulsant effect of a natural compound α,β-epoxy-carvone and its actioin on the nerve excitability. Neuroscience Letters. 443: 51-55.

de Boer H.J., Lamxay V, Björk L (2011 Dec). "Steam sauna and mother roasting in Lao PDR: practices and chemical constituents of essential oils of plant species used in postpartum recovery," BMC Complement Altern Med. 11:128.

Debersac P, Heydel JM, Amiot MJ, Goudonnet H, Artur Y, Suschetet M, Siess MH (2001 Sep). "Induction of cytochrome P450 and/or detoxication enzymes by various extracts of rosemary: description of specific patterns," Food Chem Toxicol. 39(9):907-18.

de Cássia da Silveira e Sá R, Andrade L.N., de Sousa D.P. (2013). "A review on anti-inflammatory activity of monoterpenes," Mol. Basel Switz. 18(1):1227-1254.

Deeptha K, Kamaleeswari M, Sengottuvelan M, Nalini N (2006 Nov). "Dose dependent inhibitory effect of dietary caraway on 1,2-dimethylhydrazine induced colonic aberrant crypt foci and bacterial enzyme activity in rats," Invest New Drugs. 24(6):479-88.

de la Garza, A. L., Etxeberria, U., Lostao, M. P., San Roman, B., Barrenetxe, J., Martinez, J. A., & Milagro, F. I. (2013 Dec). Helichrysum and grapefruit extracts inhibit carbohydrate digestion and absorption, improving postprandial glucose and hyperinsulinemia in rats. J Agric Food Chem, 61(49), 12012-12019.

Delaquis, P. J., Stanich, K., Girard, B., & Mazza, G. (2002 Mar). Antimicrobial activity of individual and mixed fractions of dill, cilantro, coriander and eucalyptus essential oils. Int J Food Microbiol, 74(1–2), 101-109.

DeLeo F.R., Otto M., Kreiswirth B.N., Chambers H.F. (2010) Community-associated meticillin-resistant Staphylococcus aureus. The Lancet. 375: 1557-1568.

Del Toro-Arreola S. et al (2005 May). "Effect of D-limonene on immune response in BALB/c mice with lymphoma," Int. Immunopharmacol. 5(5):829-838.

de Mendonça Rocha PM, Rodilla JM, Díez D, Elder H, Guala MS, Silva LA, Pombo EB (2012 Oct). "Synergistic antibacterial activity of the essential oil of aguaribay (Schinus molle L.)," Molecules. 17(10):12023-36.

Department of Environmental Medicine, Odense University, Denmark (1992 Dec). "Ginger (Zingiber officinale) in rheumatism and musculoskeletal disorders," Med Hypotheses. 39(4):342-8.

de Rapper S., Kamatou, G., Viljoen, A., & van Vuuren, S. (2013 Jun). The in vitro antimicrobial activity of lavandula angustifolia essential oil in combination with other aroma-therapeutic oils. Evid Based Complement Alternat Med, 2013, 1-10.

de Rapper S, Van Vuuren F, Kamatou G.P.P., Viljoen A.M., Dagne E (2012 Apr). "The additive and synergistic antimicrobial effects of select frankincense and myrrh oils – a combination from the pharaonic pharmacopoeia," Letters in Applied Microbiology. 54(4):352-358.

De S. Aguiar, R. W., Ootani, M. A., Ascencio, S. D., Ferreira, T. P., dos Santos, M. M., & dos Santos, G. R. (2014 Jan). Fumigant antifungal activity of Corymbia citriodora and Cymbopogon nardus essential oils and citronellal against three fungal species. Scientific World Journal, 2014, 1-8.

de Sant'anna J.R. et al (2009 Feb). "Genotoxicity of Achillea millefolium essential oil in diploid cells of Aspergillus nidulans," Phytother. Res. PTR. 23(2):231-235.

De Spirt S, Stahl W, Tronnier H, Sies H, Bejot M, Maurette JM, Heinrich U (2009 Feb). "Intervention with flaxseed and borage oil supplements modulates skin condition in women," Br J Nutr. 101(3):440-5.

de Sousa D.P., Goncalves J.C.R., Quintanas-Junior L., Cruz J.S., Araujo D.A.M., de Almeida R.N. (2006) Study of anticonvulsant effect of citronellol, a monoterpene alcohol, in rodents. Neuroscience Letters. 401: 231-235.

Deters A, Zippel J, Hellenbrand N, Pappai D, Possemeyer C, Hensel A (2010 Jan 8). "Aqueous extracts and polysaccharides from Marshmallow roots (Althea officinalis L.): cellular internalisation and stimulation of cell physiology of human epithelial cells in vitro," J Ethnopharmacol. 127(1):62-9.

Devika PT, Mainzen Prince PS (2008 Jan). "(-) Epigallocatechin gallate (EGCG) prevents isoprenaline-induced cardiac marker enzymes and membrane-bound ATPases," J Pharm Pharmacol. 60(1):125-33.

De Vriendt T, Moreno LA, De Henauw S (2009 Sep). "Chronic stress and obesity in adolescents: scientific evidence and methodological issues for epidemiological research," Nutr Metab Cardiovasc Dis. 19(7):511-9.

Dey, Y. N., Ota, S., Srikanth, N., Jamal, M., & Wanjari, M. (2012 Jan). A phytopharmacological review on an important medicinal plant - Amorphophallus paeoniifolius. Ayu, 33(1), 27-32.

Dhawan K, Dhawan S, Sharma A (2004 Sep). "Passiflora: a review update," Journal of Ethnopharmacology. 94(1):1-23.

Dias, F. M., Leffa, D. D., Daumann, F., Marques Sde, O., Luciano, T. F., Possato, J. C., . . . de Lira, F. S. (2014 Feb). Acerola (Malpighia emarginata DC.) juice intake protects against alterations to proteins involved in inflammatory and lipolysis pathways in the adipose tissue of obese mice fed a cafeteria diet. Lipids Health Dis, 13, 1-9.

Díaz C, Quesada S, Brenes O, Aguilar G, Cicció JF (2008). "Chemical composition of Schinus molle essential oil and its cytotoxic activity on tumour cell lines," Nat Prod Res. 22(17):1521-34.

Appendix

Diego MA, Jones NA, Field T, Hernandez-Reif M, Schanberg S, Kuhn C, McAdam V, Galamaga R, Galamaga M (1998 Dec). "Aromatherapy positively affects mood, EEG patterns of alertness and math computations," Int J Neurosci. 96(3-4):217-24.

Diggins K.C. (2008) Treatment of mild to moderate dehydration in children with oral rehydration therapy. Journal of the American Academy of Nurse Practitioners. 20: 402-406.

Dikshit A, Naqvi AA, Husain A. (1986 May). "Schinus molle: a new source of natural fungitoxicant," Appl Environ Microbiol. 51(5):1085-8.

Dimas K, Kokkinopoulos D, Demetzos C, Vaos B, Marselos M, Malamas M, Tzavaras T (1999 Mar). "The effect of sclareol on growth and cell cycle progression of human leukemic cell lines," Leuk Res. 23(3):217-34.

Dimpfel W, Pischel I, Lehnfeld R (2004 Sep 29). "Effects of lozenge containing lavender oil, extracts from hops, lemon balm and oat on electrical brain activity of volunteers," Eur J Med Res. 9(9):423-31.

Ding XF, Shen M, Xu LY, Dong JH, Chen G (2013 May). "13,14-bis(cis-3,5-di-methyl-1-piperazinyl)-beta-elemene, a novel beta-elemene derivative, shows potent antitumor activities via inhibition of mTOR in human breast cancer cells," Oncol Lett. 5(5):1554-1558.

Di Pasqua R, Betts G, Hoskins N, Edwards M, Ercolini D, Mauriello G (2007 Jun). "Membrane toxicity of antimicrobial compounds from essential oils," J. Agric. Food Chem. 55(12):4863-4870.

Djilani, A., & Dicko, A. (2012 Feb). The Therapeutic Benefits of Essential Oils. In J. Bouayed (Ed.), Nutrition, Well-Being and Health (pp. 155-178): InTech.

Do M, Martins R, Arantes S, Candeias F, Tinoco M.T., Cruz-Morais J (2014 Jan). "Antioxidant, antimicrobial and toxicological properties of Schinus molle L. essential oils," J. Ethnopharmacol. 151(1):485-92.

Dohare P, Garg P, Sharma U, Jagannathan N, Ray M (2008). "Neuroprotective efficacy and therapeutic window of curcuma oil: in rat embolic stroke model," BMC Complement. Altern. Med. 8(1):55.

Dohare P, Varma S, Ray M (2008 Aug). "Curcuma oil modulates the nitric oxide system response to cerebral ischemia/reperfusion injury," Nitric Oxide. 19(1):1-11.

Domitrović R, Jakovac H, Romić Z, Rahelić D, Tadić Z (2010 Aug 9). "Antifibrotic activity of Taraxacum officinale root in carbon tetrachloride-induced liver damage in mice," J Ethnopharmacol. 130(3):569-77.

Doran AL, Morden WE, Dunn K, Edwards-Jones V (2009 Apr). "Vapour-phase activities of essential oils against antibiotic sensitive and resistant bacteria including MRSA," Lett Appl Microbiol. 48(4):387-92.

Dorman H.J., Deans S.G. (2000 Feb). "Antimicrobial agents from plants: antibacterial activity of plant volatile oils," J. Appl. Microbiol. 88(2):308-316.

Dorow P, Weiss T, Felix R, Schmutzler H (1987 Dec). "[Effect of a secretolytic and a combination of pinene, limonene and cineole on mucociliary clearance in patients with chronic obstructive pulmonary disease]," Arzneimittelforschung. 37(12):1378-1381.

Dozmorov M.G. et al (2014). "Differential effects of selective frankincense (Ru Xiang) essential oil versus non-selective sandalwood (Tan Xiang) essential oil on cultured bladder cancer cells: a microarray and bioinformatics study," Chin Med. 9:18.

Drobiova H, Thomson M, Al-Qattan K, Peltonen-Shalaby R, Al-Amin Z, Ali M (2009 Feb 20). "Garlic increases antioxidant levels in diabetic and hypertensive rats determined by a modified peroxidase method," Evid Based Complement Alternat Med. Epub ahead of print.

Duarte MC, Leme EE, Delarmelina C, Soares AA, Figueira GM, Sartoratto A (2007 May 4). "Activity of essential oils from Brazilian medicinal plants on Escherichia coli," J Ethnopharmacol. 111(2):197-201

Duarte, Luiza C, Speakman John R (2014). "Low resting metabolic rate is associated with greater lifespan because of a confounding effect of body fatness," Age, 36:9731.

Dudai N, Weinstein Y, Krup M, Rabinski T, Ofir R (2005 May). "Citral is a new inducer of caspase-3 in tumor cell lines," Planta Med. 71(5):484-8.

Dunn C, Sleep J, Collett D (1995 Jan). "Sensing an improvement: an experimental study to evaluate the use of aromatherapy, massage and periods of rest in an intensive care unit," J Adv Nurs. 21(1):34-40.

Dunstan JA, Mori TA, Barden A, Beilin LJ, Taylor AL, Holt PG, Prescott SL (2003 Dec). "Fish oil supplementation in pregnancy modifies neonatal allergen-specific immune responses and clinical outcomes in infants at high risk of atopy: a randomized, controlled trial," J Allergy Clin Immunol. 112(6):1178-84.

Duwiejua M, Zeitlin IJ, Waterman PG, Chapman J, Mhango GJ, Provan GJ (1993 Feb). "Anti-inflammatory activity of resins from some species of the plant family Burseraceae," Planta Med. 59(1):12-6.

Dwivedi C, Abu-Ghazaleh A (1997 Aug). "Chemopreventive effects of sandalwood oil on skin papillomas in mice," Eur J Cancer Prev. 6(4):399-401.

Dwivedi C, Guan X, Harmsen WL, Voss AL, Goetz-Parten DE, Koopman EM, Johnson KM, Valluri HB, Matthees DP (2003 Feb). "Chemopreventive effects of alpha-santalol on skin tumor development in CD-1 and SENCAR mice," Cancer Epidemiol Biomarkers Prev. 12(2):151-6.

Dwivedi C, Maydew ER, Hora JJ, Ramaeker DM, Guan X. (2005 Oct) "Chemopreventive effects of various concentrations of alpha-santalol on skin cancer development in CD-1 mice," Eur J Cancer Prev. 14(5):473-6.

Dwivedi C, Valluri HB, Guan X, Agarwal R (2006 Sep). "Chemopreventive effects of alpha-santalol on ultraviolet B radiation-induced skin tumor development in SKH-1 hairless mice," Carcinogenesis. 27(9):1917-22.

Dwyer, L., Oh, A., Patrick, H., & Hennessy, E. (2015). Promoting family meals: a review of existing interventions and opportunities for future research. Adolesc Health Med Ther, 6, 115-131.

Dyer J, Cleary L, Ragsdale-Lowe M, McNeill S, Osland C (2014 Nov). "The use of aromasticks at a cancer centre: a retrospective audit," Complement. Ther. Clin. Pract. 20(4):203-206.

Ebihara T, Ebihara S, Maruyama M, Kobayashi M, Itou A, Arai H, Sasaki H (2006 Sep). "A randomized trial of olfactory stimulation using black pepper oil in older people with swallowing dysfunction," J Am Geriatr Soc. 54(9):1401-6.

Edwards-Jones V, Buck R, Shawcross SG, Dawson MM, Dunn K (2004 Dec). "The effect of essential oils on methicillin-resistant Staphylococcus aureus using a dressing model," Burns. 30(8):772-7.

Elaissi A. et al (2012). "Chemical composition of 8 eucalyptus species' essential oils and the evaluation of their antibacterial, antifungal and antiviral activities," BMC Complement. 12:81.

Ellouze I, Abderrabba M, Sabaou N, Mathieu F, Lebrihi A, Bouajila J (2012 Sep). "Season's variation impact on Citrus aurantium leaves essential oil chemical composition and biological activities," J Food Sci. 77(9):T173-80.

ElSalhy M, Sayed Zahid I, Honkala E (2012 Dec). "Effects of xylitol mouthrinse on Streptococcus mutans," J. Dent. 40(12):1151-1154.

Elson CE, Underbakke GL, Hanson P, Shrago E, Wainberg RH, Qureshi AA (1989 Aug). "Impact of lemongrass oil, an essential oil, on serum cholesterol," Lipids. 24(8):677-9.

El-Soud NH, Deabes M, El-Kassem LA, Khalil M (2015 Sep 15). "Chemical composition and antifungal activity of ocimum basilicum l. essential oil," Open Access Maced J Med Sci. 3(3):374-9.

Elwakeel HA, Moneim HA, Farid M, Gohar AA (2007 Jul). "Clove oil cream: a new effective treatment for chronic anal fissure," Colorectal Dis. 9(6):549-52.

Enan E (2001 Nov). "Insecticidal activity of essential oils: octopaminergic sites of action," Comp Biochem Physiol C Toxicol Pharmacol. 130(3):325-37.

Enshaieh S, Jooya A, Siadat AH, Iraji F (2007 Jan-Feb). "The efficacy of 5% topical tea tree oil gel in mild to moderate acne vulgaris: a randomized, double-blind placebo-controlled study," Indian J Dermatol Venereol Leprol. 73(1):22-5.

Eriksson K., Levin J.O. (1996) Gas chromatographic-mass spectrometric identification of metabolites from α-pinene in human urine after occupational exposure to sawing fumes. J. Chromatography B. 677: 85-98.

Erkkilä AT, Lichtenstein AH, Mozaffarian D, Herrington DM (2004 Sep). "Fish intake is associated with a reduced progression of coronary artery atherosclerosis in postmenopausal women with coronary artery disease," Am J Clin Nutr. 80(3):626-32.

Erkkilä AT, Schwab US, de Mello VD, Lappalainen T, Mussalo H, Lehto S, Kemi V, Lamberg-Allardt C, Uusitupa MI (2008 Sep). "Effects of fatty and lean fish intake on blood pressure in subjects with coronary heart disease using multiple medications," Eur J Nutr. 47(6):319-28.

Esfandiary, E., Karimipour, M., Mardani, M., Alaei, H., Ghannadian, M., Kazemi, M., . . . Esmaeili, A. (2014 Apr). Novel effects of Rosa damascena extract on memory and neurogenesis in a rat model of Alzheimer's disease. J Neurosci Res, 92(4), 517-530.

Evandri MG, Battinelli L, Daniele C, Mastrangelo S, Bolle P, Mazzanti G (2005 Sep). "The antimutagenic activity of Lavandula angustifolia (lavender) essential oil in the bacterial reverse mutation assay," Food Chem Toxicol. 43(9):1381-7.

Evangelista M.T.P., Abad-Casintahan F, Lopez-Villafuerte (2014 Jan). "The effect of topical virgin coconut oil on SCORAD index, transepidermal water loss, and skin capacitance in mild to moderate pediatric atopic dermatitis: a randomized, double-blind, clinical trial," Int J Dermatol. 53(1):100-108.

Evans D.L., Miller D.M., Jacobsen K.L., Bush P.B. (1987). "Modulation of immune responses in mice by d-limonene," J. Toxicol. Environ. Health. 20(1-2):51-66.

Evans J.D., Martin S.A. (2000) Effects of Thymol on Ruminal Microorganisms. Current Microbiology. 41: 336-340.

Ezoddini-Ardakani F (2010 May). "Efficacy of Miswak (salvadora persica) in preventing dental caries," Health (N. Y.). 2(5):499.

Fabio A, Cermelli C, Fabio G, Nicoletti P, Quaglio P (2007 Apr). "Screening of the antibacterial effects of a variety of essential oils on microorganisms responsible for respiratory infections," Phytother Res. 21(4):374-7.

Fan AY, Lao L, Zhang RX, Zhou AN, Wang LB, Moudgil KD, Lee DY, Ma ZZ, Zhang WY, Berman BM (2005 Oct 3). "Effects of an acetone extract of Boswellia carterii Birdw. (Burseraceae) gum resin on adjuvant-induced arthritis in lewis rats," J Ethnopharmacol. 101(1-3):104-9.

Fahn, A. (1988). Secretory tissues in vascular plants. New Phytologist, 108(3), 229-257.

Falk A.J., Bauer L., Bell C.L., Smolenski S.J. (1974 Dec). "The constituents of the essential oil from Achillea millefolium L," Lloydia. 37(4):598-602.

Fang, J. Y., Leu, Y. L., Hwang, T. L., & Cheng, H. C. (2004 Nov). Essential oils from sweet basil (Ocimum basilicum) as novel enhancers to accelerate transdermal drug delivery. Biol Pharm Bull, 27(11), 1819-1825.

Fang, Y.-Z., Yang, S., & Wu, G. (2002). Free radicals, antioxidants, and nutrition. Nutrition, 18(10), 872-879.

Farco J.A., Grundmann O. (2013). "Menthol--pharmacology of an important naturally medicinal 'cool,'" Mini Rev. Med. Chem. 13(1):124-131.

Farnsworth, N. R., & Soejarto, D. D. (1985). Potential consequence of plant extinction in the United States on the current and future availability of prescription drugs. Economic botany, 39(3), 231-240.

Farris PK (2005 Jul). "Topical vitamin C: a useful agent for treating photoaging and other dermatologic conditions," Dermatol Surg. 31(7 Pt 2):814-7

Fathiazad, F., Matlobi, A., Khorrami, A., Hamedeyazdan, S., Soraya, H., Hammami, M., . . . Garjani, A. (2012 Jan). Phytochemical screening and evaluation of cardioprotective activity of ethanolic extract of Ocimum basilicum L. (basil) against isoproterenol induced myocardial infarction in rats. Daru, 20(1), 87.

Faturi, C. B., Leite, J. R., Alves, P. B., Canton, A. C., & Teixeira-Silva, F. (2010 May). Anxiolytic-like effect of sweet orange aroma in Wistar rats. Prog Neuropsychopharmacol Biol Psychiatry, 34(4), 605-609.

Fayazi S, Babashahi M, Rezaei M (2011). "The effect of inhalation aromatherapy on anxiety level of the patients in preoperative period," Iran. J. Nurs. Midwifery Res. 16(4):278-283.

Feinblatt HM (1960 Jan). "Cajeput-type oil for the treatment of furunculosis," J Natl Med Assoc. 52:32-4.

Feng J, Zhang S, Shi W, Zubcevik N, Miklossy J, Zhang Y (2017 Oct). "Selective Essential Oils from Spice or Culinary Herbs Have High Activity against Stationary Phase and Biofilm Borrelia burgdorferi," Front Med (Lausanne). 4:169.

Fernandez, L. F., Palomino, O. M., & Frutos, G. (2014 Jan). Effectiveness of Rosmarinus officinalis essential oil as antihypotensive agent in primary hypotensive patients and its influence on health-related quality of life. J Ethnopharmacol, 151(1), 509-516.

Ferrara, L., Naviglio, D., & Armone Caruso, A. (2012). Cytological aspects on the effects of a nasal spray consisting of standardized extract of citrus lemon and essential oils in allergic rhinopathy. ISRN Pharm, 2012, 1-6.

Ferreira B.S. et al (2011 Jul). "Comparative Properties of Amazonian Oils Obtained by Different Extraction Methods," Molecules. 16(7):5875-5885.

Ferrini AM, Mannoni V, Aureli P, Salvatore G, Piccirilli E, Ceddia T, Pontieri E, Sessa R, Oliva B (2006 Jul-Sep). "Melaleuca alternifolia essential oil possesses potent anti-staphylococcal activity extended to strains resistant to antibiotics," Int J Immunopathol Pharmacol. 19(3):539-44.

Field T, Diego M, Hernandez-Reif M, Cisneros W, Feijo L, Vera Y, Gil K, Grina D, Claire He Q (2005 Feb). "Lavender fragrance cleansing gel effects on relaxation," Int J Neurosci. 115(2):207-22.

Filiptsove O.V., Gazzavi-Rogozina L.V., Timoshyna I.A., Naboka O.I., Dyomina Y.V., Ochkur A.V (2018 Mar). "The effect of the essential oils of lavender and rosemary on the human short-term memory," Alex. J. Med. 54(1):41-44.

Filoche SK, Soma K, Sissons CH (2005 Aug). "Antimicrobial effects of essential oils in combination with chlorhexidine digluconate," Oral Microbiol Immunol. 20(4):221-5.

Fine DH, Furgang D, Barnett ML, Drew C, Steinberg L, Charles CH, Vincent JW (2000 Mar). "Effect of an essential oil-containing antiseptic mouthrinse on plaque and salivary Streptococcus mutans levels," J Clin Periodontol. 27(3):157-61.

Fitzhugh DJ, Shan S, Dewhirst MW, Hale LP (2008 Jul). "Bromelain treatment decreases neutrophil migration to sites of inflammation," Clin Immunol. 128(1):66-74.

Flor-Weiler, L. B., Behle, R. W., & Stafford, K. C., 3rd. (2011 Mar). Susceptibility of four tick species, Amblyomma americanum, Dermacentor variabilis, Ixodes scapularis, and Rhipicephalus sanguineus (Acari: Ixodidae), to nootkatone from essential oil of grapefruit. J Med Entomol, 48(2), 322-326.

Force M, Sparks WS, Ronzio RA (2000 May). "Inhibition of enteric parasites by emulsified oil of oregano in vivo," Phytother Res. 14(3):213-4.

Fowke JH, Morrow JD, Motley S, Bostick RM, Ness RM (2006 Oct). "Brassica vegetable consumption reduces urinary F2-isoprostane levels independent of micronutrient intake," Carcinogenesis. 27(10):2096-102.

Franek KJ, Zhou Z, Zhang WD, Chen WY (2005 Jan). "In vitro studies of baicalin alone or in combination with Salvia miltiorrhiza extract as a potential anti-cancer agent," Int J Oncol. 26(1):217-24.

Frangou S, Lewis M, McCrone P (2006 Jan). "Efficacy of ethyl-eicosapentaenoic acid in bipolar depression: randomised double-blind placebo-controlled study," Br J Psychiatry. 188:46-50.

Frank K, Patel K, Lopez G, Willis B (2017 Jun). "Coconut Oil Research Analysis," Examine.com.

Frank M.B. et al (2009). "Frankincense oil derived from Boswellia carteri induces tumor cell specific cytotoxicity," BMC Complement Altern Med. 9:6.

Fraňková A, Marounek M, Mozrová V, Weber J, Klouček P, Lukešová D (2014 Oct). "Antibacterial activities of plant-derived compounds and essential oils toward Cronobacter sakazakii and Cronobacter malonaticus," Foodborne Pathog. Dis. 11(10):795-797.

Freires Ide, A., Murata, R. M., Furletti, V. F., Sartoratto, A., Alencar, S. M., Figueira, G. M., . . . Rosalen, P. L. (2014 Jun). Coriandrum sativum L. (Coriander) Essential Oil: Antifungal Activity and Mode of Action on Candida spp., and Molecular Targets Affected in Human Whole-Genome Expression. PLoS ONE, 9(6), 1-13.

Freise J, Köhler S (1999 Mar). "Peppermint oil-caraway oil fixed combination in non-ulcer dyspepsia--comparison of the effects of enteric preparations," Pharmazie. 54(3):210-5.

Freitas F.P., Freitas S.P., Lemos G.C.S., Vieira I.J.C., Gravina G.A., Lemos F.J.A. (2010) Comparative Larvicial Activity of Essential Oils from Three Medicinal Plants against Aedes aeypti L. Chemistry & Biodiversity. 7: 2801-2807.

Frontera WR, Meredith CN, O'Reilly KP, Knuttgen HG, Evans WJ (1988 Mar). "Strength conditioning in older men: skeletal muscle hypertrophy and improved function," J Appl Physiol. 64(3):1038-44.

Frydman-Marom, A., Levin, A., Farfara, D., Benromano, T., Scherzer-Attali, R., Peled, S., . . . Ovadia, M. (2011 Feb). Orally administered cinnamon extract reduces beta-amyloid oligomerization and corrects cognitive impairment in Alzheimer's disease animal models. PLoS ONE, 6(1), 1-11.

Fu Y. et al (2007 Oct). "Antimicrobial activity of clove and rosemary essential oils alone and in combination," Phytother. Res. PTR. 21(10):989-994.

Fu Y. et al (2009). "The antibacterial activity of clove essential oil against Propionibacterium acnes and its mechanism of action," Arch. Dermatol. 145(1):86-88.

Fukada M, Kano E, Miyoshi M, Komaki R, Watanabe T (2012 May). "Effect of 'Rose Essential Oil' Inhalation on Stress-Induced Skin-Barrier Disruption in Rats and Humans," Chemical Senses. 37(4):347-356.

Fukumoto S, Sawasaki E, Okuyama S, Miyake Y, Yokogoshi H (2006 Feb-Apr). "Flavor components of monoterpenes in citrus essential oils enhance the release of monoamines from rat brain slices," Nutr Neurosci. 9(1-2):73-80.

Furuhjelm C, Warstedt K, Larsson J, Fredriksson M, Böttcher MF, Fälth-Magnusson K, Duchén K (2009 Sep). "Fish oil supplementation in pregnancy and lactation may decrease the risk of infant allergy," Acta Paediatr. 98(9):1461-7.

Gaetani G.F., Ferraris A.M., Rolfo M., Mangerini R., Arena S., Kirkman H.N. (1996) Predominant role of catalase in the disposal of hydrogen peroxide within human erythrocytes. Blood. 87: 1595-1599.

Ganesan B, Buddhan S, Anandan R, Sivakumar R, AnbinEzhilan R. (2010 Mar). "Antioxidant defense of betaine against isoprenaline-induced myocardial infarction in rats," Mol Biol Rep. 37(3):1319-27.

Gauch L.M.R. et al (2014 Jun). "Effects of Rosmarinus officinalis essential oil on germ tube formation by Candida albicans isolated from denture wearers," Rev. Soc. Bras. Med. Trop. 47(3):389-391.

Gaunt L.F., Higgins S.C., Hughes J.F. (2005) Interaction of air ions and bactericidal vapours to control micro-organisms. Journal of Applied Microbiology. 99: 1324-1329.

Gayathri B, Manjula N, Vinaykumar KS, Lakshmi BS, Balakrishnan A (2007 Apr). "Pure compound from Boswellia serrata extract exhibits anti-inflammatory property in human PBMCs and mouse macrophages through inhibition of TNFalpha, IL-1beta, NO and MAP kinases," Int Immunopharmacol. 7(4):473-82.

Gbenou, J. D., Ahounou, J. F., Akakpo, H. B., Laleye, A., Yayi, E., Gbaguidi, F., . . . Kotchoni, S. O. (2013 Feb). Phytochemical composition of Cymbopogon citratus and Eucalyptus citriodora essential oils and their anti-inflammatory and analgesic properties on Wistar rats. Mol Biol Rep, 40(2), 1127-1134.

Gershenzon, J. (1994 Jun). Metabolic costs of terpenoid accumulation in higher plants. J Chem Ecol, 20(6), 1281-1328.

Ghelardini C, Galeotti N, Di Cesare Mannelli L, Mazzanti G, Bartolini A (2001 May-Jul). "Local anaesthetic activity of beta-caryophyllene," Farmaco. 56(5-7):387-9.

Ghelardini C, Galeotti N, Mazzanti G (2001 Aug). "Local anaesthetic activity of monoterpenes and phenylpropanes of essential oils," Planta Med. 67(6):564-6.

Ghelardini C, Galeotti N, Salvatore G, Mazzanti G (1999 Dec). "Local anaesthetic activity of the essential oil of Lavandula angustifolia," Planta Med. 65(8):700-3.

Ghersetich I, Lotti T, Campanile G, Grappone C, Dini G (1994 Feb). "Hyaluronic acid in cutaneous intrinsic aging," Int J Dermatol. 33(2):119-22.

Ghods A.A., Abforosh N.H., Ghorbani R, Asgari M.R. (2015 Jun). "The effect of topical application of lavender essential oil on the intensity of pain caused by the insertion of dialysis needles in hemodialysis patients: A randomized clinical trial," Complement. Ther. Med. 23(3):325-330.

Ghosh, V., Saranya, S., Mukherjee, A., & Chandrasekaran, N. (2013 May). Antibacterial microemulsion prevents sepsis and triggers healing of wound in wistar rats. Colloids Surf B Biointerfaces, 105, 152-157.

Gibriel, A., Al-Sayed, H., Rady, A., & Abdelaleem, M. (2013 Jun). Synergistic antibacterial activity of irradiated and nonirradiated cumin, thyme and rosemary essential oils. Journal of Food Safety, 33(2), 222-228.

Gilani, A. H., Jabeen, Q., Khan, A. U., & Shah, A. J. (2008 Feb). Gut modulatory, blood pressure lowering, diuretic and sedative activities of cardamom. J Ethnopharmacol, 115(3), 463-472.

Gillissen A, Wittig T, Ehmen M, Krezdorn H.G., de Mey C (2013 Jan). "A multicentre, randomised, double-blind, placebo-controlled clinical trial on the efficacy and tolerability of GeloMyrtol® forte in acute bronchitis," Drug Res. 63(1):19-27.

Gnatta J.R., Piason P.P., de C, Lopes L.B.C., Rogenski N.M.B., da Silva M.J.P. (2014 Jun). "[Aromatherapy with ylang ylang for anxiety and self-esteem: a pilot study]," Rev. Esc. Enferm. U P. 48(3):492-499.

Göbel H, Schmidt G, Soyka D (1994 Jun). "Effect of peppermint and eucalyptus oil preparations on neurophysiological and experimental algesimetric headache parameters," Cephalalgia. 14(3):228-34.

Goel A, Ahmad FJ, Singh RM, Singh GN (2010 Feb). "3-Acetyl-11-keto-beta-boswellic acid loaded-polymeric nanomicelles for topical anti-inflammatory and anti-arthritic activity," J Pharm Pharmacol. 62(2):273-8.

Goel N, Kim H, Lao R.P. (2005). "An olfactory stimulus modifies nighttime sleep in young men and women," Chronobiol. Int. 22(5):889-904.

Goes, T. C., Antunes, F. D., Alves, P. B., & Teixeira-Silva, F. (2012 Aug). Effect of sweet orange aroma on experimental anxiety in humans. J Altern Complement Med, 18(8), 798-804.

Golab M, Skwarlo-Sonta K (2007 Mar). "Mechanisms involved in the anti-inflammatory action of inhaled tea tree oil in mice," Exp Biol Med (Maywood). 232(3):420-6.

Goldberg, D. R. (2009). Aspirin: Turn of the Century Miracle Drug. Chemical Heritage Magazine, 27.

Gomes NM, Rezende CM, Fontes SP, Matheus ME, Fernandes PD. (2007 Feb 12). "Antinociceptive activity of Amazonian Copaiba oils," J Ethnopharmacol. 109(3):486-92.

Gómez-Rincón, C., Langa, E., Murillo, P., Valero, M. S., Berzosa, C., & López, V. (2014 May). Activity of Tea Tree (Melaleuca alternifolia) Essential Oil against L3 Larvae of Anisakis simplex. 2014, 1-6.

Appendix

Goncalves J.C.R., Alves A.M.H., de Araujo A.E.V., Cruz J.S., Araujo D.A.M. (2010) Distinct effects of carvone analogues on the isolated nerve of rats. European Journal of Pharmacology. 645: 108-112.

Goncalves J.C.R., Oliveira F.S., Benedito R.B., de Sousa D.P., de Almeida R.N., Araujo D.A.M. (2008) Antinociceptive Activity of (-)-Carvone: Evidence of Association with Decreased Peripheral Nerve Excitability. Biological and Parmaceutical Bulletin. 31: 1017-1020.

Gonzalez-Audino P, Picollo M.I., Gallardo A, Toloza A, Vassena C, Mougabure-Cueto G (2011 Jul). "Comparative toxicity of oxygenated monoterpenoids in experimental hydroalcoholic lotions to permethrin resistant adult head lice," Arch. Dermatol. 303(5):361-366.

Gonzalez-Castejon, M., Garcia-Carrasco, B., Fernandez-Dacosta, R., Davalos, A., & Rodriguez-Casado, A. (2014 May). Reduction of adipogenesis and lipid accumulation by Taraxacum officinale (Dandelion) extracts in 3T3L1 adipocytes: an in vitro study. Phytother Res, 28(5), 745-752.

González-Trujano ME, Peña EI, Martínez AL, Moreno J, Guevara-Fefer P, Déciga-Campos M, López-Muñoz FJ (2007 May 22). "Evaluation of the antinociceptive effect of Rosmarinus officinalis L. using three different experimental models in rodents," J Ethnopharmacol. 111(3):476-82.

Goodpaster, Bret H, Chomentowski, Peter, Ward, Bryan K, Rossi, Andrea, Glynn, Nancy W, Delmonico, Matthew J, Kritchevsky, Stephen B, Pahor, Marco, Newman, Anne B (2008 Sep). "Effects of physical activity on strength and skeletal muscle fat infiltration in older adults: a randomized controlled trial," J Appl Physiol, 105:1498-503.

Goodwin J.S., Atluru D., Sierakowski S., Lianos E.A. (1986) Mechanism of Action of Glucocorticosteroids: Inhibition of T Cell Proliferation and Interleukin 2 Production by Hydrocortisones Is Reversed by Leukotriene B4. Journal of Clinical Investigation. 77: 1244-1250.

Gorwitz R.J., Kruszon-Moran D., McAllister S.K., McQuillan G., McDougal L.K., Fosheim G.E., Jensen B.J., Killgore G., Tenover F.C., Kuehnert M.J. (2008) Changes in the Prevalence of Nasal Colonization with Staphylococcus aureusin the United States, 2001-2004. Journal of Infectious Diseases. 197: 1226-1234.

Gossell-Williams M, Hyde C, Hunter T, Simms-Stewart D, Fletcher H, McGrowder D, Walters CA (2011 Oct). "Improvement in HDL cholesterol in postmenopausal women supplemented with pumpkin seed oil: pilot study," Climacteric. 14(5):558-64.

Goswami, S. K., Inamdar, M. N., Jamwal, R., & Dethe, S. (2014 Jun). Effect of Cinnamomum cassia Methanol Extract and Sildenafil on Arginase and Sexual Function of Young Male Wistar Rats. J Sex Med, 11(6), 1475-1483.

Goswami, S. K., Inamdar, M. N., Jamwal, R., & Dethe, S. (2013 Dec). Efficacy of Cinnamomum cassia Blume. in age induced sexual dysfunction of rats. J Young Pharm, 5(4), 148-153.

Grassmann J, Hippeli S, Dornisch K, Rohnert U, Beuscher N, Elstner EF (2000 Feb). "Antioxidant properties of essential oils. Possible explanations for their anti-inflammatory effects," Arzneimittelforschung. 50(2):135-9.

Grassmann J, Schneider D, Weiser D, Elstner EF (2001 Oct). "Antioxidative effects of lemon oil and its components on copper induced oxidation of low density lipoprotein," Arzneimittelforschung. 51(10):799-805.

Greche, H., Hajjaji, N., Ismaïli-Alaoui, M., Mrabet, N., and Benjilali, B. (2000). "Chemical Composition and Antifungal Properties of the Essential Oil of Tanacetum annuum," J Essential Oil Research. 12(1):122-124.

Greive, K.A., & Barnes T.M. (2017 Mar. 7). "The efficacy of Australian essential oils for the treatment of head lice infestation in children: A randomised controlled trial," Australas J Dermatol. Epub ahead of print.

Grespan, R., Paludo, M., Lemos Hde, P., Barbosa, C. P., Bersani-Amado, C. A., Dalalio, M. M., & Cuman, R. K. (2012 Oct). Anti-arthritic effect of eugenol on collagen-induced arthritis experimental model. Biol Pharm Bull, 35(10), 1818-1820.

Grether -Beck, S., Muhlberg, K., Brenden, H., & Krutmann, J. (2008 Jul). [Topical application of vitamins, phytosterols and ceramides. Protection against increased expression of interstitial collagenase and reduced collagen-I expression after single exposure to UVA irradiation]. Hautarzt, 59(7), 557-562.

Grigoleit HG, Grigoleit P (2005 Aug). "Peppermint oil in irritable bowel syndrome," Phytomedicine. 12(8):601-6.

Grunebaum L.D., Murdock J, Castanedo-Tardan M.P., Basumann L.S. (2011 Jun). "Effects of lavender olfactory input on cosmetic procedures," J. Cosmet. Dermatol. 10(2):89-93.

Gonzalez, J. T., & Stevenson, E. J. (2012 Aug 3). Postprandial glycemia and appetite sensations in response to porridge made with rolled and pinhead oats. J Am Coll Nutr, 31(2), 111-116.

Gross, M., Nesher, E., Tikhonov, T., Raz, O., & Pinhasov, A. (2013 Mar). Chronic food administration of Salvia sclarea oil reduces animals' anxious and dominant behavior. J Med Food, 16(3), 216-222.

Guang, L., Li-Bin, Z., Bing-An, F., Ming-Yang, Q., Li-Hua, Y., and Ji-Hong, X. (2004). "Inhibition of growth and metastasis of human gastric cancer implanted in nude mice by d-limonene," World J. Gastroenterol. 10: 2140–2144.

Guerra-Boone L, Alvarez-Román R, Salazar-Aranda R, Torres-Cirio A, Rivas-Galindo VM, Waksman de Torres N, González González GM, Pérez-López LA (2013 Jan). "Chemical compositions and antimicrobial and antioxidant activities of the essential oils from Magnolia grandiflora, Chrysactinia mexicana, and Schinus molle found in northeast Mexico," Nat Prod Commun. 8(1):135-8.

Guillemain J, Rousseau A, Delaveau P (1989). "Neurodepressive effects of the essential oil of Lavandula angustifolia Mill," Ann Pharm Fr. 47(6):337-43.

Guimarães A.G., Quintans J.S.S., Quintans-Júnior L.J. (2013 Jan). "Monoterpenes with Analgesic ActivityA Systematic Review: MONOTERPENES WITH ANALGESIC ACTIVITY," Phytother. Res. 27(1):1-15.

Gumral, N., Doguc Kumbul, D., Aylak, F., Saygin, M., & Savik, E. (2013 Jan). Juniperus communis Linn oil decreases oxidative stress and increases antioxidant enzymes in the heart of rats administered a diet rich in cholesterol. Toxicol Ind Health.

Gundidza M (1993 Nov). "Antimicrobial activity of essential oil from Schinus molle Linn," Cent Afr J Med. 39(11):231-4.

Guo X., Longnecker M.P., Michalek J.E. (2001) Relation of serum tetrachlorodibenzo-p-dioxin concentration to diet among veterans in the Air Force health study with background-level exposure. Journal of Toxicology and Environmental Health, Part A. 63: 159-172.

Guo, X.M., Lu, Q., Liu, Z.J., Wang, L.F., & Feng, B.A. (2006 Aug.). "[Effects of D-limonene on leukemia cells HL-60 and K562 in vitro]," Zhongguo Shi Yan Xue Ye Xue Za Zhi. 14(4):692-5.

Gupta A., Myrdal P.B. (2004) Development of perillyl alcohol topical cream formulation. International Journal of Pharmaceutics. 269: 373-383.

Gurney A.M. (1994) Mechanisms of Drug-induced Vasodilation. Journal of Pharmacy and Pharmacology. 46: 242-251.

Guzmán-Gutiérrez S.L., Bonilla-Jaime H., Gómez-Cansino R., Reyes-Chilpa R (2015 May). "Linalool and βpinene exert their antidepressant-like activity through the monoaminergic pathway," Life Sci. 128:24-29.

Haag J.D., Lindstrom M.J., Gould M.N. (1992) Limonene-induced Regression of Mammary Carcinomas. Cancer Research. 52: 4021-4026.

Habashy, R. R., Abdel-Naim, A. B., Khalifa, A. E., & Al-Azizi, M. M. (2005 Feb). Anti-inflammatory effects of jojoba liquid wax in experimental models. Pharmacol Res, 51(2), 95-105.

Hadley SK, Gaarder SM (2005 Dec 15). "Treatment of irritable bowel syndrome," Am Fam Physician. 72(12):2501-6.

Hagen TM, Liu J, Lykkesfeldt J, Wehr CM, Ingersoll RT, Vinarsky V, Bartholomew JC, Ames BN. "Feeding acetyl-L-carnitine and lipoic acid to old rats significantly improves metabolic function while decreasing oxidative stress," Proc Natl Acad Sci U S A. 99(4):1870-5.

Hager K, Kenklies M, McAfoose J, Engel J, Münch G (2007). "Alpha-lipoic acid as a new treatment option for Alzheimer's disease--a 48 months follow-up analysis," J Neural Transm Suppl. (72):189-93.

Hajhashemi V, Abbasi N (2008 Mar). "Hypolipidemic activity of Anethum graveolens in rats," Phytother Res. 22(3):372-5.

Hajhashemi V, Ghannadi A, Sharif B (2003 Nov). "Anti-inflammatory and analgesic properties of the leaf extracts and essential oil of Lavandula angustifolia Mill," J Ethnopharmacol. 89(1):67-71.

Hajhashemi V, Zolfaghari B, Yousefi A (2012). "Antinociceptive and anti-inflammatory activities of Satureja hortensis seed essential oil, hydroalcoholic and polyphenolic extracts in animal models," Med Princ Pract. 21(2):178-82.

Hakim IA, Harris RB, Ritenbaugh C (2000). "Citrus peel use is associated with reduced risk of squamous cell carcinoma of the skin," Nutr Cancer. 37(2):161-8.

Hakim I.A., McClure T, Liebler D (2000 Aug). "Assessing Dietary D-Limonene Intake for Epidemiological Studies," J Food Compos. Anal. 13(4):329-336.

Halder, S., Mehta, A. K., Kar, R., Mustafa, M., Mediratta, P. K., & Sharma, K. K. (2011 May). Clove oil reverses learning and memory deficits in scopolamine-treated mice. Planta Med, 77(8), 830-834.

Halder, S., Mehta, A. K., Mediratta, P. K., & Sharma, K. K. (2011 Aug). Essential oil of clove (Eugenia caryophyllata) augments the humoral immune response but decreases cell mediated immunity. Phytother Res, 25(8), 1254-1256.

Halm M.A., Baker C, Harshe V (2014 Dec). "Effect of an Essential Oil Mixture on Skin Reactions in Women Undergoing Radiotherapy for Breast Cancer: A Pilot Study," Journal of Holistic Nursing. 32(4):290-303.

Hamada M, Uezu K, Matsushita J, Yamamoto S, Kishino Y (2002 Apr). "Distribution and immune responses resulting from oral administration of D-limonene in rats," J. Nutr. Sci. Vitaminol. (Tokyo). 48(2):155-160.

Hammer KA, Carson CF, Riley TV (2008 Aug). "Frequencies of resistance to Melaleuca alternifolia (tea tree) oil and rifampicin in Staphylococcus aureus, Staphylococcus epidermidis and Enterococcus faecalis," Int J Antimicrob Agents. 32(2):170-3.

Hammer KA, Carson CF, Riley TV (1996 Jun). "Susceptibility of transient and commensal skin flora to the essential oil of Melaleuca alternifolia (tea tree oil)," J Antimicrob Chemother. 24(3):186-9.

Hammer KA, Carson CF, Riley TV (2004 Jun). "Antifungal effects of Melaleuca alternifolia (tea tree) oil and its components on Candida albicans, Candida glabrata and Saccharomyces cerevisiae," J Antimicrob Chemother. 53(6):1081-5.

Hancianu M, Cioanca O, Mihasan M, Hritcu L (2013 Mar). "Neuroprotective effects of inhaled lavender oil on scopolamine-induced dementia via anti-oxidative activities in rats," Phytomedicine Int. J. Phytother. Phytopharm. 20(5):446-452.

Han, S. H., Hur, M. H., Buckle, J., Choi, J., & Lee, M. S. (2006 Aug). Effect of aromatherapy on symptoms of dysmenorrhea in college students: A randomized placebo-controlled clinical trial. J Altern Complement Med, 12(6), 535-541.

Han, X. Gibson, J., Eggett, D.L., & Parker, T.L. "Bergamot (Citrus bergamia) Essential Oil Inhalation Improves Positive Feelings in the Waiting Room of a Mental Health Treatment Center: A Pilot Study," Phytother. Res. 31(5):812-816.

Han X, Parker TL (2017 Feb 20). "Arborvitae (thuja plicata) essential oil significantly inhibited critical inflammation—and tissue remodeling—related proteins and genes in human dermal fibroblasts," Biochim Open. 4:56-6.

Han X, Parker TL (2017 Mar 3). "Anti-inflammatory, tissue remodeling, immuno-modulatory, and anticancer activities of oregano (origanum vulgare) essential oil in a human skin disease model," Biochim Open. 4:73-77.

Han X, Parker TL (2017 Mar 21). "Lemongrass (cymbopogon flexuosus) essential oil demonstrated anti-inflammatory effect in pre-inflamed human dermal fibroblasts," Biochim Open. 4:107-111.

Han, X., & Parker, T.L. (2017 Jul.). "Antiinflammatory Activity of Cinnamon (Cinnamomum zeylanicum) Bark Essential Oil in a Human Skin Disease Model," Phytother Res. 31(7):1034-1038.

Han, X., & Parker, T.L. (2017 Dec.). "Anti-inflammatory activity of clove (Eugenia caryophyllata) essential oil in human dermal fibroblasts," Pharm Biol. 55(1):1619-1622.

Han XJ, Wang YD, Chen YC, Lin LY, Wu QK (2013 Oct). "Transcriptome Sequencing and Expression Analysis of Terpenoid Biosynthesis Genes in Litsea cubeba," PLoS ONE. 8(10):e76890.

Hanus L.O., Rezanka T., Dembitsky V.M., Moussaieff A. (2005 Jun). "Myrrh--Commiphora chemistry," Biomed. Pap. Med. Fac. Univ. Palacký Olomouc Czechoslov. 149(1):3-27.

Haque M.M., Alsareii S.A. (2015 May). "A review of the therapeutic effects of using miswak (Salvadora Persica) on oral health," Saudi Med. J. 36(5):530-543.

Hargreaves IP, Lane A, Sleiman PM (2008 Dec 5). "The coenzyme Q(10) status of the brain regions of Parkinson's disease patients," Neurosci. Lett. 447(1):17-9.

Hart PH, Brand C, Carson CF, Riley TV, Prager RH, Finlay-Jones JJ (2000 Nov). "Terpinen-4-ol, the main component of the essential oil of Melaleuca alternifolia (tea tree oil), suppresses inflammatory mediator production by activated human monocytes," Inflamm Res. 49(11):619-26.

Harv Womens Health Watch (2013 Oct). "Staying mentally active throughout life preserves brain health," 21(2):8.

Hastak K. et al (1997). "Effect of turmeric oil and turmeric oleoresin on cytogenetic damage in patients suffering from oral submucous fibrosis," Cancer Lett. 116(2):265-269.

Hayashi N, Togawa K, Yanagisawa M, Hosogi J, Mimura D, Yamamoto Y, (2003). "Effect of sunlight exposure and aging on skin surface lipids and urate," Ex Dermatol. 12 Suppl 2:13-7.

Hay IC, Jamieson M, Ormerod AD (1998 Nov). "Randomized trial of aromatherapy. Successful treatment for alopecia areata," Arch Dermatol. 135(5):1349-52.

Hayes AJ, Markovic B (2002 Apr). "Toxicity of Australian essential oil Backhousia citriodora (Lemon myrtle). Part 1. Antimicrobial activity and in vitro cytotoxicity," Food Chem Toxicol. 40(4):535-43.

Hayflick L (1979 Jul). "The cell biology of aging," J Invest Dermatol. 73(1):8-14.

Hayouni E.A. et al (2008 Jul). "Tunisian Salvia officinalis L. and Schinus molle L. essential oils: their chemical compositions and their preservative effects against Salmonella inoculated in minced beef meat," Int. J. Food Microbiol. 125(3):242-51.

Haze S, Sakai K, Gozu Y (2002 Nov). "Effects of fragrance inhalation on sympathetic activity in normal adults," Jpn J Pharmacol 90(3):247-53.

Haze, S., Sakai, K., Gozu, Y., & Moriyama, M. (2010 Jul). Grapefruit oil attenuates adipogenesis in cultured adipocytes. Planta Med, 76(10), 950-955.

Hazgui S et al. (2008 Apr). "Epigallocatechin-3-gallate (EGCG) inhibits the migratory behavior of tumor bronchial epithelial cells," Respir Res. 9:33.

He M, Du M, Fan M, Bian Z (2007 Mar). "In vitro activity of eugenol against Candida albicans biofilms," Mycopathologia. 163(3):137-143.

Helland IB, Smith L, Saarem K, Saugstad OD, Drevon CA (2003 Jan). "Maternal supplementation with very-long-chain n-3 fatty acids during pregnancy and lactation augments children's IQ at 4 years of age," Pediatrics. 111(1):e39-44.

Herman A, Tambor K (2016 Feb). "Linalool Affects the Antimicrobial Efficacy of Essential Oils," Curr. Microbiol. 72(2):165-172.

Herman, C. P., Roth, D. A., & Polivy, J. (2003). Effects of the presence of others on food intake: a normative interpretation. Psychological Bulletin, 129(6), 873-886.

Herz, R. S., & Engen, T. (1996 Sep). Odor memory: Review and analysis. Psychon Bull Rev, 3(3), 300-313.

Heuberger, E., Hongratanaworakit, T., & Buchbauer, G. (2006 Aug). East Indian sandalwood and alpha-santalol odor increase physiological and self-rated arousal in humans. Planta Med, 72(9), 792-800.

Heydari N, Abootalebi M, Jamalimoghadam N, Kasraeian M, Emamghoreishi M, Akbarzaded M (2018 May 22). "Evaluation of aromatherapy with essential oils of rosa damascena for the management of premenstrual syndrome," Int J Gynaecol Obstet.

Hiramatsu N, Xiufen W, Takechi R, Itoh Y, Mamo J, Pal S (2004). "Antimutagenicity of Japanese traditional herbs, gennoshoko, yomogi, senburi and iwa-tobacco," Biofactors. 22(1-4):123-5.

Hirota R, Roger N.N., Nakamura H, Song HS, Sawamura M, Suganuma N (2010 Apr). "Antiinflammatory effects of limonene from yuzu (Citrus junos Tanaka) essential oil on eosinophils," J. Food Sci. 75(3):H87-92.

Hitokoto H, Morozumi S, Wauke T, Sakai S, Kurata H (1980 Apr). "Inhibitory effects of spices on growth and toxin production of toxigenic fungi," Appl Environ Microbiol. 39(4):818-22.

Ho C, Spence C (2005 Nov). "Olfactory facilitation of dual-task performance," Neurosci. Lett. 389(1):35-40.

Hojsak, I, Snovak N, Abdovic S, Szajewska H, Misak Z, Kolacek S (2009). "Lactobacillus GG in the prevention of gastrointestinal and respiratory tract infections in children who attend day care centers: A randomized, double-blind, placebo-controlled trial," Clin. Nutr. 29(3):312-6.

Holmes C, Hopkins V, Hensford C, MacLaughlin V, Wilkinson D, Rosenvinge H (2002 Apr). "Lavender oil as a treatment for agitated behaviour in severe dementia: a placebo controlled study," Int. J. 17(4):305-308.Geriatr. Psychiatry

Hölzle E (1992 Sep). "Pigmented lesions as a sign of photodamage," Br J Dermatol. 17(Suppl 41):48-50.

Hong SL et al (2014). "Essential oil content of the rhizome of Curcuma purpurascens Bl. (Temu Tis) and its antiproliferative effect on selected human carcinoma cell lines," ScientificWorldJournal. 2014:397430.

Hongratanaworakit T (2009 Feb). "Relaxing effect of rose oil on humans," Nat Prod Commun. 4(2):291-6.

Hongratanaworakit T (2011 Aug). "Aroma-therapeutic effects of massage blended essential oils on humans," Nat. Prod. Commun. 6(8):1199-1204.

Hongratanaworakit T, Buchbauer G (2004 Jul). "Evaluation of the harmonizing effect of ylang-ylang oil on humans after inhalation," Planta Med. 70(7):632-6.

Hongratanaworakit T, Buchbauer G (2006 Sep). "Relaxing effect of ylang ylang oil on humans after transdermal absorption," Phytother Res. 20(9):758-63.

Hongratanaworakit, T., Heuberger, E., & Buchbauer, G. (2004 Jan). Evaluation of the effects of East Indian sandalwood oil and alpha-santalol on humans after transdermal absorption. Planta Med, 70(1), 3-7.

Holloszy JO, (1967 May). "Biochemical adaptations in muscle. Effects of exercise on mitochondrial oxygen uptake and respiratory enzyme activity in skeletal muscle," J Biol Chem, 242(9):2278-82.

Hosseini, M., Ghasemzadeh Rahbardar, M., Sadeghnia, H. R., & Rakhshandeh, H. (2011 Oct). Effects of different extracts of Rosa damascena on pentylenetetrazol-induced seizures in mice. Zhong Xi Yi Jie He Xue Bao, 9(10), 1118-1124.

Hosseini, M., Jafarianheris, T., Seddighi, N., Parvaneh, M., Ghorbani, A., Sadeghnia, H. R., & Rakhshandeh, H. (2012 Dec). Effects of different extracts of Eugenia caryophyllata on pentylenetetrazole-induced seizures in mice. Zhong Xi Yi Jie He Xue Bao, 10(12), 1476-1481.

Hosseinzadeh, H., Karimi, G. R., & Ameri, M. (2002 Dec). Effects of Anethum graveolens L. seed extracts on experimental gastric irritation models in mice. BMC Pharmacol, 2, 1-5.

Hostanska K, Daum G, Saller R (2002 Sep-Oct). "Cytostatic and apoptosis-inducing activity of boswellic acids toward malignant cell lines in vitro," Anticancer Res. 22(5):2853-62.

Houicher A, Hechanchna H, Teldji H, Ozogul F (2016). "In vitro study of the antifungal activity of essential oils obtained from mentha spicata thymus vulgaris, and laurus nobilis," Recent Pat Food Nutr Agric. 8(2) 99-106.

Howard J., Hyman A.A. (2003) Dynamics and mechanics of the microtubule plus end. Nature. 422: 753-758.

Hoya Y, Matsumura I, Fujita T, Yanaga K. (2008 Nov-Dec). "The use of nonpharmacological interventions to reduce anxiety in patients undergoing gastroscopy in a setting with an optimal soothing environment," Gastroenterol Nurs. 31(6):395-9.

Hozumi H et al (2017 Oct). "Aromatherapies using osmanthus fragrans oil and grapefruit oil are effective complementary treatments for anxious patients undergoing colonoscopy: a randomized controlled study" Complement Ther Med. 34:165-169.

Hritcu L, Cioanca O, Hancianu M (2012 Apr). "Effects of lavender oil inhalation on improving scopolamine-induced spatial memory impairment in laboratory rats," Phytomedicine. Int. J. Phytother. Phytopharm. 19(6):529-534.

Hsieh LC, Hsieh SL, Chen CT, Chung JG, Wang JJ, Wu CC (2015). "Induction of αphellandrene on autophagy in human liver tumor cells," Am. J. Chin. Med. 43(1):121-136.

Hu L, Wang Y, Du M, Zhang J (2011 Jul). "Characterization of the volatiles and active components in ethanol extracts of fruits of Litsea cubeba (Lour.) by gas chromatography-mass spectrometry (GC-MS) and gas chromatography- olfactometry (GC-O)," JMPR. 5(14):3298-3303.

Hu, W., Zhang, N., Chen, H., Zhong, B., Yang, A., Kuang, F., Ouyang, Z., & Chun, J. (2017 Apr. 21). "Fumigant Activity of Sweet Orange Essential Oil Fractions Against Red Imported Fire Ants (Hymenoptera: Formicidae)," J Econ Entomol. [Epub ahead of print].

Huang, C. S., Yin, M. C., & Chiu, L. C. (2011 Sep). Antihyperglycemic and anti-oxidative potential of Psidium guajava fruit in streptozotocin-induced diabetic rats. Food Chem Toxicol, 49(9), 2189-2195.

Huang L, Abuhamdah S, Howes MJ, Dixon CL, Elliot MS, Ballard C, Holmes C, Burns A, Perry EK, Francis PT, Lees G, Chazot PL (2008 Nov). "Pharmacological profile of essential oils derived from Lavandula angustifolia and Melissa officinalis with anti-agitation properties: focus on ligand-gated channels," J Pharm Pharmacol. 60(11):1515-22.

Huang MT, Badmaev V, Ding Y, Liu Y, Xie JG, Ho CT (2000). "Anti-tumor and anti-carcinogenic activities of triterpenoid, beta-boswellic acid," Biofactors. 13(1-4):225-30.

Hucklenbroich J. et al (2014 Sep). "Aromatic-turmerone induces neural stem cell proliferation in vitro and in vivo," Stem Cell Res. Ther. 5(4).

Hudaib, M., Speroni, E., Di Pietra, A. M., & Cavrini, V. (2002 Jul). GC/MS evaluation of thyme (Thymus vulgaris L.) oil composition and variations during the vegetative cycle. J Pharm Biomed Anal, 29(4), 691-700.

Hunan Yi Ke Da Xue Xue Bao (1999). "Experimental study on induction of apoptosis of leukemic cells by Boswellia carterii Birdw extractive," Hunan Yi Ke Da Xue Xue Bao. 24(1):23-5.

Hudson, J., Kuo, M., & Vimalanathan, S. (2011 Dec). The antimicrobial properties of cedar leaf (Thuja plicata) oil; a safe and efficient decontamination agent for buildings. Int J Environ Res Public Health, 8(12), 4477-4487.

Hull, S., Re, R., Chambers, L., Echaniz, A., & Wickham, M. S. (2014 Sep 3). A mid-morning snack of almonds generates satiety and appropriate adjustment of subsequent food intake in healthy women. Eur J Nutr.

Hur M.H., Han SH (2004 Feb). "[Clinical trial of aromatherapy on postpartum mother's perineal healing]," Taehan Kanho Hakhoe Chi. 34(1):53-62.

Hur M.H., Park J, Maddock-Jennings W, Kim D.O., Lee M.S. (2007 Jul). "Reduction of mouth malodour and volatile sulphur compounds in intensive care patients using an essential oil mouthwash," Phytother. Res. PTR. 21(7):641-643.

Husain F.M., Ahmad I, Asif M, Tahseen Q (2013 Dec). "Influence of clove oil on certain quorumsensing-regulated functions and biofilm of Pseudomonas aeruginosa and Aeromonas hydrophila," J. Biosci. 38(5):835-844.

Hussein G, Miyashiro H, Nakamura N, Hattori M, Kakiuchi N, Shimotohno K (2000 Nov). "Inhibitory effects of sudanese medicinal plant extracts on hepatitis C virus (HCV) protease," Phytother Res. 14(7):510-6.

Hyldgaard, M., Mygind, T., & Meyer, R. L. (2012 Feb). Essential oils in food preservation: mode of action, synergies, and interactions with food matrix components. Frontiers in Microbiology, 3, 1-24.

Idaomar M, El-Hamss R, Bakkali F, Mezzoug N, Zhiri A, Baudoux D, Muñoz-Serrano A, Liemans V, Alonso-Moraga A (2002 Jan 15). "Genotoxicity and antigenotoxicity of some essential oils evaluated by wing spot test of Drosophila melanogaster," Mutat Res. 13(1-2):61-8.

Iamsaard, S., Prabsattroo, T., Sukhorum, W., Muchimapura, S., Srisaard, P., Uabundit, N., . . . Wattanathorn, J. (2013 Mar). Anethum graveolens Linn. (dill) extract enhances the mounting frequency and level of testicular tyrosine protein phosphorylation in rats. J Zhejiang Univ Sci B, 14(3), 247-252.

Ilmberger J, Heuberger E, Mahrhofer C, Dessovic H, Kowarik D, Buchbauer G (2001 Mar). "The influence of essential oils on human attention. I: alertness," Chem. Senses. 26(3):239-248.

Imai H, Osawa K, Yasuda H, Hamashima H, Arai T, Sasatsu M (2001). "Inhibition by the essential oils of peppermint and spearmint of the growth of pathogenic bacteria," Microbios. 106(Suppl 1):31-9.

Imokawa G (2009 Jul). "A possible mechanism underlying the ceramide deficiency in atopic dermatitis: expression of a deacylase enzyme that cleaves the N-acyl linkage of sphingomyelin and glucosylceramide," J Dermatol Sci. 55(1):1-9.

Imura M, Misao H, Ushijima H (2006 Mar). "The Psychological Effects of Aromatherapy-Massage in Healthy Postpartum Mothers," J. Midwifery Womens Health. 51(2):e21-e27.

Inouye S, Nishiyama Y, Uchida K, Hasumi Y, Yamaguchi H, Abe S (2006 Dec). "The vapor activity of oregano, perilla, tea tree, lavender, clove, and geranium oils against a Trichophyton mentagrophytes in a closed box," J Infect Chemother. 12(6):349-54.

Inouye S, Takizawa T, Yamaguchi H (2001 May). "Antibacterial activity of essential oils and their major constituents against respiratory tract pathogens by gaseous contact," J Antimicrob Chemother. 47(5):565-73.

Inouye S, Yamaguchi H, Takizawa T (2001 Dec). "Screening of the antibacterial effects of a variety of essential oils on respiratory tract pathogens, using a modified dilution assay method," J Infect Chemother. 7(4):251-4.

Iori A, Grazioli D, Gentile E, Marano G, Salvatore G (2005 Apr 20). "Acaricidal properties of the essential oil of Melaleuca alternifolia Cheel (tea tree oil) against nymphs of Ixodes ricinus," Vet Parasitol. 129(1-2):173-6.

Iscan G, Kirimer N, Kürkcüoğlu M, Baser K.H.C., Demirci F (2002 Jul). "Antimicrobial screening of Mentha piperita essential oils," J. Agric. Food Chem. 50(14):3943-3946.

Ishida T, Mizushina Y, Yagi S, Irino Y, Nishiumi S, Miki I, Kondo Y, Mizuno S, Yoshida H, Azuma T, Yoshida M (2012). "Inhibitory effects of glycyrrhetinic Acid on DNA polymerase and inflammatory activities," Evid Based Complement Alternat Med. 2012:650514.

Ishikawa H, Matsumoto S, Ohashi Y, Imaoka A, Setoyama H, Umesaki Y, Tanaka R, Otani T (2011 Apr). "Beneficial effects of probiotic bifidobacterium and galacto-oligosaccharide in patients with ulcerative colitis: a randomized controlled study," Digestion. 84(2):128-33.

Itai T, Amayasu H, Kuribayashi M, Kawamura N, Okada M, Momose A, Tateyama T, Narumi K, Uematsu W, Kaneko S (2000 Aug). "Psychological effects of aromatherapy on chronic hemodialysis patients," Psychiatry Clin Neurosci. 54(4):393-7.

Itai T, Amayasu H, Kuribayashi M, Kawamura N, Okada M, Momose A, Tateyama T, Narumi K, Uematsu W, Kaneko S (2000 Aug). "Psychological effects of aromatherapy on chronic hemodialysis patients," Psychiatry Clin Neurosci. 54(4):393-7.

Itkin M. et al (2016 Nov). "The biosynthetic pathway of the nonsugar, high-intensity sweetener mogroside V from Siraitia grosvenorii," Proc. Natl. Acad. Sci. U. S. A. 113(47):E7619-7628.

Ito, Y., Ohnishi, S., & Fujie, K. (1989). Chromosome aberrations induced by aflatoxin B1 in rat bone marrow cells in vivo and their suppression by green tea. Mutation Research/Genetic Toxicology, 222(3), 253-261.

Iwata, J., LeDoux, J. E., Meeley, M. P., Arneric, S., & Reis, D. J. (1986 Sep). Intrinsic neurons in the amygdaloid field projected to by the medial geniculate body mediate emotional responses conditioned to acoustic stimuli. Brain Res, 383(1-2), 195-214.

Jacob J.N., Badyal D.K. (2014 Feb). "Biological studies of turmeric oil, part 3: anti-inflammatory and analgesic properties of turmeric oil and fish oil in comparison with aspirin," Nat. Prod. Commun. 9(2):225-228.

Jacques, P. F., & Wang, H. (2014 Apr 4). Yogurt and weight management. Am J Clin Nutr, 99(5 Suppl), 1229s-1234s.

Jafarzadeh, M., Arman, S., & Pour, F. F. (2013 Aug). Effect of aromatherapy with orange essential oil on salivary cortisol and pulse rate in children during dental treatment: A randomized controlled clinical trial. Adv Biomed Res, 2, 1-10.

Jager, W., Buchbauer, G., Jirovetz, L., & Fritzer, M. (1992). Percutaneous absorption of lavender oil from a massage oil. J Soc Cosmet Chem, 43(1), 49-54.

Jager, W., Nasel, B., Nasel, C., Binder, R., Stimpfl, T., Vycudilik, W., & Buchbauer, G. (1996 Aug). Pharmacokinetic studies of the fragrance compound 1,8-cineol in humans during inhalation. Chem Senses, 21(4), 477-480.

Jamal A, Javed K, Aslam M, Jafri MA (2006 Jan 16). "Gastroprotective effect of cardamom, Elettaria cardamomum Maton. fruits in rats," J Ethnopharmacol. 103(2):149-53.

Janahmadi M, Niazi F, Danyali S, Kamalinejad M (2006 Mar 8). "Effects of the fruit essential oil of Cuminum cyminum Linn. (Apiaceae) on pentylenetetrazol-induced epileptiform activity in F1 neurones of Helix aspersa," J Ethnopharmacol. 104(1-2):278-82.

Jang M, Cai L, Udeani GO, Slowing KV, Thomas CF, Beecher CW, Fong HH, Farnsworth NR, Kinghorn AD, Mehta RG, Moon RC, Pezzuto JM (1997 Jan 10). "Cancer chemopreventive activity of resveratrol, a natural product derived from grapes," Science. 275 (5297):218-20.

Jang SE, Ryu KR, Park SH, Chung S, Teruya Y, Han MJ, Woo JT, Kim DH (2013 Nov). "Nobiletin and tangeretin ameliorate scratching behavior in mice by inhibiting the action of histamine and the activation of NF-κB, AP-1 and p38," Int Immunopharmacol. 17(3):502-7.

Jankasem M, Wuthi-udomlert M, Gritsanapan W (2013). "Antidermatophytic Properties of Ar-Turmerone, Turmeric Oil, and Curcuma longa Preparations," ISRN Dermatol. 2013:1-3.

Jayaprakasha G.K., Jena B.S., Negi P.S., Sakariah K.K. (2002 Jan). "Evaluation of Antioxidant Activities and Antimutagenicity of Turmeric Oil: A Byproduct from Curcumin Production," Z. Für Naturforschung C. 57(9-10).

Jefferies H., Coster J., Khalil A., Bot J., McCauley R.D., Hall J.C. (2003) Glutathione. ANZ Journal of Surgery. 73: 517-522.

Jenkins, D. J., Chiavaroli, L., Wong, J. M., Kendall, C., Lewis, G. F., Vidgen, E., . . . Lamarche, B. (2010 Dec 14). Adding monounsaturated fatty acids to a dietary portfolio of cholesterol-lowering foods in hypercholesterolemia. Canadian Medical Association journal, 182(18), 1961-1967.

Jeon, S., Bose, S., Hur, J., Jun, K., Kim, Y. K., Cho, K. S., & Koo, B. S. (2011 Sep). A modified formulation of Chinese traditional medicine improves memory impairment and reduces Abeta level in the Tg-APPswe/PS1dE9 mouse model of Alzheimer's disease. J Ethnopharmacol, 137(1), 783-789.

Jeong C, Han J, Cho J, Suh K, Nam G (2013 Aug). "Analysis of electrical property changes of skin by oil-in-water emulsion components," Int. J. Cosmet. Sci. 35(4):402-410.

Jeong HU, Kwon SS, Kong T.Y., Kim J.H., Lee H.S. (2014 Dec). "Inhibitory Effects of Cedrol, βCedrene, and Thujopsene on Cytochrome P450 Enzyme Activities in Human Liver Microsomes," Journal of Toxicology and Environmental Health, Part A. 77(22-24):1522-1532.

Jia S. et al (2013 Jan). "Induction of apoptosis by D-limonene is mediated by inactivation of Akt in LS174T human colon cancer cells," Oncol. Rep. 29 (1):349-54.

Jiang, J., Xu, H., Wang, H., Zhang, Y., Ya, P., Yang, C., & Li, F. (2017 Feb.). "Protective effects of lemongrass essential oil against benzo(a)pyrene-induced oxidative stress and DNA damage in human embryonic lung fibroblast cells," Toxicol Mech Methods. 27(2):121-127.

Jiang, Q., Wu, Y., Zhang, H., Liu, P., Yao, J., Chen, J., & Duan, J. (2017 Dec.). "Development of essential oils as skin permeation enhancers: penetration enhancement effect and mechanism of action," Pharm Biol. 55(1):1592-1600.

Jimenez A, Santos A, Alonso G, Vazquez D (1976 Mar 17). "Inhibitors of protein synthesis in eukarytic cells. Comparative effects of some amaryllidaceae alkaloids," Biochim Biophys Acta. 425(3):342-8.

Jiang Z, Akhtar Y, Bradbury R, Zhang X, Isman M.B. (2009 Jun). "Comparative toxicity of essential oils of Litsea pungens and Litsea cubeba and blends of their major constituents against the cabbage looper, Trichoplusia ni," J. Agric. Food Chem. 57(11): 4833-4837.

Jin M.H. et al (2014 Sep). "Cedrol Enhances Extracellular Matrix Production in Dermal Fibroblasts in a MAPK-Dependent Manner," Annals of Dermatology. 24(1):16.

Jing, L., Zhang, Y., Fan, S., Gu, M., Guan, Y., Lu, X., . . . Zhou, Z. (2013 Sep). Preventive and ameliorating effects of citrus D-limonene on dyslipidemia and hyperglycemia in mice with high-fat diet-induced obesity. Eur J Pharmacol, 715(1-3), 46-55.

Jing Y, Nakajo S, Xia L, Nakaya K, Fang Q, Waxman S, Han R (1999 Jan). "Boswellic acid acetate induces differentiation and apoptosis in leukemia cell lines," Leuk Res. 23(1):43-50.

Jing Y, Xia L, Han R (1992 Mar). "Growth inhibition and differentiation of promyelocytic cells (HL-60) induced by BC-4, an active principle from Boswellia carterii Birdw," Chin Med Sci J. 7(1):12-5.

Johannessen B (2013 Nov). "Nurses experience of aromatherapy use with dementia patients experiencing disturbed sleep patterns. An action research project," Complement. Ther. Clin. Pract. 19(4):209-213.

Johnson, K., West, T., Diana, S., Todd, J., Haynes, B., Bernhardt, J., & Johnson, R. (2017 Jun.). "Use of aromatherapy to promote a therapeutic nurse environment," Intensive Crit Care Nurs. 40:18-25.

Johnson, L. R., Ghishan, F.K., Kaunitz, J.D., Merchant, J., Said, H.M., & Wood, J. (Eds.). (2012 Jul). Physiology of the gastrointestinal tract (5th ed.). London: Elsevier.

Johnson, M., Pace, R. D., Dawkins, N. L., & Willian, K. R. (2013 Nov). Diets containing traditional and novel green leafy vegetables improve liver fatty acid profiles of spontaneously hypertensive rats. Lipids Health Dis, 12, 168.

Johny AK, Baskaran SA, Charles AS, Amalaradjou MA, Darre MJ, Khan MI, Hoagland TA, Schreiber DT, Donoghue AM, Donoghue DJ, Venkitarayanan K. (2009 Apr). "Prophylactic supplementation of caprylic acid in feed reduces Salmonella enteritidis colonization in commercial broiler chicks," J. Food Prot. 72(4):722-7.

Jolliff, G.D., Tinsley, I.J., Calhoun, W., and Crane, J.M. (1981). "Meadowfoam (Limnanthes alba): Its Research and Development as a Potential New Oilseed Crop for the Willamette Valley of Oregon," Oregon State University Agricultural Experiment Station. Station Bulletin 648.

Juergens U.R., Dethlefsen U., Steinkamp G., Gillissen A., Repges R., Vetter H. (2003) Anti-inflammatory activity of 1.8-cineol (eucalyptol) in bronchial asthma: a double-blind placebo-controlled trial. Respiratory Medicine. 97: 250-256.

Juergens UR, Stöber M, Schmidt-Schilling L, Kleuver T, Vetter H (1998 Sep 17). "Anti-inflammatory effects of euclyptol (1.8-cineole) in bronchial asthma: inhibition of arachidonic acid metabolism in human blood monocytes ex vivo," Eur J Med Res. 3(9):407-12.

Juergens UR, Stöber M, Vetter H (1998 Dec 16). "The anti-inflammatory activity of L-menthol compared to mint oil in human monocytes in vitro: a novel perspective for its therapeutic use in inflammatory diseases," Eur J Med Res. 3(12):539-45.

Juglal S, Govinden R, Odhav B (2002 Apr). "Spice oils for the control of co-occurring mycotoxin-producing fungi," J Food Prot. 65(4):683-7.

Jun, H. J., Lee, J. H., Jia, Y., Hoang, M. H., Byun, H., Kim, K. H., & Lee, S. J. (2012 Mar). Melissa officinalis essential oil reduces plasma triglycerides in human apolipoprotein E2 transgenic mice by inhibiting sterol regulatory element-binding protein-1c-dependent fatty acid synthesis. J Nutr, 142(3), 432-440.

Jung DL, Cha JY, Kim SE, Ko IG, Jee YS (2013 Apr). "Effects of Ylang-Ylang aroma on blood pressure and heart rate in healthy men," J. Exerc. Rehabil. 9(2):250-255.

Jung K, Kim IH, Han D (2004). "Effect of medicinal plant extracts on forced swimming capacity in mice," J Ethnopharmacol. 93:75-81.

Jung SH, Kang KD, Ju D, Fawcen RJ, Safa R, Kamalden TA, Osborne NN (2008 Sep). "The flavanoid baicalin counteracts ischemic and oxidative insults to retinal cells and lipid peroxidation to brain membranes," Neurochem Int.

Jung, Y. H., Kwon, S. H., Hong, S. I., Lee, S. O., Kim, S. Y., Lee, S. Y., & Jang, C. G. (2012 Dec). 5-HT(1A) receptor binding in the dorsal raphe nucleus is implicated in the anxiolytic-like effects of Cinnamomum cassia. Pharmacol Biochem Behav, 103(2), 367-372.

Kabuto, H., Tada, M., & Kohno, M. (2007 Mar). Eugenol [2-methoxy-4-(2-propenyl) phenol] prevents 6-hydroxydopamine-induced dopamine depression and lipid peroxidation inductivity in mouse striatum. Biol Pharm Bull, 30(3), 423-427.

Kadekaro AL, Kanto H, Kavanagh R, Abdel-Malek ZA (2003 Jun). "Significance of the melanocortin 1 receptor in regulating human melanocyte pigmentation, proliferation, and survival," Ann N Y Acad Sci. 994:359-65.

Kadohisa, M. (2013 Oct). Effects of odor on emotion, with implications. Front Syst Neurosci, 7, 1-6.

Kamatou G.P.P., Vermaak I, Viljoen A.M., Lawrence B.M. (2013 Dec). "Menthol: a simple monoterpene with remarkable biological properties," Phytochemistr. 96:15-25.

Kambara T, Zhou Y, Kawashima Y, Kishida N, Mizutani K, Ikeda T, Kamayama K (2003). "A New Dermatological Availability of the Flavonoid Fraction from Licorice Roots—Effect on Acne," J Soc Cosmet Chem Jpn. 37(3)179-85.

Kamiyama, M., & Shibamoto, T. (2012 Jun). Flavonoids with potent antioxidant activity found in young green barley leaves. J Agric Food Chem, 60(25), 6260-6267.

Kane FM, Brodie EE, Coull A, Coyne L, Howd A, Milne A, Niven CC, Robbins R (2004 Oct 28-Nov 10). "The analgesic effect of odour and music upon dressing change," Br J Nurs. 13(19):S4-12.

Kanehara S, Ohtani T, Uede K, Furukawa F (2007 Dec). "Clinical effects of undershirts coated with borage oil on children with atopic dermatitis: a double-blind, placebo-controlled clinical trial," J Dermatol. 34(12):811-5.

Karadog E, Samanciouglu S, Ozden D, Bakir S (2015 Jul). "Effects of aromatherapy on sleep quality and anxiety of patients," Nurs. Crit. Care.

Kasper S (2013 Nov). "An orally administered lavandula oil preparation (Silexan) for anxiety disorder and related conditions: an evidence based review," Int J Psychiatry Clin Pract. 17 Suppl 1:15-22.

Kasperczyk, S., Dobrakowski, M., Kasperczyk, J., Ostalowska, A., Zalejska-Fiolka, J., & Birkner, E. (2014 Jul). Beta-carotene reduces oxidative stress, improves glutathione metabolism and modifies antioxidant defense systems in lead-exposed workers. Toxicol Appl Pharmacol, 280(1), 36-41.

Katdare M, Singhal H, Newmark H, Osborne MP, Telang NT (1997 Jan 1). "Prevention of mammary preneoplastic transformation by naturally-occurring tumor inhibitors," Cancer Lett. 111(1-2):141-7.

Kato K., Cox A.D., Hisaka M.M., Graham S.M., Buss J.E., Der C.J. (1992) Isoprenoid addition to Ras protein is the critical modification for its membrane association and transforming activity. Proc. Natl. Sci. USA. 89: 6403-6407.

Kato T, Hancock RL, Mohammadpour H, McGregor B, Manalo P, Khaiboullina S, Hall MR, Pardini L, Pardini RS (2002 Dec). "Influence of omega-3 fatty acids on the growth of human colon carcinoma in nude mice," Cancer Lett. 187(1-2):169-77.

Kaur R, Agarwal C, Singh RP, Guan X, Dwivedi C, Agarwal R (2005 Feb). "Skin cancer chemopreventive agent, {alpha}-santalol, induces apoptotic death of human epidermoid carcinoma A431 cells via caspase activation together with dissipation of mitochondrial membrane potential and cytochrome c release," Carcinogenesis. 26(2):369-80.

Kawaski H, Morinushi T, Yakushiji M, Takigawa M (2009 Feb). "Nonlinear dynamical analysis of the effect by six stimuli on electroencephalogram," J. Clin. Neurophysiol. Off. Publ. Am. Electroencephalogr. Soc. 26(1):24-38.

Kawata S, Nagase T, Yamasaki E, Ishiguro H, Matsuzawa Y (1994 Jun). "Modulation of the mevalonate pathway and cell growth by pravastatin and d-limonene in a human hepatoma cell line (Hep G2)," Br. J. Cancer. 69(6):1015-1020.

Kee Y, Lin RC, Hsu SC, Scheller RH (1995 May). "Distinct domains of syntaxin are required for synaptic vesicle fusion complex formation and dissociation," Neuron. 14(5):991-8.

Kéita SM, Vincent C, Schmit J, Arnason JT, Bélanger A (2001 Oct). "Efficacy of essential oil of Ocimum basilicum L. and O. gratissimum L. applied as an insecticidal fumigant and powder to control Callosobruchus maculatus (Fab.)," J Stored Prod Res. 37(4):339-349.

Kennedy DO, Little W, Haskell CF, Scholey AB (2006 Feb). "Anxiolytic effects of a combination of Melissa officinalis and Valeriana officinalis during laboratory induced stress," Phytother Res. 20(2):96-102.

Kennedy DO, Wake G, Savelev S, Tildesley NT, Perry EK, Wesnes KA, Scholey AB (2003 Oct). "Modulation of mood and cognitive performance following acute administration of single doses of Melissa officinalis (Lemon balm) with human CNS nicotinic and muscarinic receptor-binding properties," Neuropsychopharmacology. 28(10):1871-81.

Keogh A, Fenton S, Leslie C, Aboyoun C, Macdonald P, Zhao YC, Bailey M, Rosenfeldt F (2003). "Randomised double-blind, placebo-controlled trial of coenzyme Q₁₀ therapy in class II and III systolic heart failure," Heart Lung Circ. 12(3):135-41.

Keshavarz Afshar M, Behboodi Moghadam Z, Taghizadeh Z, Bekhradi R, Montazeri A, Mokhtari P (2015 Apr). "Lavender fragrance essential oil and the quality of sleep in postpartum women," Iran. Red Crescent Med. J. 17(4):E25880.

Keskin, I., Gunal, Y., Alya, S., Kolbasi, B., Sakul, A., Kilc, U., Gok, O., Koroglu, K., & Ozbek, H. (2017 Apr. 20). "Effects of Foeniculum vulgare essential oil compounds, fenchone and limonene, on experimental wound healing," Biotech Histochem. 92(4):274-282.

Khachik, F., Beecher, G. R., & Smith, J. C. (1995). Lutein, lycopene, and their oxidative metabolites in chemoprevention of cancer. Journal of Cellular Biochemistry, 59(S22), 236-246.

Khalessi A.M., Pack A.R.C., Thomson W.M, Tomplins G.R. (2004 Oct). "An in vivo study of the plaque control efficacy of Persica: a commercially available herbal mouthwash containing extracts of Salvadora persica," Int. Dent. J. 54(5):279-283.

Khallouki F, Younos C, Soulimani R, Oster T, Charrouf Z, Spiegelhalder B, Bartsch H, Owen RW (2003 Feb). "Consumption of argan oil (Morocco) with its unique profile of fatty acids, tocopherols, squalene, sterols and phenolic compounds should confer valuable cancer chemopreventive effects," Eur J Cancer Prev. 12(1):67-75.

Khan AU, Gilani AH (2009 Dec 10). "Antispasmodic and bronchodilator activities of Artemisia vulgaris are mediated through dual blockade of muscarinic receptors and calcium influx," J Ethnopharmacol. 126(3):480-6.

Khatibi A, Haghparast A, Shams J, Dianati E, Komaki A, Kamalinejad M (2008 Dec 19). "Effects of the fruit essential oil of Cuminum cyminum L. on the acquisition and expression of morphine-induced conditioned place preference in mice," Neurosci Lett. 448(1):94-8.

Kheirkhah A, Casas V, Li W, Raju VK, Tseng SC (2007 May). "Corneal manifestations of ocular demodex infestation," Am J Ophthalmol. 143(5):743-749.

Kheirkhah M, Vali Pour NS, Nisani L, Haghani H (2014 Aug 17). "Comparing the effects of aromatherapy with rose oils and warm foot bath on anxiety in the first stage of labor in nulliparous women," Iran Red Crescent Med J. 16(9):e14455.

Khodabakhsh, P., Shafaroodi, H., and Asgarpanah. J. (2015). "Analgesic and anti-inflammatory activities of Citrus aurantium L. blossoms essential oil (neroli): involvement of the nitric oxide/cyclic-guanosine monophosphate pathway," J Nat Med. 69(3):324-31.

Kiecolt-Glaser JK, Graham JE, Malarkey WB, Porter K, Lemeshow S, Glaser R (2008 Apr). "Olfactory influences on mood and autonomic, endocrine, and immune function," Psychoneuroendocrinology. 33(3):328-39.

Kim D, Suh SH, Lee Y (2013 Feb). "Immune activation and antitumor response of ar-turmerone on P388D1 lymphoblast cell implanted tumors," Int. J. Mol. Med. 31(2):386-392.

Kim DS. et al (2015). "Alpha-Pinene Exhibits Anti-Inflammatory Activity Through theSuppression of MAPKs and the NF-κB Pathway in Mouse Peritoneal Macrophages," Am. J. Chin. Med. 43(4):731-742.

Kim ES, Kang SY, Kim YH, Lee YE, Choi NY, You YO, Kim KJ (2015 Apr). "Chamaecyparis obtusa Essential Oil Inhibits Methicillin-Resistant Staphylococcus aureus Biofilm Formation and Expression of Virulence Factors," J Med Food. 18(7):810-7.

Kim, H. J., Yang, H. M., Kim, D. H., Kim, H. G., Jang, W. C., & Lee, Y. R. (2003 Jun). Effects of ylang-ylang essential oil on the relaxation of rat bladder muscle in vitro and white rabbit bladder in vivo. J Korean Med Sci, 18(3), 409-414.

Kim HM, Cho SH (1999 Feb). "Lavender oil inhibits immediate-type allergic reaction in mice and rats," J Pharm Pharmacol. 51(2):221-6.

Kim, I. H., Kim, C., Seong, K., Hur, M. H., Lim, H. M., & Lee, M. S. (2012 Dec). Essential oil inhalation on blood pressure and salivary cortisol levels in prehypertensive and hypertensive subjects. Evid Based Complement Alternat Med, 2012, 1-9.

Kim J.T. et al (2007 Jul). "Treatment with lavender aromatherapy in the post-anesthesia care unit reduces opioid requirements of morbidly obese patients undergoing laparoscopic adjustable gastric banding," Obes. Surg. 17(7):920-925.

Kim JM, Marshall M, Cornell J.A., Iii J.F.P., Wei C.I (1995 Nov). "Antibacterial Activity of Carvacrol,

Citral, and Geraniol against Salmonella typhimurium in Culture Medium and on Fish Cubes," Journal of Food Science. 60(6):1364-1368.

Appendix

Kim MA, Sakong JK, Kim EJ, Kim EH, Kim EH (2005 Feb). "Effect of aromatherapy massage for the relief of constipation in the elderly," Taehan Kanho Hakhoe Chi. 35(1):56-64.

Kim MJ, Nam ES, Paik SI (2005 Feb). "The effects of aromatherapy on pain, depression, and life satisfaction of arthritis patients," Toxicol Res. 35(1):186-94.

Kim SE, Lee CM, Kim YC (2017 Jan). "Anti-Melanogenic Effect of Oenothera laciniata Methanol Extract in Melan-a Cells," Toxicol Res. 33(1):55-62.

Kim SS, Baik J.S., Oh TH, Yoon WJ, Lee N.H., Hyun CG (2008 Oct). "Biological activities of Korean Citrus obovoides and Citrus natsudaidai essential oils against acne-inducing bacteria," Biosci. Biotechnol. Biochem. 72(10):2507-2513.

Kim, T. H., Kim, H. J., Lee, S. H., & Kim, S. Y. (2012 Jun). Potent inhibitory effect of Foeniculum vulgare Miller extract on osteoclast differentiation and ovariectomy-induced bone loss. Int J Mol Med, 29(6), 1053-1059.

Kim, W., & Hur, M.H. (2016 Dec.). "Inhalation Effects of Aroma Essential Oil on Quality of Sleep for Shift Nurses after Night Work," J Korean Acad Nurs. 46(6):769-779.

Kim Y-J, Lee MS, Yang YS, Hur M-H (2011). "Self-aromatherapy massage of the abdomen for the reduction of menstrual pain and anxiety during menstruation in nurses: a placebo-controlled clinical trial," Eur J Integr Med. 3:e165–e168.

Kim Y.W. et al (2013). "Safety evaluation and risk assessment of d-Limonene," J. Toxicol. Environ. Health B Crit. 16 (1):17-38.

Kimura K, Ozeki M, Juneja LR, Ohira H (2007 Jan). "L-Theanine reduces psychological and physiological stress responses," Biol Psychol. 74(1): 39-45.

Kite SM, Maher EJ, Anderson K, Young T, Young J, Wood J, Howells N, Bradburn J (1998 May). "Development of an aromatherapy service at a Cancer Centre," Palliat Med. 12(3):171-80.

Klauke AL, Racz I, Pradier B, Markert A, Zimmer AM, Gertsch J, Zimmer A (2014 Apr). "The cannabinoid CB₂ receptor-selective phytocannabinoid beta-caryophyllene exerts analgesic effects in mouse models of inflammatory and neuropathic pain," Eur Neuropsychopharmacol. 24(4):608-20.

Klein A.H., Jpe C.L., Davoodi A., Takechi K., Carstens M.I., Carsents E (2014 Jun). "Eugenol and carvacrol excite first- and second-order trigeminal neurons and enhance their heat-evoked responses," Neuroscience. 271:45-55.

Kline RM, Kline JJ, Di Palma J, Barbero GJ (2001 Jan). "Enteric-coated, pH-dependent peppermint oil capsules for the treatment of irritable bowel syndrome in children," J Pediatr. 138(1):125-8.

Klug W.S., Cummings M.R., Spencer C., Palladino M.A. Concepts of Genetics. San Francisco: Pearson Custom Publishing, 2009.

Knott A, Reuschlein K, Mielke H, Wensorra U, Mummert C, Koop U, Kausch M, Kolbe L, Peters N, Stäb F, Wenck H, Gallinat S (2008 Dec). "Natural Arctium lappa fruit extract improves the clinical signs of aging skin," J Cosmet Dermatol. 7(4):281-9.

Kobayashi Y, Takahashi R, Ogino F (2005 Oct 3). "Antipruritic effect of the single oral administration of German chamomile flower extract and its combined effect with antiallergic agents in ddY mice," J Ethnopharmacol. 101(1-3):308-12.

Kocevski, D., Du, M., Kan, J., Jing, C., Lacanin, I., & Pavlovic, H. (2013 May). Antifungal effect of Allium tuberosum, Cinnamomum cassia, and Pogostemon cablin essential oils and their components against population of Aspergillus species. J Food Sci, 78(5), M731-737.

Kodama R, Yano T, Furukawa K, Noda K, Ide H (1976 Jun). "Studies on the metabolism of d-limonene (p- mentha-1,8-diene). IV. Isolation and characterization of new metabolites and specie differences in metabolism," Xenobiotica Fate Foreign Compd. Biol. Syst. 6(6):337-389.

Koh KJ, Pearce AL, Marshman G, Finlay-Jones JJ, Hart PH (2002 Dec). "Tea tree oil reduces histamine-induced skin inflammation," Br J Dermatol. 147(6):1212-7.

Kohlert, C., van Rensen, I., Marz, R., Schindler, G., Graefe, E. U., & Veit, M. (2000 Aug). Bioavailability and pharmacokinetics of natural volatile terpenes in animals and humans. Planta Med, 66(6), 495-505.

Komiya M, Takeuchi T, Harada E (2006 Sep 25). "Lemon oil vapor causes an anti-stress effect via modulating the 5-HT and DA activities in mice," Behav Brain Res. 172(2):240-9.

Komori T, Fujiwara R, Tanida M, Nomura J (1995 Dec). "Potential antidepressant effects of lemon odor in rats," Eur Neuropsychopharmacol. 5(4):477-80.

Komori T, Fujiwara R, Tanida M, Nomura J, Yokoyama MM (1995 May-Jun). "Effects of citrus fragrance on immune function and depressive states," Neuroimmunomodulation. 2(3):174-80.

Koo HN, Hong SH, Kim CY, Ahn JW, Lee YG, Kim JJ, Lyu YS, Kim HM (2002 Jun). "Inhibitory effect of apoptosis in human astrocytes CCF-STTG1 cells by lemon oil," Pharmacol Res. 45(6):469-73.

Koo HN, Jeong HJ, Kim CH, Park ST, Lee SJ, Seong KK, Lee SK, Lyu YS, Kim HM (2001 Dec). "Inhibition of heat shock-induced apoptosis by peppermint oil in astrocytes," J Mol Neurosci. 17(3):391-6.

Kooncumchoo P, Sharma S, Porter J, Govitrapong P, Ebadi M (2006). "Coenzyme Q(10) provides neuroprotection in iron-induced apoptosis in dopaminergic neurons," J Mol Neurosci. 28(2):125-41.

Kosalec I, Pepeljnjak S, Kustrak D. (2005 Dec). "Antifungal activity of fluid extract and essential oil from anise fruits (Pimpinella anisum L, Apiaceae)," Acta Pharm. 55(4):377-85.

Kotan R, Kordali S, Cakir A (2007 Aug). "Screening of antibacterial activities of twenty-one oxygenated monoterpenes," Z. Für Naturforschung C J. Biosci. 62(7-8):507-513.

Kothiwale S.V., Patwardham V., Ghandi M., Sohoni R., Kumar A. (2014). "A comparative study of antiplaque and antigingivitis effects of herbal mouthrinse containing tea tree oil, clove, and basil with commercially available essential oil mouthrinse," J. Indian Soc. Periodontol. 18(3):316-320.

Koto R. et al (2006 Jul). "Linalyl acetate as a major ingredient of lavender essential oil relaxes the rabbit vascular smooth muscle through dephosphorylation of myosin light chain," J. Cardiovasc. Pharmacol. 48(1):850-856.

Koutroumanidou, E., Kimbaris, A., Kortsaris, A., Bezirtzoglou, E., Polissiou, M., Charalabopoulos, K., & Pagonopoulou, O. (2013 Aug). Increased seizure latency and decreased severity of pentylenetetrazol-induced seizures in mice after essential oil administration. Epilepsy Res Treat, 2013.

Kozics, K., Srancikova, A., Sedlackova, E., Horvathova, E., Melusova, M., Melus, V., Krajcovicova, Z., & Sramkova, M. (2017). "Antioxidant potential of essential oil from Lavandula angustifolia in in vitro and ex vivo cultured liver cells," Neoplasma. 64(4):485-493.

Krishnakumar A, Abraham PM, Paul J, Paulose CS (2009 Sep 15). "Down-regulation of cerebellar 5-HT(2C) receptors in pilocarpine-induced epilepsy in rats: therapeutic role of Bacopa monnieri extract," J Neurol Sci. 284(1-2):124-8.

Krishnakumar A, Nandhu MS, Paulose CS (2009 Oct). "Upregulation of 5-HT2C receptors in hippocampus of pilocarpine-induced epileptic rats: antagonism by Bacopa monnieri," Epilepsy Behav. 16(2):225-30.

Kritsidima M, Newton T, Asimakopoulou K (2010 Feb). "The effects of lavender scent on dental patient anxiety levels: a cluster randomised-controlled trial," Community Dent. Oral Epidemiol. 38(1):83-87.

Kudryavtseva, A., Krasnov, G., Lipatova, A., Alekseev, B., Maganova, F., Shaposhnikov, M., Fedorova, M., Snexhkina, A., and Moskaley, A. (2016). "Effects of Abies sibirica terpenes on cancer- and aging-associated pathways in human cells," Oncotarget, 7(50), 83744–83754.

Kuettner A, Pieper A, Koch J, Enzmann F, Schroeder S (2005 Feb 28). "Influence of coenzyme Q(10) and cervistatin on the flow-mediated vasodilation of the brachial artery: results of the ENDOTACT study," Int J Cardiol. 98(3):413-9.

Kumar A, Malik F, Bhushan S, Sethi VK, Shahi AK, Kaur J, Taneja SC, Qazi GN, Singh J (2008 Feb 15). "An essential oil and its major constituent isointermedeol induce apoptosis by increased expression of mitochondrial cytochrome c and apical death receptors in human leukaemia HL-60 cells," Chem Biol Interact. 171(3):332-47.

Kumar, D., Nisha, S., Vinay, P. and Ali, S. (2012.) "An Insight To Pullulan: A Biopolymer in Pharmaceutical Approaches," Int J of Basic and Applied Sci. 1(3):202-219.

Kumar P, Kumar A (2003 Jun). "Possible neuroprotective effect of Withania somnifera root extract against 3-nitropropionic acid-induced behavioral, biochemical, and mitochondrial dysfunction in an animal model of Huntington's disease," J Med Food. 12(3):591-600.

Kumaran AM, D'Souza P, Agarwal A, Bokkolla RM, Balasubramaniam M (2003 Sep). "Geraniol, the putative anthelmintic principle of Cymbopogon martinii," Phytother Res. 17(8):957.

Kumari, S., & Dutta, A. (2013 Jul). Protective effect of Eleteria cardamomum (L.) Maton against Pan masala induced damage in lung of male Swiss mice. Asian Pac J Trop Med, 6(7), 525-531.

Kummer R. et al (2013). "Evaluation of Anti-Inflammatory Activity of Citrus latifolia Tanaka Essential Oil and Limonene in Experimental Mouse Models," Evid.-Based Complement. Altern. Med. 859083.

Kuroda K. et al (2005 Oct). "Sedative effects of the jasmine tea odor and (R)-(-)-linalool, one of its major odor components, on autonomic nerve activity and mood states," Eur. J. Appl. Physiol. 95(2-3):107-114.

Kuo YM, Hayflick SJ, Gitschier J (2007 Jun). "Deprivation of pantothenic acid elicits a movement disorder and azoospermia in a mouse model of pantothenate kinase-associated neurodegeneration," J Inherit Metab Dis. 30(3):310-7.

Kusuhara M. et al (2012 Feb). "Fragrant environment with α-pinene decreases tumor growth in mice," Biomed. Res. 33(1):57-61.

Kuttan R, Liju V, Jeena K (2011). An evaluation of antioxidant, anti-inflammatory, and antinociceptive activities of essential oil from Curcuma longa. L," Indian J. Pharmacol. 43(5):526.

Kuwahata, H., Komatsu, T., Katsuyama, S., Corasaniti, M. T., Bagetta, G., Sakurada, S., . . . Takahama, K. (2013 Feb). Peripherally injected linalool and bergamot essential oil attenuate mechanical allodynia via inhibiting spinal ERK phosphorylation. Pharmacol Biochem Behav, 103(4), 735-741.

Kwasniewska M, Jegier A, Kostka T, Dziankowska-Zaborszczyk E, Rebowska E, Kozinska J, Drygas W (2014 Jan). "Long-term effect of different physical activity levels on subclinical atherosclerosis in middle-aged men: a 25-year prospective study," PLoS One, 9(1):e85209.

Kwieciński J, Eick S, Wójcik K (2009 Apr). "Effects of tea tree (Melaleuca alternifolia) oil on Staphylococcus aureus in biofilms and stationary growth phase," Int J Antimicrob Agents. 33(4):343-7.

Kwon Y.S., Lee S.H., Hwang Y.C., Rosa V, Lee K.W., Min K.S. (2015 Dec). "Behaviour of human dental pulp cells cultured in a collagen hydrogel scaffold crosslinked with cinnamaldehyde," Int. Endod. J.

Labib G.S., Aldawsari H. (2015). "Innovation of natural essential oil-loaded Orabase for local treatment of oral candidiasis," Drug Des. Devel. Ther. 9:3349-3359.

Lachowicz, K., Jones, G., Briggs, D., Bienvenu, F., Wan, J., Wilcock, A., & Coventry, M. (1998). The synergistic preservative effects of the essential oils of sweet basil (Ocimum basilicum L.) against acid-tolerant food microflora. Letters in Applied Microbiology, 26(3), 209-214.

Lagouge M et al. (2006 Dec 15). "Resveratrol improves mitochondrial function and protects against metabolic disease by activating SIRT1 and PGC-1alpha," Cell. 127(6):1109-22.

Lahlou S, Figueiredo AF, Magalhães PJ, Leal-Cardoso JH (2002 Dec). "Cardiovascular effects of 1,8-cineole, a terpenoid oxide present in many plant essential oils, in normotensive rats," Can J Physiol Pharmacol. 80(12):1125-31.

Lahlou S., Interaminense L.F.L., Magalhaes P.J.C., Leal-Cardoso J.H., Duarte G.P. (2004) Cardiovascular Effects of Eugenol, a Phenolic Compound Present in Many Plant Essential Oils, in Normotensive Rats. Journal of Cardiovascular Pharmacology. 43: 250-257.

Lai F, Sinico C, De Logu A, Zaru M, Muller R.H., Fadda A.M. (2007). "SLN as a topical delivery system for Artemisia arborescens essential oil: in vitro antiviral activity and skin permeation study," Int. J. Nanomedicine. 2(3):419.

Lai Y. et al (2014 Jun). "In vitro studies of a distillate of rectified essential oils on sinonasal components of mucociliary clearance," Am. J. Rhinol. Allergy. 28(3):224-248.

Lambert R.J.W., Skandamis P.N., Coote P.J., Nychas G-J.E. (2001) A study of the minimun inhibitory concentration and mode of action of oregano essential oil, thymol and carvacrol. Journal of Applied Microbiology. 91: 453-462.

Lampronti I, Saab AM, Gambari R (2006 Oct). "Antiproliferative activity of essential oils derived from plants belonging to the Magnoliophyta division," Int J Oncol. 29(4):989-95.

Langeveld, W. T., Veldhuizen, E. J., & Burt, S. A. (2014 Feb). Synergy between essential oil components and antibiotics: a review. Crit Rev Microbiol, 40(1), 76-94.

Lantry LE, Zhang Z, Gao F, Crist KA, Wang Y, Kelloff GJ, Lubet RA, You M (1997). "Chemopreventive effect of perillyl alcohol on 4-(methylnitrosamino)-1-(3-pyridyl)-1-butanone induced tumorigenesis in (C3H/HeJ X A/J)F1 mouse lung," J Cell Biochem Suppl. 27:20-5.

Lappas C.M., Lappas N.T. (2012 Sep). "D-Limonene modulates T lymphocyte activity and viability," Cell. Immunol. 279(1):30-41.

Larder B.A., Kemp S.D., Harrigan P.R. (1995) Potential Mechanism for Sustained Antiretroviral Efficacy of AZT-3TC Combination Therapy. Science. 269: 696-699.

Laurent TC, Laurent UB, Frazer JR (1995 May). "Functions of hyaluronan," Ann Rheum Dis. 54(5):429-32.

Lawrence, H. A., & Palombo, E. A. (2009 Dec). Activity of essential oils against Bacillus subtilis spores. J Microbiol Biotechnol, 19(12), 1590-1595.

Leaf DA, Parker DL, Schaad D (1997 Sep). "Changes in Vo2max, phsical activity, and body fat with chronic exercise: effects on plasma lipids," Med Sci Sports Exerc, 29(9):1152-9.

LeDoux, J. (2003). The emotional brain, fear, and the amygdala. Cellular and molecular neurobiology, 23(4-5), 727-738.

LeDoux, J. E., Iwata, J., Cicchetti, P., & Reis, D. J. (1988 Jul). Different projections of the central amygdaloid nucleus mediate autonomic and behavioral correlates of conditioned fear. J Neurosci, 8(7), 2517-2529.

Ledoux, J. E., Romanski, L., & Xagoraris, A. (1989 Jul). Indelibility of subcortical emotional memories. J Cogn Neurosci, 1(3), 238-243.

Lee HR, Kim GH, Choi WS, Park IK (2017 Apr 1). "Repellent Activity of Apiaceae Plant Essential Oils and their Constituents Against Adult German Cockroaches," J Econ Entomol. 110(2):552-557.

Lee, H. S. (2002 Dec). Inhibitory activity of Cinnamomum cassia bark-derived component against rat lens aldose reductase. J Pharm Pharm Sci, 5(3), 226-230.

Lee HS (2005 Apr 6). "Cuminaldehyde: Aldose Reductase and alpha-Glucosidase Inhibitor Derived from Cuminum cyminum L. Seeds," J Agric Food Chem. 53(7):2446-50.

Lee, H. S., & Ahn, Y. J. (1998 Jan). Growth-Inhibiting Effects of Cinnamomum cassia Bark-Derived Materials on Human Intestinal Bacteria. J Agric Food Chem, 46(1), 8-12.

Lee IS, Lee GJ (2006 Feb). "Effects of lavender aromatherapy on insomnia and depression in women college students," Taehan Kanho Hakhoe Chi. 36(1):136-43.

Lee K, Lee JH, Kim SI, Cho M.H., Lee J (2014 Nov). "Anti-biofilm, anti-hemolysis, and antivirulence activities of black pepper, cananga, myrrh oils, and nerolidol against Staphylococcus aureus," Appl. Microbiol. Biotechnol. 98(22):9447:9457.

Lee KH et al (2011 Dec). "Essential oil of Curcuma longa inhibits Streptococcus mutans biofilm formation," J. Food Sci. 76(9):H226-230.

Lee SH, Do HS, Min KJ (2015 Dec). Effects of Essential Oil from Hinoki Cypress, Chamaecyparis obtusa, on Physiology and Behavior of Flies. PLoS One. 10(12):e0143450.

Lee SK, Zhang W, Sanderson BJ (2008 Aug). "Selective growth inhibition of human leukemia and human lymphoblastoid cells by resveratrol via cell cycle arrest and apoptosis induction," J Agric Food Chem. 56(16):7572-7.

Lee SU, Shim KS, Ryu SY, Min YK, Kim SH (2009 Feb). "Machilin A isolated from Myristica fragrans stimulates osteoblast differentiation," Planta Med. 75(2):152-7.

Lee, S. Y., Ha, S. A., Seo, J. S., Sohn, C. M., Park, H. R., & Kim, K. W. (2014). Eating habits and eating behaviors by family dinner frequency in the lower-grade elementary school students. Nutr Res Pract, 8(6), 679-687.

Lee, T., Lee, S., Ho Kim, K., Oh, K. B., Shin, J., & Mar, W. (2013 Sep). Effects of magnolialide isolated from the leaves of Laurus nobilis L. (Lauraceae) on immunoglobulin E-mediated type I hypersensitivity in vitro. J Ethnopharmacol, 149(2), 550-556.

Lee Y (2009). "Activation of apoptotic protein in U937 cells by a component of turmeric oil," BMB Rep. 42(2):96-100.

Leffa, D. D., da Silva, J., Daumann, F., Dajori, A. L., Longaretti, L. M., Damiani, A. P., . . . de Andrade, V. M. (2013 Dec). Corrective effects of acerola (Malpighia emarginata DC.) juice intake on biochemical and genotoxical parameters in mice fed on a high-fat diet. Mutat Res.

Legault J, Dahl W, Debiton E, Pichette A, Madelmont JC (2003 May). "Antitumor activity of balsam fir oil: production of reactive oxygen species induced by alpha-humulene as possible mechanism of action," Planta Med. 69(5):402-7.

Legault J, Pichette A (2007 Dec). "Potentiating effect of beta-caryophyllene on anticancer activity of alpha-humulene, isocaryophyllene and paclitaxel," J Pharm Pharmacol. 59(12):1643-7.

Leggio M, Mazza A, Cruciani G, Sgorbini L, Publiese M, Bendinin MG, Severi P, Jesi AP (2014 Jul). "Effects of exercise training on systo-diastoli ventricular dysfunction in patients with hypertension: an echocardiographic study with tissue velocity and strain imaging evaluation," Hypertens Res, 37(7):649-54.

Lehrner J, Eckersberger C, Walla P, Pötsch G, Deecke L (2000 Oct 1-15). "Ambient odor of orange in a dental office reduces anxiety and improves mood in female patients," Physiol Behav. 71(1-2):83-6.

Lehrner J, Marwinski G, Lehr S, Johren P, Deecke L. (2005 Sep 15). "Ambient odors of orange and lavender reduce anxiety and improve mood in a dental office," Physiol Behav. 86(1-2):92-5.

Lekshmi P.C., Arimboor R, Indulekha P.S., Nirmala Menon A (2012 Nov). "Turmeric (Curcuma longa L.) volatile oil inhibits key enzymes linked to type 2 diabetes," Int. J. Food Sci. Nutr. 63(7):832-834.

Letawe C, Boone M, Piérard GE (1998 Mar). "Digital image analysis of the effect of topically applied linoleic acid on acne microcomedones," Clin Exp Dermatol. 23(2):56-8.

Leung LH (1995 Jun). "Pantothenic acid deficiency as the pathogenesis of acne vulgaris," Med Hypotheses. 44(6):490-2.

Lewith GT, Godfrey AD, Prescott P (2005 Aug). "A single-blinded, randomized pilot study evaluating the aroma of Lavandula augustifolia as a treatment for mild insomnia," J Altern Complement Med. 11(4):631-7.

Li F, Tao Y, Qiao Y, Li K, Jiang Y, Cao C, Ren S, Chang X, Wang X, Wang Y, Xie Y, Dong Z, Zhao J, Liu K (2017 Sep). "Eupatilin inhibits EGF-induced JB6 cell transformation by targeting PI3K," Int J Oncol. 49(3):1148-54.

Li SP, Li P, Dont TT, Tsim KW (2001). "Anti-oxidation activity of different types of natural Cordyceps sinensis and cultured Cordyceps mycelia," Phytomedicine. 8:207-12.

Li Q, Kobayashi M, Wakayama Y, Inagaki H, Katsumata M, Hirata Y, Hirata K, Shimizu T, Kawada T, Park BJ, Ohira T, Kagawa T, Miyazaki Y. (2009 Oct). "Effect of phytoncide from trees on human natural killer cell function," Int J Immunopathol Pharmacol. 22(4):951-9

Li QQ, Lee RX, Liang H, Zhong Y (2013 Jan). "Anticancer activity of beta-elemene and its synthetic analogs in human malignant brain tumor cells," Anticancer Res. 33(1):65-76.

Li QQ, Wang G, Huang F, Li JM, Cuff CF, Reed E (2013 Mar). "Sensitization of lung cancer cells to cisplatin by beta-elemene is mediated through blockade of cell cycle progression: antitumor efficacies of beta-elemene and its synthetic analogs," Med Oncol. 30(1):488.

Li QQ, Wang G, Liang H, Li JM, Huang F, Agarwal PK, Zhong Y, Reed E (2013). "Beta element promotes cisplatin-induced cell death in human bladder cancer and other carcinomas," Anticancer Res. 33(4):1421-8.

Li, R., Liang, T., Xu, L., Li, Y., Zhang, S., & Duan, X. (2013 Jan). Protective effect of cinnamon polyphenols against STZ-diabetic mice fed high-sugar, high-fat diet and its underlying mechanism. Food Chem Toxicol, 51, 419-425.

Li WR, Shi QS, Liang Q, Xie XB, Huang XM, Chen YB (2014 Nov). "Antibacterial Activity and Kinetics of Litsea cubeba Oil on Escherichia coli," PLoS ONE. 9(11):e110983.

Li, X., Duan, S., Chu, C., Xu, J., Zeng, G., Lam, A. K., . . . Jiang, L. (2013 Aug). Melaleuca alternifolia concentrate inhibits in vitro entry of influenza virus into host cells. Molecules, 18(8), 9550-9566.

Li XJ, Yang YJ, Li YS, Zhang W.K., Tang HB (2015 Dec). "α-Pinene, linalool, and 1-octano contribute to the topical anti-inflammatory and analgesic activities of frankincense by inhibiting COX-2," J Ethnopharmacol.

Li, Y. P., Yuan, S. F., Cai, G. H., Wang, H., Wang, L., Yu, L., . . . Yun, J. (2014 May). Patchouli Alcohol Dampens Lipopolysaccharide Induced Mastitis in Mice. Inflammation.

Liakos I, Rizzello L, Scurr D.J., Pomp P.P., Bayer I.S., Athanassiou A. (2014 Mar). "All-natural composite wound dressing films of essential oils encapsulated in sodium alginate with antimicrobial properties," Int. J. Pharm. 463(2):137-145.

Liao JC, Tsai JC, Liu CY, Huang HC, Wu LY, Peng WH (2013). "Antidepressant-like activity of turmerone in behavioral despair tests in mice," BMC Complement. Altern. Med. 13(1):299.

Liapi C, Anifandis G, Chinou I, Kourounakis AP, Theodosopoulos S, Galanopoulou P (2007 Oct). "Antinociceptive properties of 1,8-Cineole and beta-pinene, from the essential oil of Eucalyptus camaldulensis leaves, in rodents," Planta Med. 73(12):1247-54.

Liju V.B., Jeena K, Kuttan R (2015 Jan). "Gastroprotective activity of essential oils from turmeric and ginger," J. Basic Clin. Physiol. Pharmacol. 26(1):95-103.

Lim W.C., Seo J.M., Lee C.I., Pyo H.B., Lee B.C. (2005 jul). "Stimulative and sedative effects of essential oils upon inhalation in mice," Arch. Pharm. Res. 28(7):770-774.

Lima CF, Azevedo MF, Araujo R, Fernandes-Ferreira M, Pereira-Wilson C (2006 Aug). "Metformin-like effect of Salvia officinalis (common sage): is it useful in diabetes prevention?," Br J Nutr. 96(2):326-33.

Appendix

487

Lima DF, Brandao MS, Moura JB, Leitao JM Carvalho FA, Miura LM, Leite JR, Sousa DP, Almeida FR (2012 Feb). "Antinociceptive activity of the monoterpene a-phellandrene in rodents: possible mechanisms of action," J Pharm Pharmacol: 64(2):283-92.

Lima N.G.P.B et al (2013 Jan). "Anxiolytic-like activity and GC-MS analysis of (R)-(+)-limonene fragrance, a natural compound found in foods and plants," Pharmacol. Biochem. Behav. 103(3):450-454.

Lin JJ et al (2013 Dec). "Alpha-phellandrene promotes immune responses in normal mice through enhancing macrophage phagocytosis and natural killer cell activities," Vivo Athens Greece. 27(6):809-814.

Lin JJ, Wu CC, Hsu SC, Weng SW, Ma YS, Huang YP, Lin JG, Chung JG (2014 May). "Alpha-phellandrene-induced DNA damage and affect DNA repair protein expression in WEHI-3 murine leukemia cells in vitro," Environ Toxicol. 30(11):1322-30.

Lin PW, Chan WC, Ng BF, Lam LC (2007 May). "Efficacy of aromatherapy (Lavandula angustifolia) as an intervention for agitated behaviours in Chinese older persons with dementia: a cross-over randomized trial," Int J Geriatr Psychiatry. 22(5):405-10.

Lin RF et al. (2014 Jun 11). "Prevention of UV radiation-induced cutaneous photoaging in mice by topical administration of patchouli oil," J Ethnopharmacol. 154(2):408-18.

Lin SC, Chung TC, Lin CC, Ueng TH, Lin YH, Lin SY, Wang LY (2000). "Hepatoprotective effects of Arctium lappa on carbon tetrachloride- and acetaminophen-induced liver damage," Am J Chin Med. 28(2):163-73.

Lin TK, Zhong L, Santiago J.L. (2017 Dec). "Anti-Inflammatory and Skin Barrier Repair Effects of Topical Application of Some Plant Oils," International Journal of Molecular Sciences. 19(1):70.

Linck V.M., da Silva A.L., Figueiro M., Piato A.L., Herrmann A.P., Birck F.D., Moreno P.R.H., Elisabetsky E. (2009) Inhaled linalool-induced sedation in mice. Phytomedicine. 16: 303-307.

Lipovac M, Chedraui P, Gruenhut C, Gocan A, Stammler M, Imhof M (2010 Mar). "Improvement of postmenopausal depressive and anxiety symptoms after treatment with isoflavones derived from red clover extracts," Maturitas. 65(3):258-61.

Lis-Balchin M, Hart S (1999 Sep). "Studies on the mode of action of the essential oil of lavender (Lavandula angustifolia P. Miller)," Phytother Res. 13(6):540-2.

Lis-Balchin M, Hart S, Wan Hang Lo B (2002 Aug). "Jasmine absolute (Jasminum grandiflora L.) and its mode of action on guinea-pig ileum in vitro," Phytother Res. 16(5):437-9.

Liu, C. T., Raghu, R., Lin, S. H., Wang, S. Y., Kuo, C. H., Tseng, Y. J., & Sheen, L. Y. (2013 Nov). Metabolomics of ginger essential oil against alcoholic fatty liver in mice. J Agric Food Chem, 61(46), 11231-11240.

Liu J, Head E, Gharib AM, Yuan W, Ingersoll RT, Hagen TM, Cotman CW, Ames BN (2002 Feb). "Memory loss in old rats is associated with brain mitochondrial decay and RNA/DNA oxidation: partial reversal by feeding acetyl-L-carnitine and/or R-alpha -lipoic acid," Proc Natl Acad Sci U S A. 99(4):2356-61.

Liu J, Killilea DW, Ames BN (2002 Feb 19). "Age-associated mitochondrial oxidative decay: improvement of carnitine acetyltransferase substrate-binding affinity and activity in brain by feeding old rats acetyl-L- carnitine and/or R-alpha-lipoic acid," Proc Natl Acad Sci U S A. 99(4):1876-81.

Liu JH, Chen GH, Yeh HZ, Huang CK, Poon SK (1997 Dec). "Enteric-coated peppermint-oil capsules in the treatment of irritable bowel syndrome: a prospective, randomized trial," J Gastroenterol. 32(6):765-8.

Liu JJ, Nilsson A, Oredsson S, Badmaev V, Duan RD (2002 Oct). "Keto- and acetyl-keto-boswellic acids inhibit proliferation and induce apoptosis in Hep G2 cells via a caspase-8 dependent pathway," Int J Mol Med. 10(4):501-5.

Liu JJ, Nilsson A, Oredsson S, Badmaev V, Zhao WZ, Duan RD (2002 Dec). "Boswellic acids trigger apoptosis via a pathway dependent on caspase-8 activation but independent on Fas/Fas ligand interaction in colon cancer HT-29 cells," Carcinogenesis. 23(12):2087-93.

Liu R, Sui X, Laditka JN, Church TS, Colabianchi N, Hussey J, Blair SN, (2012 Feb). "Cardiorespiratory fitness as a predictor of dementia mortality in men and women," Med Sci Sports Exerc, 44(2):253-9.

Liu TT, Yang TS (2012 May). "Antimicrobial impact of the components of essential oil of Litsea cubeba from Taiwan and antimicrobial activity of the oil in food systems," International Journal of Food Microbiology. 156(1):68-75.

Lobo, V., Patil, A., Phatak, A., & Chandra, N. (2010 Jul). Free radicals, antioxidants and functional foods: Impact on human health. Pharmacogn Rev, 4(8), 118-126.

Loew O. (1900) A New Enzyme of General Occurrence in Organisms. Science. 11: 701-702.

Lohidasan S, Paradkar AR, Mahadik KR (2009 Nov). "Nootropic activity of lipid-based extract of Bacopa monniera Linn. compared with traditional preparation and extracts," J Pharm Pharmacol. 61(11):1537-44.

Loizzo MR, Tundis R, Menichini F, Saab AM, Statti GA, Menichini F (2007 Sep-Oct). "Cytotoxic activity of essential oils from labiatae and lauraceae families against in vitro human tumor models," Anticancer Res. 27(5A):3293-9.

Long J, Gao F, Tong L, Cotman CW, Ames BN, Liu J (2009 Apr). "Mitochondrial decay in the brains of old rats: ameliorating effect of alpha-lipoic acid and acetyl-L-carnitine," Neurochem Res. 34(4):755-63.

Longley D.B., Harkin D.P., Johnston P.G. (2003) 5-Fluorouracil: Mechanisms of Action and Clinical Strategies. Nature Reviews. 3: 330-338.

López, V., Nielsen, B., Solas, M., Ramírez, M. J., & Jäger, A. K. (2017 May 19). "Exploring Pharmacological Mechanisms of Lavender (Lavandula angustifolia) Essential Oil on Central Nervous System Targets," Front Pharmacol. 8:280.

Loughlin R, Gilmore BF, McCarron PA, Tunney MM (2008 Apr). "Comparison of the cidal activity of tea tree oil and terpinen-4-ol against clinical bacterial skin isolates and human fibroblast cells.," Lett Appl Microbiol. 46(4):428-33.

Louis M, Kowalski S.D. (2002 Dec). "Use of aromatherapy with hospice patients to decrease pain, anxiety, and depression and to promote an increased sense of well-being," Am. J. Hosp. Palliat. Care. 19(6):381-386.

Lu J. et al (2014 Sep). "Sesquiterpene acids from Shellac and their bioactivities evaluation," Fitoterapia. 97:64-70.

Lu LJ, Cree M, Josyula S, Nagamani M, Grady JJ, Anderson KE (2000 Mar 1). "Increased urinary excretion of 2-hydroxyestrone but not 16alpha-hydroxyestrone in premenopausal women during a soya diet containing isoflavones," Cancer Res. 60(5):1299-305.

Lu M, Battinelli L, Daniele C, Melchioni C, Salvatore G, Mazzanti G (2002 Mar). "Muscle relaxing activity of Hyssopus officinalis essential oil on isolated intestinal preparations," Planta Med. 68(3):213-6.

Lu M, Xia L, Hua H, Jing Y (2008 Feb 15). "Acetyl-keto-beta-boswellic acid induces apoptosis through a death receptor 5-mediated pathway in prostate cancer cells," Cancer Res. 68(4):1180-6.

Lu, T., Sheng, H., Wu, J., Cheng, Y., Zhu, J., & Chen, Y. (2012 Jun). Cinnamon extract improves fasting blood glucose and glycosylated hemoglobin level in Chinese patients with type 2 diabetes. Nutr Res, 32(6), 408-412.

Lu X, Feng B, Zhan L, Yu Z (2003 Jul). "[D-limonene induces apoptosis of gastric cancer cells]," Zhonghua Zhong Liu Za Zhi. 25(4):325-327.

Lu XG, Zhan LB, Feng BA, Qu MY, Yu LH, Xie JH (2004 Jul). "Inhibition of growth and metastasis of human gastric cancer implanted in nude mice by d-limonene," World J. Gastroenterol. 10(14):2140-2144.

Lu XQ, Tang FD, Wang Y, Zhao T, Bian RL (2004 Feb). "Effect of Eucalyptus globulus oil on lipopolysaccharide-induced chronic bronchitis and mucin hypersecretion in rats," Zhongguo Zhong Yao Za Zhi. 29(2):168-71.

Lucas M, Asselin G, Mérette C, Poulin MJ, Dodin S (2009 Feb). "Ethyl-eicosapentaenoic acid for the treatment of psychological distress and depressive symptoms in middle-aged women: a double-blind, placebo-controlled, randomized clinical trial," Am J Clin Nutr. 89(2):641-51.

Luo M, Jiang LK, Zou GL (2005). "Acute and genetic toxicity of essential oil extracted from Litsea cubeba (Lour.) Pers.," Journal of Food Protection®. 68(3):581-588.

Luqman S, Dwivedi G.R., Darokar M.P., Kalra A, Khanuja S.P.S. (2007 Oct). "Potential of rosemary oil to be used in drug-resistant infections," Altern. Ther. Health Med. 13(5):54-59.

Lytle J, Mwatha C, Davis K.K (2014 Jan). "Effect of Lavender Aromatherapy on Vital Signs and Perceived Quality of Sleep in the Intermediate Care Unit: A Pilot Study," Am. J. Crit. Care. 23(1):24-29.

Maatta-Riihinen KR, Kahkonen MP, Torronen AR, Heinonen IM (2005 Nov 2). "Catechins and procyanidins in berries of vaccinium species and their antioxidant activity," J Agric Food Chem. 53(22):8485-91.

Mabrok HB, Klopfleisch R, Ghanem KZ, Clavel T, Blaut M, Loh G (2012 Jan). "Lignan transformation by gut bacteria lowers tumor burden in a gnotobiotic rat model of breast cancer," Carcinogenesis. 33(1):203-8.

Machado, D. G., Cunha, M. P., Neis, V. B., Balen, G. O., Colla, A., Bettio, L. E., . . . Rodrigues, A. L. (2013 Jan). Antidepressant-like effects of fractions, essential oil, carnosol and betulinic acid isolated from Rosmarinus officinalis L. Food Chem, 136(2), 999-1005.

Maddocks-Jennings W, Wilkinson JM, Cavanagh HM, Shillington D (2009 Apr). "Evaluating the effects of the essential oils Leptospermum scoparium (manuka) and Kunzea ericoides (kanuka) on radiotherapy induced mucositis: a randomized, placebo controlled feasibility study," Eur J Oncol Nurs. 13(2):87-93.

Mahboubi M (2017 Feb). "Mentha spicata as natural analgesia for treatment of pain in osteoarthritis patients," Complement Ther Clin Pract. 26:1-4.

Mahesh A, Jeyachandran R, Cindrella L, Thangadurai D, Veerapur VP, Muralidhara Rao D (2010 Jun). "Hepatocurative potential of sesquiterpene lactones of Taraxacum officinale on carbon tetrachloride induced liver toxicity in mice," Acta Biol Hung. 61(2):175-90.

Maickel, R. P., & Snodgrass, W. R. (1973 Oct). Physicochemical factors in maternal-fetal distribution of drugs. Toxicology and Applied Pharmacology, 26(2), 218-230.

Malachowska B, Fendler W, Pomykala A, Suwala S, Mlynarski W (2016 Jan). "Essential oils reduce autonomous response to pain sensation during self-monitoring of blood glucose among children with diabetes," J. Pediatr. Endocrinol. Metab. JPEM. 29(1):47-53.

Mao S, Wang K, Lei Y, Yao S, Lu B, Huang W (2017 Apr). "Antioxidant synergistic effects of Osmanthus fragrans flowers with green tea and their major contributed antioxidant compounds," Sci Rep. 7.

Maiwulanjiang M, Zhu KY, Chen J, Miernisha A, Xu SL, Du CYQ, Lau KKM, Choi, RCY, Dong TTX, Aisa HA, Tsim KWK (2013). "Song bu li decoction, a traditional uyghur medicine, protects cell death by regulation of oxidative stress and differentiation in cultured PC12 cells," Evidence-Based Complementary and Alternative Medicine.

Maiwulanjiang M, Zhu KY, Chen J, Miernisha A, Xu SL, Du CYQ, Lau KKM, Choi, RCY, Dong TTX, Aisa HA, Tsim KWK (2014 Apr). "The volatile oil of Nardostachyos radix et rhizoma inhibits the oxidative stress-induced cell injury via reactive oxygen species scavenging and Akt activation in H9c2 cardiomyocyte," J Ethnopharmacol. 153(2):491-8.

Maiwulanjiang M, Bi CW, Lee, PS, Xin G, Miernisha A, Lau KM, Xiong A, Li N, Dong TTX, Aisa HA, Tsim KWK (2014 Apr). "The volatile oil of nardostachys radix et rhizoma induces endothelial nitric oxide synthase activity in HUVEC cells," PLOS One.

Malachowska B, Fendler W, Pomykala A, Suwala S, Mlynarski W (2016 Jan). "Essential oils reduce autonomous response to pain sensation during self-monitoring of blood glucose among children with diabetes," J. Pediatr. Endocrinol. Metab. JPEM. 29(1):47-53

Malaguarnera M, Cammalleri L, Gargante MP, Vacante M, Colonna V, Motta M (2007 Dec). "L-Carnitine treatment reduces severity of physical and mental fatigue and increases cognitive functions in centenarians: a randomized and controlled clinical trial," Am J Clin Nutr. 86(6):1738-44.

Manassero C.A., Girotti J.R., Mijailovsky S, García de Bravo M, Polo M (2013). "In vitro comparative analysis of antiproliferative activity of essential oil from mandarin peel and its principal component limonene," Nat. Prod. Res. 27(16):1475-1478.

Mandel S, Stoner GD (1990 Jan). "Inhibition of N-nitrosobenzylmethylamine-induced esophageal tumorigenesis in rats by ellagic acid," Carcinogenesis. 11(1):55-61.

Manohar V, Ingram C, Gray J, Talpur NA, Echard BW, Bagchi D, Preuss HG (2001 Dec). "Antifungal activities of origanum oil against Candida albicans," Mol Cell Biochem. 228(1-2):111-7.

Manosroi J, Dhumtanom P, Manosroi A (2006 Apr). "Anti-proliferative activity of essential oil extracted from Thai medicinal plants on KB and P388 cell lines," Cancer Lett. 235(1):114-120.

Maquart FX, Siméon A, Pasco S, Monboisse JC (1999). "[Regulation of cell activity by the extracellular matrix: the concept of matrikines]," J Soc Biol. 193(4-5):423-8.

Marder M, Viola H, Wasowski C, Fernández S, Medina JH, Paladini AC (2003 Jun). "6-methylapigenin and hesperidin: new valeriana flavonoids with activity on the CNS," Pharmacol Biochem Behav. 75(3):537-45.

Margetts, L., & Sawyer, R. (2007). Transdermal drug delivery: principles and opioid therapy. Continuing Education in Anaesthesia, Critical Care & Pain, 7(5), 171-176.

Marinangeli CP, Jones PJ (2012 Aug). "Pulse grain consumption and obesity: effects on energy expenditure, substrate oxidation, body composition, fat deposition and satiety," Br J Nutr. 108 Suppl 1:246-51.

Marotti M, Piccaglia R, Giovanelli E, Deans S.G., Eaglesham E (1994 May). "Effects of planting time and mineral fertilization on peppermint (mentha x piperita l.) essential oil. 9(3):125-129.

composition and its biological activity," Flavour Fragr. J

Marounek M, Skrivanova E, Rada V, (2003). "Susceptibility of Escherichia coli to C2-C18 fatty acids," Folia Microbiol (Praha). 48(6):731-5.

Martins Mdo R, Arantes S, Candeias F, Tinoco MT, Cruz-Morais J (2013 Nov). "Antioxidant, antimicrobial and toxicological properties of Schinus molle L. essential oils," J Ethnopharmacol. 151(1):485-92.

Maruf FA, Salako BL, Akinpelu AO (2014 Jun). "Can aerobic exercise complement antihypertensive drugs to achieve blood pressure control in individuals with essential hypertension," J Cardiovasc Med (Hagerstown), 15(6):456-62.

Maruyama N, Sekimoto Y, Ishibashi H, Inouye S, Oshima H, Yamaguchi H, Abe S (2005 Feb 10). "Suppression of neutrophil accumulation in mice by cutaneous application of geranium essential oil," J Inflamm (Lond). 2(1):1.

Masago R. et al (2000 Jan). "Effects of inhalation of essential oils on EEG activity and sensory evaluation," J. Physiol. Anthropol. Appl. Human Sci. 19(1):35-42.

Masango, P. (2005). Cleaner production of essential oils by steam distillation. Journal of Cleaner Production, 13(8), 833-839.

Masukawa Y., Narita H., Sato H., Naoe A., Kondo N., Sugai Y., Oba T., Homma R., Ishikawa J., Takagi Y., Kitahara T. (2009) Comprehensive quantification of ceramide species in human stratum corneum. Journal of Lipid Research. 50: 1708-1719.

Masumoto Y, Morinushi T, Kawasaki H, Ogura T, Takigawa M (1999 Feb). "Effects of three principal constituents in chewing gum on electroencephalographic activity," Psychiatry Clin. Neurosci. 53(1):17-23.

Matsubara E et al (2012). "Volatiles emitted from the roots of Vetiveria zizanioides suppress the decline in attention during a visual display terminal task," Biomed. Res. Tokyo Jpn. 33(5):299-308.

Matsubara E., Tsunetsugu Y., Ohira T., & Sugiyama M. (2017 Jan. 21). "Essential Oil of Japanese Cedar (Cryptomeria japonica) Wood Increases Salivary Dehydroepiandrosterone Sulfate Levels after Monotonous Work," Int J Res Public Health. 14(1).

Matsumoto T, Asakura H, Hayashi T (2013). "Does lavender aromatherapy alleviate premenstrual emotional symptoms?: a randomized crossover trial," Biopsychosoc. Med. 7:12.

Matsumoto T, Kimura T, Hayashi T (2016 Apr). "Aromatic effects of a Japanese citrus fruit-yuzu (Citrus junos Sieb. ex Tanaka)-on psychoemotional states and autonomic nervous system activity during the menstrual cycle: a single-blind randomized controlled crossover study," Biopsychosoc. Med. 10:11.

Matsumoto T, Kimura T, Hayashi T (2017 May). "Does Japanese Citrus Fruit Yuzu (Citrus junos Sieb. ex Tanaka) Fragrance Have Lavender-Like Therapeutic Effects That Alleviate Premenstrual Emotional Symptoms? A Single-Blind Randomized Crossover Study," J Altern Complement Med. 23(6):461-470.

Matsuo A.L. et al (2011 Jul). "α-Pinene isolated from Schinus terebinthifolius Raddi (Anacardiaceae) induces apoptosis and confers antimetastatic protection in a melanoma model," Biochem. Biophys. Res. Commun. 411(2):449-454.

Matthys H, de Mey C, Carls C, Ryś A, Geib A, Wittig T (2000 Aug). "Efficacy and tolerability of myrtol standardized in acute bronchitis. A multi-centre, randomised, double-blind, placebo-controlled parallel group clinical trial vs. cefuroxime and ambroxol," Arzneimittelforschung. 50(8):700-711.

Maurya, A. K., Singh, M., Dubey, V., Srivastava, S., Luqman, S., Bawankule, D. U. (2014 Jun 5). "α-(-)-bisabolol reduces pro-inflammatory cytokine production and ameliorates skin inflammation," Curr Pharm Biotechnol, 15(2): 173-181.

May B, Kuntz HD, Kieser M, Köhler S (1996 Dec). "Efficacy of a fixed peppermint oil/caraway oil combination in non-ulcer dyspepsia," Arzneimittelforschung. 46(12):1149-53.

McCaffrey R, Thomas D.J., Kinzelman A.O. (2009 Apr). "The effects of lavender and rosemary essential oils on test-taking anxiety among graduate nursing students," Holist. Nurs. Pract. 23(2):88-93.

McKay D.L., Blumberg J.B. (2006 Aug). "A review of the bioactivity and potential health benefits of peppermint tea (Mentha piperita L.)," Phytother. Res. PTR. 20(8):619-633.

McCord J.M., Fridovich I. (1969) Superoxide Dismutase: an enzymic function for erytrocuprein (hemocuprein). The Journal of Biological Chemistry. 244: 6049-6055.

Meamarbashi, A., & Rajabi, A. (2013 Mar). The effects of peppermint on exercise performance. J Int Soc Sports Nutr, 10(1), 15.

Mehta S, Stone D.N. Whitehead H.F. (1998 Jul). "Use of essential oil to promote induction of anaesthesia in children," Anaesthesia. 53(7):720-721.

Meier B, Berger D, Hoberg E, Sticher O, Schaffner W, (2000). "Pharmacological Activities of Vitex agnus-castus Extracts in Vitro," Phytomedicine. 7(5):373-81.

Meier, L., Stange, R., Michalsen, A., & Uehleke, B. (2012 May). Clay jojoba oil facial mask for lesioned skin and mild acne--results of a prospective, observational pilot study. Forsch Komplementmed, 19(2), 75-79.

Meiller, T. F., Silva, A., Ferreira, S. M., Jabra-Rizk, M. A., Kelley, J. I., & DePaola, L. G. (2005 Apr). Efficacy of Listerine Antiseptic in reducing viral contamination of saliva. J Clin Periodontol, 32(4), 341-346.

Meister R, Wittig T, Beuscher N, de Mey C (1999 Apr). "Efficacy and tolerability of myrtol standardized in long-term treatment of chronic bronchitis. A double-blind, placebo-controlled study. Study Group Investigators," Arzneimittelforschung. 49(4):351-358.

Meldrum B.S. (1994) The role of glutamate in epilepsy and other CNS disorders. Neurology. 44: S14-S23.

Meldrum B.S., Akbar M.T., Chapman A.G. (1999) Glutamate receptors and transporters in genetic and acquired models of epilepsy. Epilepsy Research. 36: 189-204.

Melo, F. H., Venancio, E. T., de Sousa, D. P., de Franca Fonteles, M. M., de Vasconcelos, S. M., Viana, G. S., & de Sousa, F. C. (2010 Aug). Anxiolytic-like effect of Carvacrol (5-isopropyl-2-methylphenol) in mice: involvement with GABAergic transmission. Fundam Clin Pharmacol, 24(4), 437-443.

Melov S., Ravenscroft J., Malik S., Gill M.S., Walker D.W., Clayton P.E., Wallace D.C., Malfroy B., Doctrow S.R., Lithgow G.J. (2000) Extension of Life-Span with Superoxide Dismutase/Catalase Mimetics. Science. 289: 1567-1569.

Mercier B., Prost J., Prost M. (2009) The Essential Oil of Turpentine and Its Major Volatile Fraction (α- and β-Pinenes): A Review. International Journal of Occupational Medicine and Environmental Health. 22: 331-342.

Metwalli K.H., Khan S.A., Krom B.P., Jabra-Rizk M.A. (2013 Oct). "Streptococcus mutans, Candida albicans, and the Human Mouth: A Sticky Situation," PLoS Pathog. 9(10).

Michie C.A., Cooper E (1991). "Frankincense and myrrh as remedies in children," J. R. Soc. Med. 84(10):602-605.

Miguel, M. G. (2010 Dec). Antioxidant and anti-inflammatory activities of essential oils: a short review. Molecules, 15(12), 9252-9287.

Mikhaeil B.R., Maatooq G.T., Badria F.A., Amer M.M.A. (2003 Apr). "Chemistry and immunomodulatory activity of frankincense oil," Z. Naturforsch., C, J. Biosci. 58(3-4):230-238.

Miller J.A. et al (2013 Jun). "Human breast tissue disposition and bioactivity of limonene in women with earlystage breast cancer," Cancer Prev. Res. 6(6):557-84.

Miller J.A. et al (2015 Jan). "Plasma metabolomic profiles of breast cancer patients after short-term limonene intervention," Cancer Prev. Res. 8(1):86-93.

Miller J.A., Hakin I.A., Chew W, Thompson P, Thomson C.A., Chow HS (2010). "Adipose tissue accumulation of d-limonene with the consumption of a lemonade preparation rich in d-limonene content," Nutr. Cancer. 62(6):783-788.

Mills JJ, Chari RS, Boyer IJ, Gould MN, Jirtle RL (1995 Mar 1). "Induction of apoptosis in liver tumors by the monoterpene perillyl alcohol," Cancer Res. 55(5):979-83.

Mimica-Dukić N, Bozin B, Soković M, Mihajlović B, Matavulj M (2003 May). "Antimicrobial and antioxidant activities of three Mentha species essential oils," Planta Med. 69(5):413-9.

Minaiyan, M., Ghannadi, A. R., Afsharipour, M., & Mahzouni, P. (2011 Jan). Effects of extract and essential oil of Rosmarinus officinalis L. on TNBS-induced colitis in rats. Res Pharm Sci, 6(1), 13-21.

Miocinovic R et al. (2005 Jan). "In vivo and in vitro effect of baicalin on human prostate cancer cells," Int J Oncol. 26(1):241-6.

Mishra, A., Bhatti, R., Singh, A., & Singh Ishar, M. P. (2010 Mar). Ameliorative effect of the cinnamon oil from Cinnamomum zeylanicum upon early stage diabetic nephropathy. Planta Med, 76(5), 412-417.

Mishra S, Palanivelu K (2008) "The effect of curcumin (turmeric) on Alzheimer's disease: An overview," Ann. Indian Acad. Neurol. 11(1):13-19.

Misharina TA, Bulakova EB, Fatkullina LD, Terinina MB, Krikunova NI, Vorob'eva AK, Erokhin VN, Goloshchapov AN (2011 Nov–Dec). "Changes in fatty acid composition in the brain and liver in aging mice of high cancer risk AKR strain and effect of savory essential oil administration on leukemic process," biomed Khim. 57(6):604-14.

Appendix

Mix, J. A., & Crews, W. D., Jr. (2000 Jun). An examination of the efficacy of Ginkgo biloba extract EGb761 on the neuropsychologic functioning of cognitively intact older adults. J Altern Complement Med, 6(3), 219-229.

Miyazawa M, Shindo M, Shimada T (2002 May). "Metabolism of (+)- and (-)-limonenes to respective carveols and perillyl alcohols by CYP2C9 and CYP2C19 in human liver microsomes," Drug Metab. Dispos. Biol. Fate Chem. 30(5):602-607.

Mkolo MN, Magano SR (2007 Sep). "Repellent effects of the essential oil of Lavendula angustifolia against adults of Hyalomma marginatum rufipes," J S Afr Vet Assoc. 78(3):149-52.

Mogosan, C., Vostinaru, O., Operean, R., Heghes, C., Filip, L., Balica, G., & Moldovan R.I. (2017 Feb. 10). "A Comparative Analysis of the Chemical Composition, Anti-Inflammatory, and Antinociceptive Effects of the Essential Oils from Three Species of Mentha Cultivated in Romania," Molecules. 22(2).

Mohamed A.G., Abbas H.M., Kassem J.M., Gafour W.A., Attalah A.G. (2016 Feb). "Impact of Myrrh Essential Oil as a Highly Effective Antimicrobial Agent in Processed Cheese Spreads," Int. J. Dairy Sci. 11(2):41-51.

Mohamed S.A., Khan J.A. (2013 Feb). "Antioxidant capacity of chewing stick miswak Salvadora persica," BMC Complement. Altern. Med. 13:40.

Mohsenzadeh M (2007 Oct 15). "Evaluation of antibacterial activity of selected Iranian essential oils against Staphylococcus aureus and Escherichia coli in nutrient broth medium," Pak J Biol Sci. 10(20):3693-7.

Mondello F, De Bernardis F, Girolamo A, Cassone A, Salvatore G (2006 Nov 3). "In vivo activity of terpinen-4-ol, the main bioactive component of Melaleuca alternifolia Cheel (tea tree) oil against azole-susceptible and -resistant human pathogenic Candida species," BMC Infect Dis. 6:158.

Monfalouti HE, Guillaume D, Denhez C, Charrouf Z (2010 Dec). "Therapeutic potential of argan oil: a review," J Pharm Pharmacol. 62(12):1669-75.

Monsefi, M., Zahmati, M., Masoudi, M., & Javidnia, K. (2011 Dec). Effects of Anethum graveolens L. on fertility in male rats. Eur J Contracept Reprod Health Care, 16(6), 488-497.

Moon HJ, Park KS, Ku MJ, Lee MS, Jeong SH, Imbs TI, Zvyagintseva TN, Ermakova SP, Lee YH (2009 Oct). "Effect of Costaria costata fucoidan on expression of matrix metalloproteinase-1 promoter, mRNA, and protein," J Nat Prod. 72(10):1731-4.

Moon SE, Kim HY, Cha JD (2011 Sep). "Synergistic effect between clove oil and its major compounds and antibiotics against oral bacteria," Arch. Oral Biol. 56(9):907-916.

Moon T, Wilkinson JM, Cavanagh HM (2006 Nov). "Antiparasitic activity of two Lavandula essential oils against Giardia duodenalis, Trichomonas vaginalis and Hexamita inflata," Parasitol Res. 99(6):722-8.

Moore LE, Brennan P, Karami S, Hung RJ, Hsu C, Boffetta P, Toro J, Zaridze D, Janout V, Bencko V, Navratilova M, Szeszenia-Dabrowska N, Mates D, Mukeria A, Holcatova I, Welch R, Chanock S, Rothman N, Chow WH (2007 Sep). "Glutathione S-transferase polymorphisms, cruciferous vegetable intake and cancer risk in the Central and Eastern European Kidney Cancer Study," Carcinogenesis. 28(9):1960-4.

Moraes T.M. et al (2009 Aug). "Effects of limonene and essential oil from Citrus aurantium on gastric mucosa: role of prostaglandins and gastric mucus secretion," Chem. Biol. Interact. 180(3):499-505.

Moreno S, Scheyer T, Romano CS, Vojnov AA (2006 Feb). "Antioxidant and antimicrobial activities of rosemary extracts linked to their polyphenol composition," Free Radic Res. 40(2):223-31.

Moretti MD, Sanna-Passino G, Demontis S, Bazzoni E (2002). "Essential oil formulations useful as a new tool for insect pest control," AAPS PharmSciTech. 3(2):E13.

Mori TA, Bao DQ, Burke V, Puddey IB, Beilin LJ (1999 Aug). "Docosahexaenoic acid but not eicosapentaenoic acid lowers ambulatory blood pressure and heart rate in humans," Hypertension. 34(2):253-60.

Morris N (2002 Dec). "The effects of lavender (Lavendula angustifolium) baths on psychological well-being: two exploratory randomised control trials," Complement. Ther. Med. 10(4):223-228.

Morinobu A et al. (2008 Jul). "-Epigallocatechin-3-gallate suppresses osteoclast differentiation and ameliorates experimental arthritis in mice," Arthritis Rheum. 58(7):2012-8.

Morowitz, M. J., Carlisle, E. M., & Alverdy, J. C. (2011). Contributions of intestinal bacteria to nutrition and metabolism in the critically ill. Surg Clin North Am, 91(4), 771-785, viii.

Morris MC, Sacks F, Rosner B (1993 Aug). "Does fish oil lower blood pressure? A meta-analysis of controlled trials," Circulation. 88(2):523-33.

Morris N (2002 Dec). "The effects of lavender (Lavendula angustifolium) baths on psychological well-being: two exploratory randomised control trials," Complement. Ther. Med. 10(4):223-228.

Morse M.A., Stoner G.D. (1993) Cancer chemoprevention: principles and prospects. Carcinogenesis. 14: 1737-1746.

Mosaffa F, Behravan J, Karimi G, Iranshahi M (2006 Feb). "Antigenotoxic effects of Satureja hortensis L. on rat lymphocytes exposed to oxidative stress," Arch Pharm Res. 29(2):159-64.

Moss M, Cook J, Wesnes K, Duckett P (2003 Jan). "Aromas of rosemary and lavender essential oils differentially affect cognition and mood in healthy adults," Int J Neurosci. 113(1):15-38.

Moss M, Hewitt S, Moss L, Wesnes K (2008 Jan). "Modulation of cognitive performance and mood by aromas of peppermint and ylang-ylang," Int J Neurosci. 118(1):59-77.

Moss M, Oliver L (2012). "Plasma 1, 8-cineole correlates with cognitive performance following exposure to rosemary essential oil aroma," Ther. Adv. Psychopharmacol. 2(3):103-113.

Motomura N, Sakurai A, Yotsuya Y (2001 Dec). "Reduction of mental stress with lavender odorant," Percept Mot Skills. 93(3):713-8.

Moussaieff A. et al (2008 Aug). "Incensole acetate, an incense component, elicits psychoactivity by activating TRPV3 channels in the brain," FASEB J. 22(8):3024-3034.

Moussaieff A, Rimmerman N, Bregman T, Straiker A, Felder CC, Shoham S, Kashman Y, Huang SM, Lee H, Shohami E, Mackie K, Caterina MJ, Walker JM, Fride E, Mechoulam R (2008 Aug). "Incensole acetate, an incense component, elicits psychoactivity by activating TRPV3 channels in the brain," FASEB J. 22(8):3024-34.

Moussaieff A, Shein NA, Tsenter J, Grigoriadis S, Simeonidou C, Alexandrovich AG, Trembovler V, Ben-Neriah Y, Schmitz ML, Fiebich BL, Munoz E, Mechoulam R, Shohami E (2008 Jul). "Incensole acetate: a novel neuroprotective agent isolated from Boswellia carterii," J Cereb Blood Flow Metab. 28(7):1341-52.

Moustafa, A. H., Ali, E. M., Moselhy, S. S., Tousson, E., & El-Said, K. S. (2012 Oct). Effect of coriander on thioacetamide-induced hepatotoxicity in rats. Toxicol Ind Health, 1-10.

Moy KA, Yuan JM, Chung FL, Wang XL, Van Den Berg D, Wang R, Gao YT, Yu MC (2009 Dec 1). "Isothiocyanates, glutathione S-transferase M1 and T1 polymorphisms and gastric cancer risk: a prospective study of men in Shanghai, China," Int J Cancer. 125(11):2652-9.

Mugnaini, L., Nardoni, S., Pinto, L., Pistelli, L., Leonardi, M., Pisseri, F., & Mancianti, F. (2012 Jun). In vitro and in vivo antifungal activity of some essential oils against feline isolates of Microsporum canis. J Mycol Med, 22(2), 179-184.

Muhlbauer, R. C., Lozano, A., Palacio, S., Reinli, A., & Felix, R. (2003 Apr). Common herbs, essential oils, and monoterpenes potently modulate bone metabolism. Bone, 32(4), 372-380.

Mukherjee P.K., Chandra J., Kuhn D.M., Ghannoum M.A. (2003) Mechanism of Fluconazole Resistance in Candida albicansBiofilms: Phase-Specific Role of Efflux Pumps and Membrane Sterols. Infection and Immunity. 71: 4333-4340.

Mumcuoglu KY, Magdassi S, Miller J, Ben-Ishai F, Zentner G, Helbin V, Friger M, Kahana F, Ingber A (2004 Dec). "Repellency of citronella for head lice: double-blind randomized trial of efficacy and safety," Isr Med Assoc J. 6(12):756-9.

Munzel T., Feil R., Mulsch A., Lohmann S.M., Hofmann F., Walter U. (2003) Physiology and Pathophysiology of Vascular Signaling Controlled by Cyclic Guanosine 3',5' –Cyclic Monophospate—Dependent Protein Kinase. Circulation. 108: 2172-2183.

Muzzarelli L, Force M, Sebold M (2006 Dec). "Aromatherapy and reducing preprocedural anxiety: A controlled prospective study," Gastroenterol. Nurs. Off. J. Soc. Gastroenterol. Nurses Assoc. 29(6):466-471.

Na HJ, Koo HN, Lee GG, Yoo SJ, Park JH, Lyu YS, Kim HM (2001 Dec). "Juniper oil inhibits the heat shock-induced apoptosis via preventing the caspase-3 activation in human astrocytes CCF-STTG1 cells," Clin Chim Acta. 314(1-2):215-20.

Nadeem M, Anjum FM, Kah MI, Tehseen S, El-Ghorab A, sultan JI (2013 May). "Nutritional and medicinal aspects of coriander (Coriandrum sativum L.)," British Food Journal. 115(5):743-55.

Nadim M.M., Malink A.A., Ahmad J, Bakshi S.K. (2011). "The essential oil composition of Achillea millefolium L. cultivated under tropical condition in India," World J Agric Sci. 7(5):561-565.

Nagashyana N, Sankarankutt P, Nampoothiri MRV, Moahan P, Mohan Kumar P (2000). "Association of L-dopa with recovery following Ayurvedic medication in Parkinson's disease," J Neurol Sci. 176:1121-7.

Naguib YM (2000 Apr). "Antioxidant activities of astaxanthin and related carotenoids," J Agric Food Chem. 48(4):1150-4.

Nair B (2001). "Final report on the safety assessment of Mentha Piperita (Peppermint) Oil, Mentha Piperita (Peppermint) Leaf Extract, Mentha Piperita (Peppermint) Leaf, and Mentha Piperita (Peppermint) Leaf Water," Int J Toxicol. 20(Suppl 3):61-73..

Nair MK, Joy J, Vasudevan P, Hinckley L, Hoagland TA, Venkitanarayanan KS (2009 Mar 30). "Antibacterial effect of caprylic acid and monocaprylin on major bacterial mastitis pathogens," Vet Microbiol. 135(3-4):358-62.

Nair, V., Singh, S., & Gupta, Y. K. (2012 Mar). Evaluation of disease modifying activity of Coriandrum sativum in experimental models. Indian J Med Res, 135, 240-245.

Nakayama, S., Kishimoto, Y., Saita, E., Sugihara, N., Toyozaki, M., Taguchi, C., . . . Kondo, K. (2015 Jan). Pine bark extract prevents low-density lipoprotein oxidation and regulates monocytic expression of antioxidant enzymes. Nutr Res, 35(1), 56-64.

Nanthakomon T, Pongrojpaw D (2006 Oct). "The efficacy of ginger in prevention of postoperative nausea and vomiting after major gynecologic surgery," J Med Assoc Thai. 89(4):S130-6.

Nardoni, S., Mugnaini, L., Pistelli, L., Leonardi, M., Sanna, V., Perrucci, S., . . . Mancianti, F. (2014 Apr). Clinical and mycological evaluation of an herbal antifungal formulation in canine Malassezia dermatitis. J Mycol Med.

Nascimento CM, Pereira JR, de Andrade LP, Garuffi M, Talib LL, Forlenza OV, Cancela JM, Cominetti MR, Stella F, (2014). "Physical exercise in MCI elderly promotes reduction of pro-inflammatory cytokines and improvements on cognition and BDNF peripheral levels," Curr Alzheimer Res, 11(8):799-805.

Narishetty S.T.K., Panchagnula R. (2004) Transdermal delivey of zidovudine: effect of terpenes and their mechanism of action. Journal of Controlled Release. 95: 367-379.

Narishetty S.T.K., Panchagnula R. (2005) Effects of L-menthol and 1,8-cineole on phase behavior and molecular organization of SC lipids and skin permeation of zidovudine. Journal of Controlled Release. 102: 59-70.

Nasel C, Nasel B, Samec P, Schindler E, Buchbauer G (1994 Aug). "Functional imaging of effects of fragrances on the human brain after prolonged inhalation," Chem Senses. 19(4):359-64.

Naseri, M., Mojab, F., Khodadoost, M., Kamalinejad, M., Davati, A., Choopani, R., . . . Emtiazy, M. (2012 Nov). The Study of Anti-Inflammatory Activity of Oil-Based Dill (Anethum graveolens L.) Extract Used Topically in Formalin-Induced Inflammation Male Rat Paw. Iran J Pharm Res, 11(4), 1169-1174.

Nasiri, A., Mahmodi, M.A., & Nobakht, Z. (2016 Nov.). "Effect of aromatherapy massage with lavender essential oil on pain in patients with osteoarthritis of the knee: A randomized controlled clinical trial," Complement Ther Clin Pract. 25:75-80.

Navarra M., Mannucci C., Delbò M, Calapai G (2015 Mar). "Citrus bergamia essential oil: from basic research to clinical application," Front Pharmacol. 6.

Navarra, M., Ursino, M. R., Ferlazzo, N., Russo, M., Schumacher, U., & Valentiner, U. (2014 Jun). Effect of Citrus bergamia juice on human neuroblastoma cells in vitro and in metastatic xenograft models. Fitoterapia, 95, 83-92.

Navarro SL, Chang JL, Peterson S, Chen C, King IB, Schwarz Y, Li SS, Li L, Potter JD, Lampe JW (2009 Nov). "Modulation of human serum glutathione S-transferase A1/2 concentration by cruciferous vegetables in a controlled feeding study is influenced by GSTM1 and GSTT1 genotypes," Cancer Epidemiol Biomarkers Prev. 18(11):2974-8.

Navarro SL, Peterson S, Chen C, Makar KW, Schwarz Y, King IB, Li SS, Li L, Kestin M, Lampe JW. (2009 Apr). "Cruciferous vegetable feeding alters UGT1A1 activity: diet- and genotype-dependent changes in serum bilirubin in a controlled feeding trial," Cancer Prev Res (Phila Pa). 2(4):345-52.

Nayak P.A., Nayak U.A., Khandelwal (2014 Nov). "The effect of xylitol on dental caries and oral flora," Clin. Cosmet. Investig. Dent. 6:89-94.

Nevin K.G., Rajamohan T (2010). "Effect of topical application of virgin coconut oil on skin components and antioxidant status during dermal wound healing in young rats," Skin Pharmacol Physiol. 23(6):290-297.

Ngan A, Conduit R (2011 Aug). "A double-blind, placebo-controlled investigation of the effects of Passiflora incarnata (passionflower) herbal tea on subjective sleep quality," Phytother Res. 25(8):1153-9.

Ni X et al (2012). "Frankincense essential oil prepared from hydrodistillation of Boswellia sacra gum resins induces human pancreatic cancer cell death in cultures and in a xenograft murine model," BMC complementary and alternative medicine. 12(1):253.

Nielsen FH, Hunt CD, Mullen LM, Hunt JR (1987 Nov). "Effect of dietary boron on mineral, estrogen, and testosterone metabolism in postmenopausal women," FASEB J. 1(5):394-7.

Nikolaevski VV, Kononova NS, Pertsovski AI, Shinkarchuk IF (1990 Sep-Oct). "Effect of essential oils on the course of experimental atherosclerosis," Patol Fiziol Eksp Ter. (5):52-3.

Ninomiya K, Matsuda H, Shimoda H, Nishida N, Kasajima N, Yoshino T, Morikawa T, Yoshikawa M (2004 Apr 19). "Carnosic acid, a new class of lipid absorption inhibitor from sage," Bioorg Med Chem Lett. 14(8):1943-6.

Ni Raghallaigh S, Bender K, Lacey N, Brennan L, Powell FC (2012 Feb). "The fatty acid profile of the skin surface lipid layer in papulopustular rosacea," Br J Dermatol. 166(2):279-87.

Nishio M, Kawmata H, Fujita K, Ishizaki T, Hayman R, Idemi T (2004). "A new enamel restoring agent for use after PMTC," Journal of Dental Research 83(1920):SpclIssueA.

Nomicos E.Y.H. (2007 Dec). "Myrrh: medical marvel or myth of the Magi?," Holist. Nurs. Pract. 21(6):308-323.

Noori, S., Hassan, Z. M., & Salehian, O. (2013 Mar). Sclareol reduces CD4+ CD25+ FoxP3+ Treg cells in a breast cancer model in vivo. Iran J Immunol, 10(1), 10-21.

Norazmir M. N., Jr., & Ayub, M. Y. (2010 Apr). Beneficial lipid-lowering effects of pink guava puree in high fat diet induced-obese rats. Malays J Nutr, 16(1), 171-185.

Noreikaitė, A., Ayupova, R., Satbayeva, E., Seitaliyeva, A., Amirkulova, M., Pichkhadze, G., Datkhayev, U., and Stankevičius, E. (2017). "General Toxicity and Antifungal Activity of a New Dental Gel with Essential Oil from Abies Sibirica L.," Med Sci Monit. 23:521-527.

Nord D, Belew J (2009 Oct). "Effectiveness of the essential oils lavender and ginger in promoting children's comfort in a perianesthesia setting," J. Perianesthesia Nurs. Off. J. Am. Soc. PeriAnesthesia Nurses Am. Soc. PeriAnesthesia Nurses. 24(5):307-312.

Nostro A, Bisignano G, Angela Cannatelli M, Crisafi G, Paola Germanò M, Alonzo V (2001 Jun). "Effects of Helichrysum italicum extract on growth and enzymatic activity of Staphylococcus aureus," Int J Antimicrob Agents. 17(6):517-20.

Nostro A, Blanco AR, Cannatelli MA, Enea V, Flamini G, Morelli I, Sudano Roccaro A, Alonzo V (2004 Jan 30). "Susceptibility of methicillin-resistant staphylococci to oregano essential oil, carvacrol and thymol," FEMS Microbiol Lett. 230(2):191-5.

Nostro A, Cannatelli MA, Marino A, Picerno I, Pizzimenti FC, Scoglio ME, Spataro P (2003 Jan). "Evaluation of antiherpesvirus-1 and genotoxic activities of Helichrysum italicum extract," New Microbiol. 26(1):125-8.

Nothlings U, Murphy SP, Wilkens LR, Henderson BE, Kolonel LN (2007 Oct). "Flavonols and pancreatic cancer risk: the multiethnic cohort study," Am J Epidemiol. 166(8):924-31.

Nuñez L, Aquino M.D. (2012). "Microbicide activity of clove essential oil (Eugenia caryophyllata)," Braz. J. Microbiol. 43(4):1255-1260.

Nyadjeu P., Nguelefack-Mbuyo, E. P., Atsamo, A. D., Nguelefack, T. B., Dongmo, A. B., & Kamanyi, A. (2013 Feb). Acute and chronic antihypertensive effects of Cinnamomum zeylanicum stem bark methanol extract in L-NAME-induced hypertensive rats. BMC Complement Altern Med, 13, 1-10.

Oboh, G., Olasehinde, T. A., & Ademosun, A. O. (2014 Mar). Essential oil from lemon peels inhibit key enzymes linked to neurodegenerative conditions and pro-oxidant induced lipid peroxidation. J Oleo Sci, 63(4), 373-381.

O'Bryan C.A., Crandall P.G., Chalova V.I., Ricke S.C. (2008 Aug). "Orange Essential Oils Antimicrobial Activities against Salmonella spp.," J. Food Sci. 73(6):M264-M267.

Ogeturk, M., Kose, E., Sarsilmaz, M., Akpinar, B., Kus, I., & Meydan, S. (2010 Oct). Effects of lemon essential oil aroma on the learning behaviors of rats. Neurosciences (Riyadh), 15(4), 292-293.

Oh M.J. (2017 Sep). "Novel phytoceramides containing fatty acids of diverse chain lengths are better than a single C18-ceramide N-stearoyl phytosphingosine to improve the physiological properties of human stratum corneum," Clin Cosmet Investig Dermatol. 10:363-371.

Oh S. et al (2014 Jul). "Suppression of Inflammatory cytokine production by ar-Turmerone isolated from Curcuma phaeocaulis," Chem. Biodivers. 11(7):1034-1041.

Ohkawara S, Tanaka-Kagawa T, Furukawa Y, Nishimura T, Jinno H (2010). "Activation of the Human Transient Receptor Potential Vanilloid Subtype 1 by Essential Oils," Biological and Pharmaceutical Bulletin. 33(8):1434-1437.

Ohno T, Kita M, Yamaoka Y, Imamura S, Yamamoto T, Mitsufuji S, Kodama T, Kashima K, Imanishi J (2003 Jun). "Antimicrobial activity of essential oils against Helicobacter pylori," Helicobacter. 8(3):207-15.

Ohta T, Imagawa T, Ito S (2009 Feb). "Involvement of Transient Receptor Potential Vanilloid Subtype 1 in Analgesic Action of Methylsalicylate," Mol. Pharmacol. 75(2):307-317.

Okugawa, H., Ueda, R., Matsumoto, K., Kawanishi, K., & Kato, K. (2000 Oct). Effects of sesquiterpenoids from Oriental incenses on acetic acid-induced writhing and D2 and 5-HT2A receptors in rat brain. Phytomedicine, 7(5), 417-422.

Olajide OA, Ajayi FF, Ekhelar AI, Awe SO, Makinde JM, Alada AR (1999 Jun). "Biological effects of Myristica fragrans (nutmeg) extract," Phytother Res. 13(4):344-5.

Olapour, A., Behaeen, K., Akhondzadeh, R., Soltani, F., Al Sadat Razavi, F., & Bekhradi, R. (2013 Nov). The Effect of Inhalation of Aromatherapy Blend containing Lavender Essential Oil on Cesarean Postoperative Pain. Anesth Pain Med, 3(1), 203-207.

Onawunmi GO, Yisak WA, Ogunlana EO (1984 Dec). "Antibacterial constituents in the essential oil of Cymbopogon citratus (DC.) Stapf.," J Ethnopharmacol. 12(3):279-86.

Onocha, P., Oloyede, G., & Afolabi, Q. (2011). Chemical composition, cytotoxicity and antioxidant activity of essential oils of Acalypha hispida flowers. Inter J Pharm, 7(1), 144-148.

Opalchenova G, Obreshkova D (2003 Jul). "Comparative studies on the activity of basil—an essential oil from Ocimum basilicum L.—against multidrug resistant clinical isolates of the genera Staphylococcus, Enterococcus and Pseudomonas by using different test methods," J Microbiol Methods. 54(1):105-10.

Orafidiya LO, Agbani EO, Abereoje OA, Awe T, Abudu A, Fakoya FA (2003 Oct). "An investigation into the wound-healing properties of essential oil of Ocimum gratissimum linn," J Wound Care. 12(9):331-4.

Orav A, Arak E, Raal A (2006 Oct). "Phytochemical analysis of the essential oil of Achillea millefolium L. from various European Countries," Nat. Prod. Res. 20(12):1082-1088.

Orellana-Paucar A.M. et al (2013 Dec). "Insights from Zebrafish and Mouse Models on the Activity and Safety of Ar-Turmerone as a Potential Drug Candidate for the Treatment of Epilepsy," PLoS ONE. 8(12):e81634.

Ornano L. et al (2013 Aug). "Chemopreventive and Antioxidant Activity of the Chamazulene-Rich Essential Oil Obtained from Artemisia arborescens L. Growing on the Isle of La Maddalena, Sardinia, Italy," Chem. Biodivers. 10(8):1464-1474.

Osawa K, Saeki T, Yasuda H, Hamashima H, Sasatsu M, Araj T (1999). "The Antibacterial Activities of Peppermint Oil and Green Tea Polyphenols, Alone and in Combination, against Enterohemorrhagic <I>Escherichia coil</I>," Biocontrol Sci. 4(1):1-7.

Osher Y, Bersudsky Y, Belmaker RH (2005 Jun). "Omega-3 eicosapentaenoic acid in bipolar depression: report of a small open-label study," J Clin Psychiatry. 66(6):726-9.

Ostad SN, Soodi M, Shariffzadeh M, Khorshidi N, Marzban H (2001 Aug). "The effect of fennel essential oil on uterine contraction as a model for dysmenorrhea, pharmacology and toxicology study," J Ethnopharmacol. 76(3):299-304.

Ou M. C., Hsu, T. F., Lai, A. C., Lin, Y. T., & Lin, C. C. (2012 May). Pain relief assessment by aromatic essential oil massage on outpatients with primary dysmenorrhea: a randomized, double-blind clinical trial. J Obstet Gynaecol Res, 38(5), 817-822.

Ou-Yang, D.W., Wu, L., Li, Y.L., Yang, P.M., Kong, D.Y., Yang, X.W., and Zhang, W.D. (2011). "Miscellaneous terpenoid constituents of Abies nephrolepis and their moderate cytotoxic activities," Phytochemistry. 72(17):2197-204.

Palmefors H, DuttaRoy S, Rundqvist B, Borjesson M (2014 Jul). "The effect of physical activity or exercise on key biomarkers in atherosclerosis—a systematic review," Atherosclerosis, 235(1):150-61.

Paliwal S, J Sundaram and S Mitragotri (2005). "Induction of cancer-specific cytotoxicity towards human prostate and skin cells using quercetin and ultrasound," British Journal of Cancer. 92:499-502.

Palozza P, Krinsky NI (1992 Sep). "Astaxanthin and canthaxanthin are potent antioxidants in a membrane model," Arch Biochem Biophys. 297(2):291-5.

Pandey, A., Bigoniya, P., Raj, V., & Patel, K. K. (2011 Jul). Pharmacological screening of Coriandrum sativum Linn. for hepatoprotective activity. J Pharm Bioallied Sci, 3(3), 435-441.

Appendix

Paoletti P., Neyton J. (2007) NMDA receptor subunits: functions and pharmacology. Current Opinion in Pharmacology. 7: 39-47.

Pardridge, W. M. (2003 Mar). Blood-brain barrier drug targeting: the future of brain drug development. Mol Interv, 3(2).

Pardridge, W. M. (2009 Sep). Alzheimer's disease drug development and the problem of the blood-brain barrier. Alzheimers Dement, 5(5), 427-432.

Parimoo, H. A., Sharma, R., Patil, R. D., Sharma, O. P., Kumar, P., & Kumar, N. (2014 Apr). Hepatoprotective effect of Ginkgo biloba leaf extract on lantadenes-induced hepatotoxicity in guinea pigs. Toxicon, 81, 1-12.

Park, G., Kim, H. G., Kim, Y. O., Park, S. H., Kim, S. Y., & Oh, M. S. (2012 Feb). Coriandrum sativum L. protects human keratinocytes from oxidative stress by regulating oxidative defense systems. Skin Pharmacol Physiol, 25(2), 93-99.

Park, H. J., Kim, S. K., Kang, W. S., Woo, J. M., & Kim, J. W. (2014 Feb). Effects of essential oil from Chamaecyparis obtusa on cytokine genes in the hippocampus of maternal separation rats. Can J Physiol Pharmacol, 92(2), 95-101.

Park H.M., Lee J.H., Yaoyao J, Jun H.J., Lee S.J. (2011 Jan). "Limonene, a natural cyclic terpene, is an agonistic ligand for adenosine A(2A) receptors," Biochem. Biophys. Res. Commun. 404(1):345-348.

Park S.Y., Kim HS, Cho EK, Kwon BY, Phark S, Hwang KW, Sul D (2008 Aug). "Curcumin protected PC12 cells against beta-amyloid-induced toxicity through the inhibition of oxidative damage and tau hyperphosphorylation," Food Chem Toxicol. 46(8):2881-7.

Park S.Y., Kim Y.H., Kim Y, Lee SJ (2012 Dec). "Aromatic-turmerone attenuates invasion and expression of MMP-9 and COX-2 through inhibition of NF-κB activation in TPA-induced breast cancer cells," J. Cell. Biochem. 113(12):3653-3662.

Park S.Y., Jin M.L., Kim Y.H., Kim Y, Lee S.J. (2012 Sep). "Anti-inflammatory effects of aromatic-turmerone through blocking of NF-κB, JNK, and p38 MAPK signaling pathways in amyloid β-stimulated microglia," Int. Immunopharmacol. 14(1):13-20.

Patel, B. P., Bellissimo, N., Luhovyy, B., Bennett, L. J., Hurton, E., Painter, J. E., & Anderson, G. H. (2013 Jun 29). An after-school snack of raisins lowers cumulative food intake in young children. J Food Sci, 78 Suppl 1, A5-A10.

Patrick L (2011 Jun). "Gastroesophageal reflux disease (GERD): a review of conventional and alternative treatments," Altern. Med. Rev. J. Clin. Ther. 16(2):116-133.

Pattnaik S, Subramanyam V.R., Bapaji M, Kole C.R. (1997). "Antibacterial and antifungal activity of aromatic constituents of essential oils," Microbios. 89(358):39-46.

Pattnaik S, Subramanyam V.R., Kole C.R., Sahoo S (1995). "Antibacterial activity of essential oils from Cymbopogon: inter- and intra-specific differences," Microbios. 84(341):239-245.

Pause, B. M., Raack, N., Sojka, B., Goder, R., Aldenhoff, J. B., & Ferstl, R. (2003 Mar). Convergent and divergent effects of odors and emotions in depression. Psychophysiology, 40(2), 209-225.

Pavela R (2005 Dec). "Insecticidal activity of some essential oils against larvae of Spodoptera littoralis," Fitoterapia. 76(7-8):691-6.

Pavela R (2008 Feb). "Insecticidal properties of several essential oils on the house fly (Musca domestica L.)," Phytother Res. 22(2):274-8.

Peana AT, D'Aquila PS, Panin F, Serra G, Pippia P, Moretti MD (2002 Dec). "Anti-inflammatory activity of linalool and linalyl acetate constituents of essential oils," Phytomedicine. 9(8):721-6.

Peana A.T., D'Aquila P.S., Chessa M. L., Moretti M.D.L., Serra G., Pippia P. (2003) (-)-Linalool produces antinociception in two experimental models of pain. European Journal of Pharmacology. 460: 37-41.

Peana A.T., Marzocco S, Popola A, Pinto A (2006 Jan). "(-)-Linalool inhibits in vitro NO formation: Probable involvement in the antinociceptive activity of this monoterpene compound," Life Sci. 78(7):719-723.

Pearce AL, Finlay-Jones JJ, Hart PH (2005 Jan). "Reduction of nickel-induced contact hypersensitivity reactions by topical tea tree oil in humans," Inflamm Res. 54(1):22-30.

Pemberton E, Turpin PG (2008 Mar-Apr). "The effect of essential oils on work-related stress in intensive care unit nurses," Holist Nurs Pract. 22(2):97-102.

Penalvo JL, Lopez-Romero P (2012 Feb 29). "Urinary enterolignan concentrations are positively associated with serum HDL cholesterol and negatively associated with serum triglycerides in U.S. adults," J Nutr. [Epub ahead of print].

Peng SM, Koo M, Yu ZR (2009 Jan). "Effects of music and essential oil inhalation on cardiac autonomic balance in healthy individuals," J Altern Complement Med. 15(1):53-7.

Pengelly, A. (2004). The Constituents of Medicinal Plants (2nd ed.). Singapore: Allen and Unwin.

Perry N, Perry E (2006). "Aromatherapy in the management of psychiatric disorders: clinical and neuropharmacological perspectives," CNS Drugs. 20(4):257-80.

Peters G.J., Backus H.H.J., Freemantle S., van Triest B., Codacci-Pisanelli G., van der Wilt C.L., Smid K., Lunec J., Calvert A.H., Marsh S., McLeod H.L., Bloemena E., Meijer S., Jansen G., van Groeningen C.J., Pinedo H.M. (2002) Induction of thymidylate synthase as a 5-fluorouracil resistance mechanism. Biochimica et Biophysica Acta. 1587: 194-205.

Pevsner J, Hsu SC, Braun JE, Calakos N, Ting AE, Bennett MK, Scheller RH (1994 Aug). "Specificity and regulation of a synaptic vesicle docking complex," Neuron. 13(2):353-61.

Philippe M, Garson JC, Gilard P, Hocquaux M, Hussler G, Leroy F, Mahieu C, Semeria D, Vanlerberghe G (1994 Aug). "Synthesis of 2-N-oleoylamino-octadecane-1,3-diol: a new ceramide highly effective for the treatment of skin and hair," Int J Cosmet Sci. 17(4):133-46.

Phillips L.R., Malspeis L, Supko J.G. (1995 Jul.) "Pharmacokinetics of active drug metabolites after oral administration of perillyl alcohol, an investigational antineoplastic agent, to the dog," Drug Metab. Dispos. Biol. Fate Chem. 23(7):676-680.

Piazza GA, Ritter JL, Baracka CA (1995 Jan). "Lysophosphatidic acid induction of transforming growth factors alpha and beta: modulation of proliferation and differentiation in cultured human keratinocytes and mouse skin," Exp Cell Res. 216(1):51-64.

Piccinelli A.C. et al "Antihyperalgesic and antidepressive actions of (R)-(+)-limonene, αphellandrene, and essential oil from Schinus terebinthifolius fruits in a neuropathic pain model," Nutr. Neurosci. 18(5):217-224.

Pichette A, Larouche PL, Lebrun M, Legault J (2006 May). "Composition and antibacterial activity of Abies balsamea essential oil," Phytother Res. 20(5):371-3.

Pietruck F, Busch S, Virchow S, Brockmeyer N, Siffert W (1997 Jan). "Signalling properties of lysophosphatidic acid in primary human skin fibroblasts: role of pertussis toxin-sensitive GTP-binding proteins," Naunyn Schmiedebergs Arch Pharmacol. 355(1):1-7.

Pinker, S. (2010 May). Colloquium paper: the cognitive niche: coevolution of intelligence, sociality, and language. Proc Natl Acad Sci USA, 107 Suppl 2, 8993-8999.

Pina-Vaz C, Gonçalves Rodrigues A, Pinto E, Costa-de-Oliveira S, Tavares C, Salgueiro L, Cavaleiro C, Gonçalves MJ, Martinez-de-Oliveira J (2004 Jan). "Antifungal activity of Thymus oils and their major compounds," J Eur Acad Dermatol Venereol. 18(1):73-8.

Ping H, Zhang G, Ren G (2010 Aug-Sep). "Antidiabetic effects of cinnamon oil in diabetic KK-Ay mice," Food Chem Toxicol. 48(8-9):2344-9.

Pinto E, Vale-Silva L, Cavaleiro C, Salgueiro L (2009 Nov). "Antifungal activity of the clove essential oil from Syzygium aromaticum on Candida, Aspergillus and dermatophyte species," J. Med. Microbiol. 58(11):1454-62.

Pistone G, Marino A, Leotta C, Dell'Arte S, Finocchiaro G, Malaguarnera M (2003). "Levocarnitine administration in elderly subjects with rapid muscle fatigue: effect on body composition, lipid profile and fatigue," Drugs Aging. 20(10):761-7.

P. M. de Mendonça Rocha et al. (2012 Oct). "Synergistic antibacterial activity of the essential oil of aguaribay (Schinus molle L.)," Mol. Basel Switz., vol. 17(10):12023-12036.

Porres-Martínez M, González-Burgos E, Carretero M.E., Gómez-Serranillos M.P. (2015 Jun). "Major selected monoterpenes α-pinene and 1,8-cineole found in Salvia lavandulifolia (Spanish sage) essential oil as regulators of cellular redox balance," Pharm Biol. 53(6):921-929.

Portincasa P et al (2016 June). "Curcumin and fennel essential oil improve symptoms and quality of life," J Gastrointestin Liver Dis. 25(2):151-7.

Pouresalmi H.R., Makarem A, Mojab F (2007). "Paraclinical Effects of Miswak Extract on Dental Plaque," Dent. Res. J. 4(2):5.

Pouvreau L, Gruppen H, Piersma SR, van den Broek LA, van Koningsvend GA, Voragen AG (2001 Jun). "Relative abundance and inhibitory distribution of protease inhibitors in potato juice from cv. Elkana," J Agric Food Chem. 49(6):2864-74.

Prabuseenivasan S, Jayakumar M, Ignacimuthu S (2006). "In vitro antibacterial activity of some plant essential oils," BMC Complement. Altern. Med. 6(1):39.

Prakash P. et al (2011 Feb). "Anti-platelet effects of Curcuma oil in experimental models of myocardial ischemia-reperfusion and thrombosis," Thromb. Res. 127(2):111-118.

Pramod K., Ansari S.H., Ali J (2010 Dec). "Eugenol: a natural compound with versatile pharmacological actions," Nat. Prod. Commun. 5(12):1999-2006.

Prasad M. et al 2016 May "The Clinical Effectiveness of Post-Brushing Rinsing in Reducing Plaque and Gingivitis: A Systematic Review," J. Clin. Diagn. 10(5):ZE01-ZE07.

Preuss HG, Echard B, Enig M, Brook I, Elliott TB (2005 Apr). "Minimum inhibitory concentrations of herbal essential oils and monolaurin for gram-positive and gram-negative bacteria," Mol Cell Biochem. 272(1-2):29-34.

Prins, C. L., Vieira, I. J., & Freitas, S. P. (2010). Growth regulators and essential oil production. Brazilian Journal of Plant Physiology, 22(2), 91-102.

Prottey C, Hartop C.J., Press M (1975 Apr). "Correction of the cutaneous manifestations of essential fatty acid deficiency in man by application of sunflower-seed oil to the skin," J. Invest. Dermatol. 64(4):228-234.

Puatanachokchai R, Kishida H, Denda A, Murata N, Konishi Y, Vinitketkumnuen U, Nakae D (2002 Sep 8). "Inhibitory effects of lemon grass (Cymbopogon citratus, Stapf) extract on the early phase of hepatocarcinogenesis after initiation with diethylnitrosamine in male Fischer 344 rats," Cancer Lett. 183(1):9-15.

Qiu Y, Du GH, Qu ZW, Zhang JT (1995). "Protective effects of ginsenoside on the learning and memory impairment induced by transient cerebral ischemia-reperfusion in mice," Chin Pharmacol Bull. 11:299-302.

Quiroga P.R., Asensio C.M., Nepote V (2015 Feb). "Antioxidant effects of the monoterpenes carvacrol, thymol and sabinene hydrate on chemical and sensory stability of roasted sunflower seeds," J. Sci. Food Agric. 95(3):471-479.

Qureshi A.A., Mangels W.R., Din A.A., Elson C.E. (1988) Inhibition of Hepatic Mevalonate Biosynthesis by the Monoterpene, d-Limonene. J. Agric. Food Chem. 36: 1220-1224.

Ragho R., Postlethwaite AE, Keski-Oja J, Moses HL, Kang AH (1987 Apr). "Transforming growth factor-beta increases steady state levels of type I procollagen and fibronectin messenger RNAs posttranscriptionally in cultured human dermal fibroblasts," J Clin Invest. 79(4):1285-8.

Rahimikian F, Rahimi R, Golzareh P, Bekhradi R, Mehran A (2017 Sep). "Effect of Foeniculum vulgare Mill. (fennel) on menopausal symptoms in postmenopausal women: a randomized, triple-blind, placebo-controlled trial," Menopause. 24(9):1017-1021.

Rahman MM, Ichiyanagi T, Komiyama T, Sato S, Konishi T (2008 Aug). "Effects of anthocyanins on psychological stress-induced oxidative stress and neurotransmitter status," J Agric Food Chem. 56(16):7545-50.

Raisi Dehkordi Z, Hosseini Baharanchi F.S., Bekhardi R (2014 Apr). "Effect of lavender inhalation on the symptoms of primary dysmenorrhea and the amount of menstrual bleeding: A randomized clinical trial," Complement. Ther. Med. 22(2):212-219.

Ra Kovi, A., Milanovi, I., Pavlovi, N. A., Ebovi, T., Vukmirovi, S. A., & Mikov, M. (2014 Jul). Antioxidant activity of rosemary (Rosmarinus officinalis L.) essential oil and its hepatoprotective potential. BMC Complement Altern Med, 14(1), 1-20.

Raman A, Weir U, Bloomfield SF (1995 Oct). "Antimicrobial effects of tea-tree oil and its major components on Staphylococcus aureus, Staph. epidermidis and Propionibacterium acnes," Lett Appl Microbiol. 21(4):242-5.

Ramezani, R., Moghimi, A., Rakhshandeh, H., Ejtehadi, H., & Kheirabadi, M. (2008 Mar). The effect of Rosa damascena essential oil on the amygdala electrical kindling seizures in rat. Pak J Biol Sci, 11(5), 746-751.

Rana I.S., Rana A.S., Rajak R.C. (2011 Oct). "Evaluation of antifungal activity in essential oil of the Syzygium aromaticum (L.) by extraction, purification and analysis of its main component eugenol," Braz. J. Microbiol. Publ. Braz. Soc. Microbiol. 42(4):1269-1277.

Ranasinghe L, Jayawardena B, Abeywickrama K (2002 Sep). "Fungicidal activity of essential oils of Cinnamomum zeylanicum (L.) and Syzygium aromaticum (L.) Merr et L.M.Perry against crown rot and anthracnose pathogens isolated from banana," Lett. Appl. Microbiol. 35(3):208-211.

Ranzato, E., Martinotti, S., & Burlando, B. (2011 Mar). Wound healing properties of jojoba liquid wax: an in vitro study. J Ethnopharmacol, 134(2), 443-449.

Rao S., Krauss N.E., Heerding J.M., Swindell C.S., Ringel I., Orr G.A., Horwitz S.B. (1994) 3'-(p-Azidobenzamido)taxol Photolabels the N-terminal 31 AminoAcids of β-Tubulin. The Journal of Biological Chemistry. 269: 3132-3134.

Rao S., Orr G.A., Chaudhary A.G., Kingston D.G.I., Horwitz S.B. (1995) Characterization of the Taxol Binding Site on the Microtubule. The Journal of Biological Chemistry. 270: 20235-20238.

Raphael T.J., Kuttan G (2003 May). "Immunomodulatory activity of naturally occurring monoterpenes carvone, limonene, and perillic acid," Immunopharmacol. Immunotoxicol. 25(2):285-294.

Rashidi-Fakari F, Tabatabaeichehr M, Mortazavi H (2015 Dec). "The effect of aromatherapy by essential oil of orange on anxiety during labor: A randomized clinical trial," Iran J Nurs Midwifery Res. 20(6):661-664.

Rasooli I, Fakoor MH, Yadegarinia D, Gachkar L, Allameh A, Rezaei MB (2008 Feb 29). "Antimycotoxigenic characteristics of Rosmarinus officinalis and Trachyspermum copticum L. essential oils," Int J Food Microbiol. 122(1-2):135-9.

Rasooli I, Shayegh S, Taghizadeh M, Astaneh SD (2008 Sep). "Phytotherapeutic prevention of dental biofilm formation," Phytother Res. 22(9):1162-7.

Rates, S. M. K. (2001). Plants as source of drugs. Toxicon, 39(5), 603-613.

Rathi, B., Bodhankar, S., Mohan, V., & Thakurdesai, P. (2013 Jun). Ameliorative Effects of a Polyphenolic Fraction of Cinnamomum zeylanicum L. Bark in Animal Models of Inflammation and Arthritis. Sci Pharm, 81(2), 567-589.

Raudenbush B, Meyer B, Eppich B (2002). "The Effects of Odors on Objective and Subjective Measures of Athletic Performance," Int. Sports J. 6(1):14.

Raut J.S., Shinde R.B., Chauhan N.M., Karuppayil S.M. (2013). "Terpenoids of plant origin inhibit morphogenesis, adhesion, and biofilm formation by Candida albicans," Biofouling. 29(1):87-96.

Reddy AC, Lokesh BR (1994). "Studies on anti-inflammatory activity of spice principles and dietary n-3 polyunsaturated fatty acids on carrageenan-induced inflammation in rats," Ann Nutr Metab. 38(6):349-58.

Reddy BS, Wang CX, Samaha H, Lubet R, Steele VE, Kelloff GJ, Rao CV (1997 Feb 1). "Chemoprevention of colon carcinogenesis by dietary perillyl alcohol," Cancer Res. 57(3):420-5.

Rekka E.A., Kourounakis A.P., Kourounakis P.N. (1996 Jun). "Investigation of the effect of chamazulene on lipid peroxidation and free radical processes," Res. Commun. Mol. Pathol. Pharmacol. 92(3):361-364.

Rees WD, Evans BK, Rhodes J (1979 Oct 6). "Treating irritable bowel syndrome with peppermint oil," Br Med J. 2(6194):835-6.

Reeve, V. E., Allanson, M., Arun, S. J., Domanski, D., & Painter, N. (2010 Apr). Mice drinking goji berry juice (Lycium barbarum) are protected from UV radiation-induced skin damage via antioxidant pathways. Photochem Photobiol Sci, 9(4), 601-607. Reichling J, Fitzi J, Hellmann K, Wegener T, Bucher S, Saller R (2004 Oct). "Topical tea tree oil effective in canine localised pruritic dermatitis--a multi-centre randomised double-blind controlled clinical trial in the veterinary practice," Dtsch Tierarztl Wochenschr. 111(10):408-14.

Reichling J, Koch C, Stahl-Biskup E, Sojka C, Schnitzler P (2005 Dec). "Virucidal activity of a beta-triketone-rich essential oil of Leptospermum scoparium (manuka oil) against HSV-1 and HSV-2 in cell culture," Planta Med. 71(12):1123-7.

Renimel I, Andre P (Inventors) (1995). "Method for treatment of allergic disorders and cosmetic compositions using cucurbitine," USPTO 5714164.

Rhee SG (2006 Jun). "Cell signaling. H2O2, a necessary evil for cell signaling," Science. 312(5782):1882-3.

Rigano L, Dell'Acqua G, Leporatti R (2000). "Benefits of Trimethylglycine (Betaine) in Personal-Care Formulations," Cosm Toil. 115(12):47-54.

Ritschel, W. A., Brady, M. E., & Tan, H. S. (1979 Mar). First-pass effect of coumarin in man. Int J Clin Pharmacol Biopharm, 17(3), 99-103.

Rivas da Silva A.C., Lopes P.M., Barros de Azevedo M.M, Costa D.C.M., Alviano C.S., Alviano D.S. (2012). "Biological activities of α-pinene and β-pinene enantiomers," Molecules. 17(6):6305-6316.

Rivero-Cruz B, Rojas MA, Rodríguez-Sotres R, Cerda-García-Rojas CM, Mata R (2005 Apr). "Smooth muscle relaxant action of benzyl benzoates and salicylic acid derivatives from Brickellia veronicaefolia on isolated guinea-pig ileum," Planta Med. 71(4):320-5.

Rocha, N. F., Rios, E. R., Carvalho, A. M., Cerqueira, G. S., Lopes Ade, A., Leal, L. K., . . . de Sousa, F. C. (2011 Aug 27). "Anti-nociceptive and anti-inflammatory activities of (-)-alpha-bisabolol in rodents," Naunyn Schmiedebergs Arch Pharmacol, 384(6): 525-533.

Rochel I.D. et al (2011). "Effect of experimental xylitol and fluoride-containing dentifrices on enamel erosion with or without abrasion in vitro," J. Oral Sci. 53(2):163-168.

Rodriguez J, Yáñez J, Vicente V, Alcaraz M, Benavente-García O, Castillo J, Lorente J, Lozano JA (2002 Apr). "Effects of several flavonoids on the growth of B16F10 and SK-MEL-1 melanoma cell lines: relationship between structure and activity," Melanoma Res. 12(2):99-107.

Rombolà, L., Tridico, L., Scuteri, D., Sakurada, T., Sakurada, S., Mizoquchi, H., Avato, P., Corasaniti, M.T., Bagetta, G., & Morrone, L.A. (2017 Apr. 11). "Bergamot Essential Oil Attenuates Anxiety-Like Behaviour in Rats," Molecules. 22(4).

Romero-Jiménez M, Campos-Sánchez J, Analla M, Muñoz-Serrano A, Alonso-Moraga A (2005 Aug 1). "Genotoxicity and anti-genotoxicity of some traditional medicinal herbs," Mutat Res. 585(1-2):147-55.

Romijn JA, Coyle EF, Sidossis LS, Gastaldelli A, Horowitz JF, Endert E, Wolfe RR (1993 Sep.). "Regulation of endogenous fat and carbohydrate metabolism in relation to exercise intensity and duration," Am J Physiol, 265(3 Pt 1):E380-91.

Rosa A, Deiana M, Atzeri A, Corona G, Incani A, Melis MP, Appendino G, Dessì MA (2007 Jan 30). "Evaluation of the antioxidant and cytotoxic activity of arzanol, a prenylated alpha-pyrone-phloroglucinol etherodimer from Helichrysum italicum subsp.microphyllum," Chem Biol Interact. 165(2):117-26.

Rose JE, Behm FM (1994 Feb). "Inhalation of vapor from black pepper extract reduces smoking withdrawal symptoms," Drug Alcohol Depend. 34(3):225-9.

Ross R, Freeman JA, Janssen J (2000 Oct). "Exercise alone is an effective strategy for reducing obesity and related comorbidities," Exerc Sport Sci Rev, 28(4):165-70.

Rowinsky E.K., Donehower R.C. (1995) Paclitaxel (Taxol). The New England Journal of Medicine. 332: 1004-1014.

Roy S, Khanna S, Krishnaraju AV, Subbaraju GV, Yasmin T, Bagchi D, Sen CK (2006 Mar-Apr). "Regulation of vascular responses to inflammation: inducible matrix metalloproteinase-3 expression in human microvascular endothelial cells is sensitive to antiinflammatory Boswellia," Antioxid Redox Signal. 8(3-4):653-60.

Roy S, Khanna S, Shah H, Rink C, Phillips C, Preuss H, Subbaraju GV, Trimurtulu G, Krishnaraju AV, Bagchi M, Bagchi D, Sen CK (2005 Apr). "Human genome screen to identify the genetic basis of the anti-inflammatory effects of Boswellia in microvascular endothelial cells," DNA Cell Biol. 24(4):244-55.

Roy S, Khanna S, Alessio HM, Vider J, Bagchi D, Bagchi M, Sen CK (2002 Sep). "Anti-angiogenic property of edible berries," Free Radic Res. 36(9):1023-31.

Rozza, A. L., Moraes Tde, M., Kushima, H., Tanimoto, A., Marques, M. O., Bauab, T. M., . . . Pellizzon, C. H. (2011 Jan). Gastroprotective mechanisms of Citrus lemon (Rutaceae) essential oil and its majority compounds limonene and beta-pinene: involvement of heat-shock protein-70, vasoactive intestinal peptide, glutathione, sulfhydryl compounds, nitric oxide and prostaglandin E(2). Chem Biol Interact, 189(1-2), 82-89.

Ruthig DJ, Meckling-Gill KA (1999 Oct). "Both (n-3) and (n-6) fatty acids stimulate wound healing in the rat intestinal epithelial cell line, IEC-6," J Nutr. 129(10):1791-8.

Sabzghabaee AM, Davoodi N, Ebadian B, Aslani A, Ghannadi A (2012 Mar). "Clinical evaluation of the essential oil of "Saturejo hortensis" for the treatment of denture stomatitis," Dent Res J (isfahan). 9(2):198-202.

Sacchetti G. et al (2005 Aug). "Comparative evaluation of 11 essential oils of different origin as functional antioxidants, antiradicals and antimicrobials in foods," Food Chem. 91(4):621-632.

Sadraei, H., Asghari, G., & Emami, S. (2013 Jan). Inhibitory effect of Rosa damascena Mill flower essential oil, geraniol and citronellol on rat ileum contraction. Res Pharm Sci, 8(1), 17-23.

Sadraei H, Asghari GR, Hajhashemi V, Kolagar A, Ebrahimi M. (2001 Sep). "Spasmolytic activity of essential oil and various extracts of Ferula gummosa Boiss. on ileum contractions," Phytomedicine. 8(5):370-6.

Saeed M.A., Sabir A.W. (2004 Mar). "Antibacterial activities of some constituents from oleo-gumresin of Commiphora mukul," Fitoterapia. 75(2):204-208.

Saeed SA, Gilani AH (1994 May). "Antithrombotic activity of clove oil," J Pak Med Assoc. 44(5):112-5.

Saeedi M, Morteza, Semnani K, Ghoreishi MR (2003 Sep). "The treatment of atopic dermatitis with licorice gel," J Dermatol Treat. 14(3):153-7.

Saeki Y, Ito Y, Shibata M, Sato Y, Okuda K, Takazoe I (1989 Aug). "Antimicrobial action of natural substances on oral bacteria," Bull. Tokyo Dent. Coll. 30(3):129-135.

Saerens KM, Zhang J, Saey L, Van Bogaert IN, Soetaert W (2011 Apr). "Cloning and functional characterization of the UDP-glucosyltransferase UgtB1 involved in sophorolipid production by Candida bombicola and creation of a glucolipid-producing yeast strain," Yeast. 28(4):279-92.

Safayhi H, Sabieraj J, Sailer ER, Ammon HP (1994 Oct). "Chamazulene: an antioxidant-type inhibitor of leukotriene B4 formation," Planta Med. 60(5):410-3.

Appendix

Saha SS, Ghosh M (2009 Jul 18). "Comparative study of antioxidant activity of alpha-eleosteraric acid and punicic acid against oxidative stress generated by sodium arsenite," Food Chem Toxicol. [Epub ahead of print].

Saharkhiz M.J., Motamedi M, Zomorodian K, Pakshir K, Miri R, Hemyari K (2012). "Chemical Composition, Antifungal and Antibiofilm Activities of the Essential Oil of Mentha piperita L," ISRN Pharm. 2012:718645.

Said T, Dutot M, Martin C, Beaudeux JL, Boucher C, Enee E, Baudouin C, Warnet JM, Rat P (2007 Mar). "Cytoprotective effect against UV-induced DNA damage and oxidative stress: role of new biological UV filter," Eur J Pharm Sci. 30(3-4):203-10.

Saikia, D., Parveen, S., Gupta, V. K., & Luqman, S. (2012 Dec). Anti-tuberculosis activity of Indian grass KHUS (Vetiveria zizanioides L. Nash). Complement Ther Med, 20(6), 434-436.

Saiyudthong, S., & Marsden, C. A. (2011 Jun). Acute effects of bergamot oil on anxiety-related behaviour and corticosterone level in rats. Phytother Res, 25(6), 858-862.

Saiyudthong S, Pongmayteegul S, Marsden C.A., Phansuwan-Pujito P (2015 Nov). "Anxiety-like behaviour and c-fos expression in rats that inhaled vetiver essential oil," Nat. Prod. Res. 29(22):2141-2144.

Salmalian, H., Saghebi, R., Moghadamnia, A. A., Bijani, A., Faramarzi, M., Nasiri Amiri, F., . . . Bekhradi, R. (2014 Apr). Comparative effect of thymus vulgaris and ibuprofen on primary dysmenorrhea: A triple-blind clinical study. Caspian J Intern Med, 5(2), 82-88.

Samani Keihan, G., Gharib M.H., Momeni, A., Hemati Z., & Sedighin R. (2017 Jan. 24). "A Comparison Between the Effect of Cuminum Cyminum and Vitamin E on the Level of Leptin, Paraoxonase 1, HbA1c and Oxidized LDL in Diabetic Patients," Int J Mol Cel Med. 5(4):229-235.

Samarth RM (2007 Nov). "Protection against radiation induced hematopoietic damage in bone marrow of Swiss albino mice by Mentha piperita (Linn)," J Radiat Res (Tokyo). 48(4):523-8.

Samarth RM, Goyal PK, Kumar A (2004 Jul). "Protection of swiss albino mice against whole-body gamma irradiation by Mentha piperita (Linn.).," Phytother Res. 18(7):546-50.

Samarth RM, Kumar A (2003 Jun). "Radioprotection of Swiss albino mice by plant extract Mentha piperita (Linn.)," J Radiat Res (Tokyo). 44(2):101-9.

Samarth RM, Panwar M, Kumar M, Kumar A (2006 May). "Radioprotective influence of Mentha piperita (Linn) against gamma irradiation in mice: Antioxidant and radical scavenging activity," Int J Radiat Biol. 82(5):331-7.

Samarth RM, Samarth M (2009 Apr). "Protection against radiation-induced testicular damage in Swiss albino mice by Mentha piperita (Linn.).," Basic Clin Pharmacol Toxicol. 104(4):329-34.

Samber N, Khan A, Varma A, Manzoor (2015). "Synergistic anti-candidal activity and mode of action of Mentha piperita essential oil and its major components," Pharm. Biol. 53(10):1496-1504.

Samman S, Naghii MR, Lyons Wall PM, Verus AP (1998 Winter). "The nutritional and metabolic effects of boron in humans and animals," Biol Trace Elem Res. 66(1-3):227-35.

Sándor Z et al (2018 Apr 5). "Evidence support tradition: the in vitro effects of roman chamomile on smooth muscles," Front Pharmacol. 9:323.

Sanguinetti, M., Posteraro, B., Romano, L., Battaglia, F., Lopizzo, T., De Carolis, E., & Fadda, G. (2007 Feb). In vitro activity of Citrus bergamia (bergamot) oil against clinical isolates of dermatophytes. J Antimicrob Chemother, 59(2), 305-308.

Santamaria, M., Jr., Petermann, K. D., Vedovello, S. A., Degan, V., Lucato, A., & Franzini, C. M. (2014 Feb). Antimicrobial effect of Melaleuca alternifolia dental gel in orthodontic patients. Am J Orthod Dentofacial Orthop, 145(2), 198-202.

Santos AO, Ueda-Nakamura T, Dias Filho BP, Veiga Junior VF, Pinto AC, Nakamura CV (2008 May). "Antimicrobial activity of Brazilian copaiba oils obtained from different species of the Copaifera genus," Mem Inst Oswaldo Cruz. 103(3):277-81.

Santos AO, Ueda-Nakamura T, Dias Filho BP, Veiga Junior VF, Pinto AC, Nakamura CV (2008 Nov 20). "Effect of Brazilian copaiba oils on Leishmania amazonensis," J Ethnopharmacol. 120(2):204-8.

Santos FA, Rao VS (2000 Jun). "Anti-inflammatory and antinociceptive effects of 1,8-cineole a terpenoid oxide present in many plant essential oils," Phytother Res. 14(4):240-4.

Santos, R.C., dos Santos Alves, C.F., Schneider, T., Lopes, L.Q., Aurich, C., Giongo, J.L., Brandelli, A., and de Almeida Vaucher, R. (2012). "Antimicrobial activity of Amazonian oils against Paenibacillus species," J Invertebr Pathol. 109(3):265-8.

Sarahroodi, S., Esmaeili, S., Mikaili, P., Hemmati, Z., & Saberi, Y. (2012 Apr). The effects of green Ocimum basilicum hydroalcoholic extract on retention and retrieval of memory in mice. Anc Sci Life, 31(4), 185-189.

Sarrau E, Chatzopoulou P, Dimassi-Theriou K, Therios I (2013). "Volatile constituents and antioxidant activity of peel, flowers, and leaf oils of Citrus aurantium L. growing in Greece," Molecules 18:10639-47.

Sasannejad, P., Saeedi, M., Shoeibi, A., Gorji, A., Abbasi, M., & Foroughipour, M. (2012 Apr). Lavender essential oil in the treatment of migraine headache: a placebo-controlled clinical trial. Eur Neurol, 67(5), 288-291.

Satchell AC, Saurajen A, Bell C, Barnetson RS (2002 Aug). "Treatment of interdigital tinea pedis with 25% and 50% tea tree oil solution: a randomized, placebo-controlled, blinded study," Australas J Dermatol. 43(3):175-8.

Satou, T., Takahashi, M., Kasuya, H., Murakami, S., Hayashi, S., Sadamoto, K., & Koike, K. (2013 Feb). Organ accumulation in mice after inhalation of single or mixed essential oil compounds. Phytother Res, 27(2), 306-311.

Savelev SU, Okello EJ, Perry EK (2004 Apr). "Butyryl- and acetyl-cholinesterase inhibitory activities in essential oils of Salvia species and their constituents," Phytother Res. 18(4):315-24.

Savino F, Cresi F, Castagno E, Silvestro L, Oggero R (2005 Apr). "A randomized double-blind placebo-controlled trial of a standardized extract of Matricariae recutita, Foeniculum vulgare and Melissa officinalis (ColiMil) in the treatment of breastfed colicky infants," Phytother Res. 19(4):335-40.

Sayorwan W (2013). "Effects of Inhaled Rosemary Oil on Subjective Feelings and Activities of the Nervous System," Sci. Pharm. 81(2):531-542.

Sayorwan W, Siripornpanich V, Piriyapunyaporn T, Hongratanaworakit T, Kotchabhakdi N, Ruangrungsi N (2012 Apr). "The effects of lavender oil inhalation on emotional states, autonomic nervous system, and brain electrical activity," J. Med. Assoc. Thail. Chotmaihet Thangphaet. 95(4):598-606.

Sayyah M, Nadjafnia L, Kamalinejad M (2004 Oct). "Anticonvulsant activity and chemical composition of Artemisia dracunculus L. essential oil," J Ethnopharmacol. 94(2-3):283-7.

Sayyah M, Saroukhani G, Peirovi A, Kamalinejad M (2003 Aug). "Analgesic and anti-inflammatory activity of the leaf essential oil of Laurus nobilis Linn," Phytother Res. 17(7):733-6.

Sayyah M, Valizadeh J, Kamalinejad M (2002 Apr). "Anticonvulsant activity of the leaf essential oil of Laurus nobilis against pentylenetetrazole- and maximal electroshock-induced seizures," Phytomedicine. 9(3):212-6.

Scalbert A, Johnson IT, and Saltmarsh M (2005 Jan). "Polyphenols: antioxidants and beyond," Presented at the 1st International Conference on Polyphenols and Health, Vichy, France. Am J Clin Nut. 81(1):215S-7S.

Schecter A., Birnbaum L., Ryan J.J., Constable J.D. (2006) Dioxins: An overview. Environmental Research. 101: 419-428.

Scheinfeld NS, Mones J (2005 May). "Granular parakeratosis: pathologic and clinical correlation of 18 cases of granular parakeratosis," J Am Acad Dermatol. 52(5):863-7.

Schellack, G. (2011). Series on nursing pharmacology and medicine management part 3: drug dosage forms and the routes of drug administration. Profession Nurse Today, 15(6), 10-15.

Schelz Z, Molnar J, Jojmann J (2006 Jun). "Antimicrobial and antiplasmid activities of essential oils," Fitoterapia. 77(4):279-285.

Schillaci D, Arizza V, Dayton T, Camarda L, Di Stefano V (2008 Nov). "In vitro anti-biofilm activity of Boswellia spp. oleogum resin essential oils," Lett. Appl. Microbiol. 47(5):433-438.

Schlachterman A et al. (2008 Mar). "Combined resveratrol, quercetin, and catechin treatment reduces breast tumor growth in a nude mouse model," Transl Oncol. 1(1):19-27.

Schmid, D., Schürch, C., and Zülli, F. (2006.) "Mycosporine-like Amino Acids from Red Algae Protect against Premature Skin-Aging," Euro Cosmetics.

Schmitt, S., Schaefer, U. F., Doebler, L., & Reichling, J. (2009 Oct). Cooperative interaction of monoterpenes and phenylpropanoids on the in vitro human skin permeation of complex composed essential oils. Planta Med, 75(13), 1381-1385.

Schnitzler P, Schön K, Reichling J (2001 Apr). "Antiviral activity of Australian tea tree oil and eucalyptus oil against herpes simplex virus in cell culture," Pharmazie. 56(4):343-7.

Schnitzler P, Schuhmacher A, Astani A, Reichling J (2008 Sep). "Melissa officinalis oil affects infectivity of enveloped herpesviruses," Phytomedicine. 15(9):734-40.

Schreckinger, M. E., Lotton, J., Lila, M. A., & de Mejia, E. G. (2010 Apr). Berries from South America: a comprehensive review on chemistry, health potential, and commercialization. J Med Food, 13(2), 233-246.

Schroter A., Kessner D., Kiselev M.A., Haub T., Dante S., Neubert R.H.H. (2009) Basic Nanostructure of Stratum Corneum Lipid Matrices Based on Ceramides [EOS] and [AP]: A Neutron Diffraction Study. Biophysical Journal. 97: 1104-1114.

Schuhmacher A, Reichling J, Schnitzler P (2003). "Virucidal effect of peppermint oil on the enveloped viruses herpes simplex virus type 1 and type 2 in vitro," Phytomedicine. 10(6-7):504-10.

Scott, Sophie (2015). "Peanut allergies: Australian study into probiodics offers hope for possible cure," abc.net.au.

Seifi Z, Beikmoradi A, Oshvandi K, Poorolajal J, Araghchian M, Safiaryan R (2014 Nov). "The effect of lavender essential oil on anxiety level in patients undergoing coronary artery bypass graft surgery: A double-blinded randomized clinical trial," Iran. J. Nurs. Midwifery Res. 19(6):574-580.

Selim, S. A., Adam, M. E., Hassan, S. M., & Albalawi, A. R. (2014). Chemical composition, antimicrobial and antibiofilm activity of the essential oil and methanol extract of the Mediterranean cypress (Cupressus sempervirens L.). BMC Complement Altern Med, 14(1), 1-8.

Sell, C. (Ed.). (2006). The Chemistry of Fragrances From Perfumer to Consumer (2nd ed.). Dorchester, UK: The Royal Society of Chemistry.

Senapati S, Banerjee S, Gangopadhyay DN (2008 Sep-Oct). "Evening primrose oil is effective in atopic dermatitis: a randomized placebo-controlled trial," Indian J Dermatol Venereol Leprol. 74(5):447-52.

Senni K, Gueniche F, Foucault-Bertaud A, Igondjo-Tchen S, Fioretti F, Colliec-Jouault S, Durand P, Guezennec J, Godeau G, Letourneur D (2006 Jan 1). "Fucoidan a sulfated polysaccharide from brown algae is a potent modulator of connective tissue proteolysis," Arch Biochem Biophys. 445(1):56-64.

Seo Y.M., Jeong S.H. (2015 Jun). "[Effects of Blending Oil of Lavender and Thyme on Oxidative Stress, Immunity, and Skin Condition in Atopic Dermatitis Induced Mice]," J. Korean Acad. Nurs. 45(3):367-377.

Seol, G. H., Shim, H. S., Kim, P. J., Moon, H. K., Lee, K. H., Shim, I., . . . Min, S. S. (2010 Jul). Antidepressant-like effect of Salvia sclarea is explained by modulation of dopamine activities in rats. J Ethnopharmacol, 130(1), 187-190.

Serafino, A., Sinibaldi Vallebona, P., Andreola, F., Zonfrillo, M., Mercuri, L., Federici, M., . . . Pierimarchi, P. (2008 Apr). Stimulatory effect of eucalyptus essential oil on innate cell-mediated immune response. BMC Immunol, 9, 17.

Shaikh IA, Brown I, Schofield AC, Wahle KW, Heys SD (2008 Nov). "Docosahexaenoic acid enhances the efficacy of docetaxel in prostate cancer cells by modulation of apoptosis: the role of genes associated with the NF-kappaB pathway," Prostate. 68(15):1635-46.

Shaltiel-Karyo, R., Davidi, D., Frenkel-Pinter, M., Ovadia, M., Segal, D., & Gazit, E. (2012 Oct). Differential inhibition of alpha-synuclein oligomeric and fibrillar assembly in parkinson's disease model by cinnamon extract. Biochim Biophys Acta, 1820(10), 1628-1635.

Sharma N., Tripathi A. (2008 May). "Effects of Citrus sinensis (L.) Osbeck epicarp essential oil on growth and morphogenesis of Aspergillus niger (L.) Van Tieghem," Microbiol. Res. 163(3):337-344.

Shankar GM, Li S, Mehta TH, Garcia-Munoz A, Shepardson NE, Smith I, Brett FM, Farrell MA, Rowan MJ, Lemere CA, Regan CM, Walsh DM, Sabatini BL, Selkoe DJ (2008 Jun 22). "Amyloid-protein dimers isolated directly from Alzheimer's brains impair synaptic plasticity and memory," Nat Med. 14(8):837-42.

Shankar S, Ganapathy S, Hingorani SR, Srivastava RK (2008 Jan). "EGCG inhibits growth, invasion, angiogenesis and metastasis of pancreatic cancer," Front Biosci. 13:440-52.

Shimada K. et al (2011 Feb). "Aromatherapy alleviates endothelial dysfunction of medical staff after night-shift work: preliminary observations," Hypertens. Res. Off. J. Jpn. Soc. Hypertens. 34(2):264-267.

Santha S, Dwivedi C (2015 Jun). "Anticancer Effects of Sandalwood (Santalum album)," Anticancer Res. 35(6):3137-45.

Shapiro S., Guggenheim B. (1995) The action of thymol on oral bacteria. Oral Microbiology and Immunology. 10: 241-246.

Shapiro S, Meier A, Guggenheim B (1994 Aug). "The antimicrobial activity of essential oils and essential oil components towards oral bacteria," Oral Microbiol Immunol. 9(4):202-8.

Shao Y, Ho CT, Chin CK, Badmaev V, Ma W, Huang MT (1998 May). "Inhibitory activity of boswellic acids from Boswellia serrata against human leukemia HL-60 cells in culture," Planta Med. 64(4):328-31.

Sharma JN, Srivastava KC, Gan EK (1994 Nov). "Suppressive effects of eugenol and ginger oil on arthritic rats," Pharmacology. 49(5):314-8.

Sharma M et al (2014 June). "Suppression of lipopolysaccharide-stimulated cytokine/chemokine production in skin cells by sandalwood oils and purified α-santalol and β-santalol," Phytother Res. 28(6):925-32.

Sharma PR, Mondhe DM, Muthiah S, Pal HC, Shahi AK, Saxena AK, Qazi GN (2009 May 15). "Anticancer activity of an essential oil from Cymbopogon flexuosus," Chem Biol Interact. 179(2-3):160-8.

Shaw D, Norwood K, Leslie J.C. (2011 Oct). "Chlordiazepoxide and lavender oil alter unconditioned anxiety-induced c-fos expression in the rat brain," Behav. Brain Res. 224(1):1-7.

Shayegh S, Rasooli I, Taghizadeh M, Astaneh SD (2008 Mar 20). "Phytotherapeutic inhibition of supragingival dental plaque," Nat Prod Res. 22(5):428-39.

Sheikhan F, Jahdi D, Khoei E.M., Shamsalizadeh N, Sheikhan M, Haghani H (2012 Feb). "Episiotomy pain relief: Use of Lavender oil essence in primiparous Iranian women," Complement. Ther. Clin. Pract. 18(1):66-70.

Shen J, Niijima A, Tanida M, Horii Y, Maeda K, Nagai K (2005 Jun 3). "Olfactory stimulation with scent of grapefruit oil affects autonomic nerves, lipolysis and appetite in rats," Neurosci Lett. 380(3):289-94.

Shen J, Niijima A, Tanida M, Horii Y, Maeda K, Nagai K (2005 Jul 22-29). "Olfactory stimulation with scent of lavender oil affects autonomic nerves, lipolysis and appetite in rats," Neurosci Lett. 383(1-2):188-93.

Sherry E, Boeck H, Warnke PH (2001). "Percutaneous treatment of chronic MRSA osteomyelitis with a novel plant-derived antiseptic," BMC Surg. 1:1.

Shetty AV, Thirugnanam S, Dakshinamoorthy G, Samykutty A, Zheng G, Chen A, Bosland MC, Kajdacsy-Balla A, Gnanasekar M (2011 Sep). "18α-glycyrrhetinic acid targets prostate cancer cells by down-regulating inflammation-related genes," In J Oncol. 39(3):635-40.

Shibata M., Ohkubo T., Takahashi H., Inoki R. (1989) Modified formalin test: characteristic biphasic pain response. Pain. 38: 347-352.

Shieh PC, Tsao CW, Li JS, et. al (2008). "Rp;e pf [otiotaru ademu;ate cuc;ase=actovatomg [p;u[e[tode){ACA{ om tje actopm pf gomsempsode Rj2 agaomst beta=a,u;pod=omdiced omjobotopm pf rat braom astrpcutes. Meirpsco :ett/ 434"1=5/

Shiina Y et al (2008 Sep). "Relaxation effects of lavender aromatherapy improve coronary flow velocity reserve in healthy men evaluated by transthoracic Doppler echocardiography," Int. J. Cardiol. 129(2):193-197.

Shimada K. et al (2011 Feb). "Aromatherapy alleviates endothelial dysfunction of medical staff after night-shift work: preliminary observations," Hypertens. Res. Off. J. Jpn. Soc. Hypertens. 34(2):264-267.

Shimizu K. et al (2008 Jul). "Essential oil of lavender inhibited the decreased attention during a long-term task in humans," Biosci. Biotechnol. Biochem. 72(7):1944-1947.

Shinohara, K., Doi, H., Kumagai, C., Sawano, E., & Tarumi, W. (2017 Jan.). "Effects of essential oil exposure on salivary estrogen concentration in perimenopausal women," Neuro Endocrinol Lett. 37(8):567-572.

Shirazi M et al (2017 Jan). "The effect of topical rosa damascena (rose) oil on pregnancy-related low back pain: a randomized controlled clinical trial," J Evid Based Complementary Altern Med. 22(1):120-126.

Shrivastav P, George K, Balasubramaniam N, Jasper MP, Thomas M, Kanagasabhapathy AS (1988 Feb). "Suppression of puerperal lactation using jasmine flowers (Jasminum sambac)," Aust N Z J Obstet Gynaecol. 28(1):68-71.

Shoskes DA, Zeitlin SI, Shahed A, Rajfer J (1999 Dec). "Quercetin in men with category III prostatitis: a preliminary prospective, double-blind, placebo-controlled trial," Urology. 54(6):960-3.

Shukla, V., Vashistha, M., & Singh, S. N. (2009 Jan). Evaluation of antioxidant profile and activity of amalaki (Emblica officinalis), spirulina and wheat grass. Indian J Clin Biochem, 24(1), 70-75.

Shukla, Y. M., Dhruve, J. J., Patel, N. J., Bhatnagar, R., Talati, J. G., & Kathiria, K. B. (2009). Plant Secondary Metabolites. New Delhi, India: New India Publishing Agency.

Shyam, R., Singh, S. N., Vats, P., Singh, V. K., Bajaj, R., Singh, S. B., & Banerjee, P. K. (2007 Aug). Wheat grass supplementation decreases oxidative stress in healthy subjects: a comparative study with spirulina. J Altern Complement Med, 13(8), 789-791.

Si L. et al (2012 Jun). "Chemical Composition of Essential Oils of Litsea cubeba Harvested from Its Distribution Areas in China," Molecules. 17(12):7057-7066.

Sienkiewicz M, Glowacka A, Poznańska-Kurowska K, Kaszuba A, Urbaniak A, Kowalczyk E (2015 Feb). "The effect of clary sage oil on staphylococci responsible for wound infections," Postepy Dermatol Alergol. 32(1):21-6.

Sies H (1997). "Oxidative stress: oxidants and antioxidants," Exp Physiol. 82(2):291–5.

Sikkema J., de Bont J.A.M., Poolman B. (1995) Mechanisms of Membrane Toxicity of Hydrocarbons. Microbiological Reviews. 59: 201-222.

Sikora, E., & Bodziarczyk, I. (2012). Composition and antioxidant activity of kale (Brassica oleracea L. var. acephala) raw and cooked. Acta Sci Pol Technol Aliment, 11(3), 239-248.

Silva Brum L.F., Emanuelli T., Souza D.O., Elisabetsky E. (2001) Effects of Linalool on Glutamate Release and Uptake in Mouse Cortical Synaptosomes. Neurochemical Research. 26: 191-194

Silva Brum L.F., Elisabetsky E., Souza D. (2001) Effects of Linalool on [3H] MK801 and [3H] Muscimol Binding in Mouse Cortical Membranes. Phytotherapy Research. 15: 422-425.

Silva J, Abebe W, Sousa SM, Duarte VG, Machado MI, Matos FJ (2003 Dec). "Analgesic and anti-inflammatory effects of essential oils of Eucalyptus," J Ethnopharmacol. 89(2-3):277-83.

Siméon A, Monier F, Emonard H, Gillery P, Birembaut P, Hornebeck W, Maquart FX (1999 Jun). "Expression and activation of matrix metalloproteinases in wounds: modulation by the tripeptide-copper complex glycyl-L-histidyl-L-lysine-Cu2+," J Invest Dermatol. 112(3):957-64.

Singh, D., Rao, S. M., & Tripathi, A. K. (1984 May). Cedarwood oil as a potential insecticidal agent against mosquitoes. Naturwissenschaften, 71(5), 265-266.

Singh G, Maurya S, deLampasona M.P., Catalan C.A.N. (2007 Sep). "A comparison of chemical, antioxidant and antimicrobial studies of cinnamon leaf and bark volatile oils, oleoresins and their constituents," Food Chem. Toxicol. 45(9):1650-1661.

Singh HB, Srivastava M, Singh AB, Srivastava AK (1995 Dec). "Cinnamon bark oil, a potent fungitoxicant against fungi causing respiratory tract mycoses," Allergy. 50(12):995-9.

Singh, K. K., Mridula, D., Rehal, J., & Barnwal, P. (2011). Flaxseed: a potential source of food, feed and fiber. Crit Rev Food Sci Nutr, 51(3), 210-222.

Singh N, Bhalla M, deJager P, Gilca M (2011). "An overview on ashwagandha: a rasayana (rejuvenator) of ayurveda," Afr J Tradit Complement Altern Med. 8(s):208-13.

Singh RH, Udupa KN (1993). "Clinical and experimental studies on rasayana drugs and rasayana therapy," Special Research Monograph, Central Council for Research in Ayurveda and Siddha (CCRAS), Ministry of Health and Family Welfare, New Delhi.

Singh V. et al (2013 Aug). "Curcuma oil ameliorates hyperlipidaemia and associated deleterious effects in golden Syrian hamsters," Br. J. Nutr. 110(3):437-446.

Singletary K, MacDonald C, Wallig M (1996 Jun 24). "Inhibition by rosemary and carnosol of 7,12-dimethylbenz[a]anthracene (DMBA)-induced rat mammary tumorigenesis and in vivo DMBA-DNA adduct formation," Cancer Lett. 104(1):43-8.

Siqueira H.D.S. et al (2016 Sep). "α-Phellandrene, a cyclic monoterpene, attenuates inflammatory response through neutrophil migration inhibition and mast cell degranulation," Life Sci. 160:27-33.

Siu KM, Mak DH, CHiu PY, Poon MK, Du Y, Ko KM "2004). "Pharmacological basis of "Yin-nourishing" and "Yang-invigorating" actions of Cordyceps, a Chinese tonifying herb," Life Sci. 76:385-95.

Siurin SA (1997). "Effects of essential oil on lipid peroxidation and lipid metabolism in patients with chronic bronchitis," Klin Med (Mosk). 75(10):43-5.

Siveen K.S., Kuttan G. (2011 Dec). "Augmentation of humoral and cell mediated immune responses by Thujone," Int. Immunopharmacol. 11(12):1967-1975.

Skocibusić M, Bezić N (2004 Dec). "Phytochemical analysis and in vitro antimicrobial activity of two Satureja species essential oils," Phytother Res. 18(12):967-70.

Skold M., Borje A., Matura M., Karlberg A-T. (2002) Studies on the autoxidation and sensitizing capacity of the fragrance chemical linalool, identifying a linalool hydroperoxide. Contact Dermatitis. 46: 267-272.

Skrivanova E., Savka OG, Marounek M (2004). "In vitro effect of C2-C18 fatty acids on Salmonellas," Folia Microbiol (Praha). 49(2):199-202.

Appendix

Slamenova D, Kuboskova K, Horvathova E, Robichova S. (2002 Mar 28). "Rosemary-stimulated reduction of DNA strand breaks and FPG-sensitive sites in mammalian cells treated with H2O2 or visible light-excited Methylene Blue," Cancer Lett. 177(2):145-53.

Slima, A. B., Ali, M. B., Barkallah, M., Traore, A. I., Boudawara, T., Allouche, N., & Gdoura, R. (2013 Mar). Antioxidant properties of Pelargonium graveolens L'Her essential oil on the reproductive damage induced by deltamethrin in mice as compared to alpha-tocopherol. Lipids Health Dis, 12(1), 30.

Smith DG, Standing L, de Man A (1992 Apr). "Verbal memory elicited by ambient odor," Percept Mot Skills. 74(2):339-43.

Smith-Palmer A, Stewart J, Fyfe L (2004 Oct). "Influence of subinhibitory concentrations of plant essential oils on the production of enterotoxins A and B and alpha-toxin by Staphylococcus aureus," J Med Microbiol. 53(Pt 10):1023-7.

Smith PJ, Potter GG, McLaren ME, Blumenthal JA (2013 Oct). "Impact of aerobic exercise on neurobehavioral outcomes," Ment Health Phys Act, 6(3):139-53.

Soares SF, Borges LM, de Sousa Braga R, Ferreira LL, Louly CC, Tresvenzol LM, de Paula JR, Ferri PH (2009 Oct 7). "Repellent activity of plant-derived compounds against Amblyomma cajennense (Acari: Ixodidae) nymphs," Vet Parasitol. Epub ahead of print.

Soković M, Glamočlija J, Marin P.D., Brkić D, van Griensven L.J.L.D (2010 Nov). "Antibacterial effects of the essential oils of commonly consumed medicinal herbs using an in vitro model," Mol. Basel Switz. 15 (11):7532-7546.

Soltani R, Soheilipour S, Hajhashemi V, Asghari G, Bagheri M, Molavi M (2013 Sep). "Evaluation of the effect of aromatherapy with lavender essential oil on post-tonsillectomy pain in pediatric patients: a randomized controlled trial," Int. J. Pediatr. Otorhinolaryngol. 77(9):1579-1581.

Sorentino S., Landmesser U. (2005) Nonlipid-lowering Effects of Statins. Current Treatment Options to Cardiovascular Medicine. 7: 459-466.

Spirduso WW (1975 Jul). "Reaction and movement time as a function of age and physical activity level," J Gerontol, 30(4):435-40.

Sriram N, Kalayarasan S, Sudhandiran G (2008 Jul). "Enhancement of antioxidant defense system by epigallocatechin-3-gallate during bleomycin induced experimental Pulmonary Fibrosis," Biol Pharm Bull. 31(7):1306-11.

Stanzl K, Zastrow L, Röding J, Artmann C (1996 Jun). "The effectiveness of molecular oxygen in cosmetic formulations," Int J Cosmet Sci. 18(3):137-50.

Stefanick ML, Mackey S, Sheehan M, Ellsworth N, Haskell WL, Wood PD (1998 Jul). "Effects of diet and exercise in men and postmenopausal women with low levels of HDL cholesterol and high levels of LDL cholesterol," N Engl J Med, 339(1):12-20.

Stefanovits-Bányai E, Tulok M.H., Hegedûs A, Renner C, Varga I.S. (2003). "Antioxidant effect of various rosemary (Rosmarinus officinalis L.) clones," Acta Biol. Szeged. 47(1-4):111-113.

Steiner M, Priel I, Giat J, Levy J, Sharoni Y, Danilenko M (2001). "Carnosic acid inhibits proliferation and augments differentiation of human leukemic cells induced by 1,25-dihydroxyvitamin D3 and retinoic acid," Nutr Cancer. 41(1-2):135-44.

Steiner JL, Murphy EA, McClellan JL, Carmichael MD, Davis JM (2011 Oct). "Exercise training increases mitochondrial biogenesis in the brain," J Appl Physiol. 111(4):1066-71.

Strati A, Papoutsi Z, Lianidou E, Moutsatsou P (2009 Sep). "Effect of ellagic acid on the expression of human telomerase reverse transcriptase (hTERT) alpha+Beta+ transcript in estrogen receptor-positive MCF-7 breast cancer cells," Clin Biochem. 42(13-14):1358-62.

Stratton S.P., Alberts D.S., Einspahr J.G. (2010) A Phase 2a Study of Topical Perillyl Alcohol Cream for Chemoprevention of Skin Cancer. Cancer Prevention Research. 3: 160-169.

Stratton S.P., Saboda K.L., Myrdal P.B., Gupta A., McKenzie N.E., Brooks C., Salasche S.J., Warneke J.A., Ranger-Moore J., Bozzo P.D., Blanchard J., Einspahr J.G. (2008) Phase 1 Study of Topical Perillyl Alcohol Cream for Chemoprevention of Skin Cancer. Nutrition and Cancer. 60: 325-330.

Su KP, Huang SY, Chiu TH, Huang KC, Huang CL, Chang HC, Pariante CM (2008 Apr). "Omega-3 fatty acids for major depressive disorder during pregnancy: results from a randomized, double-blind, placebo-controlled trial," J Clin Psychiatry. 69(4):644-51.

Subash Babu P, Prabuseenivasan S, Ignacimuthu S. (2007 Jan). "Cinnamaldehyde--a potential antidiabetic agent," Phytomedicine.14(1):15-22.

Subramenium G.A., Vijayakumar K, Pandian S.K. (2015 Aug). "Limonene inhibits streptococcal biofilm formation by targeting surface-associated virulence factors," J. Med. Microbiol. 64(8):879-890.

Südhof TC (1995 Jun 22). "The synaptic vesicle cycle: a cascade of protein-protein interactions," Nature. 375(6533):645-53.

Sugimoto, H., Watanabe, K., Toyama, T., Takahashi, S. S., Sugiyama, S., Lee, M. C., & Hamada, N. (2015 Feb). Inhibitory effects of French pine bark extract, pycnogenol((R)), on alveolar bone resorption and on the osteoclast differentiation. Phytother Res, 29(2), 251-259.

Suhail M.M. et al (2011). "Boswellia sacra essential oil induces tumor cell-specific apoptosis and suppresses tumor aggressiveness in cultured human breast cancer cells," BMC Complement Altern Med. 11:129.

Suneetha, W. J., & Krishnakantha, T. P. (2005 May). Cardamom extract as inhibitor of human platelet aggregation. Phytother Res, 19(5), 437-440.

Sun J (2007 Sep). "D-Limonene: safety and clinical applications," Altern. Med. Rev. J. Clin. Ther. 12(3):259-64.

Sun J, Qian J, Zhao J, Liu L (2011 Oct). "[Clinical observation of mucoregulatory agents' application after chronic rhinosinusitis surgery]," Lin Chuang Er Bi

Yan Hou Tou Jing Wai Ke Za Zhi J. Clin. Otorhinolaryngol. Head Neck Surg. 25(20):922-24.

Sun L et al (2016 Dec 24). "The essential oil from the twigs of cinnamomum cassia presl alleviates pain and inflammation in mice," J Ethnopharmacol. 194:904-912.

Svoboda, K. P., Svoboda, T. G., & Syred, A. (2001). A Closer Look: Secretory Structures of Aromatic and Medicinal Plants HerbalGram: The Journal of the Amercian Botanical Council (53), 34-43.

Taavoni S, Darsareh F, Jooalee S, Haghani H (2013 Jun). "The effect of aromatherapy massage on the psychological symptoms of postmenopausal Iranian women," Complement. Ther. Med. 21(3):158-63.

Tabanca, N., Wang, M., Avonto, C., Chittiboyina, A. G., Parcher, J. F., Carroll, J. F., . . . Khan, I. A. (2013 May). Bioactivity-guided investigation of geranium essential oils as natural tick repellents. J Agric Food Chem, 61(17), 4101-4107.

Tadtong S, Suppawat S, Tintawee A, Saramas P, Jareonvong S, Hongratanaworakit T (2012 Oct). "Antimicrobial activity of blended essential oil preparation," Nat. Prod. Commun. 7(10):1401-1404.

Taguchi Y, Hasumi Y, Hayama K, Arai R, Nishiyama Y, Abe S (2012). "Effect of cinnamaldehyde on hyphal growth of C. albicans under various treatment conditions," Med. Mycol. J. 53(3):199-204.

Taher Y.A. et al (2015). "Experimental evaluation of anti-inflammatory, antinociceptive and antipyretic activities of clove oil in mice," Libyan J. Med. 10:28685.

Taherian, A. A., Vafaei, A. A., & Ameri, J. (2012 Apr). Opiate System Mediate the Antinociceptive Effects of Coriandrum sativum in Mice. Iran J Pharm Res, 11(2), 679-688.

Takahashi M, et al (2012 Nov). "Effects of inhaled lavender essential oil on stress-loaded animals: changes in anxiety-related behavior and expression levels of selected mRNAs and proteins," Nat. Prod. Commun. 7(11):1539-1544.

Takahashi M, Satou T, Ohashi M, Hayahi S, Sadamoto K, Koike K (2011 Nov). "Interspecies comparison of chemical composition and anxiolytic-like effects of lavender oils upon inhalation," Nat. Prod. Commun. 6(11):1769-1774.

Takahashi, N., Yao, L., Kim, M., Sasako, H., Aoyagi, M., Shono, J., . . . Kawada, T. (2013 Jul). Dill seed extract improves abnormalities in lipid metabolism through peroxisome proliferator-activated receptor-alpha (PPAR-alpha) activation in diabetic obese mice. Mol Nutr Food Res, 57(7), 1295-1299.

Takaki I, Bersani-Amado LE, Vendruscolo A, Sartoretto SM, Diniz SP, Bersani-Amado CA, Cuman RK (2008 Dec). "Anti-inflammatory and antinociceptive effects of Rosmarinus officinalis L. essential oil in experimental animal models," J Med Food. 11(4):741-6.

Takarada K, Kimizuka R, Takahashi N, Honma K, Okuda K, Kato T (2004 Feb). "A comparison of the antibacterial efficacies of essential oils against oral pathogens," Oral Microbiol Immunol. 19(1):61-4.

Tan P, Zhong W, Cai W (2000 Sep). "Clinical study on treatment of 40 cases of malignant brain tumor by elemene emulsion injection," Zhongguo Zhong Xi Yi Jie He Za Zhi. 20(9):645-8.

Tan X.C., Chua K.H., Ravishankar Ram M, Kuppusamy U.R. (2016 Apr). "Monoterpenes: Novel insights into their biological effects and roles on glucose uptake and lipid metabolism in 3T3-L1 adipocytes," Food Chem. 196:242-250.

Tang J, Wingerchuk DM, Crum BA, Rubin DI, Demaerschalk BM (2007 May). "Alpha-lipoic acid may improve symptomatic diabetic polyneuropathy," Neurologist. 12(3):164-7.

Tanida M, Niijima A, Shen J, Nakamura T, Nagai K (2005 Oct 5). "Olfactory stimulation with scent of essential oil of grapefruit affects autonomic neurotransmission and blood pressure," Brain Res. 1058(1-2):44-55.

Tanida M, Niijima A, Shen J, Nakamura T, Nagai K (2006 May 1). "Olfactory stimulation with scent of lavender oil affects autonomic neurotransmission and blood pressure in rats," Neurosci Lett. 398(1-2):155-60.

Tanida M, Niijima A, Shen J, Nakamura T, Nagai K (2008 Jul). "Day-night difference in thermoregulatory responses to olfactory stimulation," Neurosci. Lett. 439(2):192-197.

Tanida M. et al (2008 May). "Effects of olfactory stimulations with scents of grapefruit and lavender oils on renal sympathetic nerve and blood pressure in Clock mutant mice," Auton. Neurosci. Basic Clin. 139(1-2):1-83.

Tantaoui-Elaraki A, Beraoud L (1994). "Inhibition of growth and aflatoxin production in Aspergillus parasiticus by essential oils of selected plant materials," J Environ Pathol Toxicol Oncol. 13(1):67-72.

Tao L, Zhou L, Zheng L, Yao M (2006 Jul). "Elemene displays anti-cancer ability on laryngeal cancer cells in vitro and in vivo," Cancer Chemother Pharmacol. 58(1):24-34.

Tare V, Deshpande S, Sharma RN (2004 Oct). "Susceptibility of two different strains of Aedes aegypti (Diptera: Culicidae) to plant oils," J Econ Entomol. 97(5):1734-6.

Tavares AC, Gonçalves MJ, Cavaleiro C, Cruz MT, Lopes MC, Canhoto J, Salgueiro LR (2008 Sep 2). "Essential oil of Daucus carota subsp. halophilus: composition, antifungal activity and cytotoxicity," J Ethnopharmacol. 119(1):129-34.

Tayarani-Najaran, Z., Talasaz-Firoozi, E., Nasiri, R., Jalali, N., & Hassanzadeh, M. (2013 Jan). Antiemetic activity of volatile oil from Mentha spicata and Mentha x piperita in chemotherapy-induced nausea and vomiting. Ecancermedicalscience, 7, 1-6.

Terzi V, Morcia C, Faccioli P, Valè G, Tacconi G, Malnati M (2007 Jun). "In vitro antifungal activity of the tea tree (Melaleuca alternifolia) essential oil and its major components against plant pathogens," Lett Appl Microbiol. 44(6):613-8.

Thavara U, Tawatsin A, Bhakdeenuan P, Wongsinkongman P, Boonruad T, Bansiddhi J, Chavalittumrong P, Komalamisra N, Siriyasatien P, Mulla MS (2007 Jul).

"Repellent activity of essential oils against cockroaches (Dictyoptera: Blattidae, Blattellidae, and Blaberidae) in Thailand," Southeast Asian J Trop Med Public Health. 38(4):663-73.

Thompson, J. D., Chalchat, J. C., Michet, A., Linhart, Y. B., & Ehlers, B. (2003). Qualitative and quantitative variation in monoterpene co-occurrence and composition in the essential oil of Thymus vulgaris chemotypes. Journal of Chemical Ecology, 29(4), 873.

Thukham-Mee, W., & Wattanathorn, J. (2012). Evaluation of Safety and Protective Effect of Combined Extract of Cissampelos pareira and Anethum graveolens (PM52) against Age-Related Cognitive Impairment. Evid Based Complement Alternat Med, 2012, 1-10.

Tian X, Sun L, Gou L, Ling X, Feng Y, Wang L, Yin X, Liu Y (2013 Mar 29). "Protective effect of l-theanine on chronic restraint stress-induced cognitive impairments in mice," Brain Res. 1503:24-32.

Tiano L, Belardinelli R, Carnevali P, Principi F, Seddaiu G, Littarru GP (2007 Sep). "Effect of coenzyme Q10 administration on endothelial function and extracellular superoxide dismutase in patients with ischaemic heart disease: a double-blind, randomized controlled study," Eur Heart J. 28(18):2249-55.

Tildesley NT, Kennedy DO, Perry EK, Ballard CG, Wesnes KA, Scholey AB (2005 Jan 17). "Positive modulation of mood and cognitive performance following administration of acute doses of Salvia lavandulaefolia essential oil to healthy young volunteers," Physiol Behav. 83(5):699-709.

Tipton DA, Hamman NR, Dabbous MKh (2006 Mar). "Effect of myrrh oil on IL-1beta stimulation of NF-kappaB activation and PGE(2) production in human gingival fibroblasts and epithelial cells," Toxicol In Vitro. 20(2):248-55.

Tipton DA, Lyle B, Babich H, Dabbous MKh (2003 Jun). "In vitro cytotoxic and anti-inflammatory effects of myrrh oil on human gingival fibroblasts and epithelial cells," Toxicol In Vitro. 17(3):301-10.

Tisserand, R. & Young, R. (2014). Essential oil safety a guide for health care professionals (2nd ed.). China: Churchill Livingstone Elsevier.

Tognolini M, Ballabeni V, Bertoni S, Bruni R, Impicciatore M, Barocelli E (2007 Sep). "Protective effect of Foeniculum vulgare essential oil and anethole in an experimental model of thrombosis," Pharmacol Res. 56(3):254-60.

Thompson A. et al (2013). "Comparison of the antibacterial activity of essential oils and extracts of medicinal and culinary herbs to investigate potential new treatments for irritable bowel syndrome," BMC Complement. Altern. Med. 13:338.

Thompson, Dixie L, Rakow, Jennifer, Perdue, Sara M (2004 May). "Relationship between Accumulated Walking and Body Composition in Middle-Aged Women," Med Sci Sports Exerc, 36(5):911-4.

Toda M, Morimoto K (2008 Oct). "Effect of lavender aroma on salivary endocrinological stress markers," Arch. Oral Biol. 53(10):964-968.

Todd J, Friedman M, Patel J, Jaroni D, Ravishankar S (2013 Aug). "The antimicrobial effects of cinnamon leaf oil against multi-drug resistant Salmonella Newport on organic leafy greens," Int. J. Food Microbiol. 166(1):193-199.

Tortora G.J., Funke B.R., Case C.L. Microbiology: An Introduction. 9th ed. San Francisco: Pearson Benjamin Cummings, 2007.

Traka M, Gasper AV, Melchini A, Bacon JR, Needs PW, Frost V, Chantry A, Jones AM, Ortori CA, Barrett DA, Ball RY, Mills RD, Mithen RF (2008 Jul 2). "Broccoli consumption interacts with GSTM1 to perturb oncogenic signalling pathways in the prostate," PLoS One. 3(7):e2568.

Tran KT, Griffith L, Wells A (2004 May-Jun). "palmitoyl-glycyl-histidyl-lysine," Wound Repair Regen. 12(3):262-8.

Trautmann M, Peskar BM, Peskar BA (1991 Aug 16). "Aspirin-like drugs, ethanol-induced rat gastric injury and mucosal eicosanoid release," Eur J Pharmacol. 201(1):53-8.

Trigg JK (1996 Jun). "Evaluation of a eucalyptus-based repellent against Anopheles spp. in Tanzania," J Am Mosq Control Assoc. 12(2 Pt 1):243-6.

Tripathi, P., Tripathi, R., Patel, R. K., & Pancholi, S. S. (2013 Jan). Investigation of antimutagenic potential of Foeniculum vulgare essential oil on cyclophosphamide induced genotoxicity and oxidative stress in mice. Drug Chem Toxicol, 36(1), 35-41.

Trisonthi P, Sato A, Nishiwaki H, Tamura H (2014 May). "A New Diterpene from Litsea cubeba Fruits: Structure Elucidation and Capability to Induce Apoptosis in HeLa Cells," Molecules. 19(5):6838-6850.

Trongtokit Y, Rongsriyam Y, Komalamisra N, Apiwathnasorn C (2005 Apr). "Comparative repellency of 38 essential oils against mosquito bites," Phytother Res. 19(4):303-9.

Trovato, A., Taviano, M. F., Pergolizzi, S., Campolo, L., De Pasquale, R., & Miceli, N. (2010 Apr). Citrus bergamia Risso & Poiteau juice protects against renal injury of diet-induced hypercholesterolemia in rats. Phytother Res, 24(4), 514-519.

Truan JS, Chen JM, Thompson LU (2012). "Comparative effects of sesame seed lignan and flaxseed lignan in reducing the growth of human breast tumors (MCF-7) at high levels of circulating estrogen in athymic mice," Nutr Cancer. 64(1):65-71.

Tsiri, D., Graikou, K., Poblocka-Olech, L., Krauze-Baranowska, M., Spyropoulos, C., & Chinou, I. (2009 Nov). Chemosystematic value of the essential oil composition of Thuja species cultivated in Poland-antimicrobial activity. Molecules, 14(11), 4707-4715.

Tso MOM, Lam TT (1994 Oct 27). "Method of retarding and ameliorating central nervous system and eye damage," University of Illinois: USPatent #5527533.

Tsuda H et al (2004 Aug). "Cancer prevention by natural compounds," Drug Metab. Pharmacokinet. 19(4):245-263.

Tumen, I., Suntar, I., Eller, F. J., Keles, H., & Akkol, E. K. (2013 Jan). Topical wound-healing effects and phytochemical composition of heartwood essential oils of

Juniperus virginiana L., Juniperus occidentalis Hook., and Juniperus ashei J. Buchholz. J Med Food, 16(1), 48-55.

Turley, S.M. (2009). Understanding pharmacology for health professionals (4th ed.). Prentice Hall.

Turrens J.F. (2003) Mitochondrial formation of reactive oxygen species. Journal of Physiology.552: 335-344.

Tuzcu M, Sahin N, Karatepe M, Cikim G, Kilinc U, Sahin K (2008 Sep). "Epigallocatechin-3-gallate supplementation can improve antioxidant status in stressed quail," Br Poult Sci. 49(5):643-8.

Tyagi, A., & Malik, A. (2010). Antimicrobial action of essential oil vapours and negative air ions against Pseudomonas fluorescens. Int J Food Microbiol, 143(3), 205-210.

Tyagi, A. K., & Malik, A. (2012). Bactericidal action of lemon grass oil vapors and negative air ions. Innovative Food Science & Emerging Technologies, 13(0), 169-177.

Tysoe P (2000). "The effect on staff of essential oil burners in extended care settings," Int. J. Nurs. Pract. 6(2):110-112.

Uchida, N., Silva-Filho, S.E., Aguiar, R.P., Wiirzler, L.A.M., Cardia, G.F.E., Cavalcante, H.A.O., Silva-Comar, F.M.S., Becker, T.C.A., Silva E.L., Bersani-Amado, C.A., & Cuman, R.K.N. (2017). "Title: Protective Effect of Cymbopogon citratus Essential Oil in Experimental Model of Acetaminophen-Induced Liver Injury," Am J Chin Med. 45(3):515-532.

Ueno-Iio, T., Shibakura, M., Yokota, K., Aoe, M., Hyoda, T., Shinohata, R., ... Kataoka, M. (2014 Jun). Lavender essential oil inhalation suppresses allergic airway inflammation and mucous cell hyperplasia in a murine model of asthma. Life Sci.

Ulusoy S, Boşgelmez-Tinaz G, Seçilmiş-Canbay H (2009 Nov). "Tocopherol, carotene, phenolic contents and antibacterial properties of rose essential oil, hydrosol and absolute," Curr Microbiol. 59(5):554-8.

Umezu T (2000 Jun). "Behavioral effects of plant-derived essential oils in the geller type conflict test in mice," Jpn J Pharmacol. 83(2):150-3.

Umezu T (1999 Sep). "Anticonflict effects of plant-derived essential oils," Pharmacol Biochem Behav. 64(1):35-40.

Umezu T (2012 Jun). "Evaluation of the Effects of Plant-derived Essential Oils on Central Nervous System Function Using Discrete Shuttle-type Conditioned Avoidance Response in Mice: ESSENTIAL OILS AND AVOIDANCE RESPONSE," Phytother. Res. 26(6):884-891.

Umezu T, Ito H, Nagano K, Yamakoshi M, Oouchi H, Sakaniwa M, Morita M (2002 Nov 22). "Anticonflict effects of rose oil and identification of its active constituents," Life Sci. 72(1):91-102.

Uribe S., Ramirez J., Pena A. (1985) Effects of β-Pinene on Yeast Membrane Functions. Journal of Bacteriology. 161: 1195-1200.

Urso, M. L., & Clarkson, P. M. (2003). Oxidative stress, exercise, and antioxidant supplementation. Toxicology, 189(1), 41-54.

Vakilian K, Atarha M, Bekhradi R, Chaman R (2011 Feb). "Healing advantages of lavender essential oil during episiotomy recovery: a clinical trial," Complement. Ther. Clin. Pract. 17(1):50-53.

Valente J. et al (2013 Dec). "Antifungal, antioxidant and anti-inflammatory activities of Oenanthe crocata L. essential oil," Food Chem. Toxicol. 62:349-354.

Vallianou, I., Peroulis, N., Pantazis, P., & Hadzopoulou-Cladaras, M. (2011 Nov). Camphene, a plant-derived monoterpene, reduces plasma cholesterol and triglycerides in hyperlipidemic rats independently of HMG-CoA reductase activity. PLoS ONE, 6(11), e20516.

Vanderhoof, J.A. (1999). "Lactobacillus GG in the prevention of antibiotic-associated diarrhea in children," The Journal of Pediatrics. 135:564-8.

van Lieshout E.M., Posner G.H., Woodard B.T., Peters W.H. (1998 Mar). "Effects of the sulforaphane analog compound 30, indole-3-carbinol, D-limonene or relafen on glutathione S-transferases and glutathione peroxidase of the rat digestive tract," Biochim. Biophys. 1379(3): 325-336.

van Poppel G, Verhoeven DT, Verhagen H, Goldbohm RA (1999). "Brassica vegetables and cancer prevention. Epidemiology and mechanisms," Adv Exp Med Biol. 472:159-68.

van Tol RW, Swarts HJ, van der Linden A, Visser JH (2007 May). "Repellence of the red bud borer Resseliella oculiperda from grafted apple trees by impregnation of rubber budding strips with essential oils," Pest Manag Sci. 63(5):483-90.

Van Vuuren S.F., Kamatou G.P.P., Viljoen A.M (2010 Oct). "Volatile composition and antimicrobial activity of twenty commercial frankincense essential oil samples," South African Journal of Botany. 76(4):686-691.

Varga J, Jimenez SA (1986 Jul 31). "Stimulation of normal human fibroblast collagen production and processing by transforming growth factor-beta," Biochem Biophys Res Commun. 138(2):974-80.

Vazquez JA, Arganoza MT, Boikov D, Akins RA, Vaishampayan JK (2000 Jun). "In vitro susceptibilities of Candida and Aspergillus species to Melaleuca alternafolia (tea tree) oil," Rev Iberoam Micol. 17(2):60-3.

Velaga, M. K., Yallapragada, P. R., Williams, D., Rajanna, S., & Bettaiya, R. (2014 Jun). Hydroalcoholic Seed Extract of Coriandrum sativum (Coriander) Alleviates Lead-Induced Oxidative Stress in Different Regions of Rat Brain. Biol Trace Elem Res, 159(1-3), 351-363.

Venegas C, Cabrera-Vique C, Garcia-Corzo L, Escames G, Acuna-Castroviejo D, Lopez LC (2011 Nov). "Determination of coenzyme Q10, coenzyme Q9, and melatonin contents in virgin argan oils: comparison with other edible vegetable oils," J Agric Food Chem. 59(22):12102-8.

Veratti E, Rossi T, Giudice S, Benassi L, Bertazzoni G, Morini D, Azzoni P, Bruni E, Giannnetti A, MaqnoniC. (2011 Jun). "18beta-glycyrrhetinic acid and glabridin pre-

Appendix

vent oxidative DNA fragmentation in UVB-irradiated human keratinocyte cultures," Anticancer Res. 31(6):2209-15.

Verma, S. K., Jain, V., & Katewa, S. S. (2009 Dec). Blood pressure lowering, fibrinolysis enhancing and antioxidant activities of cardamom (Elettaria cardamomum). Indian J Biochem Biophys, 46(6), 503-506.

Vertuani S, Angusti A, Manfredini S (2004). "The antioxidants and pro-antioxidants network: an overview," Curr Pharm Des. 10(14):1677–94.

Vigo E, Cepeda A, Gualillo O, Perez-Fernandez R (2005 Mar). "In-vitro anti-inflammatory activity of Pinus sylvestris and Plantago lanceolata extracts: effect on inducible NOS, COX-1, COX-2 and their products in J774A.1 murine macrophages," J Pharm Pharmacol. 57(3):383-91.

Victor Antony Santiago J, Jayachitra J, Shenbagam M, Nalini N (2012 Feb). "Dietary d-limonene alleviates insulin resistance and oxidative stress-induced liver injury in high-fat diet and L-NAME-treated rats," Eur. J. Nutr. 51(1):57-68.

Vigo E, Cepeda A, Gualillo O, Perez-Fernandez R (2004 Feb). "In-vitro anti-inflammatory effect of Eucalyptus globulus and Thymus vulgaris: nitric oxide inhibition in J774A.1 murine macrophages," J Pharm Pharmacol. 56(2):257-63.

Vigushin DM, Poon GK, Boddy A, English J, Halbert GW, Pagonis C, Jarman M, Coombes RC (1998). "Phase I and pharmacokinetic study of D-limonene in patients with advanced cancer. Cancer Research Campaign Phase I/II Clinical Trials Committee," Cancer Chemother Pharmacol. 42(2):111-7.

Villareal MO, Ikeya A, Sasaki K, Arfa AB, Neffatic M, Isoda H (2017 Dec 22). "Anti-stress and neuronal cell differentiation induction effects of rosmarinus officinalis l. essential oil," BMC Complement Altern Med. 17(1):549.

Votava-Rai A. et al (2003). "ACTA DERMATOVENEROLOGICA CROATICA".

Vujosević M, Blagojević J (2004). "Antimutagenic effects of extracts from sage (Salvia officinalis) in mammalian system in vivo," Acta Vet Hung. 52(4):439-43.

Vuković-Gacić B, Nikcević S, Berić-Bjedov T, Knezević-Vukcević J, Simić D (2006 Oct). "Antimutagenic effect of essential oil of sage (Salvia officinalis L.) and its monoterpenes against UV-induced mutations in Escherichia coli and Saccharomyces cerevisiae," Food Chem Toxicol. 44(10):1730-8.

Vutyavanich T, Kraisarin T, Ruangsri R (2001 Apr). "Ginger for nausea and vomiting in pregnancy: randomized, double-masked, placebo-controlled trial," Obstet Gynecol. 97(4):577-82.

Walker AF, Bundy R, Hicks SM, Middleton RW (2002 Dec). "Bromelain reduces mild acute knee pain and improves well-being in a dose-dependent fashion in an open study of otherwise healthy adults," Phytomedicine. 9(8):681-6.

Walker TB, Smith J, Herrera M, Lebegue B, Pinchak A, Fischer J (2010 Oct). "The influence of 8 weeks of whey-protein and leucine supplementation on physical and cognitive performance," Int J Sport Nutr Exerc Metab. 20(5):409-17.

Wallerius S, Rosmond R, Ljung T, Holm G, Björntorp P (2003 Jul). "Rise in morning saliva cortisol is associated with abdominal obesity in men: a preliminary report," J Endocrinol Invest. 26(7):616-9. Walter BM, Bilkei G (2004 Mar 15). "Immunostimulatory effect of dietary oregano etheric oils on lymphocytes from growth-retarded, low-weight growing-finishing pigs and productivity," Tijdschr Diergeneeskd. 129(6):178-81.

Wang H, Liu Y (2010 Jan). "Chemical composition and antibacterial activity of essential oils from different parts of Litsea cubeba," Chem. Biodivers. 7(1):229-235.

Wang, K., & Su, C. Y. (2000 Oct). Pharmacokinetics and disposition of beta-elemene in rats. Yao Xue Xue Bao, 35(10), 725-728.

Wang, L., Li, W. G., Huang, C., Zhu, M. X., Xu, T. L., Wu, D. Z., & Li, Y. (2012 Nov). Subunit-specific inhibition of glycine receptors by curcumol. J Pharmacol Exp Ther, 343(2), 371-379.

Wang L. et al (2017 Dec). "Analysis of the main active ingredients and bioactivities of essential oil from Osmanthus fragrans Var. thunbergii using a complex network approach," BMC Syst Biol. 11.

Wang, W., Zu, Y., Fu, Y., Reichling, J., Suschke, U., Nokemper, S., & Zhang, Y. (2009 Feb). In vitro antioxidant, antimicrobial and anti-herpes simplex virus type 1 activity of Phellodendron amurense Rupr. from China. Am J Chin Med, 37(1), 195-203.

Wang, Y.W., Zeng, W.C., Xu, P.Yp., Lan, Y.J., Zhu, R.X., Zhong, K., Huang, Y.N., and Gao, H. (2012). "Chemical composition and antimicrobial activity of the essential oil of kumquat peel," Int J Molecular Sci. 13:3382-3393.

Warskulat U, Brookmann S, Felsner I, Brenden H, Grether-Beck S, Haussinger D (2008 Dec). "Ultraviolet A induces transport of compatible organic osmolytes in human derman fibroblasts," Exp Dermatol. 17(12):1031-6.

Warskulat U, Reinen A, Grether-Beck S, Krutmann J, Haussinger D (2004 Sep). "The osmolyte strategy of normal human keratinocyts in maintaining cell homeostasis," J Invest Dermatol. 123(3):516-21.

Watanabe, S., Hara, K., Ohta, K., Iino, H., Miyajima, M., Matsuda, A., ... Matsushima, E. (2013 Jan). Aroma helps to preserve information processing resources of the brain in healthy subjects but not in temporal lobe epilepsy. Seizure, 22(1), 59-63.

Weaver CM, Martin BR, Jackson GS, McCabe GP, Nolan JR, McCabe LD, Barnes S, Reinwald S, Boris ME, Peacock M (2009 Oct). "Antiresorptive effects of phytoestrogen supplements compared with estradiol or risedronate in postmenopausal women using (41)Ca methodology," J Clin Endocrinol Metab. 94(10):3798-805.

Weaver R.F. Molecular Biology. 4th ed. New York: McGraw Hill, 2008.

Wee, JJ, Park, KM, Chug A (2011). "Biological Activities of Ginseng and Its Application to Human Health," Herbal Medicine: Biomolecular and Clinical Aspects. 2nd ed.

Wei A, Shibamoto T (2007). "Antioxidant activities of essential oil mixtures toward skin lipid squalene oxidized by UV irradiation," Cutan Ocul Toxicol. 26(3):227-33.

Whitehouse PJ, Rajcan JL, Sami SA, Patterson MB, Smyth KA, Edland SD, George DR (2006 Oct). "ADCS Prevention Instrument Project: pilot testing of a book club

as a psychosocial intervention and recruitment and retention strategy," Alzheimer Dis Assoc Disord, 20(4 Suppl 3):S203-8.

Wierniuk, A., & Wlodarek, D. (2013). Estimation of energy and nutritional intake of young men practicing aerobic sports. Rocz Panstw Zakl Hig, 64(2), 143-148.

Wiig, H., & Swartz, M. A. (2012). Interstitial fluid and lymph formation and transport: physiological regulation and roles in inflammation and cancer. Physiological Reviews, 92(3), 1005-1060.

Wilkinson JM, Hipwell M, Ryan T, Cavanagh HM (2003 Jan 1). "Bioactivity of Backhousia citriodora: antibacterial and antifungal activity," J Agric Food Chem. 51(1):76-81.

Wilkinson S, Aldridge J, Salmon I, Cain E, Wilson B (1999 Sep). "An evaluation of aromatherapy massage in palliative care," Palliat Med. 13(5):409-17.

Wilkinson, S. M., Love, S. B., Westcombe, A. M., Gambles, M. A., Burgess, C. C., Cargill, A., . . . Ramirez, A. J. (2007 Feb). Effectiveness of aromatherapy massage in the management of anxiety and depression in patients with cancer: a multicenter randomized controlled trial. Journal of Clinical Oncology, 25(5), 532-539.

Wille JJ, Kydonieus A (2003 May-Jun). "Palmitoleic acid isomer (c15:1delta6) in human skin sebum is effective against gram-positive bacteria," Ski Pharmacol Appl Skin Physiol. 16(3):176-87.

Williams R.M. (2004 Apr). "Fragrance Alters Mood and Brain Chemistry," Townsend Lett. Dr. Patients. 249:36-38

Williamson EM, Priestley CM, Burgess IF (2007 Dec). "An investigation and comparison of the bioactivity of selected essential oils on human lice and house dust mites," Fitoterapia. 78(7-8):521-5.

Winkler-Stuck K, Wiedemann FR, Wallesch CW, Kunz WS (2004 May 15). "Effect of coenzyme Q10 on the mitochondrial function of skin fibroblasts from Parkinson patients," J Neurol Sci. 220(1-2):41-8.

Witvrouw E, Danneels L, Asselman P, D'Have T, Cambier D (2003). "Muscle flexibility as a risk factor for developing muscle injuries in male professional soccer players. A prospective study," Am J Sports Med, 31(1):41-46.

Woelk H, Schläfke S (2010 Feb). "A multi-center, double-blind, randomised study of the Lavender oil preparation Silexan in comparison to Lorazepam for generalized anxiety disorder." Phytomedicine. 17 (2):94-9.

Woodruff J (2002 Mar). "Improving Hair Strength," Cosm Toil. :33-5.

Woollard A.C., Tatham K.C., Barker S (2007 Jun). "The influence of essential oils on the process of wound healing: a review of the current evidence," J. Wound Care. 16(6):255-257.

Wu LL, Wang KM, Liao PI, Kao YH, Huang YC (2015 Jul). "Effects of an 8-Week Outdoor Brisk Walking Program on Fatigue in Hi-Tech Industry Employees: A Randomized Control Trial," Workplace Health Saf.

Wu Y. et al (2012). "The metabolic responses to aerial diffusion of essential oils," PloS One. 7(9):e44830.

Xia L, Chen D, Han R, Fang Q, Waxman S, Jing Y (2005 Mar). "Boswellic acid acetate induces apoptosis through caspase-mediated pathways in myeloid leukemia cells," Mol Cancer Ther. 4(3):381-8.

Xiao D, Powolny AA, Barbi de Moura M, Kelley EE, Bommareddy A, Kim SH, Hahm ER, Normolle D, Van Houten B, Singh SV (2010 Jun 22). "Phenethyl isothiocyanate inhibits oxidative phosphorylation to trigger reactive oxygen species-mediated death of human prostate cancer cells," J Biol Chem Epub ahead of print. Epub ahead of print.

Xie P, Lu J, Wan H, Hao Y (2010 Aug). "Effect of toothpaste containing d-limonene on natural extrinsic smoking stain: a 4-week clinical trial," Am. J. Dent. 23(4):196-200.

Xiufen W, Hiramatsu N, Matsubara M (2004). "The antioxidative activity of traditional Japanese herbs," Biofactors. 21(1-4):281-4.

Xu F. et al (2008 Oct). "Pharmaco-physio-psychologic effect of Ayurvedic oil-dripping treatment using an essential oil from Lavendula angustifolia," J. Altern. Complement. Med. N. Y. N. 14(8):947-956.

Xu, J., Guo, Y., Zhao, P., Xie, C., Jin, D. Q., Hou, W., & Zhang, T. (2011 Dec). Neuroprotective cadinane sesquiterpenes from the resinous exudates of Commiphora myrrha. Fitoterapia, 82(8), 1198-1201.

Xu J., Zhou F., Ji B-P., Pei R-S., Xu N. (2008) The antibacterial mechanism of carvacrol and thymol against Escherichia coli. Letters in Applied Microbiology. 47: 174-179.

Xu, P., Wang, K., Lu, C., Dong, L., Gao, L., Yan, M., Aibai, S., Yang, Y., & Liu, X. (2017). "The Protective Effect of Lavender Essential Oil and Its Main Component Linalool against the Cognitive Deficits Induced by D-Galactose and Aluminum Trichloride in Mice," Evid Based Complement Alternat Med. 2017:7426538.

Xu X, Duncan AM, Merz BE, Kurzer MS (1998 Dec). "Effects of soy isoflavones on estrogen and phytoestrogen metabolism in premenopausal women," Cancer Epidemiol Biomarkers Prev. 7(12):1101-8.

Xu X, Duncan AM, Wangen KE, Kurzer MS (2000 Aug). "Soy consumption alters endogenous estrogen metabolism in postmenopausal women," Cancer Epidemiol biomarkers Prev. 9(8):781-6.

Yamada, K., Mimaki, Y., & Sashida, Y. (2005 Feb). Effects of inhaling the vapor of Lavandula burnatii super-derived essential oil and linalool on plasma adrenocorticotropic hormone (ACTH), catecholamine and gonadotropin levels in experimental menopausal female rats. Biol Pharm Bull, 28(2), 378-379.

Yamaguchi M, Tahara Y, Kosaka S (2009 Oct). "Influence of concentration of fragrances on salivary alphaamylase," Int. J. Cosmet. Sci. 31(5):391-395.

Yan, H., Sun, X., Sun, S., Wang, S., Zhang, J., Wang, R., ... Kang, W. (2011 Jun). Anti-ultraviolet radiation effects of Coptis chinensis and Phellodendron amurense glycans by immunomodulating and inhibiting oxidative injury. Int J Biol Macromol, 48(5), 720-725.

Yang E.J., Kim, S.S., Moon, Y.J., Oh, T.H., Baik, J.S., Lee, N.H., and Hyun, C.G. (2010). "Inhibitory effects of Fortunella japonica var. margarita and Citrus sunki essential oils on nitric oxide production and skin pathogens," Acta Microbiol Immunol Hung. 57(1):15-27.

Yang F. et al. (2005 Feb 18). "Curcumin inhibits formation of amyloid beta oligomers and fibrils, binds plaques, and reduces amyloid in vivo," J Biol Chem. 280(7):5892-901.

Yang GY, Wang W (1994 Sep). "Clinical studies on the treatment of coronary heart disease with Valeriana officinalis var latifolia," Zhongguo Zhong Xi Yi Jie He Za Zhi. 14(9):540-2.

Yang L, Hao J, Zhang J (2009). "Ginsenoside Rg3 promotes beta-amyloid peptide degradation by enhancing gene expression of neprilysin," J Pharm Pharmacol. 61:375-80.

Yang SA, Jeon SK, Lee EJ, Im NK, Jhee KH, Lee SP, Lee IS (2009 May). "Radical Scavenging Activity of the Essential Oil of Silver Fir (Abies alba)," J Clin Biochem Nutr. 44(3):253-9.

Yang SA, Jeon SK, Lee EJ, Shim CH, Lee IS (2010 Jan). "Comparative study of the chemical composition and antioxidant activity of six essential oils and their components," Nat. Prod. Res. 24(2):140-151.

Yano H, Tatsuta M, Iishi H, Baba M, Sakai N, Uedo N (1999 Aug). "Attenuation by d-limonene of sodium chloride-enhanced gastric carcinogenesis induced by N-methyl-N'-nitro-N-nitrosoguanidine in Wistar rats," Int. J. Cancer. 82(5):665-668.

Yap, P. S., Krishnan, T., Yiap, B. C., Hu, C. P., Chan, K. G., & Lim, S. H. (2014 May). Membrane disruption and anti-quorum sensing effects of synergistic interaction between Lavandula angustifolia (lavender oil) in combination with antibiotic against plasmid-conferred multi-drug-resistant Escherichia coli. J Appl Microbiol, 116(5), 1119-1128.

Yates, D. (2014). Study: Many in U.S. have poor nutrition, with the disabled doing worst [Press release]. Retrieved from http://news.illinois.edu/news/14/1023DisabledNutrition_RuopengAn.html

Yavari Kia, P., Safajou, F., Shahnazi, M., & Nazemiyeh, H. (2014 Mar). The effect of lemon inhalation aromatherapy on nausea and vomiting of pregnancy: a double-blinded, randomized, controlled clinical trial. Iran Red Crescent Med J, 16(3).

Yazdanparast R, Shahriyary L (2008 Jan). "Comparative effects of Artemisia dracunculus, Satureja hortensis and Origanum majorana on inhibition of blood platelet adhesion, aggregation and secretion," Vascul Pharmacol. 48(1):32-7.

Yazdkhasti, M., & Pirak, A. (2016 Nov.). "The effect of aromatherapy with lavender essence on severity of labor pain and duration of labor in primiparous women," Complement Ther Clin Pract. 25:81-86.

Yiengprugsawan, V., Banwell, C., Takeda, W., Dixon, J., Seubsman, S. A., & Sleigh, A. C. (2015). Health, Happiness and Eating Together: What Can a Large Thai Cohort Study Tell Us? Glob J Health Sci, 7(4), 270-277.

Yip YB, Tam AC. (2008 Jun). "An experimental study on the effectiveness of massage with aromatic ginger and orange essential oil for moderate-to-severe knee pain among the elderly in Hong Kong," Complement Ther Med. 16(3):131-8.

Yip YB, Tse S. H. M. (2006 Feb). "An experimental study on the effectiveness of acupressure with aromatic lavender essential oil for sub-acute, non-specific neck pain in Hong Kong," Complement. Ther. Clin. Pract. 12(1):18-26.

Yip YB, Tse S. H. M. (2004 Mar). "The effectiveness of relaxation acupoint stimulation and acupressure with aromatic lavender essential oil for non-specific low back pain in Hong Kong: a randomised controlled trial," Complement. Ther. Med. 12(1):28-37.

Yoo, C. B., Han, K. T., Cho, K. S., Ha, J., Park, H. J., Nam, J. H., . . . Lee, K. T. (2005 Jul). Eugenol isolated from the essential oil of Eugenia caryophyllata induces a reactive oxygen species-mediated apoptosis in HL-60 human promyelocytic leukemia cells. Cancer Lett, 225(1), 41-52.

Yoshizaki N, Hashizume R, Masaki H. (2017 Jun). "A polymethoxyflavone mixture extracted from orange peels, mainly containing nobiletin, 3,3',4',5,6,7,8-heptamethoxyflavone and tangeretin, suppresses melanogenesis through the acidification of cell organelles, including melanosomes," J Dermatol Sci. S0923-1811(16)31097-0.

Yosipovitch G, Szolar C, Hui X.Y., Maibach H (1996 May). "Effect of topically applied menthol on thermal, pain and itch sensations and biophysical properties of the skin," Arch. Dermatol. Res. 288(5-6):245-248.

Youdim KA, Deans SG (1999 Sep 8). "Dietary supplementation of thyme (Thymus vulgaris L.) essential oil during the lifetime of the rat: its effects on the antioxidant status in liver, kidney and heart tissues," Mech Ageing Dev. 109(3):163-75.

Youdim KA, Deans SG (2000 Jan). "Effect of thyme oil and thymol dietary supplementation on the antioxidant status and fatty acid composition of the ageing rat brain," Br J Nutr. 83(1):87-93.

Youn L.J., Yoon J.W., Hovde C.J. (2010) A Brief Overview of Escherichia coli O157:H7 and Its Plasmid O157. Journal of Microbiology and Biotechnology. 20: 1-10.

Younis F, Mirelman D, Rabinkov A, Rosenthal T (2010 Jun). "S-allyl-mercapto-captopril: a novel compound in the treatment of Cohen-Rosenthal diabetic hypertensive rats," J Clin Hypertens (Greenwich) 12(6):451-5.

Yu B.P. (1994) Cellular Defenses Against Damage From Reactive Oxygen Species. Physiological Reviews. 74: 139-162.

Yu D, Wang J, Shao X, Xu F, Wang H (2015 Nov). "Antifungal modes of action of tea tree oil and its two characteristic components against Botrytis cinerea," J. Appl. Microbiol. 119(5):1253-1262.

Yu YM, Chang WC, Wu CH, Chiang SY (2005 Nov). "Reduction of oxidative stress and apoptosis in hyperlipidemic rabbits by ellagic acid," J Nutr Biochem. 16(11):675-81.

Yu Z, Wang R, Xu L, Xie S, Dong J, Jing Y (2011 Jan 25). "β-Elemene piperazine derivatives induce apoptosis in human leukemia cells through downregulation of c-FLIP and generation of ROS," PLos One 6(1)e15843.

Yuan HQ, Kong F, Wang XL, Young CY, Hu XY, Liu HX (2008 Jun 1). "Inhibitory effect of acetyl-11-keto-beta-boswellic acid on androgen receptor by interference of Sp1 binding activity in prostate cancer cells," Biochem Pharmacol. 75(11):2112-21.

Yuan YV, Walsh NA (2006 Jul). "Antioxidant and antiproliferative activities of extracts from a variety of edible seaweeds," Food Chem Toxicol. 44(7):1144-50.

Yüce, A., Turk, G., Ceribasi, S., Guvenc, M., Ciftci, M., Sonmez, M., . . . Aksakal, M. (2014 Apr). Effectiveness of cinnamon (Cinnamomum zeylanicum) bark oil in the prevention of carbon tetrachloride-induced damages on the male reproductive system. Andrologia, 46(3), 263-272.

Yue G.G.L. et al (2012 Mar). "The Role of Turmerones on Curcumin Transportation and P-Glycoprotein Activities in Intestinal Caco-2 Cells," J. Med. Food. 15(3):242-252.

Yue G.G.L. et al (2010 Aug). "Evaluation of in vitro anti-proliferative and immunomodulatory activities of compounds isolated from Curcuma longa," Food Chem. Toxicol. 48(8-9):2011-2020.

Yun, J. (2014 Jan). Limonene inhibits methamphetamine-induced locomotor activity via regulation of 5-HT neuronal function and dopamine release. Phytomedicine. Retrieved from http://dx.doi.org/10.1016/j.phymed.2013.12.004

Zabirunnisa M, Gadagi J.S., Gadde P, Myla N, Koneru J, Thatimatla C (2014 Jul). "Dental patient anxiety: Possible deal with Lavender fragrance," J. Res. Pharm. Pract. 3(3):100-103.

Zaim, A., Benjelloun, M., El Harchli, E.H., Farah, A., Meni Mahzoum, A., Alaoui Mhamdi, M., and El Ghadraoui, L. (2015). "Chemical Composition And Acrididcid Properties Of The Morrocan Tanacetum Annuum L. Essential Oils," Int J Eng and Sci. 5(5):13-19.

Zeidán-Chuliá F. et al (2012 Jun). "Bioinformatical and in vitro approaches to essential oil-induced matrix metalloproteinase inhibition," Pharm. Biol. 50(6):675-686.

Zembron-Lacny A, Szyszka K, Szygula Z (2007 Dec). "Effect of cysteine derivatives administration in healthy men exposed to intense resistance exercise by evaluation of pro-antioxidant ratio," J Physiol Sci. 57(6):343-8.

Zha C., Brown G.B., Brouillette W.J. (2004) Synthesis and Structure-Activity Relationship Studies for Hydantoins and Analogues as Voltage-Gasted Sodium Channel Ligands. Journal of Medicinal Chemistry. 47: 6519-6528.

Zhan L. et al (2012 Jul). "Effects of Xylitol Wipes on Cariogenic Bacteria and Caries in Young Children," J. Dent. Res. 91(7):S85-S90.

Zhao J, Zhang J, Yang B, Lv GP, Li SP (2010 Oct). "Free Radical Scavenging Activity and Characterization of Sesquiterpenoids in Four Species of Curcuma Using a TLC Bioautography Assay and GC-MS Analysis," Molecules. 15(11):7547-7557.

Zhang, J., Kang, M. J., Kim, M. J., Kim, M. E., Song, J. H., Lee, Y. M., & Kim, J. I. (2008 Jan). Pancreatic lipase inhibitory activity of taraxacum officinale in vitro and in vivo. Nutr Res Pract, 2(4), 200-203.

Zhang, L.L., Lv, S., Xu, J.G., and Xhang, L.F. (2017) "Influence of drying methods on chemical compositions, antioxidant and antibacterial activity of essential oil from lemon peel," Natural Product Research. 0(0):1-5.

Zhang, R., Wang, B., Zhao, H., Wei, C., Yuan, G., & Guo, R. (2009). Tissue distribution of curcumol in rats after intravenous injection of zedoary turmeric oil fat emulsion. Asian Journal of Pharmacodynamics and Pharmacokinetics, 1608, 51-57.

Zhang W, Wang X, Liu Y, Tian H, Flickinger B, Empie MW, Sun SZ (2008 Jun). "Dietary flaxseed lignan extract lowers plasma cholesterol and glucose concentrations in hypercholesterolaemic subjects," Br J Nutr. 99(6):1301-9.

Zhang X, Zhang Y, Li Y (2013 Aug). "Beta-element decreases cell invasion by upregulating E-cadherin expression in MCF-7 human breast cancer cells," Oncol Rep. 30(2):745-50.

Zhang X-Z., Wang L, Liu D.W., Tang G.Y., Zhang H.Y. (2014 Sep). "Synergistic inhibitory effect of berberine and d-limonene on human gastric carcinoma cell line MGC803," J. Med. 17(9):955-962.

Zhang Z, Li Y, Zhang Y, Song J, Wang Q, Zheng L, Liu D. (2013). "Beta-element blocks epithelial mesenchymal transition in human breast cancer cell line MCF-7 through Smad3-mediated down-regulation of nuclear transcription factors," PLoS One 8(3):e58719.

Zhang, Z., Liu, X., Zhang, X., Liu, J., Hao, Y., Yang, X., & Wang, Y. (2011 May). Comparative evaluation of the antioxidant effects of the natural vitamin C analog 2-O-beta-D-glucopyranosyl-L-ascorbic acid isolated from Goji berry fruit. Arch Pharm Res, 34(5), 801-810.

Zhao W, Entschladen F, Liu H, Niggemann B, Fang Q, Zaenker KS, Han R (2003). "Boswellic acid acetate induces differentiation and apoptosis in highly metastatic melanoma and fibrosarcoma cells," Cancer Detect Prev. 27(1):67-75.

Zheng GQ, Kenney PM, Lam LK. (1992 Aug). "Anethofuran, carvone, and limonene: potential cancer chemopreventive agents from dill weed oil and caraway oil," Planta Med. 58(4):338-41.

Zheng GQ, Kenney PM, Zhang J, Lam LK (1993). "Chemoprevention of benzo[a]pyrene-induced forestomach cancer in mice by natural phthalides from celery seed oil," Nutr Cancer. 19(1):77-86.

Zhou BR, Luo D, Wei FD, Chen XE, Gao J (2008 Jul). "Baicalin protects human fibroblasts against ultraviolet B-induced cyclobutane pyrimidine dimers formation," Arch Dermatol Res. 300(6):331-4.

Appendix

Zhou J, Ma X, Qiu BH, Chen J, Bian L, Pan L (2013 Jan). "Parameters optimization of supercritical fluid-CO2 extracts of frankincense using response surface methodology and its pharmacodynamics effects," J Sep Sci. 36(2):383-390.

Zhou, J., Tang F., Bian R. (2004) Effect of α-pinene on nuclear translocation of NF-κB in THP-1 cells. Acta Pharmacol Sin. 25: 480-484.

Zhou J, Zhou S, Tang J, Zhang K, Guang L, Huang Y, Xu Y, Ying Y, Zhang L, Li D (2009 Mar 15). "Protective effect of berberine on beta cells in streptozotocin- and high-carbohydrate/high-fat diet-induced diabetic rats," Eur J Pharmacol. 606(1-3):262-8.

Zhou W, Fukumoto S, Yokogoshi H (2009 Apr). "Components of lemon essential oil attenuate dementia induced by scopolamine," Nutr. Neurosci. 12(2):57-64.

Zhou, X. M., Zhao, Y., He, C. C., & Li, J. X. (2012 Feb). Preventive effects of Citrus reticulata essential oil on bleomycin-induced pulmonary fibrosis in rats and the mechanism. Zhong Xi Yi Jie He Xue Bao, 10(2), 200-209.

Zhu BC, Henderson G, Chen F, Fei H, Laine RA (2001 Aug). "Evaluation of vetiver oil and seven insect-active essential oils against the Formosan subterranean termite," J Chem Ecol. 27(8):1617-25.

Zhu BC, Henderson G, Yu Y, Laine RA (2003 Jul 30). "Toxicity and repellency of patchouli oil and patchouli alcohol against Formosan subterranean termites Coptotermes formosanus Shiraki (Isoptera: Rhinotermitidae)," J Agric Food Chem. 51(16):4585-8

Zhu JS, Halpern GM, Jones K (1998). "The scientific rediscovery of a precious ancient Chinese herbal regimen: Cordyceps sinensis. Part I," J Altern Complement Med. 4:289-303.

Ziegler D, Ametov A, Barinov A, Dyck PJ, Gurieva I, Low PA, Munzel U, Yakhno N, Raz I, Novosadova M, Maus J, Samigullin R (2006 Nov). "Oral treatment with alpha-lipoic acid improves symptomatic diabetic polyneuropathy: the SYDNEY 2 trial," Diabetes Care. 29(11):2365-70.

Ziegler G, Ploch M, Miettinen-Baumann A, Collet W (2002 Nov 25). "Efficacy and tolerability of valerian extract LI 156 compared with oxazepam in the treatment of non-organic insomnia--a randomized, double-blind, comparative clinical study," Eur J Med Res. 7(11):480-6.

Zore G.B., Thakre A.D., Jadhav S., Karuppayil S.M. (2011) Terpenoids inhibit Candida albicans growth by affecting membrane integrity and arrest of cell cycle. Phytomedicine. doi: 10.1016/j.phymed.2011.03.008.

Zou B, Li QQ, Zhao J, Li JM, Cuff CF, Reed E (2013 Mar). "Beta-Elemene and taxanes synergistically induce cytotoxicity and inhibit proliferation in ovarian cancer and other tumor cells," Anticancer Res. 33(3):929-40.

Zu Y. et al (2010 Apr). "Activities of Ten Essential Oils towards Propionibacterium acnes and PC-3, A-549 and MCF-7 Cancer Cells," Molecules. 15(5):3200-3210.

Bibliography

Balch, M.D., James, and Phyllis Balch, C.N.C. *Prescription for Nutritional Healing.* Garden City Park, NY: Avery Publishing Group, 1990.

Başer, Kemal Hüsnü Can & Gerhard Buchbauer. *Handbook of Essential Oils: Science, Technology, and Applications.* Florida: CRC Press, 2010. Print.

Bear, M. F., Connors, B. W., Paradiso, M. A. (2007). Neuroscience: Exploring the Brain (3rd ed.). Baltimore, MD: Lippincott Williams & Wilkins.

Bendich, A., & Deckelbaum, R. J. (Eds.). (2010). Preventive Nutrition: The Comprehensive Guide for Health Professionals (4th ed.). New York, NY: Springer Science & Business Media.

Berg, J. M., Tymoczko, J. L., Stryer, L. (2002). Biochemistry (Section 30.2, Each Organ Has a Unique Metabolic Profile) (5th ed.). New York, NY: W H Freeman.

Becker, M.D., Robert O. *The Body Electric.* New York, NY: Wm. Morrow, 1985.

Brown, J. E. (1991). Everywoman's Guide to Nutrition. Minneapolis, MN: University of Minnesota Press.

Brown T.L., LeMay H.E., Bursten B.E. *Chemistry: The Central Science. 10th ed.* Upper Saddle River: Pearson Prentice Hall, 2006.

Burroughs, Stanley. *Healing for the Age of Enlightenment.* Auburn, CA: Burroughs Books, 1993.

Burton Goldberg Group, The. *Alternative Medicine: The Definitive Guide.* Fife, WA: Future Medicine Publishing, Inc., 1994.

Can Baser, K Husnu, Buchbauer, Gerhard. Handbood of Essential Oils: Science Technology, and Applications. Boca Raton, FL: Taylor & Francis Group, 2010.

Carter, Howard. *The Tomb of Tutankhamen.* Washington, D.C.: National Geographic Society, 2003. Print.

Chemical Engineering Research Trends. (2007). (L. P. Berton Ed.). New York, New York: Nova Science Publishers, Inc.

Chevallier, Andrew. *Encyclopedia of Herbal Medicine*, 2nd Ed.. New York, NY: Dorling Kindersley Limited, 2000.

"Chilblains." Mayo Clinic, Mayo Foundation for Medical Education and Research, 17 Aug. 2017.

Clark, Micheal A; Sutton, Brian G; and Lucett, Scott C. *NASM Essentials of Personal Fitness Training.* Burlington, MA: Jones & Bartlett Learning, 2014.

Clark, Micheal A; Lucett, Scott C; and Sutton, Brian G. *NASM Essentials of Corrective Exercise Training.* Burlington, MA: Jones & Bartlett Learning, 2014.

Cowan M.K., Talaro K.P. *Microbiology: A Systems Approach. 2nd ed.* New York: McGraw Hill, 2009.

Fischer-Rizzi, Suzanne. *Complete Aromatherapy Handbook.* New York, NY: Sterling Publishing, 1990.

Gattefosse, Rene-Maurice. *Gattefosse's Aromatherapy.* Essex, England: The C.W. Daniel Company Ltd., 1937 English translation.

Gawronski, Donald. *Medical Choices.* Lincoln, Nebraska: Authors Choice Press, 2002. Print.

Guyton A.C., Hall J.E. *Textbook of Medical Physiology. 10th ed.* Philadelphia: W.B. Saunders Company, 2000.

Green, Mindy. *Natural Perfumes: Simple Aromatherapy Recipes.* Loveland CO: Interweave Press Inc., 1999.

Hill, David K. *Frankincense.* Spanish Fork, UT: AromaTools, 2010.

Integrated Aromatic Medicine. Proceedings from the First International Symposium, Grasse, France. Essential Science Publishing, March 2000.

Kraak, V. I., Liverman, C. T., & Koplan, J. P. (Eds.). (2005). Preventing Childhood Obesity: Health in the Balance. Washington, DC: National Academies Press.

Keville, Kathi. "A History of Fragrance." Healthy.net. 1995. Web. 9 Aug. 2012.

Lis-Balchin, Maria. *Aromatherapy Science: A Guide for Healthcare Professionals.* London, UK: Pharmaceutical Press, 2006.

Lawless, Julia. *The Encyclopaedia of Essential Oils.* Rockport, MA: Element, Inc., 1992.

L. H. Bailey and E. Z. Bailey, Hortus Third: A Concise Dictionary of Plants Cultivated in the United States and Canada, 1 edition. New York: Macmillan, 1976.

Maughan, R. J., Burke L. M. (Eds.). (2002). Sports Nutrition: Handbook of Sports Medicine and Science. Bodmin, England: Blackwell Science Publishing.

Maury, Marguerite. *Marguerite Maury's Guide to Aromatherapy.* C.W. Daniel, 1989.

McArdle, William D.; Katch, Frank I.; and Katch, Victor L. *Exercise Physiology: Nutrition, Energy, and Human Performance, Eighth Edition.* Baltimore, MD: Wolters Kluwer Health, 2015.

Muscolino, Joseph E. Kinesiology: *The Skeletal System and Muscle Function, 2nd Edition.* St. Louis, MO: Elsevier Mosby, 2011.

Pènoël, M.D., Daniel and Pierre Franchomme. L'aromatherapie exactement. Limoges, France: Jollois, 1990.

Petrovska, Biljana Bauer. "Historical Review of Medicinal Plants' Usage." *Pharmacognosy Reviews* 2012 (6:11): 1–5. Print.

Porter, Stephen. *The Great Plague.* Stroud, Gloucestershire: Amberly Publishing, 2009. Print.

Price, Shirley, and Len Price. *Aromatherapy for Health Professionals.* New York, NY: Churchill Livingstone Inc., 1995.

Price, Shirley, and Penny Price Parr. *Aromatherapy for Babies and Children.* San Francisco, CA: Thorsons, 1996.

Rose, Jeanne. *375 Essential Oils and Hydrosols.* Berkeley, CA: North Atlantic Books, 1999.

Rose, Jeanne. *The Aromatherapy Book: Applications and Inhalations.* Berkeley, CA: North Atlantic Books, 1992.

Ryman, Danièle. *Aromatherapy: The Complete Guide to Plant & Flower Essences for Health and Beauty.* New York: Bantam Books, 1993.

Seigler, D. (2002). Plant Secondary Metabolism (Second Printing ed.). Norwell, Massachusetts: Kluwer Academic Publishers.

Sheppard-Hanger, Sylla. *The Aromatherapy Practitioner Reference Manual.* Tampa, FL: Atlantic Institute of Aromatherapy, Twelfth Printing February 2000.

Singh, M. A. F. (Ed.). (2000). Exercise, Nutrition, and the Older Woman: Wellness for Women over Fifty. Boca Raton, FL: CRC Press.

Sizer, F. S. & Whitney, E. (2014). Nutrition: Concepts and Controversies (13th ed.). Belmont, CA: Wadsworth, Cengage Learning.

Tisserand, Maggie. *Aromatherapy for Women: a Practical Guide to Essential Oils for Health and Beauty.* Rochester, VT: Healing Arts Press, 1996.

Tisserand, Robert. *Aromatherapy: to Heal and Tend the Body.* Wilmot, WI: Lotus Press, 1988.

Tisserand, Robert. *The Art of Aromatherapy.* Rochester, VT: Healing Arts Press, 1977.

Tisserand, Robert, and Tony Balacs. *Essential Oil Safety: A Guide for Health Care Professionals.* New York, NY: Churchill Livingstone, 1995.

Tortora G.J., Funke B.R., Case C.L. *Microbiology: An Introduction. 9th ed.* San Francisco: Pearson Benjamin Cummings, 2007.

Valnet, M.D., Jean. *The Practice of Aromatherapy: a Classic Compendium of Plant Medicines and their Healing Properties.* Rochester, VT: Healing Arts Press, 1980.

Valnet, Jean. *The Practice of Aromatherapy.* Rochester Vermont: Healing Arts Press, 1982. Print.

Watson, Franzesca. *Aromatherapy Blends & Remedies.* San Francisco, CA: Thorsons, 1995.

Weaver R.F. *Molecular Biology. 4th ed.* New York: McGraw Hill, 2008.

Wilson, Roberta. *Aromatherapy for Vibrant Health and Beauty: a practical A-to-Z reference to aromatherapy treatments for health, skin, and hair problems.* Honesdale, PA: Paragon Press, 1995.

Worwood, Valerie Ann. *The Complete Book of Essential Oils & Aromatherapy.* San Rafael, CA: New World Library, 1991.

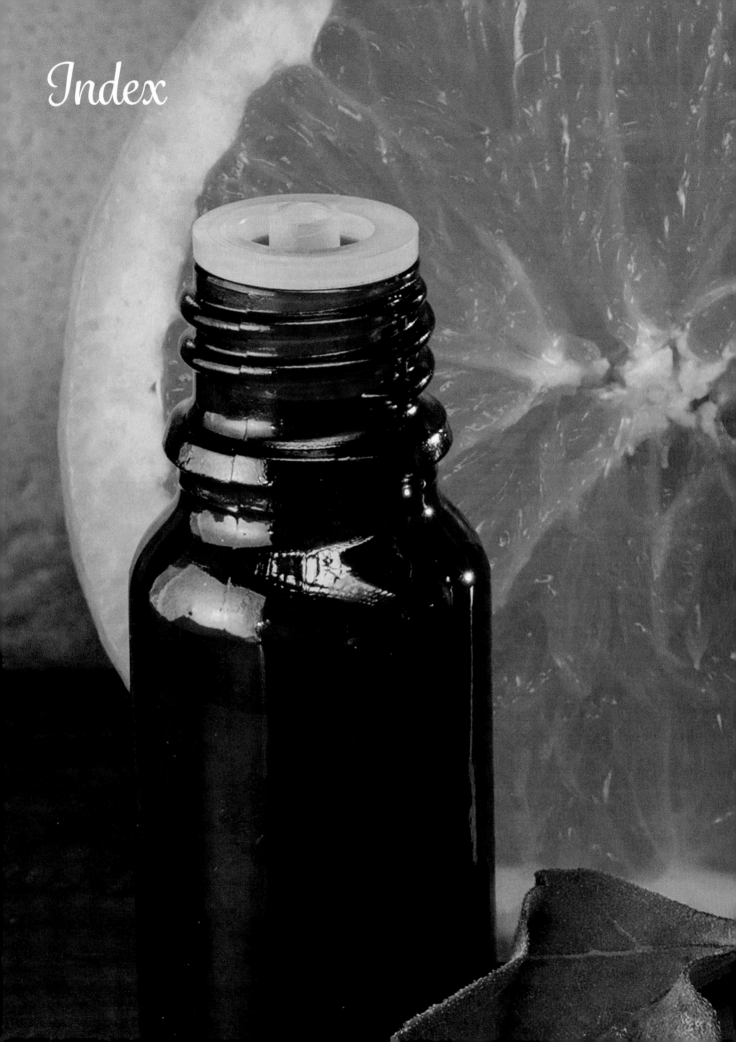

Index

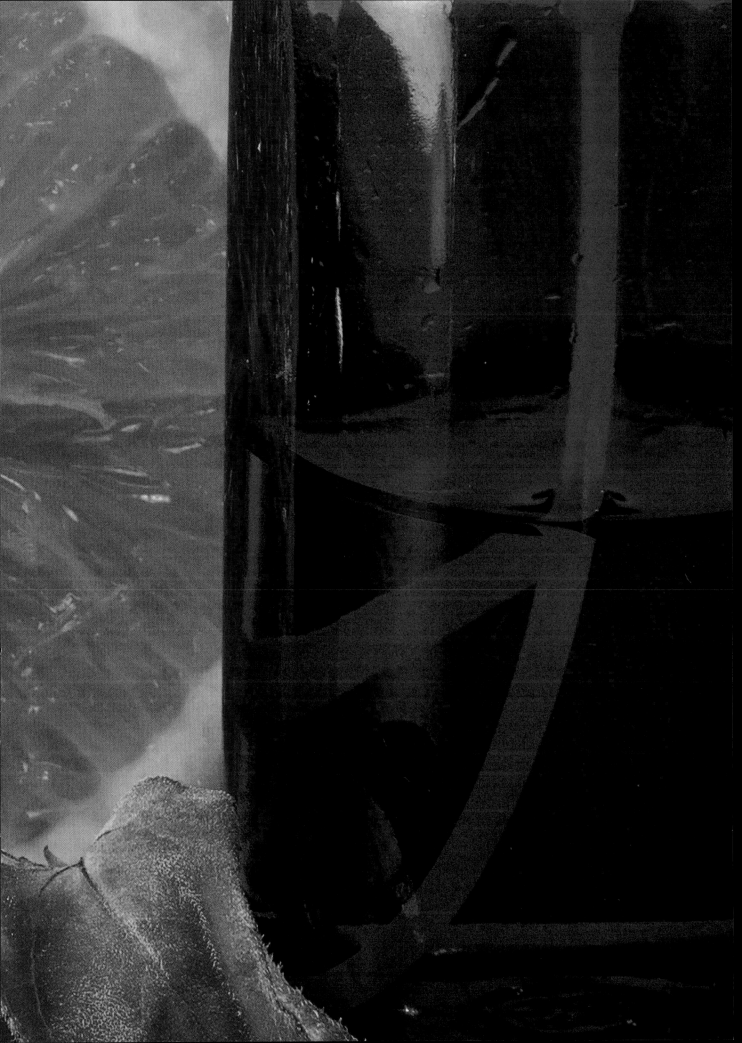

Index

Symbols

A

B

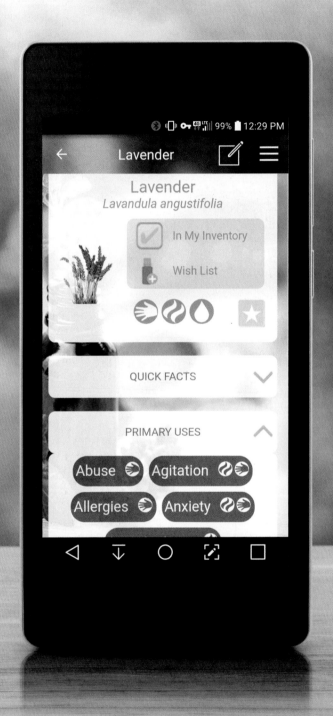

MODERN *Essentials*
On the Go!

Download the new ME Plus app
from your app store today!

Essential Oils *Quick Reference*

Single Oil Name	Topical			Aromatic			Internal			Common Uses (see the Single Oils chapter for additional uses)
	Adult	Child/Sensitive	Pregnancy	Adult	Child	Pregnancy	Adult	Child (6+)	Pregnancy	
Arborvitae	●	●	●	●	●	●	✗	✗	✗	Antibacterial, Antifungal, Calming, Repellent
Basil	●	●	●	●	●	●	●	●	✗	Autism, Bronchitis, Earache, Cramps/Spasms, Bug Bites, Wounds
Bergamot**	●	●	●	●	●	●	●	●	●	Brain Injury, Colic, Depression, Respiratory Infection, Stress
Birch	●	●	✗	●	●	✗	✗	✗	✗	Muscle Aches, Pain
Black Pepper	●	●	●	●	●	●	●	●	●	Addictions, Cooking, Circulation
Blue Tansy	●	●	●	●	●	●	✗	✗	✗	Anxiety, Calming, Wounds
Cardamom	●	●	●	●	●	●	●	●	●	Coughs, Inflammation, Muscle Aches, Nausea, Respiratory Ailments
Cassia	●	●	✗	●	●	●	●	●	✗	Antibacterial, Antiviral, Disinfectant, Warming
Cedarwood	●	●	●	●	●	●	✗	✗	✗	Calming, Tension, Tuberculosis, Urinary Infection, Yoga
Cilantro	●	●	●	●	●	●	●	●	●	Anxiety, Cooking
Cinnamon	●	●	✗	●	●	●	●	●	✗	Antibacterial, Antifungal, Diabetes, Mold, Respiratory Infection, Warming
Clary Sage	●	●	●	●	●	●	●	●	●	Cholesterol, Cramps, Hot Flashes, PMS, Respiratory Infection
Clove	●	●	●	●	●	●	●	●	●	Antifungal, Antioxidant, Antiviral, Corns, Hypothyroidism, Toothache
Copaiba	●	●	●	●	●	●	●	●	●	Acne, Antioxidant, Anxiety, Inflammation, Muscle Aches/Pain
Coriander	●	●	●	●	●	●	●	●	●	Cartilage Injury, Muscle Aches, Muscle Development, Whiplash
Cypress	●	●	●	●	●	●	✗	✗	✗	Aneurysm, Carpal Tunnel, Concussion, Muscle Fatigue, Pain, Stroke
Dill	●	●	●	●	●	●	●	●	●	Cholesterol, Cooking, Flavoring
Douglas Fir	●	●	●	●	●	●	✗	✗	✗	Asthma, Bronchitis, Congestion, Coughs, Flu, Focus, Infection
Eucalyptus	●	●	●	●	●	●	✗	✗	✗	Inflammation, Neuralgia, Pain, Respiratory Issues, Shingles
Fennel	●	●	●	●	●	●	●	●	●	Blood Clots, Bruises, Digestive Support, Skin, Wrinkles
Frankincense	●	●	●	●	●	●	●	●	●	Arthritis, Inflammation, Mental Fatigue, Respiratory Issues, Skin, Warts
Geranium	●	●	●	●	●	●	●	●	●	Air Purification, Bleeding, Diabetes, Dry Skin, Vertigo, Wrinkles
Ginger*	●	●	●	●	●	●	●	●	●	Digestive Issues, Morning Sickness, Nausea, Rheumatic Fever
Grapefruit	●	●	●	●	●	●	●	●	●	Anorexia, Appetite Suppressant, Cellulite, Hangover
Green Mandarin**	●	●	●	●	●	●	●	●	●	Nausea, Calming, GERD, Skin (Toning), Soothing
Helichrysum	●	●	●	●	●	●	●	●	●	Antiviral, Bleeding, Cholesterol, Earache, Herpes, Sciatica, Wounds
Hinoki	●	●	●	●	●	●	✗	✗	✗	Calming, Cleaning, Colds, Cuts/Scrapes, Rashes
Jasmine	●	●	●	●	●	●	●	●	●	Hoarse Voice, Pink Eye, Sensitive Skin, Uplifting
Juniper Berry	●	●	●	●	●	●	●	●	●	Acne, Alcoholism, Dermatitis/Eczema, Kidney Stones, Tinnitus
Lavender	●	●	●	●	●	●	●	●	●	Allergies, Boils, Burns, Calming, Itching, Pain, Skin, Sleep, Wrinkles
Lemon*	●	●	●	●	●	●	●	●	●	Anxiety, Cleansing, Depression, Disinfectant, Grease, Heartburn, Stress
Lemon Myrtle	●	●	●	●	●	●	●	●	●	Antibacterial, Antifungal, Candida, Staph MRSA
Lemongrass	●	●	●	●	●	●	●	●	●	Air Purification, Cholesterol, Cramps, Joint Injuries, Tissue Repair
Lime*	●	●	●	●	●	●	●	●	●	Bacterial Infections, Fever, Gum/Grease Removal, Skin
Litsea	●	●	●	●	●	●	●	●	●	Bacterial Infections, Cleaning, Energizing, Flavoring, Meditation, Yoga
Magnolia	●	●	●	●	●	●	✗	✗	✗	Anxiety, Calming, Soothing (Skin)
Manuka	●	●	●	●	●	●	✗	✗	✗	Respiratory Infections, Arthritis, Rheumatism, Skin
Marjoram	●	●	●	●	●	●	●	●	●	Arthritis, Cramps, Muscle Ache/Spasm, Neuralgia, Whiplash
Melaleuca	●	●	●	●	●	●	●	●	●	Acne, Antifungal, Boils, Cold Sores, Disinfectant, Sore Throat, Wounds